AF531003

Proceedings of an
International Symposium/Workshop

Biological Interaction of Inhaled Mineral Fibers and Cigarette Smoke

Held at the Battelle Seattle Conference Center
April 10-14, 1988, Seattle, Washington

Alfred P. Wehner, D.M.D., Sc.D., Cand. Med., D.A.T.S.
Editor

Dvara-Lee Felton, B.A.
Associate Editor

Battelle, Pacific Northwest Laboratories
Richland, WA 99352

Sponsored by

R. J. Reynolds Tobacco Company
Winston-Salem, NC 27102

and

Electric Power Research Institute
Palo Alto, CA 94303

Library of Congress Cataloging-in-Publication Data

Biological interaction on inhaled mineral fibers and
cigarette smoke/edited by Alfred P. Wehner.
618 pp.

Based on a symposium and workshop held April 10-14, 1988
at the Battelle Seattle Conference Center.

ISBN 0-935470-44-1
1. Lungs—Dust diseases—Pathogenesis—Congresses.
2. Cigarette smoke—Health aspects—Congresses.
3. Inorganic fibers—Health aspects—Congresses.
4. Asbestosis—Congresses. I. Wehner, Alfred P.

[DNLM: 1. Minerals—adverse effects—congresses.
2. Respiratory Systems—pathology—congresses. 3. Smoke—
adverse effects—congresses. 4. Tobacco—congresses. WF
101 B615 1988]
RC773.B54 1988
616.2′44—dc 19
DNLM/DLC
for Library of Congress 88-22240
CIP

Printed in the United States of America

Battelle Press
505 King Avenue
Columbus, Ohio 43201-2693
614-424-6393; 1-800-451-3543

Contents

Preface

Clinical Studies

Deposition and Clearance of Inhaled Particles: Macrophages

Preface

Much is known about the biological effects of inhaled mineral fibers and about the biological effects of tobacco smoke. Some 20 years ago it was first recognized that there appears to be a synergism between these two agents. However, very little information exists on the mechanisms of their biological interaction.

Many people smoke, and mineral fibers are ubiquitous in our environment. Litigation involving health effects of smoking and mineral fibers, both singly and in combination, is making the news. Given the synergistic biological effects of this combination and their potential health consequences, it is important to elucidate the mechanisms of this interaction.

The primary purpose of the symposium/workshop was to *develop* knowledge in this field. I endeavored this by bringing together, in a relaxed, think-tank-like atmosphere, invited scientists from six countries and from various topic-related disciplines. The participants represented academia, government agencies, independent research laboratories, and industry. The symposium/workshop format comprised both formal presentations of research findings and new hypotheses as well as extensive discussions, with emphasis on the latter. The formal presentations served as catalysts for animated argumentation among the multidisciplinary mix of scientists representing different interests. Free expression of new ideas and reasonable speculation were encouraged by deliberately not identifying the discussants in the Proceedings.

The Proceedings present both the prepared manuscripts and the edited discussions, with up-to-date views of the biological interaction of inhaled mineral fibers and cigarette smoke. They include hypotheses and models for this complex phenomenon; clinical studies; new *in vitro* test systems; deposition and clearance of inhaled particles; the role of macrophages; differences between lesions induced by erionite and asbestos fibers; identification of factors whose effects on the interaction of inhaled mineral fibers and cigarette smoke remain to be determined; and lessons learned from the past. As such, the Proceedings reflect the latest thinking by experts in this field, including their sometimes sharply divergent opinions. They are, therefore, suitable as a current reference not only for the symposium participants but for all those professionally involved in the consequences of the biological interaction of inhaled mineral fibers and cigarette smoke.

Alfred P. Wehner, D.M.D., Sc.D.,
Cand. Med., D.A.T.S.
Symposium Organizer and Chairman

GENERAL PRESENTATIONS

Biological Interactions: Important Things We Do Not Know

Francis J. C. Roe

19 Marryat Road, Wimbledon Common, London SW19 5BB, England

KEY WORDS: animal models, biological interactions, tobacco smoke, mineral fibers, asbestos, lung neoplasia

---

ABSTRACT

Human mortality data suggest that, on average, smoking increases the risk of death from lung cancer by a factor of 10. Inhalation exposure to asbestos increases the risk by a factor of 5, and a combination of smoking and asbestos exposure increases the risk by a factor of 50. This implies multiplicative interaction between smoking and asbestos but throws no light on the mechanisms involved. It has been suggested that the basis of the interaction is "physical": that the adsorption of genotoxic carcinogens from cigarette smoke onto asbestos particles leads to prolonged contact between DNA-damaging electrophiles and lung cells. Alternatively, it has been suggested that one of the two agents (probably in cigarette smoke) is a genotoxic initiator, while the other (probably the asbestos) acts as a promoter because it causes prolonged cellular proliferation. Many experiments involve the introduction, by intratracheal instillation, of particulate material (e.g., ferric oxide, carbon black, as a surrogate for asbestos particles) along with benzo[a]pyrene or another carcinogen (as a surrogate for cigarette smoke) into the lungs of laboratory rodents. These studies have been undertaken on the assumption that the presence of supposedly inert particles in the lung is necessary for and/or greatly increases the chances of tumor development in response to the carcinogen. In fact, the evidence for this is somewhat equivocal. A second problem is that the neoplastic lung lesions most commonly produced in rodents (e.g., nonfatal, peripherally located bronchioloalveolar adenomatous lesions or highly keratinized, seemingly benign, squamous lesions) may have little relevance to the undoubtedly malignant, often centrally arising, and usually fatal lung cancers of man. A third problem is that cigarette smoke is itself largely composed of particulates. Therefore, why should one expect the presence of other particulate matter in the lungs to enhance its carcinogenic activity? So far, attempts to enhance respiratory tract carcinogenesis in smoke-exposed rodents by prior or concomitant exposure to asbestos or other particulate materials have not produced impressive evidence of multiplicative interaction comparable with that seen by epidemiologists for human lung-cancer mortality.

A critical reevaluation is needed of the results of animal studies and of the likely relevance of producing particular kinds of lesions in the lungs of laboratory rodents to mechanisms involved in human lung carcinogenesis. Only then can one hope to obtain meaningful answers to the many topical and important questions concerning the physical and chemical characteristics of fibrous materials which determine whether or not they contribute to lung-cancer risk in smokers and nonsmokers.

Even if one accepts the epidemiological evidence for a multiplicative interaction between tobacco smoke and asbestos in relation to lung cancer risk, many important questions remain. Must exposure be concomitant, or is an ex-smoker more susceptible to asbestos-induced lung cancer than a lifelong nonsmoker? Also, is a retired asbestos worker more likely than a retired office worker to develop lung cancer if he takes up smoking for the first time? Can we exclude the possibility that irritants in the vapor phase of tobacco smoke (e.g., oxides of nitrogen) may have the effect of enhancing pulmonary carcinogenesis by asbestos? Does smoking enhance the retention of radon more in the lungs of asbestos workers than in those of other workers? These and many other questions apply not only to risks from asbestos exposure but also to risks from exposure to other fibrous dusts.

INTRODUCTION

The starting point of this symposium is the widely held view that cigarette-smoking and exposure to asbestos fibers by inhalation act synergistically in relation to lung-cancer risk in man. Table 1, based on the findings of Hammond et al. (1979), illustrates the epidemiological basis for this view. According to Berry et al. (1985), the observed relative risk of developing lung cancer (after allowing for smoking) that is associated with asbestos exposure is greater in nonsmokers than in smokers. However, Doll and Peto (1985) thought that this might be due to methodological defects, the most important of which is the misclassifying of some current or ex-smokers as nonsmokers. Presently, the position is that the carcinogenic effects of asbestos dust and cigarette-smoking on the human lung are approximately multiplicative.

Table 1. Mortality ratios based on age-standardized death rates from lung cancer in cigarette smokers and nonsmokers, with or without occupational exposure to asbestos dust (from Hammond et al., 1979).

Asbestos Exposure	Cigarette-Smoke Exposure	Mortality Ratios
+	+	53
+	–	5
–	+	11
–	–	1

Laboratory evidence that particulate matter enhances lung-cancer induction by known carcinogens has tempted some investigators to assume that an animal model exists for asbestos/smoking interaction in humans. They therefore apply the terms tumor initiator and tumor promoter to asbestos dust and cigarette smoke. This symposium provides, among other opportunities, the chance to review the appropriateness of using such terms in light of the available evidence.

LACK OF A SUITABLE ANIMAL MODEL

A serious hurdle in investigating the basis of the synergism between asbestos dust and cigarette-smoking in relation to lung-cancer risk in man is the lack of any really suitable animal model for inducing lung cancer by tobacco-smoke inhalation. In the absence of such a model, a variety of far less appropriate model systems that depend on surrogates have been used. However, surrogation can easily be pushed beyond the point of credibility, particularly when multiple surrogates are incorporated into a single model system. Some of the surrogates that have been used are:

- rat, mouse or hamster lung for human lung
- intratracheal instillation of tobacco tar or suspended dust for inhalation exposure

- intrapleural injection instead of inhalation exposure
- carcinogenic polycyclic aromatic hydrocarbons for cigarette smoke
- a seemingly inert dust (e.g., ferric oxide, India ink) for a biologically active dust (e.g., asbestos)
- doubtful neoplastic end points arising in alveoli or bronchioles instead of the squamous or small-cell carcinomas that arise mainly in large airways
- short-term *in vitro* studies with non-neoplastic end points (e.g., chromosomal aberrations) instead of long-term *in vivo* studies with neoplastic end points.

POSSIBLE MECHANISMS

There is, in fact, no dearth of possible explanations for the interaction between asbestos dust and smoking in the genesis of lung cancer. As an armchair exercise, I have listed some of them. Following are factors that may be determinants of lung-cancer risk in response to a potential carcinogen:

- genetic susceptibility
- dose (airborne concentration, respiratory rate, period of exposure)
- time since first exposure
- particle size, deposition and distribution
- penetration from surface into lung tissue
- clearance rate
- metabolic activation
- detoxification
- tissue damage (irritation, necrosis, cell turnover)
- repair of tissue damage
- immune competence
- other diseases
- nutrition (calories, fat, vitamin A).

In the following list, I postulate a variety of ways in which inhaled cigarette smoke may enhance response to a particulate carcinogen, such as asbestos:

- effect on particle deposition or distribution

- effect on particle penetration into tissues
- effect on particle clearance (e.g., because of ciliotoxicity, destruction of cilia, replacement of ciliated epithelium by squamous epithelium, blockage of lymph drainage, etc.)
- induction of metabolically activating enzymes or inhibition of detoxifying enzymes
- stimulated proliferation of mutant cells (tumor promotion)
- interference with immune competence
- effect on nutritional (including vitamin) status.

Listed below are various ways in which chemically inert non-genotoxic particles that are retained in the lungs may enhance carcinogenesis by cigarette smoke:

- adsorption of smoke carcinogens onto particles might increase the number of cells with which they interact and/or delay their clearance
- effect on clearance of smoke carcinogens in the absence of adsorption onto particles
- proliferation of target cells when exposed to smoke carcinogens
- stimulated proliferation of smoke-damaged mutant cells (tumor promotion)
- Interference with immune competence.

These lists are by no means exhaustive, and another philosopher, sitting in another armchair, could doubtless add to all three lists. The point is that, given the wide variety of possibilities, it would be unwise to plump for one without excluding the others. And it would be very unwise to assume that any of the available animal models is reliable for predicting human lung-cancer risk from exposure to tobacco smoke or dusts such as asbestos.

Among the more popular theoretical causes advanced to explain asbestos/tobacco-smoke interaction in lung carcinogenesis are: (1) the adsorption onto asbestos particles of carcinogens present in tobacco smoke; (2) the slowing of asbestos particle clearance by cigarette smoke; and (3) the slowing of smoke-particle clearance by asbestos. The first two of these explanations seem unlikely, insofar as all observers agree that smoking is wholly without effect on the incidence of mesotheliomas in persons exposed to asbestos. This is not what one would expect if asbestos adsorbed smoke carcinogens, and there is no reason why slowing the clearance of asbestos particles from the lung should not result in an increased risk of mesotheliomas along with the increased risk of lung cancer. Since smoking is not, by itself, associated with increased risk of mesothelioma, the third of these three possible explanations is the only one that is at all plausible.

IF THE TWO-STAGE THEORY OF CARCINOGENESIS APPLIES, WHICH IS THE INITIATOR AND WHICH IS THE PROMOTER?

According to the two-stage theory of carcinogenesis, a genotoxic (initiating) agent and a nongenotoxic, hyperplasia-stimulating (promoting) agent may operate sequentially in causing neoplasia. However, for each of the two kinds of agent to complement the activity of the other in this way, exposure to the genotoxin must either precede or occur at the same time as exposure to the promoter.

In the case of the combined effects of cigarette smoke and asbestos, most investigators have looked to cigarette smoke to provide the genotoxins, because asbestos has proved inactive in virtually all laboratory tests for genotoxicity. In other words, asbestos is usually cast in the role of tumor promoter, with cigarette smoke possessing all the initiating activity and, perhaps, contributing to the promoting activity as well. Notwithstanding this, Kobayashi et al. (1974) claimed to have shown that inhaled tobacco smoke acted as a tumor promoter and/or co-carcinogen for the upper respiratory tract, including the larynx, of hamsters previously given a large dose of 7,12-dimethylbenz[a]anthracene (DMBA).

In recent years, the two-stage theory of carcinogenesis has been increasingly questioned (Iversen and Astrup, 1984). However, whether it is true or not, the following question arises: For asbestos dust and cigarette smoke to interact in causing lung cancer, does exposure have to be concomitant or in a particular sequence? Thus, are ex-smokers more likely than nonsmokers to develop lung cancer if they are subsequently exposed to asbestos dust? Also, are persons who have previously been exposed to asbestos dust more susceptible than persons who have not if they take up smoking later in life? At present, the answers to these questions are not known, and no one seems to be seeking the answers.

DO NOT LET US FORGET THAT TOBACCO SMOKE IS PARTLY PARTICULATE

It is interesting to compare theories about tobacco-smoke/asbestos interaction and environmental tobacco-smoke/radon interaction in relation to lung-cancer risk. In the case of the former, asbestos is the particulate material which, perhaps, adsorbs carcinogens from tobacco smoke so that they are not so readily cleared from the lungs.

However, in the case of radon and environmental tobacco smoke, it is the latter that is cast in the role of the particulate material onto which genotoxic radon is adsorbed! The foundations of both theories would seem to be a little shaky, to say the least!

IS ENHANCING PENETRATION OF ASBESTOS PARTICLES INTO LUNG TISSUES BY TOBACCO SMOKE IMPORTANT?

Simani et al. (1974) demonstrated that cigarette smoke opens up intercellular junctions in the tracheal epithelium of guinea pigs, thereby allowing relatively large particles to penetrate between epithelial cells and find their way more deeply into the epithelium. Although it seems unlikely that this is an important mechanism in lung carcinogenesis induced by combined exposure to asbestos and cigarette smoke, I am not sure that evidence exists to disprove the theory.

DO ASBESTOSIS, FIBROSIS AND/OR SCARRING OF THE LUNG PREDISPOSE TO LUNG CANCER

According to many groups of investigators, asbestosis is not a prerequisite for the development of lung cancer in persons exposed to asbestos (Selikoff et al., 1964; Enterline, 1965; Jacob and Anspach, 1965). However, Parkes (1974) pointed out that, in many cases, this conclusion was based simply on the absence of radiological evidence of asbestosis (Edge, 1976) and was not backed-up by postmortem data.

Several investigators have reported that lung cancers arising in persons exposed to asbestos tend to occur in the lower lobes, that is to say, the parts of the lung most affected by the deposition of dust and by the consequent fibrosis (Jacob and Anspach, 1965). However, the fact that dust deposition, fibrosis, and cancer development tend to take place in the same area of the lung does not establish that fibrosis predisposes to cancer risk in the case of asbestos.

The picture is confused; firstly, by historical epidemiological data for asbestosis and lung cancer, secondly, because of conflicting data for the association between lung cancer and other pneumoconiotic diseases; and thirdly, by the reported association between local scarring in the lung and cancer development.

A strong association has long been known to exist between asbestosis and lung cancer. Thus, Merewether (1949) reported that 14.7% of workers with asbestosis later developed lung cancer. By 1963, the percentage had, according to Buchanan (1965), risen to over 50. A plausible explanation of this steep rise was that a decrease in ambient asbestos dust concentrations led to delayed and slower development of asbestosis. In these circumstances, men had more time to develop lung cancer before they died of asbestosis. In any case, evidence of association is not evidence of causation, so that even a 50% risk of lung cancer in a person with asbestosis does not establish that asbestosis predisposes to lung cancer in a causal sense.

The absence of any apparently increased risk of lung cancer in association with pneumoconiotic fibrosis due to other dusts (e.g., coal, amorphous silicates, talc, etc.) suggests that pulmonary fibrosis *per se* is, in fact, not a risk factor for lung cancer. On the other hand, there is good evidence that, in the lung, cancers tend to arise in the vicinity of localized scars (e.g., secondary to tuberculosis), and when they do so, they are mostly adenocarcinomas (Auerbach et al., 1979; Carroll, 1962).

Laboratory studies have not really resolved the matter. Wagner et al. (1974) reported increased incidences of both adenocarcinoma and squamous carcinoma of the lung in rats exposed to asbestos. They stated that there was a positive association between asbestosis and lung tumors. However, all their rats were heavily exposed to asbestos dust, and it remains unclear whether the asbestosis was a prerequisite for tumor development.

There would seem, therefore, still to be some unanswered questions concerning the association between fibrosis, scarring, and lung-cancer risk.

ARE THE LUNG CANCERS THAT ARISE IN RESPONSE TO ASBESTOS AND CIGARETTE SMOKE SIMILAR IN PATHOGENESIS AND HISTOLOGICAL TYPE?

According to Auerbach et al. (1956, 1961), the beginnings of most smoking-associated lung cancers in men are to be found in the epithelium of main airways in the form of basal cell hyperplasia, loss of cilia, nuclear atypia, squamous metaplasia and carcinoma *in situ*. Progression from these changes results in the development of mostly squamous and small-cell cancers that arise, for the most part, close to the center of the chest, near the tracheal bifurcation. Originally, it was thought that the risk of adenocarcinoma development from small airways or from alveolar epithelium, more peripherally in the lung, was only rarely associated with smoking. However, it is clear now, especially in women, that this is not true. By contrast, a seemingly greater proportion of the lung cancers arising in men exposed to asbestos dust are adenocarcinomas than in men not so exposed. If this is so, then it suggests that fibrosis and scarring may really be of some importance.

Kannerstein and Churg (1972) compared 50 cases of asbestos-associated lung cancer and 50 cases of lung cancer not associated with exposure to asbestos. In the former cases, they confirmed that a majority of the cancers arose in the lower lobes, where the asbestosis was most severe. They also recorded more severe pleural involvement in the asbestos-associated cases. However, they saw no significant difference between the two groups in the location of cancers within lung lobes (i.e., central versus peripheral), in the incidence of different types of lung cancer (squamous, small cell, adenocarcinoma, etc.), or in the incidence or pattern of metastasis. They regarded their findings as consistent with asbestos being a weak carcinogen which augments the effect of another potent carcinogen, namely, cigarette smoke.

All in all, it seems likely that the answer to the question posed in the heading of this section is yes. However, whether it is reasonable to regard asbestos as a weak carcinogen and cigarette smoke as a potent carcinogen is certainly open to debate, as is the question as to which agent augments the other.

ASBESTOS, SMOKING, AND CANCER OF THE LARYNX

It is easy to think of possible mechanisms for the interaction of asbestos dust and smoking in relation to lung-cancer risk, even if the plausibility of some of the proposed mechanisms is reduced by the lack of evidence of interaction in relation to mesothelioma, as discussed before. On the other hand, claims that asbestos and smoking interact in the genesis of cancer of the larynx (U.S. Surgeon General, 1979) are more difficult to reconcile with any plausible mechanism. A direct carcinogenic effect of cigarette smoke on the risk of cancer of the larynx has been demonstrated both epidemiologically (U.S. Surgeon General, 1979) and experimentally, in hamsters (Dontenwill et al., 1973). However, no effect of asbestos dust alone on the larynx has ever been described either in man or animals, and it is difficult to imagine what sort of biological activity asbestos dust could exhibit at this site.

Kobayashi et al. (1974) demonstrated that cigarette smoke exacerbates epithelial changes in the larynx of hamsters exposed to DMBA by intratracheal instillation. This adds confusion rather than enlightenment, insofar as tobacco smoke was cast by these investigators in the role of tumor promoter. (See also Kannerstein and Churg, 1972, who considered tobacco smoke a potent carcinogen.)

DATA BASE FOR EFFECTS OF MINERAL DUSTS OTHER THAN ASBESTOS IN RELATION TO ENHANCEMENT OF LUNG-CANCER RISK BY SMOKING

In 1987, the International Agency for Research on Cancer (IARC, 1987) reviewed the available data from animal and epidemiological studies for exposure to silica and various silicates. Unfortunately, none of the data reviewed shed any light on mineral-dust/smoking interactions in relation to lung-cancer risk.

Marked fibrosis as well as lung cancers have been induced in rats, but not in hamsters, by inhalation exposure to crystalline silica (e.g., quartz). However, there is no information on whether exposure to tobacco smoke, in addition, enhances the risk of cancer development. For exposure to amorphous silica, the position is even more unsatisfactory. The epidemiological evidence for increased lung-cancer risk in ore miners, quarriers, coal miners, and persons working in the ceramics industry is either equivocal or negative. Coal miners with pneumoconiosis are seemingly not at as much increased risk of developing lung cancer as asbestos workers with asbestosis. A higher than expected incidence of lung cancer in granite workers and others in the stone-cutting industry might well be due to exposure to radon rather than to silicates. Overall, there seems to be a somewhat higher incidence of lung cancer among persons with silicosis, but even this is not certain because of the failure to collect information about smoking habits. Particularly for this reason, it is impossible to assess whether there is any interaction between exposure to silica and smoking in the causation of lung cancer.

In the case of talc, there is evidence of increased lung-cancer risk for workers exposed to talc that is contaminated with asbestos, but not for workers exposed to talc that is not so contaminated. In the former, there is no information on whether smoking enhances the risk, and no informative inhalation studies in animals have been performed.

Erionite, a fibrous aluminosilicate dust, produces fibrosis of the lung and mesotheliomas in high incidence following exposure by inhalation, both in humans and in laboratory animals. Lung-cancer risk, however, is seemingly not influenced and, in the case of humans, there is no evidence to suggest that smoking has any influence.

DOES INHALED PARTICULATE MATTER REALLY ENHANCE LUNG-CANCER RISK UNDER CONDITIONS OF PRIOR, SIMULTANEOUS, OR SUBSEQUENT EXPOSURE TO GENOTOXIC CARCINOGENS?

This question is fundamental to the subject of this symposium. Although it is traditional to think that inhaled or intratracheally instilled particulate matter enhances the risk of lung cancer in animals exposed, by the same route, to carcinogens such as DMBA or benzo[a]pyrene (BaP), the evidence is, in fact, equivocal (Farrell and Davis, 1974). Certainly it is not true that a particulate vehicle is *necessary* for experimental lung carcinogenesis induced by carcinogenic polycyclic aromatic hydrocarbons (Staub et al., 1965; Feron, 1972).

Pylev et al. (1969) reported that asbestos particles significantly increased the retention of radioactivity in the lungs of hamsters 21 days after the intratracheal instillation of a 10% aminosol vitrum* suspension of [3H] BaP mixed with asbestos dust, as compared with a suspension of [3H] BaP in 10% aminosol vitrum only. The inclusion of asbestos in the instilled material was associated with an increase in the number of macrophages that could be recovered from the lungs. However, the radioactivity per macrophage was higher in hamsters given BaP only.

Davis et al. (1975) reported that the repeated intratracheal instillation of BaP in infusine gave rise to more squamous neoplasms in the lungs of rats than did the repeated intratracheal instillation of BaP plus carbon-black particles in infusine. In other words, the addition of the particulate matter to the instillate *reduced* the risk of lung-tumor development. These findings were in line with those of Herrold and Dunham (1962), Feron et al. (1973) and Henry et al. (1973, 1974), who reported that a particulate vehicle is not necessary for lung-tumor production by instilled BaP in hamsters.

Wehner et al. (1975a) exposed male hamsters either to chrysotile asbestos dust alone, cigarette smoke alone, or both asbestos dust and cigarette smoke. Lung disease, diagnosed as asbestosis, led to early death in the asbestos-exposed animals. This may explain why the animals exposed to both asbestos and cigarette smoke exhibited a lower incidence of laryngeal lesions than was seen in animals exposed to cigarette smoke only. The incidence of lung adenomas was slightly but not significantly higher (7/51) in the asbestos-plus-smoke-exposed group than in the asbestos-only group (3/51). There were no lung adenomas in hamsters exposed to smoke only (0/51) and only one in a control animal (1/51).

In similar studies involving the exposure of male hamsters to nickel oxide dust and/or cigarette smoke (Wehner et al., 1975b), the main effects of exposure to cigarette smoke alone were reduced body-weight gain, delayed onset of amyloid disease, prolonged survival, and an increased incidence of various pathological changes in the larynx. Exposure to nickel oxide only also increased the

*An aqueous preparation of 10% amino acid and low-molecular-weight peptide derived by enzymatic hydrolysis of animal proteins and marketed by the Vitrum Company, Stockholm, Sweden.

incidence of laryngeal lesions. However, there was no evidence of synergism in animals exposed to both agents. A variety of effects on the lungs, though no lung tumors, were seen in animals exposed to nickel oxide dust, but exposure to tobacco smoke in addition had little or no effect on the incidence or severity of these lesions.

The answer to the question posed in the heading of this section seems to be sometimes yes and sometimes no. The size and composition of particles clearly are important, but so are the chemical and physical natures of genotoxic carcinogens. *Clearly, the results of experiments involving combined exposure to a particular genotoxic carcinogen and a particular dust is not a reliable model for any other carcinogen or any other dust.*

CONCLUSIONS

There is persuasive evidence that smoking and occupational exposure to asbestos act in a multiplicative way in increasing the risk of lung cancer in humans. However, there is no meaningful animal model for investigating the mechanism underlying this phenomenon. Attempts to explain the synergism in terms of the two-stage hypothesis are based on muddled thinking and a lack of persuasive supportive evidence. It is not clear whether the multiplicative effect depends on concomitant exposure to both agents, or whether it would be seen in a retired asbestos worker who took up smoking or in an ex-smoker whose exposure to asbestos dust began only in later life.

In the absence of a better understanding of mechanisms, it is uncertain whether the multiplicative effect applies to very low levels of exposure to both agents. There is persuasive evidence that the long thin shape of asbestos particles, coupled with their other physical and chemical characteristics, is highly relevant to their biological activity. However, the part played by physical and chemical characteristics other than shape is still uncertain (Pott, 1987). Thus, it is not possible to predict, with any confidence, how combined exposure to other dusts and to cigarette smoke might interact in relation to lung-cancer risk.

REFERENCES

Auerbach, O, TG Petrick, AP Stout, AL Stalsingel, GE Muelhsam, JB Forman, and JB Gere. **1956.** The anatomical approach to the study of smoking and bronchogenic carcinoma. Cancer 9:76-83.

Auerbach, O, AP Stout, EC Hammond, and L Garfinkel. **1961.** Changes in the bronchial epithelium in relation to cigarette smoking and in relation to lung cancer. N Engl J Med 265:253-267.

Auerbach, O, L Garfinkel, and VR Parks. **1979.** Scar cancer of the lung: Increase over a 21 year period. Cancer 43:636-642.

Berry, G, ML Newhouse, and P Antonis. **1985.** Combined effects of asbestos and smoking on mortality from lung cancer and mesothelioma in factory workers. Br J Ind Med 49:364-372.

Buchanan, WD. **1965.** Asbestos and primary intrathoracic neoplasms. Ann NY Acad Sci 132:507-518.

Carroll, R. **1962.** The influence of lung scars on primary lung cancer. J Pathol Bacteriol 83:293-297.

Davis, BR, JK Whitehead, ME Gill, PN Lee, AD Butterworth, and FJC Roe. **1975.** Response of rat lung to 3,4-benzpyrene administered by intratracheal instillation in infusine with or without carbon black. Br J Cancer 31:443-452.

Doll, R and J Peto. **1985.** *Asbestos: Effects on Health of Exposure to Asbestos, pp. 1-58.* Health and Safety Commission, Her Majesty's Stationery Office, London, UK.

Dontenwill, W, H-J Chevalier, H-P Harke, U Lafrenz, G Reckzeh, and B Schneider. **1973.** Investigations on the effects of chronic cigarette smoke inhalation in Syrian Golden hamsters. J Natl Cancer Inst 51:1781-1806.

Edge, JR. **1976.** Asbestos related disease in Barrow-in-Furness. Environ Res 11:244-247.

Enterline, PE. **1965.** Mortality among asbestos products workers in the United States. Ann NY Acad Sci 132:156-165.

Farrell, RL and GW Davis. **1974.** Effect of particulate benzo(a)pyrene carrier on carcinogenesis in the respiratory tract of hamsters, pp. 186-198 and 219-233. In: *Experimental Lung Cancer: Carcinogenesis and Bioassays,* E Karbe and JF Park (eds.). Springer-Verlag, Berlin.

Feron, VJ. **1972.** Respiratory tract tumors in hamsters after intratracheal instillation of benzo(a)pyrene alone or with furfural. Cancer Res 32:28-36.

Feron, VJ, D de Jong, and P Emmelot. **1973.** Dose-response correlation for the induction of respiratory-tract tumours in Syrian Golden hamsters by intratracheal instillations of benzo(a)pyrene. Eur J Cancer 9:387-393.

Hammond, EC, IJ Selikoff, and H Seidman. **1979.** Asbestos exposure, cigarette smoking and death rates. Ann NY Acad Sci 330:473-490.

Henry, MC, CD Port, RR Bates, and DG Kaufman. **1973.** Respiratory tract tumours in hamsters induced by benzo(a)pyrene. Cancer Res 33:1585-1592.

Henry, MC, CD Port, and DG Kaufman. **1974.** Role of particles in respiratory carcinogenesis bioassay, pp. 175-185. In: *Experimental Lung Cancer: Carcinogenesis and Bioassays,* E Karbe and JF Park (eds.). Springer-Verlag, Berlin.

Herrold, KM and LJ Dunham. **1962.** Induction of carcinoma and papilloma of the tracheobronchial mucosa of Syrian hamsters by intratracheal instillation of benzo(a)pyrene. J Natl Cancer Inst 28:467-491.

IARC (International Agency for Research on Cancer). **1987.** *Monograph on the Evaluation of the Carcinogenic Risk of Chemicals to Humans: Silica and Some Silicates,* Vol. 42. IARC, Lyon, France, 289 p.

Iversen, OH and EG Astrup. **1984.** The paradigm of two-stage carcinogenesis: A critical attitude. Cancer Invest 2:51-60.

Jacob, G and M Anspach. **1965.** Pulmonary neoplasia among Dresden asbestos workers. Ann NY Acad Sci 132:536-548.

Kannerstein, M and J Churg. **1972.** Pathology of carcinoma of the lung associated with asbestos exposure. Cancer 30:14-21; 1972.

Kobayashi, N, D Hoffmann, and EL Wynder. **1974.** A study of tobacco carcinogenesis. XII. Epithelial changes induced in the upper respiratory tracts of Syrian Golden hamsters by cigarette smoke. J Natl Cancer Inst 53:1085-1089.

Merewether, ERA. **1949.** *Annual Report Chief Inspector of Factories, 1947.* His Majesty's Stationery Office, London, UK.

Parkes, WR. **1974.** *Occupational Lung Disorders.* Butterworths, Edinburgh, Scotland.

Pott, F. 1987. Problems in defining carcinogenic fibres. Ann Occup Hyg 31:799-802.

Pylev, LN, FJC Roe, and GP Warwick. **1969.** Elimination of radioactivity after intratracheal instillation of initiated 3,4-benzopyrene in hamsters. Br J Cancer 23:103-115.

Selikoff, IJ, J Churg, and EC Hammond. **1964.** Asbestos exposure and neoplasia. J Am Med Assoc 188:22-66.

Simani, AS, S Inoue, and JC Hogg. **1974.** Penetration of the respiratory epithelium of guinea pigs following exposure to cigarette smoke. Lab Invest 31:75-81.

Staub, EW, R Eisenstein, G Hass, EJJ Beattie. **1965.** Bronchogenic carcinoma produced experimentally in the normal dog. Thorac Cardiovasc Surg 49:364-372.

U.S. Surgeon General. 1979. *Smoking and Health: A Report to the Surgeon General,* DHEW Publication No. (PHS) 79-50066. U.S. Government Printing Office, Washington, DC.

Wagner, JC, G Berry, JW Skidmore, and V Timbrell. **1974.** The effects of the inhalation of asbestos in rats. Br J Cancer 29:252-269.

Wehner, AP, RH Busch, RJ Olson, and DK Craig. **1975a.** Chronic inhalation of asbestos and cigarette smoke by hamsters. Environ Res 10:368-383.

Wehner, AP, RH Busch, RJ Olson, and DK Craig. **1975b.** Chronic inhalation of nickel oxide and cigarette smoke by hamsters. Am Ind Hyg Assoc J 36:801-810.

Inhalation Exposure of Rodents to Mineral Fibers and Cigarette Smoke: What Did We Learn?

Alfred P. Wehner

Battelle, Pacific Northwest Laboratories, P. O. Box 999, Richland, WA 99352

KEY WORDS: inhalation exposures, rodents, mineral fibers, cigarette smoke

---

ABSTRACT

Based on experience with inhalation exposures in our laboratory, caution is advisable in formulating a suitable experimental protocol, in selecting a valid animal model, and in interpreting experimental results. Confounding factors should be kept at a minimum.

Underexposing experimental animals will seriously undermine a study's value for risk assessment; overexposing animals might induce "artifact" effects which, in turn, would lead to erroneous conclusions. The route of administration and exposure regimen should simulate human exposure conditions as closely as practical. Species-specific characteristics, not necessarily known before the start of an experiment, can interfere with the objectives of a study. Agents generally recognized as harmful at higher concentrations might not be noxious at very low concentrations; they may, in fact, have certain "beneficial" effects (hormesis). The time of onset of a lesion may be as important as its final incidence in evaluating experimental results. The significantly higher incidences of respiratory tract lesions observed, in our laboratory, in cigarette-smoke-exposed hamsters would make a fairly strong case for cigarettes being the causative agent, had not the exposed hamsters had a 28% longer life span than their controls, thus raising the possibility of age-related lesions. Age-specific comparisons are, therefore, important. If a test agent significantly affects body weight, another confounding factor will be introduced, one which might make it difficult to differentiate between biological effects of the test agent and weight-related effects. And what does squamous metaplasia of the respiratory tract, experimentally induced in an inhalation study, mean for human risk assessment?

It behooves a skipper to steer carefully in these troubled waters to avoid the many shoals and mines.

INTRODUCTION

Over a period of 20 years we have conducted several inhalation bioassays of cigarette smoke in the hamster (Wehner et al., 1974a,b, 1976a, manuscript in preparation) and in the rat (Wehner et al., 1979b, 1981, manuscript in preparation; Loscutoff et al., 1982; Phelps et al., 1984). We have also performed inhalation bioassays of asbestos (Wehner et al., 1974a, 1975b; Wehner ,1980; Dagle and Wehner, 1985) and asbestos cement in the hamster (Wehner et al., 1978a,b, 1979a). Combined exposures of hamsters to cigarette smoke and other substances (Wehner et al., 1974a,b, 1975a, 1976b, 1977), including asbestos (Wehner et al., 1975b), and exposures of beagle dogs to radon daughters, uranium ore dust, and cigarette smoke (Cross et al., 1982; Gies et al., 1987) have also been conducted in our laboratory. What did we learn from these studies relative to the topic and objectives of this symposium?

Most of all, we learned caution: caution in formulating an experimental protocol designed to best meet the objectives of a given study (e.g., selecting a sensible exposure regimen, rational exposure concentrations, and suitable equipment); caution in selecting a proper animal model, based on the priorities assigned to the various criteria chosen to evaluate the biological effects of a given test article; and, last but not least, caution in interpreting the results of a study. While this might sound cogent and compellingly simple, reality is, unfortunately, more complex, because each step requires value judgments. Seasoned investigators have argued, are arguing, and will continue to argue—and I expect to see them argue at this symposium—about what constitutes a "sensible" exposure regimen, "rational" exposure conditions, "suitable" equipment, an "appropriate" animal model, and how to interpret results. In a maze with few absolutes I can offer only my humble opinion.

THE EXPERIMENTAL PROTOCOL

Route of Administration

Considerable energy has been spent debating the merits and demerits of various routes of administering air pollutants to be experimentally tested for biological effects. Each route of administration has advantages and disadvantages that determine its principal applications. Skin painting, for example, is widely used as a screening test to determine the relative toxicity of tobacco-smoke condensates. Intratracheal instillation and intrapleural implantation are common screening tests for dusts as well as tobacco-smoke condensates. These tests are relatively inexpensive and do not require sophisticated facilities and highly trained personnel. However, the predictive value of results from these tests for risk assessment of an air pollutant for humans is lower than that of an inhalation bioassay. Dose at the deposition site, dose distribution in target tissues, and dose administered over time simulate human exposure conditions much more closely in an inhalation bioassay than in any other test. Inhalation studies, however, are expensive because they are labor-intensive and require special facilities and equipment as well as specially trained personnel. Given these circumstances, inhalation bioassays are called for if the potential hazard and the size of the population at risk are deemed significant enough to warrant the effort. I am, perhaps, prejudiced by my 21 years in inhalation toxicology: When massive doses of an implanted or instilled air pollutant eventually produce some tumors and publications, I take note but tend to avoid enthusiastic chants of "Eureka!"

Exposure Regimen

The exposure regimen should be determined by the objective(s) of the study. If risk assessment for humans is contemplated, the exposure regimen—like the route of administration—should simulate human exposure as closely as practical.

In the case of cigarette smoke, ideally this would call for multiple 10-minute exposures of animals to fresh cigarette smoke, produced under standard smoking conditions, 16 hours/day, 7 days/week, for life. This statement is based on the observation that a given quantity of a test material, administered as a single, relatively high dose, does not necessarily have the same biological effects as when it is administered in multiple smaller doses. Some target cells might be more resistant to the challenge because of the lower dose of each of the multiple applications; other cells might become less resistant over a period of multiple exposures (even to relatively low doses) with continued suppression of repair processes. In either case, conditions and events at the cellular and molecular levels could be markedly different from those experienced by cells receiving a single, high-dose exposure, and different conditions can lead to different biological consequences. Likewise, interruption of exposures during weekends might permit tissue repair, which might prevent or attenuate the progression of lesions that might have taken place under conditions of uninterrupted exposure.

Occupational exposure to mineral fibers can be simulated in the laboratory more conveniently than cigarette-smoke exposures; animals need be exposed only for 6 to 8 hours/day, 5 days/week, for life.

Any study attempting to investigate long-term biological effects—especially such endpoints as malignant tumors—generally calls for lifespan exposures. In a "chronic" study conducted quite a number of years ago, the client specified, despite our recommendations to the contrary, that exposures end after only X number of months, when more than 50% of the animals were still alive. The client then requested that I present the results of this study at an international symposium. I still remember the painfully embarrassing moment when the first question that I received from the audience after my presentation was: "Why did you truncate the experiment after only X months?" Other worthwhile findings of that study notwithstanding, the results were nearly useless for evaluating the carcinogenicity of the test material.

Cross et al. (1982) exposed dogs chronically to radon (105 nCi/L air), radon daughters (605 working levels* [WL]), uranium ore dust (13 mg/m^3) for 4 hours/day, 5 days/ week and to cigarette smoke (10 or 20 cigarettes/day, 7 days/week). Tumors in the dogs exposed to the radioactive agents were observed only after about 50 months of exposure, while no tumors were observed in the dogs exposed to cigarette smoke.

EXPOSURE CONCENTRATIONS

Defining or determining "rational" exposure concentrations presents a vexing problem. Owing to obvious logistic and budgetary limitations, we cannot conduct "megamouse" experiments to investigate and confirm in laboratory animals, for example, epidemiological findings in hundreds of thousands of people on a one-animal-to-one-human basis. An alternative, accepted by most investigators, is to conduct laboratory experiments with a considerably smaller number of animals and a compensatory increase in dose. This "compensatory" increase is quite often interpreted as the maximally tolerated dose, administered to the animal for life, regardless of the usually very much lower concentrations to which humans are exposed. These dose differences between human and animal exposures can lead to different results, both quantitatively (incidence and severity of resultant lesions) and qualitatively (type

*Working level (WL) is defined as any combination of the short-lived radon daughters in 1 L of air that will result in the ultimate emission of 1.3×10^5 MeV of potential α-energy.

of resultant lesions). Paul Morrow has for years criticized the "overloading" of animals in inhalation studies, with their potentially misleading conclusions. He sets an upper limit of 2 to 3 mg/m^3 for exposures to any test agent, concentrations that, he says, do not overwhelm the animals' clearance mechanisms. Muhle et al. (1987) determined the maximal dose of a pigmented polymer powder that could be functionally tolerated as a lung burden for which macrophage-mediated clearance was not significantly impaired. These investigators exposed Fischer-344 (F-344) rats to $^{59}FeO_2$-spiked test material at concentrations of 0, 1, 4, 16, or 64 mg/m^3, 6 hours/day, 5 days/week, for 13 weeks. Some indications of slightly impaired clearance were observed in the 16-mg/m^3 group after 13 weeks of exposure. Significant clearance impairment occurred at 30, 60, and 90 days of exposure in the 64-mg/m^3 group.

In the previously mentioned study by Cross et al. (1982), the authors found that exposure of dogs to cigarette smoke had a mitigating effect on radon-daughter-induced tumors. Exposure to 10 cigarettes/day produced no significant respiratory tract lesions, but exposures to 20 cigarettes/day resulted in pulmonary emphysema, fibrosis, chronic bronchitis, and bronchiolitis.

"Proper" dose selection presents a dilemma for which I see no solution on the horizon, especially with the various professional, commercial, political, and emotional forces pulling in different directions. All we can do is to steer away from extremes and use good professional judgment, and experience, in an attempt to determine a "rational" concentration range for a given test agent.

In a cocarcinogenicity study sponsored by the National Cancer Institute, we exposed 102 Syrian Golden hamsters in an intended lifespan study to a mean chrysotile aerosol concentration of 23 mg/m^3, 7 hours/day, 5 days/week. Half of the animals were also exposed, in modified Hamburg II smoking machines, to smoke from Kentucky 1R1 research cigarettes, 10 minutes/exposure, three exposures/day, 5 days/week. Another group of 102 hamsters served as controls. Half of the controls received smoke exposures (smoke controls), the other half received sham dust and sham smoke exposures. Asbestos exposure resulted in earlier and more severe lung lesions than those observed in identical groups of the same study that had received lifespan exposures to aerosols of NiO (53 mg/m^3) and CoO (10 mg/m^3), or that were treated with diethylnitrosamine (12 x 0.25 mg, by subcutaneous injection). Asbestosis developed in all animals and forced discontinuation of the asbestos exposures after 11 months. Of 12 lung adenomas found in 510 hamsters, 10 occurred among the 102 animals of the asbestos-exposed groups, indicating an early neoplastic response. The incidence of laryngeal lesions and of malignant tumors was significantly lower in the asbestos-plus-smoke-exposed group than in the smoke control group, probably because of their significantly shorter life span as a result of asbestosis. Neither a carcinogenic effect of asbestos nor a cocarcinogenic effect of cigarette smoke was observed. Cigarette-smoke inhalation resulted in significantly lower mean body weights (~20%) and *longer* life spans in the smoke-exposed groups. In hindsight—i.e., about 10 months into the exposures—it became apparent that the concentration of 23 mg asbestos/m^3 was too high, a fact that would not have been revealed even if we had been authorized to conduct a subchronic range-finding study before the chronic exposures. I will comment on the longer life span when I discuss interpretation of results, later in this presentation.

In another study (again, many years ago), we were requested by a client to expose animals for a few minutes/day to low concentrations of a rather innocuous substance. Such experimental protocols certainly can provide answers to specific scientific questions, but their predictive value for assessing risks to human populations is next to nil.

THE ANIMAL MODEL

I have previously commented on animal models for inhalation bioassays of cigarette smoke (Wehner, 1983) in a contribution to the book *Comparative Respiratory Tract Carcinogenesis* (Reznik-Schüller, 1983). With permission from CRC Press I repeat these comments here, with a few updates.

Various animal models, including chickens, cats, sheep, rabbits, several rodent species, dogs, donkeys, and primates, have been used to investigate biological effects of cigarette smoke. However, for inhalation bioassays to determine carcinogenicity, interest has focused mainly on rats, hamsters, mice, and dogs.

Each of the species has advantages and disadvantages. Laskin and Sellakumar (1974), for example, comment on animal models in chemical carcinogenesis: "...the present state of our knowledge finds the animal that most closely meets the requirements of the ideal model (as postulated by Roe, 1966) to be the common laboratory rat." The rat and mouse, of course, were selected as animal models of choice by the National Toxicology Program. The positive response of the Syrian Golden hamster to a variety of carcinogens has been reported by a number of investigators. Among them are Dontenwill (1964, 1970), Dontenwill et al. (1973), Dontenwill and Mohr (1961), Herrold and Dunham (1963), Montesano et al. (1970), Montesano and Saffiotti (1968, 1970), and Mohr et al. (1966a,b). In developing an experimental animal model for the study of the pathogenesis of lung cancer, Montesano et al. (1970) used this species extensively and reported that the Syrian Golden hamster was "markedly susceptible to various respiratory carcinogens and conveniently refractory to chronic pulmonary infections." Dontenwill (1970) reported precancerous and cancerous lesions in the respiratory tract of hamsters exposed to cigarette smoke in Hamburg II smoking machines. Auerbach et al. (1967,1968,1969,1970) and Frasca et al. (1971,1974) are among the investigators who have used the dog repeatedly. In our laboratory, all four species have been used in inhalation studies.

The rat is the most extensively investigated laboratory animal and the one for which the most complete and best database is available. In addition, the rat is large enough for the convenient measurement of a variety of physiological parameters, yet it is small enough to conduct a study using several hundred animals without the logistic problems one would encounter with the same number of a larger species, such as the dog. Furthermore, lifespan studies can be completed in 3 years. In addition, the rat is inexpensive and readily available. On the other hand, the rat is probably more prone to intercurrent lung lesions than the hamster. Such lesions of the primary target organ might mask changes produced by the inhaled test material and/or interfere with interpretation of the (histo)pathologic and/or physiological findings. This problem can be controlled by using Cesarean-derived, specific-pathogen-free animals and maintaining them for the duration of the experiment (i.e., often for 24 or more months) under barrier conditions designed to exclude murine pathogens. However, such procedures require considerable effort as well as facilities that are not available in many laboratories.

The mouse is also well-researched, inexpensive, and readily available. Owing to its small size, large numbers of animals can be conveniently handled in a given experiment, but because of its small size, the blood available for hematology and clinical chemistry tests is severely limited.

The primary advantage of the hamster is its "clean" lung. Lifespan exposures can be completed in less than 2 years; and, like the rat, the hamster is inexpensive, and studies with a large number of animals can be conducted without logistic problems. On the other hand, its relatively small size can be a disadvantage. While recent developments permit respiratory-function measurements to be made on hamsters, these state-of-the-art techniques are not readily available in many laboratories. In addition, hematology and clinical chemistry tests are more limited than in the rat because of the smaller quantities of blood that can be safely collected. Major disadvantages are the hamster's susceptibility to proliferative ileitis (wet-tail disease) and amyloidosis, and the limited availability of hamsters that are free of common viral pathogens.

The dog—usually the beagle—resembles man in size much more closely than the rat, the hamster, or the mouse. Smoke-exposure conditions can simulate those of human smokers rather closely by having dogs inhale the smoke through appropriate mask/valve systems (Bair et al., 1969), or tracheostomized dogs can be used (Auerbach et al., 1970; Zwicker et al., 1978). Both approaches would be impractical, if not impossible, in rodents. Blood samples can be collected from the dog without negative effects, and in larger quantities, more frequently than from the rat, the hamster, or the mouse. However, dogs are more expensive to obtain and maintain and are not as readily available from well-controlled, "clean" stock as rats or mice. Aside from budgetary considerations, the dog's size poses logistic problems that limit the number of dogs that can be used in an experiment. Results from lifespan studies take considerable time (and thus money) to develop in view of the beagle's mean life span of more than 12 years.

Each of the four species—rat, mouse, hamster, and dog—has been shown to develop cancer of the respiratory tract in response to challenge by an appropriate carcinogen. However, this specific response to cigarette smoke administered by inhalation is rather rare in all four species. Whether manifestation of respiratory tract cancer in an animal model is necessary, or whether dose-dependent and potentially precancerous lesions in the respiratory tract suffice as predictive indicators for relative pathogenicity—and, more specifically, carcinogenicity—of a given cigarette remains a matter of animated debate among disciples of different schools of thought.

Regarding our own experience, I would like to refer in addition to the aforementioned cocarcinogenicity study of cigarette smoke and dusts in hamsters—to an inhalation bioassay of cigarette smoke in rats (Wehner et al., 1979b, 1981). This study was conducted for the National Cancer Institute with the objective of determining whether inhalation bioassays of cigarette smoke in the rat are a suitable technique to determine biological effects of cigarette smoke and whether this bioassay is sensitive enough to differentiate between the biological effects of three different types of research cigarettes.

In summary, groups of 80 female F-344 rats were exposed to cigarette smoke from three types (Code 13 = high tar, low nicotine; Code 27 = low tar, medium nicotine; Code 32 = high tar, high nicotine) of research cigarettes in Maddox-ORNL smoking machines (Maddox et al., 1978) eight times/day, 7 days/week, for up to 24 months. An additional group received sham exposures, and a fifth group served as untreated controls. Various physiological measurements were made periodically and before serial sacrifices to evaluate acute and chronic effects of exposure to cigarette smoke. Acute effects observed during smoke exposure included irregular breathing and a decrease in total inhaled volume to 25% of the sham-exposed controls' volume. Body weight (lower in smoke-exposed animals), blood pressure (higher in smoke-exposed animals) and heart rate (lower in smoke-exposed animals) showed consistent and significant differences between smoke-exposed and control groups. Body weight and survival parameters were sensitive enough to reflect the two dose groups indicated by *in vivo* dosimetry measurements (Code 13 versus Codes 27 and 32). Survival of Code 13 animals was similar to that of the sham-exposed and untreated control groups; survival rates of Codes 27 and 32 animals were lower. Smoke-induced histopathologic lesions consisted primarily of pulmonary smoke granulomas. Additional changes included alveolar epithelial hyperplasia, basal cell hyperplasia, interstitial reaction, and squamous metaplasia of laryngeal and tracheal epithelium. Differences in the severity of the smoke granulomas made it possible to differentiate between the Code 27 exposure group (less-severe granulomas) and the groups exposed to smoke from Codes 13 or 32 cigarettes. One primary epidermoid carcinoma was found in the lung of a Code 27 rat.

To my knowledge, no other species has shown a pronounced susceptibility to cigarette-smoke-induced cancer of the respiratory tract in inhalation studies, with the exception of the tracheostomized dogs of Auerbach et al. (1970) and the inbred BIO 15.16 hamster strain (Bernfeld et al., 1979), which appears to be difficult to obtain.

Recently, we conducted two almost identical 3-month exposures of Sprague-Dawley-derived (Crl:CD) rats and Syrian Golden hamsters to smoke from the Kentucky 1R4F reference cigarette and a newly developed cigarette that only heats but does not burn tobacco (manuscripts to be submitted for publication). These studies provided a unique opportunity to compare the response of the rat and the hamster to cigarette smoke under very similar experimental conditions. While there were no dramatic differences in response, the results suggested that the rat appears to be a somewhat more responsive model in terms of smoke-induced lesions of the respiratory tract; the hamster appears to be somewhat more sensitive in its body-weight response. Histopathologic changes are, without doubt, the most important criterion in such studies. We therefore consider the rat the model of choice for inhalation bioassays of cigarette smoke, and the hamster an acceptable choice as a second species. This opinion is based on the sum of our experience with both species over a period of 20 years. It should be noted that neither species responds to cigarette-smoke inhalation with a significant incidence of primary malignant tumors of the respiratory tract. As stated before, it remains a matter of debate whether such a response is necessary, or whether dose-dependent benign respiratory tract lesions, such as severe squamous metaplasia with atypical cell nuclei, suffice as reasonably valid predictive indicators for potential carcinogenicity in humans.

The hamster model failed to show a potentiating effect of cigarette smoke on asbestos exposures, as reported in man by Selikoff et al. (1968). However, in the absence of appropriate experiments, we do not know whether the rat would have been more responsive under the same experimental conditions. Based on our results, we do know that the hamster is unacceptable for bioassays of cigarette smoke in which survival is the chief criterion, because species-specific characteristics significantly increase survival in cigarette-smoke-exposed hamsters (see below). Renne et al. (1985) investigated the fibrogenic potential of intratracheally deposited quartz and other materials in the hamster. While these materials did cause pulmonary fibrosis, the authors noted that "the dense fibrous tissue present in the lungs in classical human silicosis and in experimental silicosis of rats was not observed." The authors conclude that the hamster is therefore not a suitable model for quartz-induced pulmonary fibrosis.

INTERPRETATION OF RESULTS

Sometimes, things are not what they seem. Obscure factors can interfere with experimental procedures and affect results of a study. It then takes caution, experience and intuition to avoid a potentially embarrassing misinterpretation of experimental findings.

For example, we were dumbfounded, at first, when the mortality in all five smoke-exposed hamster groups of our previously mentioned cocarcinogenicity study was significantly lower than in the sham-exposed controls (Wehner et al., 1974a, 1976a). These findings contradicted everything that had been published about the effects of tobacco smoke on the survival of both humans and experimental animals. The fact that the phenomenon occurred in all five smoke-exposed groups proved that this was not a spurious event. After many hours of examining and re-examining our data, we discovered that the *onset* of amyloidosis was delayed in the smoke-exposed hamsters even though the final incidence of amyloidosis showed no significant differences among the various treatment groups (Wehner et al., 1976a). Amyloidosis is a common degenerative disease in aging hamsters and was frequently the cause of death in the animals of that experiment. Obviously, if a given agent manages to delay the onset of a potentially fatal disease, the exposed animals can be expected to live longer. As to the mode of action by which amyloidosis was delayed in the smoke-exposed groups, two explanations appear plausible. Cigarette smoke could enhance the immune response of the exposed animals or attenuate the production and/or activity of the amyloid-enhancing factor (Franklin and Zucker-Franklin, 1972). In both cases, amyloid deposition would be retarded. The second possibility would be an indirect effect of cigarette smoke associated with reduced body weight, whereby reduced weight might affect the immune system. Widdowson and Kennedy (1962) found that rats maintained at reduced body weight by hypocaloric feeding had a longer life span and a lower incidence of age-related degenerative diseases than rats maintained at normal body weight by *ad libitum* feeding. Berg and Simms (1961) reported that rats whose feed intake was restricted lived longer and experienced a delay in the onset of disease (e.g., tumors, cardiac, renal, and vascular lesions).

Another example of a confounding variable faced us in the same experiment. The group of 51 hamsters exposed only to cigarette smoke (smoke controls) experienced a significantly increased incidence of the following lesions, compared to the 51 sham-exposed control hamsters:

Incidence of all tumors	=	28% versus 6% (P <0.05)
Malignant tumors	=	18% versus 2% (P <0.05)
Epithelial lesions of the larynx	=	22% versus 0% (P <0.01).

However, the increased incidence of lesions in the smoke-exposed hamsters is not necessarily a direct effect of the exposures to cigarette smoke. It might be explained by the significantly longer mean life span (19.6 months) of the smoke-exposed group, compared to 15.3 months for the sham-exposed controls (+28%). We will never know what the lesion incidence in the sham-exposed hamsters would have been if they had lived as long as the smoke-exposed hamsters. This dilemma emphasizes the importance of age-specific comparisons.

An agent generally considered toxic or pathogenic is not necessarily so under all conditions and at all concentrations. Paracelsus (1493-1541) stated some 400 years ago, "*Dosis solum venenum facit.*" (Only the dose makes a poison.) Extrapolation from observed effects at higher doses to effects at very low doses, based on an assumption of a linear, no-threshold dose-response relationship, might be contraindicated for more agents than is generally realized. Active immunization is a splendid example of agents that are protective ("beneficial") at very low doses but harmful at higher doses. Certainly, the linear no-threshold assumption does not apply here, nor does it in many other cases. This "pharmacological inversion" (Furst, 1987) as a function of dose is called hormesis. Hormetic effects have been observed even for agents of such ill repute as ionizing radiation. Last year, the prestigious journal Health Physics devoted an entire issue to radiation hormesis. Dr. Leonard A. Sagan's guest editorial in that issue (1987) should be required reading for all scientists concerned with these issues. As reviewed by Sterling (1983), there is some evidence suggesting that low doses of cigarette smoke stimulate defensive mechanisms (e.g., immune system, accumulation of pulmonary alveolar macrophages, stimulation of mucus production, accelerated respiratory tract clearance), thereby exerting a "beneficial" effect of one kind or another. The mitigating effect of cigarette smoke on radon-daughter-induced tumors in dogs (Cross et al., 1982) has already been mentioned. The underexposure of experimental animals to cigarette smoke, compared to human exposure, and the possibility of resultant hormetic effects might explain why inhalation exposure generally does not induce a significant incidence of malignant respiratory tract tumors in these animals.

Regarding interpretation of results, what does squamous metaplasia really mean? Is it a carcinoma waiting to happen, or is it merely a reversible, nonspecific reaction to a very high or repeatedly administered dose of some agent?

Some of us tend to make value judgments based on our perception of a test agent. It was somewhat sobering, but perhaps altogether not too surprising, to find that we could induce squamous metaplasia of the larynx—albeit of only minimal to mild severity—in rats exposed for 2 weeks to very high concentrations (4 mg/L) or for 13 weeks to 0.66 mg/L glycerol, a substance generally recognized as safe (GRAS compound; manuscript in preparation). *Dosis solum venenum facit!*

Confounding variables that contributed to the complexity of the data analysis in our chronic inhalation bioassay of cigarette smoke in rats (and, probably, to similar studies) included: (1) body weight, (2) age at final sacrifice, and possibly (3) selection of the "fittest" animals.

(1) Significant differences among the body weights of the experimental groups were observed. It is therefore necessary to consider the possibility that the cardiovascular effects reported in that study might not be a primary consequence of smoke exposure but might be secondary to the significant weight differences among the exposure groups. While it appears unlikely that changes in body weight alone could account for the observed cardiovascular effects, other physiological functions could be directly affected by weight loss. They, in turn, could then exert some effects on cardiovascular functions. Some form of matched-feeding protocol would be one approach to minimizing this problem, although not necessarily solving it: the animals whose feed intake is restricted to match the lower *ad-libitum* feed intake of the smoke-exposed animals might be stressed by feeling hungry. This would introduce another confounding variable with intangible effects, but only for the control animals.

(2) The most detailed cardiovascular-function measurements of that study were made before each of three scheduled serial sacrifices. To ensure survival of an adequate number of animals to final (24-month) sacrifice, only five animals per treatment group were invasively tested before the serial (12- and 18-month) sacrifices. Natural biological variability, combined with a small test population, resulted in diminished statistical sensitivity for detecting differences by what might otherwise have been more powerful tests. At the time of final sacrifice, the statistically useful number of surviving animals might have been so old as to show age-related cardiovascular changes, confounded by the changes resulting from smoke exposure. Age-related changes in cardiovascular functions are well documented (Berg, 1955; Berg and Harmison, 1955; Tuttle, 1966).

(3) The smoke-exposed rats tested before the final sacrifice had lived for 2 years under adverse conditions. These conditions might have functioned as a selection process in which only the fittest survived. It is therefore conceivable that data obtained from smoke-exposed animals during the final months of the study are not necessarily representative of values observed in a normal, unselected population of animals.

Results of that study also show that the probability of discovering subtle physiological changes is low when physiological measurements are merely an ancillary part rather than the main objective of the investigation. A physiologically oriented experimental protocol should provide for a sufficiently large number of animals to be tested before aging can mask treatment-related physiological effects.

As to the interpretation of cardiorespiratory findings, it must be remembered that nicotine and carbon monoxide (CO) are the two most important components of cigarette smoke known to affect cardiovascular function (Goodman and Gillman, 1975; Ball and Turner, 1974). At concentrations normally encountered during exposure to cigarette smoke, the principal pharmacological action of nicotine is to cause the release of catecholamines, both from adrenergic nerve endings and from the adrenal medulla. Nicotine also stimulates carotid and aortic body chemoreceptors. The net effect of these actions is to cause an increase in heart rate, blood pressure, and myocardial contractility with a concomitant increase in myocardial oxygen demand. Carbon monoxide has also been implicated as a causative agent in smoking-related cardiovascular disease. It binds to hemoglobin 250 to 300 times more efficiently than O_2. In doing so, CO decreases the O_2 content of the arterial blood and impairs the release of oxygen to the tissues. Thus, at a time when oxygen demands are increased by the actions of nicotine, the ability to supply the needed oxygen is impaired. The resulting tissue hypoxia might ultimately contribute to the effects on cardiovascular function associated with chronic exposure to cigarette smoke.

CLOSING COMMENTS

Santayana's maxim that those who do not learn from the mistakes of the past are doomed to relive them is not restricted to political history. It is a generally applicable truism that includes scientific research. Caution and experience are good companions on the difficult road toward elucidating the biological interaction of inhaled mineral fibers and cigarette smoke.

REFERENCES

Auerbach, O, EC Hammond, D Kirman, and L Garfinkel. **1967.** Emphysema produced in dogs by cigarette smoking. J Am Med Assoc 199:241-246.

Auerbach, O, EC Hammond, D Kirman, et al. **1968.** The effect of direct cigarette smoke inhalation on the respiratory tree of dogs. Natl Cancer Inst Monogr 28:65-77.

Auerbach, O, EC Hammond, D Kirman, L Garfinkel, and AP Stout. **1969.** Histologic changes in bronchial tubes of cigarette-smoking dogs. Cancer 20:2055-2066.

Auerbach, O, EC Hammond, D Kirman, et al. **1970.** Effects of cigarette smoking in dogs: II. Pulmonary neoplasms. Arch Environ Health 21:754-768.

Bair, WJ, NS Porter, DP Brown, and AP Wehner. **1969.** Apparatus for direct inhalation of cigarette smoke by dogs. J Appl Physiol 26:847-850.

Ball, K and R Turner. **1974.** Smoking and the heart. The basis for action. Lancet 2:822-826.

Berg, BN. **1955.** The electrocardiogram in aging rats. J Gerontol 10:420-423.

Berg, BN and CR Harmison. **1955.** Blood pressure and heart size in aging rats. J Gerontol 10:416-419.

Berg, BN and HS Simms. **1961.** Nutrition and longevity in the rat: III. Food restriction beyond 800 days. J Nutr 74:23-32.

Bernfeld, P, F Homburger, and AB Russfield. **1979.** Cigarette smoke-induced cancer of the larynx in hamsters (CINCH): A method to assay the carcinogenicity of cigarette smoke, pp. 315-319. In: *The Syrian Hamster in Toxicology and Carcinogenesis Research,* F Homburger (ed.), *Progress in Experimental Tumor Research,* Vol. 24. S. Karger, New York, NY.

Cross, FT, RF Palmer, R.E Filipy, GE Dagle, and BO Stuart, **1982.** Carcinogenic effects of radon daughters, uranium ore dust and cigarette smoke in beagle dogs. Health Phys 42:33-52.

Dagle, GE and AP Wehner. **1985.** Asbestosis in hamsters, pp. 183-185. In: *The Respiratory System,* TC Jones, V Mohr, and RD Hunt (eds.), *Monographs on Pathology of Laboratory Animals.* Springer-Verlag, New York, NY.

Dontenwill, W. **1964.** Experimentelle Untersuchungen zur Genese des Lungencarcinoms. Arzneim Forsch 14:774.

Dontenwill, W. **1970.** Experimental investigations on the effect of cigarette smoke inhalation on small laboratory animals, pp. 389-409. In: *Inhalation Carcinogenesis,* MG Hanna, Jr, P Nettesheim, and JR Gilbert (eds.). CONF-691001, NTIS, Springfield, VA.

Dontenwill, W, HJ Chevalier, HP Harke, U LaFrenz, and G Reckzeh. **1973.** Spontantumoren des syrischen Goldhamsters. Z Krebsforsch 80:127.

Dontenwill, W and U Mohr. **1961.** Carcinome des Respirationstrakts nach Behandlung von Goldhamstern mit Diäthylnitrosamin. Z Krebsforsch 64:305.

Franklin, EC and D Zucker-Franklin. **1972.** Current concepts of amyloid. Adv Immunol 15:249-304.

Frasca, JM, O Auerbach, VR Parks, and JD Jamieson. **1971.** Electron microscopic observations on pulmonary fibrosis and emphysema in smoking dogs. Exp Mol Pathol 15:108-125.

Frasca, JM, O Auerbach, VR Parks, and JD Jamieson. **1974.** Alveolar cell hyperplasia in the lungs of smoking dogs. Exp Mol Pathol 21:300-312.

Furst, A. **1987.** Hormetic effects in pharmacology: Pharmacological inversions as prototypes for hormesis. Health Phys 52:527-530.

Gies, RA, FT Cross, and GE Dagle. **1987.** A histologic study of the influence of cigarette smoking in suppressing Rn daughter carcinogenesis in dogs. Health Phys 53:527-529.

Goodman, LS and A Gillman (eds.). **1975.** *The Pharmacological Basis of Therapeutics,* 5th Edition. MacMillan Publishing Co., New York, NY.

Herrold, KM and LJ Dunham. **1963.** Induction of tumors in the Syrian hamster with diethylnitrosamine (N-nitrosodiethylamine). Cancer Res 23:773-777.

Laskin, S and A Sellakumar. **1974.** Models in chemical respiratory carcinogenesis, pp. 7-19. In: *Experimental Lung Cancer. Carcinogenesis and Bioassays,* E Karbe and JF Park (eds.). Springer-Verlag, New York, NY.

Loscutoff, SM, RA Jaffe, DI Hilton, DW Phelps, DB Carr, and AP Wehner. **1982.** Dosimetry and cardiopulmonary function in rats chronically exposed to cigarette smoke. Toxicol Appl Pharmacol 64:335-352.

Maddox, WL, WE Dalbey, MR Guerin, JR Stokeley, DA Cresia, and J Kendrick. **1978.** A tobacco smoke inhalation exposure device for rodents. Arch Environ Health 33:64-71.

Mohr, U, J Althoff, and A Authaler. **1966a.** Diaplacental effect of the carcinogen diethylnitrosamine in the golden hamster. Cancer Res 26:2349-2352.

Mohr, U, O Wieser, and K Pielsticker. **1966b.** Die Minimaldosis für die Wirkung von Diäthylnitrosamin auf die Trachea beim Goldhamster. Naturwissenschaften 53:229.

Montesano, R and U Saffiotti. **1968.** Carcinogenic response of the respiratory tract of Syrian golden hamsters to different doses of diethylnitrosamine. Cancer Res 28:2197-2210.

Montesano, R and U Saffiotti. **1970.** Carcinogenic response of the hamster respiratory tract to single subcutaneous administrations of diethylnitrosamine at birth. J Natl Cancer Inst 44:413-417.

Montesano, R, U Saffiotti, and P Shubik. **1970.** The role of topical and systemic factors in experimental respiratory carcinogenesis, pp. 353-368. In: *Inhalation Carcinogenesis,* MG Hanna, Jr, P Nettesheim, and JR Gilbert (eds.). CONF-691001, NTIS, Springfield, VA.

Muhle, H, B Bellmann, O Creutzenberg, R Klipper, and R Mermelstein. **1987.** Pulmonary deposition, retention, and clearance of pigmented polymer in rats. In: *The Design and Interpretation of Inhalation Studies and Their Use in Risk Assessments,* International Life Sciences Institute Symposium, March 23-27, 1987, Hannover, Federal Republic of Germany. Institute of Experimental Pathology, Hannover Medical School, Hannover, Federal Republic of Germany (abstract).

Phelps, DW, JT Veal, RL Buschbom, RE Filipy, and AP Wehner. **1984.** Tobacco smoke inhalation studies: A dosimetric comparison of different cigarette types. Arch Environ Health 39:359-363.

Renne, RA, SR Eldridge, TR Lewis, and DL Stevens. **1985.** Fibrogenic potential of intratracheally instilled quartz, ferric oxide, fibrous glass, and hydrated alumina in hamsters. Toxicol Pathol 13:306-314.

Reznik-Schüller, HM (ed.). **1983.** *Comparative Respiratory Tract Carcinogenesis,* CRC Press, Boca Raton, FL.

Roe, FJC. **1966.** The relevance and value of studies of lung tumors in laboratory animals in research on cancer of the human lung, pp. 101-126. In: *Lung Tumors in Animals,* L Severi, (ed.), Proceedings of the Third Quad. Conference on Cancer, University of Perugia.

Sagan, LA **1987.** What is hormesis and why haven't we heard about it before? Health Phys 52:521-525.

Selikoff, IJ, EC Hammond, and J Churg. **1968.** Asbestos exposure, smoking and neoplasia. J Am Med Assoc 204:104-110.

Sterling, TD. **1983.** Possible effects on occupational lung cancer from smoking related changes in the mucus content of the lung. J Chron Dis 36:669-676.

Tuttle, RS. **1966.** Age-related changes in the sensitivity of rat aortic strips to norepinephrine and associated chemical and structural alterations. J Gerontol 21:510-516.

Wehner, AP. **1980.** Effects of inhaled asbestos, asbestos plus cigarette smoke, asbestos cement, and talc baby powder in hamsters, pp. 373-376. In: *Biological Effects of Mineral Fibers,* JC Wagner and W Davis (eds.), IARC Scientific Publication No. 30, World Health Organization. IARC, Lyon, France.

Wehner, AP. **1983.** Cigarette smoke-induced alterations in the respiratory tract of man and experimental animals. In: *Comparative Respiratory Tract Carcinogenesis,* HM Reznik-Schüller (ed.). CRC Press, Boca Raton, FL.

Wehner, AP, et al. **1974a.** *Investigation of Cocarcinogenicity of Asbestos, Cobalt Oxide (CoO), Nickel Oxide (NiO), Diethylnitrosamine and Cigarette Smoke,* Technical Report to National Cancer Institute, Bethesda, MD. Battelle, Pacific Northwest Laboratories, Richland, WA.

Wehner, AP, RH Busch, and RJ Olson. **1974b.** Effect of chronic exposure to cigarette smoke on tumor incidence in the Syrian Golden hamster, pp. 360-368. In: *Experimental Lung Cancer. Carcinogenesis and Bioassays,* E Karbe and JF Park (eds.). Springer-Verlag, New York, NY.

Wehner, AP, RH Busch, RJ Olson, and DK Craig. **1975a.** Chronic inhalation of nickel oxide and cigarette smoke by hamsters. Am Ind Hyg Assoc J 36:801-810.

Wehner, AP, RH Busch, RJ Olson, and DK Craig. **1975b.** Chronic inhalation of asbestos and cigarette smoke by hamsters. Environ Res 10:368-383.

Wehner, AP, RJ Olson, and RH Busch. **1976a.** Increased life span and decreased body weight in cigarette-smoke-exposed hamsters. Arch Environ Health 31:146-153.

Wehner, AP, RH Busch, and RJ Olson. **1976b.** Effects of diethylnitrosamine and cigarette smoke in hamsters. J Natl Cancer Inst 56:749-756.

Wehner, AP, RH Busch, RJ Olson, and DK Craig. **1977.** Chronic inhalation of cobalt oxide and cigarette smoke by hamsters. Am Ind Hyg Assoc J 38:338-346.

Wehner, AP, GE Dagle, and WC Cannon. **1978a.** Development of an animal model, techniques, and an exposure system to study the effects of asbestos cement dust inhalation. Environ Res 16:393-407.

Wehner, AP, GE Dagle, WC Cannon, and RL Buschbom. **1978b.** Biological effects of inhaled asbestos cement dust in the Syrian Golden hamster. Environ Res 17:367-389.

Wehner, AP, GE Dagle, WC Cannon, and RL Buschbom. **1979a.** Biological effects of inhaled asbestos cement dust in the Syrian Golden hamster, pp. 97-108. In: *Dust and Diseases,* R Lemen and JM Dement (eds.). Pathotox Publications, Inc., Park Forest South, IL.

Wehner, AP, EM Milliman, DB Carr, and JR Decker. **1979b.** *Inhalation Bioassay of Cigarette Smoke in Rats,* Technical Report to Enviro Control, Inc., Rockville, MD. Battelle, Pacific Northwest Laboratories, Richland, WA.

Wehner, AP, GE Dagle, EM Milliman, DW Phelps, DB Carr, JR Decker, and RE Filipy. **1981.** Inhalation bioassay of cigarette smoke in rats. Toxicol Appl Pharmacol 61:1-17.

Widdowson, EM and GC Kennedy. **1962.** Rate of growth, mature weight and life span. Proc R Soc Lond (Ser B) 156:96-108.

Zwicker, GM, RE Filipy, JF Park, SM Loscutoff, HA Ragan, and DL Stevens. **1978.** Clinical and pathological effects of cigarette smoke exposure in beagle dogs. Arch Pathol Lab Med 102:623-628.

INTERACTION OF FIBERS AND CIGARETTE SMOKE: HYPOTHESES, MODELS AND FACTORS

Model for the Joint Influence of Occupational Exposure to Carcinogenic Dust and to Cigarette Smoke and Occupational Lung Cancer

Theodor D. Sterling

Faculty of Applied Sciences, School of Computing Science, Simon Fraser University, Burnaby, B.C., V5A 1S6, Canada

KEY WORDS: inhaled carcinogens, occupational lung cancer, cigarette smoke, increased mucus layer, mitigating effect

---

ABSTRACT

The model seeks to explain the substantial number of occupational health studies that find that the relative risk for lung cancer for carcinogen-exposed versus unexposed smokers is less than the relative risk for exposed versus unexposed nonsmokers or those who have never smoked. The model is built on the assumption that the smoking-induced mucus layer in the respiratory tract reduces the risk of exposure to inhaled occupational carcinogens in the lung by reducing the probability of contact between inhaled particles and the underlying lung tissue. Relevant evidence and support for the model come from a wide range of observations. These include: (1) findings of great difference in the mucus content of the lung between smokers and nonsmokers; (2) magnetometric manipulations of inhaled magnetized particles and fibers, which show that particles migrate differently in the lungs of smokers than in those of nonsmokers; (3) simulation of particle movements in mucus-like medium; and (4) animal studies that have shown that the effect of inhaled carcinogens (radon) on animals' lungs is reduced by simultaneous smoke inhalation. The important implication of the model is that the increased mucus content of the lungs and, possibly, the thickening of lung tissue may mitigate the effect of occupational exposures to carcinogens.

INTRODUCTION

The idea that smoking-induced biological processes may protect lungs against environmental hazards is not entirely new. A comparable hypothesis was suggested in the 1950s to explain the fact that coal miners with cigarette-smoke-induced bronchitis appeared to develop pneumoconiosis less often than miners without bronchitis. It has also been suggested that occupationally induced asthma is found less frequently among smokers than among nonsmokers (Ortmeyer et al., 1974).* Again, there is a possibility that this might be due to increased mucus in the lungs of smokers. There is anecdotal evidence that workers in dusty occupations sometimes claim they smoke (or chew) tobacco because it helps them eliminate dust from their lungs. Thomson and Pavia (1973) speculated that an increase in the viscosity of the mucus or a change in the thickness of the mucus sol layer (the less viscous layer of the mucus blanket in which the cilia beat) might affect the rate of particle removal and, thus, cancer incidence. The same idea has been suggested by other investigators (Axelson and Sundell, 1978; Weiss, 1980).

A number of years ago I accumulated evidence that suggested that smoking-related changes in the mucus content of the lung had a possible mitigating effect on occupational lung cancer (Sterling, 1983, 1984). The evidence has increased, since then, in support of a hypothesis that increased mucus and, possibly, other tissue changes in the lungs of workers exposed to dusts and fumes may, to some extent, protect them against occupational lung disease. Verification of these findings could have important consequences for preventive occupational measures. Various methods of increasing mucus flow of workers exposed to carcinogens could be devised. Also, verification of this hypothesis might elucidate the complex interaction between the effects of smoking and occupational (and, by extension, environmental) exposures to various irritants.

DO SMOKING-RELATED CHANGES IN THE LUNG PROTECT SMOKERS AGAINST EXPOSURE TO CARCINOGENS?

The hypothesis that smoking-related changes in the lung offer some protection from exposure to carcinogenic particles is difficult to test in a single, experimental setting. It depends on a large

*Also: Personal communication, 1982, S. Grzybowski, Director, Respiratory Clinic, University of British Columbia, Department of Medicine, Vancouver, B.C., Canada.

amount of data that have been reported by various investigators. Of special interest are answers to a number of questions:

1. Is the relative risk for occupational exposure greater for exposed compared to unexposed nonsmokers than that for exposed compared to unexposed smokers?
2. Do smokers and nonsmokers differ with respect to the mucus content of their lungs?
3. Do inhaled particles move differently in smokers' versus nonsmokers' lungs?
4. Does smoking inhibit or promote the elimination of particles from the lung?
5. What is the role of particles in producing malignancies?
6. To what extent can animal studies support this hypothesis?
7. What other differences between smokers and nonsmokers might throw light on this hypothesis?

This report is based on a literature search for data that can help answer these questions.

IS THE RELATIVE RISK FOR OCCUPATIONAL EXPOSURE GREATER FOR EXPOSED COMPARED TO UNEXPOSED NONSMOKERS THAN THAT FOR EXPOSED COMPARED TO UNEXPOSED SMOKERS?

A search was conducted through available computer-accessible abstracting services, using keywords "lung or pulmonary" and "cancer or carcino?"; "tobacco or smoke?"; and "occupation? or employ?" (The "?" represents all possible suffixes to a keyword, so that, for instance, "smoke?" stands for the words "smoke," "smoking," "smoker," and "smokers.")

The search produced 18 potentially usable studies that calculated risks separately for smokers and nonsmokers (or those who have never smoked; hereafter called "never-smokers"). Fifteen of these studies computed these separate risks for exposed workers compared to unexposed workers. Three other studies compared workers with high concentrations with workers exposed to low concentrations. The studies and their relevant results are summarized in Table 1.

For only three studies is the relative risk of exposed smokers versus that of unexposed or less-exposed smokers greater than the relative risk of exposed nonsmokers versus that of unexposed or

Table 1. Comparison of occupational lung-cancer relative risks for smokers and nonsmokers*

Study Type	Number of Subjects		Substance	Relative Risk	
(Archer et al., 1973)**					
Cohort		1,269	Uranium	Nonsmokers[a]	6.46
				Smokers	9.59
(Blot & Fraumeni, 1981)**[b]					
Case control		2,551	Asbestos	Nonsmokers[a]	2.2
				Ex-smokers	0.81
				0.5 pack/day	1.08
				0.5 to 1.5 pack/day	1.42
				>2 packs/day	2.11
(Damber & Larsson, 1982)**					
Case control	All Ages		Radon	All Ages	
	Cases	589		Nonsmokers[c]	2.4
	Controls	582		Smokers	2.7
	Ages ≤80			Ages ≤80	
	Cases	456		Nonsmokers[d]	7.0
	Controls	899		Smokers	2.17
(Damber & Larsson, 1985b)**					
Case control	All Ages		Radon	All Ages	
	Cases	69		Nonsmokers[c]	5.4
	Controls	67		Smokers	4.7
	Ages ≤80			Ages ≤80	
	Cases	60		Nonsmokers[c]	3.9
	Controls	118		Smokers	2.90
(Damber & Larsson, 1985a)**					
Case control	Cases	604	Fossil fuel	Nonsmokers[c]	
	Controls	1,071	by-products	Drivers in general	2.9
				Truck Drivers	5.4
				Smokers	
				Drivers in general	1.01
				Truck Drivers	0.95
(Hall & Wynder, 1984)**					
Case control	Cases	502	Diesel exhaust	Nonsmokers[d]	1.46
	Controls	1,502		Smokers	1.18

*This table compares the relative risks of occupationally exposed to unexposed nonsmokers (those who have never smoked) with the relative risk of occupationally exposed to unexposed smokers.
**(Reference)

[a]Definite "never-smokers"
[b]Data from four Atlantic coastal surveys
[c]Includes smokers of <1 year in a lifetime
[d]Includes ex-smokers

Table 1. (Continued)

Study Type	Number of Subjects		Substance	Relative Risk	
(Hammond et al., 1979)*					
Cohort	Cases	17,800	Asbestos	Nonsmokers[a]	5.17
	Controls	73,763		Smokers	4.91
(Levin et al., 1955)*					
Case control	Cases	137	Occupations	Nonsmokers[b]	3.2
	Controls	396	with high	Other	2.3
			lung-cancer	<20 cigarettes/day	4.3
			risk	≥20 cigarettes/day	1.5
(Liddell et al., 1984)*					
Case control	Cases	223	Asbestos	Nonsmokers[c]	2.98
	Controls	715		Smokers	1.66
(Pastorino et al., 1984)*					
Case control	Cases	204	Known	0 cigarette/day[d]	2.5
	Controls	351	carcinogens	1-9 cigarettes/day	1.4
				10-19 cigarettes/day	2.3
				20-29 cigarettes/day	2.1
				30+ cigarettes/day	1.8
(Pershagen et al., 1981)*					
Case control	Cases	76	Arsenic SO_2	Nonsmokers[e]	2.58
	Controls	152		Smokers	1.69
(Pershagen, 1985)*					
Case control	Cases	212	Arsenic	Nonsmokers[f]	6.46
	Controls	424	compounds	(<lend, f)	
				2>Smokers	2.65
(Radford & Renard, 1984)*[g]					
Cohort		1,415	Radon	Nonsmokers[h]	10
				Smokers	2.9
(Rothschild & Mulvey, 1982)*					
Case control	Cases	284	Sugarcane	Nonsmokers	0.94
	Controls	284	farming	Smokers	2.63

*(Reference)

[a]Never smoked regularly
[b]Never cigarette smokers but includes pipe and cigar smokers
[c]Includes smokers of <5 cigarettes/day
[d]Definite "never smokers"
[e]Age-adjusted relative risk; includes smokers of <2 years in a lifetime
[f]Includes ex-smokers who quit at least 15 years prior to death
[g]Age- and smoking-adjusted lung-cancer deaths are based on the national rates for Swedish men
[h]Includes ex-smokers of >10 years

Table 1. (Continued)

Study Type	Number of Subjects		Substance	Relative Risk	
(Selikoff et al., 1980)*[a]					
Cohort		933	Asbestos	Nonsmokers[b]	15
				Smokers	5.73
(Stellman & Garfinkel, 1984)*[c]					
Cohort	Cases	10,322	Wood dust	0 cigarette/day[d]	
	Controls	406,798		Woodworkers	1.4
				Carpentry & joinery	1
				1-19 cigarettes/day	
				Woodworkers	0.8
				Carpentry & joinery	0.8
				20 cigarettes/day	
				Woodworkers	1.23
				Carpentry & joinery	1.42
				21-39 cigarettes/day	
				Woodworkers	1.5
				Carpentry & joinery	1.6
				40+ cigarettes/day	
				Woodworkers	1.0
				Carpentry & joinery	1.3
(Tenkanen et al., 1985)*[e]					
Cohort		4,475	Dust/ agriculture	Nonsmokers[f]	
				Agriculture	0.8
				Dusty Occupations	1.2
				Smokers	
				Agriculture	3.0
				Dusty Occupations	3.6
(Weiss, 1980)*[g]					
Cohort		51	Chloromethyl ether	Nonsmokers	2,702.7
				Smokers	35.5

*(Reference)

[a]Observed deaths are based on the best available evidence. Age- and smoking-adjusted expected lung-cancer rates are based on the American Cancer Society study (Hammond, 1966).
[b]Never smoked regularly
[c]Standard mortality ratios estimated from a graph. Age- and smoking-adjusted expected lung-cancer deaths are based on nonwoodworker death rates.
[d]Definite "never smokers"
[e]Cohort-adjusted relative risks estimated from a graph
[f]Includes ex-smokers
[g]Standard mortality ratio. Age- and smoking-adjusted expected lung-cancer deaths, based on Kahn (1966).

less-exposed nonsmokers (Archer et al., 1973; Rothschild and Mulvey, 1982; Tenkanen et al., 1985). Three of the studies have mixed results, that is, they report multiple comparisons for different categories of smokers and/or workers, of which some show a higher and some a lower risk ratio for exposed versus unexposed smokers compared to exposed versus unexposed nonsmokers. The remaining 12 studies show a consistently higher risk ratio for exposed nonsmokers to unexposed or less-exposed nonsmokers than that of exposed smokers to unexposed or less-exposed smokers.

The probability of obtaining such a distribution of differences can be calculated directly for the assumption that the difference in relative risk between exposed and unexposed smokers, and exposed and unexposed nonsmokers, is independent of the smoking characteristics. Therefore, the expectation is that in 50% of the comparisons, the relative risk for smokers versus smokers would be larger than that for nonsmokers versus nonsmokers. The probability of obtaining the observed distribution of differences in relative risks under this assumption is extremely small ($P \leq 0.001$).

Altogether, then, the results of Table 1 strongly support the hypothesis that, in general, the relative lung-cancer risk for nonsmokers from occupational exposure to carcinogens is greater than the relative risk for smokers.

DO SMOKERS AND NONSMOKERS DIFFER WITH RESPECT TO THE MUCUS CONTENT IN THEIR LUNGS?

There is general agreement among results of cytological studies that smokers produce much greater quantities of respiratory secretion than nonsmokers (Poppius et al., 1965; Jahn, 1968; Brille, 1969; Cohen et al., 1979; Evans et al., 1969; Herzog, 1969; Holland et al., 1969; Ashford et al., 1970; Comstock et al., 1970; Ulmer, 1970; Ulmer and Reichel, 1970; Higgins et al., 1971; Miller and Ashcroft, 1971; Nikodemowicz, 1971; Seely et al., 1971; Wallace and Langlands, 1971; Woolf and Suero, 1971; de Hamel and O'Donnell, 1972; Feureisl, 1972; Woolf, 1974; El-Sewefy, 1970; Freedman et al., 1972; Guyatt et al., 1970; Howard, 1970; Huhti et al., 1970; Islam et al., 1970; Jancik, 1970; Reichel et al., 1970a,b; Reichel and Ulmer, 1970a,b). Not only do many smokers spontaneously produce adequate amounts of sputum, but even when heated aerosols or other means are used to aid in the production of sputum specimens for subjects with low sputum levels, smokers respond much more satisfactorily than nonsmokers (Olsen et al., 1961; Rome and Olson, 1961; Woolf, 1974; Woolf and Suero, 1971).

There seems to be no doubt that evidence from cytological examinations consistently shows that smokers' lungs contain relatively large amounts of mucus compared to the lungs of nonsmokers.

DO INHALED PARTICLES MOVE DIFFERENTLY IN SMOKERS' VERSUS NONSMOKERS' LUNGS?

Differences in the patterns of movement of inhaled particulates in lungs of smokers and nonsmokers have been demonstrated in magnetometric dust-clearance experiments. Cohen et al. (1981) had 12 human subjects inhale small ferromagnetic particles (magnetites). The relative amounts of these particles remaining in the lung at any time during the experiment was detected through magnetometric techniques. Subjects were exposed to strong external magnetic fields that caused the ferromagnetic particles to align themselves with the field (i.e., become magnetized). The particles retained some of their magnetization (remanence) when the applied field was removed. The remanence field was then measured outside the body by a sensitive superconducting magnetometer (SQUID). The investigations then measured the rate (called the relaxation rate) at which the magnetic field in a defined area lost strength.

Two observations reported by Cohen et al. (1979) are of particular relevance.

(1) Relaxation rates for smokers depended on the area of the lung where they were measured, in contrast to the relatively uniform rates of relaxation over the lungs of nonsmokers.

(2) The relaxation rates for smokers were significantly higher than those for nonsmokers.

Both observations indicate a heterogeneous distribution of magnetized materials in the lungs of smokers but not in the lungs of nonsmokers (Sterling, 1981). Magnetized particles in the lungs of smokers appeared to form clusters or clumps, but this did not occur in the lungs of nonsmokers. The hypothesis that magnetite particles clustered because of high concentrations of mucus was further tested experimentally by Reinstein et al. (1981). They found that magnetite particles clustered in mucus-like medium when subjected to an external magnetic force.

Magnetometric dust experiments support the conclusion that inhaled particles travel in different patterns in the lungs of smokers and nonsmokers.

DOES SMOKING INHIBIT OR PROMOTE THE ELIMINATION OF PARTICLES FROM THE LUNG?

Long-term dust elimination rates in human lungs are very difficult to determine. For the most part, radioactive particles with a short half-life have been used in short-term studies of terminally ill patients.

Luchsinger et al. (1968) found that the fastest lung clearance time (determined from the rate of removal of radioactive chromium) was observed among the heaviest smokers. Thomson and Pavia (1973) found no difference in clearance rates of smokers, nonsmokers and ex-smokers. Camner and Philipson (1971) reported on tracheobronchial clearance of fluorinated ethylene propylene tagged with ^{18}F and ^{99}Tc. They reported ". . . no tendency to reduce clearance in connection with acute exposure to tobacco smoke, indeed, two persons show a striking increase." Lourenco et al. (1971) reported on the tracheobronchial clearance of iron oxide labeled with ^{198}Au. In smokers, tracheobronchial clearance was delayed for 1 to 4 hours, depending on the individual. Nonsmokers, on the other hand, were found to clear their lungs at a relatively rapid pace at first, followed by a slower phase. However, by 24 hours there was no significant difference in particle retention for smokers and nonsmokers. Delayed onset of clearance among smokers was also noted by Sanchis et al. (1971). Here again, smokers as a group showed some delay before clearance started, but the overall rate of clearance was faster for smokers than for nonsmokers. In fact, while cigarette smoke might be expected to impair ciliary action (Filipy et al., 1980), Binns (1975) reviewed available studies and concluded that ciliary impairment is transitory, and that the net effect of smoke exposure is to increase clearance. Albert et al. (1971) found no differences in average clearance time between smokers and nonsmokers. Albert et al. (1971) took special note of the interaction between increased mucus flow and coughing to clear dust from smokers' lungs. Similarly, Cross et al. (1982) concluded that results are contradictory from experiments that investigated the effect of cigarette smoke on mucociliary clearance.

In short, data on the effect of cigarette smoke on pulmonary clearance are contradictory. While some investigators observed that cigarette-smoking inhibits dust clearance, others reported that it may accelerate clearance under certain conditions, or that it did not affect clearance.

WHAT IS THE ROLE OF PARTICLES IN PRODUCING MALIGNANCIES?

Carcinogenic particles have a definite role in the etiology of lung cancer. However, their major role may be as carriers of chemical carcinogens. There is sound experimental evidence to support this hypothesis. Campbell (1934, 1937) demonstrated that lung cancer could be induced in mice by exposing them to dust obtained from highways. Primary lung tumors appeared in the exposed mice, earlier, and with greater frequency, and they were larger than the tumors in a control group. In view of the importance of Campbell's experiment, it is surprising that it has not been replicated by other investigators.

In a number of experiments, a significant increase in tumor production was achieved by intratracheal injection or inhalation of carcinogens (Miller et al., 1965; Henry and Kaufman, 1973 [on hamsters]; Pylev, 1972; Pylev and Shabab, 1973; Wagner et al., 1974 [on rats]; and Cross et al., 1982 [on beagle dogs]). Also, Gross (1980) cites a number of studies in which instilled or inhaled beryllium compounds have led to cancer formation in rats and monkeys. It should be noted that respiratory tumors have also been produced in animals by inhalation of carcinogenic vapors (rather than particles), such as bis(chloromethyl)ether (Laskin et al., 1971, 1975; Kushner et al., 1975).

It is of interest that, according to the 1982 Surgeon General's report (U.S. Department of Health and Human Services, 1982), inhalation experiments using fresh tobacco smoke have generally failed to produce lung cancer in animals.

In all animal studies that used either ferric oxide or asbestos, lung cancers were produced in profusion when combined with carcinogens adsorbed to the particles. The carcinogen usually used to measure carcinogenic potential was benzo[a]pyrene (BaP), and both ferric oxide and asbestos with adsorbed BaP have proven to be potent carcinogens. (See, for instance, Mossman and Craighead, 1981.) McDonald (1985) has suggestd that there is a difference in carcinogenicity, particularly for mesothelioma, between groups of asbestos fibers that is related to their ability to adsorb BaP. However, no firm conclusions have been reached for lung cancer, because the estimated risks, even for the same type of asbestos fiber, vary widely (McDonald, 1985; Liddell and Hanley, 1985). There is some evidence that asbesto particles may, by themselves, produce malignant tumors.

TO WHAT EXTENT CAN ANIMAL STUDIES SUPPORT THIS HYPOTHESIS?

Human-type lung cancer has been produced by inhalation or instillation of particles into animals' lungs. Animal experiments are now needed to test for the effect of mucus; the first step may have been taken already. Cross et al. (1982) reported that they observed a mitigating effect of tobacco smoke on the formation of respiratory cancer in beagle dogs exposed to radon, radon daughters, and uranium dust. Four exposure groups were compared: (1) exposure to radon, radon daughters, uranium dust and tobacco smoke;

(2) exposure to radon, radon daughters and uranium dust but not to tobacco smoke; (3) exposure to tobacco smoke only; and (4) sham-exposed controls.

There were seven lung and two nasal carcinomas in beagles exposed to radon, radon daughters, and uranium dust but not to tobacco smoke [(2) above]. Only one lung and one nasal carcinoma were observed in beagles exposed to these materials plus tobacco smoke [(1) above]. No carcinomas occurred in the control group. Unfortunatley, Cross et al. (1982) did not compare the amounts of dust or mucus in the lungs of individual dogs. However, other studies have found that tobacco smoke increases mucus secretion in rats (Jones et al., 1973), in sheep (Mawdesley-Thomas and Healey, 1973), and in dogs (Frasca et al., 1968).

In summary, animal experiments have been performed that support the hypothesis that smoke-generated mucus can mitigate the effect of inhaled carcinogenic agents in animals.

WHAT OTHER DIFFERENCES BETWEEN SMOKERS AND NONSMOKERS MIGHT THROW LIGHT ON THIS HYPOTHESIS?

One interesting observation that emerges from studies of occupational asbestos exposure is that there is a difference in the percentages of smokers and nonsmokers who died, on the one hand from lung cancer and, on the other, from mesothelioma. Table 2 compares the proportion of deaths from lung cancer and from mesotheliomas that were reported in four studies. Smokers (including those who formerly smoked) have a higher proportion of death from lung cancer than do never-smokers. However, for studies that give the necessary information, the number of never-smokers who died from mesothelioma is two to three times greater than the number of smokers who died from mesothelioma. This may be due to differences in the movement of asbestos particles in the lungs of smokers and nonsmokers. Perhaps the thicker pleura observed in smokers also aided in decreasing the number of mesotheliomas among them. In contrast, in the absence of that protection, mesotheliomas may be more frequent among nonsmokers (Axelson and Sundell, 1978). A related observation concerns the extent to which smokers and nonsmokers die from different cancers, with different proportions. Hammond and Selikoff (1973) showed that, apparently, in their large insulation-workers study, 45.2% of the nonsmokers and 44.5% of the smokers died from cancer at all sites. Insofar as 2.7% of the nonsmokers and 22.5% of the smokers died from lung cancer, the number of nonsmokers who died from causes other than lung cancer was consistently greater than that of smokers (Sterling, 1979).

Table 2. Deaths (%) from lung cancer and from mesotheliomas among smokers[a] and nonsmokers[b] reported in 13 studies.

Study	Smokers	Nonsmokers
Berry et al., 1985[c]		
Lung cancer	14.5	9.7
Mesothelioma	7.2	16.1
Hammond et al., 1979[d]		
Lung cancer	26.9	5.3
Mesothelioma	1.4	3.2
Selikoff et al., 1980[d]		
Lung cancer	25.7	7.4
Mesothelioma	4.2	7.9

[a]Includes those who formerly smoked
[b]Includes only those who have never smoked
[c]Females only
[d]Males only

Kotin et al. (1966) observed that the stimulus for tissue repair brought on by embedded foreign particles is, by itself, conducive to carcinogenic response. Kotin et al. also indicated that a repeated sequence of insult and repair can lead by stages to abnormal repair, with a lesion progressing from hyperplasia to metaplasia, and with atypical changes ultimately leading to cancer. In fact, one study found such a progression, caused by particles of soot retained in rabbits exposed to synthetic smog (Miller et al., 1965).

DISCUSSION

Particulate air pollutants deposited and retained in the respiratory tract might present an increased risk because of carcinogens adsorbed on them. The greater the number of particles and the longer they are retained, the greater the risk. Taken together, the evidence supports the hypothesis that smokers might gain some degree of protection against particulate carcinogens from the improved clearance mechanism that is represented by smoking-induced mucus. A thicker mucus layer in the respiratory tract presumably better protects the underlying epithelial cells from the action of carcinogenic particles than a thin mucus layer. In addition, it might increase the clearance rate of potentially hazardous particles. Part of the protection may also occur because irritation from smoking may lead to tissue changes and, possibly, to increased thickness (and, therefore better protection) of the pleura.

So far, the hypothesis that increased mucus in the lungs of workers exposed to hazardous particulate air pollutants may protect them against lung disease is based on indirect evidence. It now needs experimental verification in appropriate animal and human studies. If the protection qualities of smoking-induced lung and mucus changes can be verified, ways need to be found to induce these changes by means other than smoking in nonsmoking (and smoking) workers at risk.

REFERENCES

Albert, RE, M Lippman, and HT Peterson. **1971.** The effects of cigarette smoking on the kinetics of bronchial clearance in humans and donkeys, pp. 165-182. In: *Inhaled Particles,* WH Walton (ed.). Unwin, Old Woking, England.

Archer, VE, JK Wagoner, and FE Lundin. **1973.** Uranium mining and cigarette smoking effects on man. J Occup Med 15:204-211.

Ashford, JR, DC Morgan, S Rae, and RR Sowden. **1970.** Respiratory symptoms in British coal miners. Am Rev Respir Dis 102:370-381.

Axelson, O and I Sundell. **1978.** Mining, smoking and lung cancer. Scand J Work Environ Health 41:46.

Berry, G, ML Newhouse, and P Antonis. **1985.** Combined effect of asbestos and smoking on mortality from lung cancer and mesothelioma in factory workers. Br J Ind Med 42:12-18.

Binns, R. **1975.** Animal inhalation studies with tobacco smoke. Rev Environ Health 2:81.

Blot, WJ and JF Fraumeni. **1981.** Cancer among shipyard workers, p. 37. In: *Banbury Report 9: Quantification of Occupational Cancer,* R Peto and M. Schneiderman (eds.). Cold Spring Harbor Laboratory, Cold Spring Harbor, New York, NY.

Brille, D. **1969.** Fréquence de la bronchité chronique chez la femme: Rôle du tabac. Rev Tuberc 33:794-796.

Camner, P and K Philipson. **1971.** Intra-individual studies of tracheobronchial clearance in man using fluorocarbon resin particles tagged with ^{18}F and ^{99m}Tc, pp. 157-180. In: *Inhaled Particles,* WH Walton (ed.). Unwin, Old Woking, England.

Campbell, JA. **1934.** Cancer of skin and increase in incidence of primary tumours of lung in mice exposed to dust obtained from tarred roads. Br J Exp Pathol 15:287.

Campbell, JA. **1937.** The effects of road dust "freed" from tar products upon the incidence of primary lung tumours of mice. Br J Exp Pathol 18:215.

Cohen, D, SF Arai, and JD Brain. **1979.** Smoking impairs long-term dust clearance from the lung. Science 204:514.

Cohen, D, TS Crowther, GW Gibbs, and MR Becklake. **1981.** Magnetic lung measurements in relation to occupational exposure in asbestos miners and millers of Quebec. Environ Res 26:535.

Comstock, GW, WJ Brownlow, RW Stone, and PE Sartwell. **1970.** Cigarette smoking and change in respiratory findings. Arch Environ Health 21:50-57.

Cross, FT, RF Palmer, RE Filipy, GE Dagle, and BO Stuart. **1982.** Carcinogenic effects or radon daughters, uranium ore dust and cigarette smoke in beagle dogs. Health Phys 42:32.

Damber, L and LG Larsson. **1982.** Combined effects of mining and smoking in the causation of lung carcinoma. A case control study in Northern Sweden. Acta Radiol Oncol 21:305-313.

Damber, L and LG Larsson. **1985a.** Professional driving; smoking and lung cancer: A case referent study. Br J Ind Med 42:246-252.

Damber, L and LG Larsson. **1985b.** Underground mining; smoking; and lung cancer: A case-control study in the iron ore municipalities of Northern Sweden. J Natl Cancer Inst 74:1207-1213.

de Hamel, EA and TV O'Donnell. **1972.** Smoking habits and respiratory symptoms of Dunedin public servants. N Z Med J 76:1-4.

El-Sewefy, AZ. **1970.** Chest symptomatology in a Sheffield Steel Works (S.P.T.). J. Egypt Med Assoc 52:578-581.

Evans, SM, E Wilkes, and D Dalrymple-Smith. **1969.** Presymptomatic diagnosis. A study in country practice. J R Coll Gen Practitioners 17:237-246.

Feureisl, R. **1972.** Effect of smoking on the cardiopulmonary function. Klin Med (Moscow) 50:82-84.

Filipy, RE, JL Pappin, DL Stevens, and SG Irby. **1980.** Effects of cigarette smoke exposure on pulmonary clearance of $^{239}PuO_2$ in rats, p. 128. In: *Pacific Northwest Laboratory Annual Report for 1979 to the DOE Assistant Secretary for Environment,* Part 1, Biomedical Sciences, PNL-3300. NTIS, Springfield, VA.

Frasca, JM, O Auerbach, VR Perks, and JD Jamieson. **1968.** Electron microscopic observations of the bronchial epithelium of dogs. J Exp Pathol 9:380.

Freedman, S, CM Fletcher, and GB Field. **1972.** Effects of smoking modified cigarettes on respiratory symptoms and ventilatory capacity. J Natl Cancer Inst 48:1805-1810.

Gross, DH. **1980.** Carcinogenicity of beryllium: Review of the literature. Environ Res 21:56.

Guyatt, AR, B Berry, JH Alpers, AC Braniley, and CM Fletcher. **1970.** Relationship of airway conductance and its immediate change on smoking habits and symptoms of chronic bronchitis. Am Rev Respir Dis 101:44-54.

Hall, NL and EL Wynder. **1984.** Diesel exhaust exposure and lung cancer: A case control study. Environ Res 34:77-86.

Hammond, EC. **1966.** Smoking in relation to the death rates of one million men and women. J Natl Cancer Inst 19:127-204.

Hammond, EC and IF Selikoff. **1973.** Relation of cigarette smoking to risk of death from asbestos-associated disease among insulation workers in the U.S.: Biological effects of asbestos. IARC, Scientific Publication 8:312-316. International Agency for Research in Cancer,

Lyon, France. Also published as: Hammond, EC and IF Selikoff. 1975. Multiple risk factors in environmental cancer. In: *Persons at High Risk of Cancer,* JF Fraumeni (ed.). Academic Press, New York, NY.

Hammond, E, I Selikoff, and H Seidman. **1979.** Asbestos exposure; cigarette smoking; and death rates. Ann NY Acad Sci 33:473-489.

Henry, MC and DG Kaufman. **1973.** Clearance of benzo(a)pyrene from hamster lungs after administration of coated particles. J Natl Cancer Inst 51:1961.

Herzog, H. **1969.** Chronisch-obstruktive Lungenerkrankungen. Fortschr Med 87:1426-1436.

Higgins, ITT, MW Higgins, JC Gilson, et al. **1971.** Smoking and chronic respiratory disease: Findings in surveys carried out in 1957 and 1966 in Staveley, England. Chest 59:345-355.

Holland, WW, HS Kasap, JRT Colley, and W Cormack. **1969.** Respiratory symptoms and ventilatory function: A family study. Br J Soc Prevent Med 23:77-84.

Howard, PA. **1970.** A long-term follow-up of respiratory symptoms in a group of working men. Br J Ind Med 27:326-333.

Huhti, E, P Ryhanen, U Vuopala, and J Takkunen. **1970.** Chronic respiratory disease among pulp workers in an arctic area in Northern Finland. Acta Med Scand 187:433-444.

Islam, MS, PK Datta, DK Mitra, and MK Chakraborty. **1970.** Changes of ventilatory function among smokers and non-smokers. Indian J Physiol Pharmacol 14:165-173.

Jahn, E. **1968.** Bronchitishäufigkeit in einer Grosstadtbevölkerung bei Rauchern und Nichtrauchern. Arbeitsmed Sozialmed Arbeitshyg 22:229-236.

Jancik, E. **1970.** Quelques données et correlations provenant d'une étude épidémiologique sur l'incidence des symptomes characteristiques des maladies respiratoires chroniques nonspecifiques. Rev Tuberc Pneumol 34:794-752.

Jones, R, P Bolduc, and L Reid. **1973.** Goblet cells glycoprotein and tracheal gland hypertrophy in rat airways. Br J Exp Pathol 54:229.

Kahn, H. **1966.** Dorn study of smoking and mortality among U.S. veterans: Report on eight and one-half years of observations, pp. 1-25. In: *Epidemiological Approaches to the Study of Cancer and Other Diseaes,* W Haenszel (ed.). National Cancer Institute Monograph 19. U.S. Government Printing Office, Washington, DC.

Kotin, P, D Courington, and HL Falk. **1966.** Pathogenesis of cancer in a ciliated mucus-secreting epithelium. Am Rev Respir Dis 93:115.

Kuschner, M, S Laskin, RT Drew, V Cappiello, and N Nelson. **1975.** Inhalation carcinogenicity of alpha halo ethers. III. Lifetime and limited period inhalation studies with bis(chloromethyl)ether at 0.1 ppm. Arch Environ Health 30:73.

Laskin, S, M Kuschner, RT Drew, VP Cappiello, and N Nelson. **1971.** Tumors of the respiratory tract induced by inhalation of bis(chloromethyl)ether. Arch Environ Health 23:135.

Laskin, S, RT Drew, V Cappiello, M Kuschner, and N Nelson. **1975.** Inhalation carcinogenicity of alpha halo ethers. II. Chronic inhalation studies with chloromethyl methyl ether. Arch Environ Health 30:70.

Levin, ML, AS Kraus, ID Goldberg, and PR Gerhardt. **1955.** Problems in the study of occupation and smoking in relation to lung cancer. Cancer 8:932-936.

Liddell, FDK and JA Hanley. **1985.** Relations between asbestos exposure and lung cancer SMRs in occupational cohort studies. Br J Ind Med 42:389-396.

Liddell, F, D Thomas, G Gibbs, et al. **1984.** Fibre exposure and mortality from pneumoconiosis; respiratory and abdominal malignancies in chrysotile production in Quebec; 1926-1975. Singapore Ann Acad Med 13:339-344.

Lourenco, RV, MF Klimek, and CJ Borowski. **1971.** Deposition and clearance of 2m particles in the tracheobronchial tree of normal subjects—smokers and nonsmokers. J Clin Invest 50:1411.

Luchsinger, PC, B La Garde, and JE Kilfeather. **1968.** Particle clearance from the human tracheobronchial tree. Am Rev Respir Dis 97:1046.

Mawdesley-Thomas, LE and P Healey. **1973.** Experimental bronchitis in lambs exposed to cigarette smoke. Arch Environ Health 27:248.

McDonald, JC. **1985.** Health implications of environmental exposure to asbestos. Environ Health Perspect 62:319-328.

Miller, GJ and MT Ashcroft. **1971.** A community survey of respiratory disease among East Indian and African adults in Guyana. Thorax 26:331-338.

Miller, L, WE Smith, and SW Berlinger. **1965.** Tests for effect of asbestos on benzo(a)pyrene carcinogenesis in the respiratory tract. Ann NY Acad Sci 132:489.

Mossman, BT and JE Craighead. **1981.** Mechanisms of asbestos carcinogenesis. Environ Res 25:269-280.

Nikodemowicz, E. **1971.** Pulmonary tuberculosis and expectoration in inhabitants of Krakow. Gruzlica 39:595-603.

Olsen, CR, HF Froeb, and LA Palmer. **1961.** Sputum cytology after inhalation of heated propylene glycol. J Am Med Assoc 178:668-680.

Ortmeyer, CE, J Costello, WKC Morgan, et al. **1974.** The mortality of Appalachian coal miners. Arch Environ Health 29:67-72.

Pastorino, U, F Berrino, A Gervasio, V Presenti, E Riboli, and F Crosignani. **1984.** Proportion of lung cancers due to occupational exposure. Int J Cancer 33:231-237.

Pershagen, G. **1985.** Lung cancer mortality among men living near an arsenic-emitting smelter. Am J Epidemiol 122:684-694.

Pershagen, G, S Wall, A Taube, and L Linnman. **1981.** On the interaction between occupational arsenic exposure and smoking and its relationship to lung cancer. Scand J Work Environ Health 7:302-309.

Poppius, H, M Lehtinen, and J Patiala. **1965.** Kroonisen bronkiitin esiintyminen metsatyomiehilla suomessa. Duodecim 81:881-894.

Pylve, LN. **1972.** Morphological lesions in rat lungs induced by intratracheal injection of chrysotile asbestos alone and with benzo(a)pyrene. Vopr Onkol 18:40.

Pylev, LN and LM Shabab. **1973.** Some results of experimental studies in asbestos carcinogenesis, p. 99. In: *Proceedings of the Conference on Biologial Effects of Asbestos,* P Bogovski, JC Bilson, B Timbrell, and JC Wagner (eds.). IARC, Lyon, France.

Radford, EP and KGS Renard. **1984.** Lung cancer in Swedish iron miners exposed to low doses of radon daughters. N Engl J Med 310:1384-1494.

Reichel, G and WT Ulmer. **1970a.** Einfluss des jahreszeitlichen Wechsels der Luftverunreinigung unter den Wetterfaktoren auf die Häufigkeit chronischer unspezifischer Atemwegserkrankungen. Int Arch Arbeitsmed 27:130-154.

Reichel, G and WT Ulmer. **1970b.** Berufliche Belastung und Häufigkeit unspezifischer Atemwegserkrankungen. Int Arch Arbeitsmed 27:155-184.

Reichel, G, WT Ulmer, and SF Ikonomides. **1970a.** Einflüsse des örtlich unterschiedlichen Verschmutzungsgrades im Stadtgebiet von Duisburg auf die Häufigkeit unspezifischer Atemwegserkrankungen. Mitteilung. Int Arch Arbeitsmed 27:110-129.

Reichel, G, WT Ulmer, and SF Ikonomides. **1970b.** Einflüsse der Rauchergewohnheiten auf die Häufigkeite unspezifischer Atemwegserkrankungen. Int Arch Arbeitsmed 27:49-72.

Reinstein, LE, L. Robinson, and AS Glicksman. **1981.** Formation of iron clusters in a mucus-like medium. J Appl Phys 52:2572-2574.

Rome, DS and KB Olson. **1961.** A direct comparison of natural and aerosol produced sputum collected from 776 asymptomatic men. Acta Cytol 5:173-176.

Rothschild, H and JJ Mulvey. **1982.** An increased risk for lung cancer mortality associated with sugarcane farming. J Natl Cancer Inst 68:755-760.

Sanchis, J, M Dolovich, R Chalmers, and MT Newhouse. **1971.** Regional distribution and lung clearance mechanisms in smokers and nonsmokers, pp. 183-191. In: *Inhaled Particles,* WH Walton (ed.). Unwin, Old Woking, England.

Seely, JE, E Zuskin, and A Bouhuys. **1971.** Cigarette smoking: objective evidence for lung damage among teenagers. Science 172: 741-743.

Selikoff, I, H Seidman, and E Hammond. **1980.** Mortality effects of cigarette smoking among amosite asbestos factory workers. J Natl Cancer Inst 65:507-513.

Stellman, SD and L Garfinkel. **1984.** Cancer mortality among woodworkers. Am J Ind Med 5:343-357.

Sterling, TD. **1979.** Statistical problems in multi-variate (etiological) surveys. Can J Statist 7:205-215.

Sterling, TD. **1981.** Possible risks to human lungs from magnetometric dust clearance experiments. J Appl Phys 52:2575-2577.

Sterling, TD. **1983.** Possible effects on occupational lung cancer from smoking related changes in the mucus content of the lung. J Chron Dis 36:669-676.

Sterling, TD, **1984.** Second thoughts: Filtering information about occupation smoking and disease. J Chron Dis 37:227-230.

Tenkanen, L, T Hakulinen, M Hakama, E Saxen, and T Sauna. **1985.** Dust and migration as risk factors in lung cancer among smoking and non-smoking males in Finland. Int J Cancer 35:637-642.

Thomson, ML and D Pavia. **1973.** Long-term tobacco smoking and mucociliary clearance. Arch Environ Health 26:86.

Ulmer, WT. **1970.** Lung function studies in epidemiologic investigations of respiratory diseases. Bull Physiopathol Respir 6:605-616.

Ulmer, WT and G Reichel. **1970.** Der Einfluss von Alter Geschlecht und Gewicht auf die Häufigkeite unspezifischer Atemwegserkrankungen. Int Arch Arbeitsmed 27:27-48.

U.S. Department of Health and Human Services. 1982. *The Health Consequences of Smoking.* U.S. Public Health Service, Office of Smoking and Health, Rockville, MD.

Wagner, JC, G Berry, JW Skidmore, and V Timbrell. **1974.** The effects of the inhalation of asbestos in rats. Br J Cancer 29:252.

Wallace, WFM and JHM Langlands. **1971.** Insulation workers in Belfast. Br J Ind Med 28:211-216.

Weiss, W. **1980.** The cigarette factor in lung cancer due to chloromethyl ethers. J Occup Med 22:527-529.

Woolf, CR. **1974.** Clinical findings, sputum examinations and pulmonary function tests related to the smoking habit of 500 women. Chest 66:652-659.

Woolf, CR and JT Suero. **1971.** The respiratory effects of regular cigarette smoking in women. Am Rev Respir Dis 103:26-37.

A Hypothesis for Explaining the Syncarcinogenic Effect of Cigarette Smoke and Asbestos

Friedrich Pott

Medical Institute for Environmental Hygiene, University of Düsseldorf, Federal Republic of Germany

KEY WORDS: asbestos, cigarette smoke, mineral fibers, synergism, lung cancer

---

ABSTRACT

Some rationales for the biological mechanism for the epidemiologically proven syncarcinogenicity of cigarette smoke and asbestos maintain that asbestos fibers carry polycyclic aromatic hydrocarbons (PAH) into the cells and influence their metabolism. However, in this function, asbestos is only a cocarcinogen. These can be termed "PAH carrier hypotheses." An alternative hypothesis proposes that asbestos acts as a complete carcinogen when it is chronically retained in the bronchial wall.

The irritants and cytotoxins contained in tobacco smoke serve as efficient cocarcinogens by damaging the bronchial mucosa and the bronchial clearance mechanism. It is reasonable to assume that such impairments can enhance, manyfold, the number of asbestos fibers that may be implanted in the basal layer of the bronchial epithelium and persist there for many years. This can be termed the "fiber-implantation hypothesis." If the hypothesized mechanism does, indeed, occur, it would also apply to other natural and man-made mineral fibers that remain intact and chronically lodged in the bronchial wall.

The latter hypothesis also leads to other conclusions, e.g.: the location of the persisting fibers is much more important for carcinogenic risk than the total number of fibers retained in the lung; and that the latter is related instead to the severity of fibrosis.

INTRODUCTION

Since Selikoff et al., in 1968, reported a synergistic effect of cigarette smoke and asbestos exposure, hypotheses have developed on the possible mechanism for this phenomenon. Meanwhile, those first findings have been confirmed by several studies. Adsorption of simultaneously inhaled polycyclic aromatic hydrocarbons (PAH) on the surface of asbestos fibers may affect their carcinogenicity, and the fibers may influence PAH metabolism (Mossman, 1983; Bastie-Sigeac et al., 1983; Gerde, 1987). In the rationales for these hypotheses, asbestos fibers are proposed as the carriers of PAH into the cells, functioning only as cocarcinogens. These can be called the "PAH carrier hypotheses." In an alternative hypothesis (Pott, 1984; Pott et al., 1984), described more extensively in this paper, asbestos fibers are considered a complete carcinogen, and the irritants and cytotoxic substances in tobacco smoke serve as efficient cocarcinogens by damaging the bronchial mucosa. They act independently of the carcinogens and promoters contained in tobacco smoke.

Some preconditions for tumor induction by fibers, described here, may help to explain the hypothesized mechanism of the syncarcinogenic effect.

PRECONDITIONS FOR TUMOR INDUCTION BY FIBERS

Fiber Properties

In 1972 and 1973 the first experimental results on the tumor-inducing effect of mineral fibers other than asbestos were published. The results strongly supported the old hypothesis that the elongated shape of asbestos particles, rather than their chemical composition, might be the true cause of their carcinogenicity (Nordmann, 1938; Linzbach and Wedler, 1941; Stanton and Wrench 1972; Pott and Friedrichs, 1972; Wagner et al., 1973). The same general conclusion has been drawn in recent reviews of many additional experiments (Davis, 1986; Doll, in press). Up to now, the relationships between fiber length, diameter, and aspect ratio and expected tumor incidence have not been well understood. According to our working hypothesis, which is supported by the results of several experiments, there is a continuous transition from these fibers, which are too short or too thick to be carcinogenic, to the maximal carcinogenicity of fibers that have the optimal length and diameter for cancer induction. Based on carcinogenicity studies in rats after intrapleural or intraperitoneal administration of different fiber types, fibers longer than 20 μm and thinner than 0.2 μm are very carcinogenic. Fibers shorter than 5 μm and thicker than 2 μm

have only low carcinogenic potential (Stanton and Layard, 1978; Pott, 1978). However, it is not known which dimensions of durable fibers result in maximal carcinogenic potency of elongated particles and which fiber dimensions are not capable of inducing any carcinogenic risk. Moreover, the possible differences between the carcinogenic reaction of the bronchial mucosa and that of the serosa to the same fiber size must be considered. Data are sparse, but the differences could be small.

Studies also show that, apart from their dimensions, the durability of fibers (i.e., their ability to remain intact by resisting dissolution) in the body is important for tumor response (Pott et al., 1987). This durability depends on the fibers' chemical composition and crystalline structure. The half-life of different fiber types *in vivo* differs widely (Bellmann et al., 1987). Although chemical composition influences the effectiveness of the carcinogenic agent, it cannot be the true cause of the biological reactions that lead to the malignant growth of cells.

Other fiber properties may also affect their carcinogenicity. In several publications on *in vitro* studies, surface properties are assumed to have causative significance. This conclusion is based mainly on results showing that altered dust surfaces influence certain cytotoxic effects . But caution is required for extrapolating from cytotoxic effects *in vitro* to carcinogenicity *in vivo.* A much greater analogy may exist between carcinogenicity in rats and genotoxicity *in vitro* (Jaurand, in press).

Behavior of Fibers in the Body and Effect of Location on Carcinogenic Risk

Intraperitoneally administered fibers of little durability (e.g., gypsum, HCl-treated chrysotile, and HCl-treated glass microfibers) did not induce tumors (Pott et al., 1987). This suggests that intact fibers must remain for a certain length of time in the serosa to induce tumors. Although we do not know how long this period is, it seems reasonable to assume that the longer the fibers persist, the greater the carcinogenic risk. A fiber must, of course, be durable to remain at a given target cell site, but durability alone does not necessarily ensure that a fiber will chronically persist at a certain location, because it can be removed by pulmonary clearance mechanisms, or it can be translocated inside the body.

After intraperitoneal injection in rats, short fibers migrated easily to the lymph nodes, while the longer ones settled predominantly in the serosa and remained there for a long time unless they dissolved. No clearance mechanism exists in the abdominal cavity such as that in the lung. Therefore, it is not surprising that intraperitoneal injection of only 10 μg of actinolite increased tumor incidence from 2% in the control group to 23% in the treated group (Pott et al., in press). We calculated that the dose comprised a total of approximately 4 million fibers with lengths of more than 5 μm.

In contrast, most fibers deposited in the airways by inhalation will be cleared into the esophagus. The alveolar clearance rate for long fibers is much slower than that for short fibers. However, so far as is known, only 5% of primary lung cancers in humans are bronchioloalveolar carcinomas (Greenberg, 1987), even though the surface area of the nonciliated airways in humans (like that of rats) amounts to about 99% of the total surface area of the airways (Yu and Xu, 1987; Figure 1). The data are remarkable because, under physiological conditions, the cells of the bronchial wall are protected from "insoluble" carcinogenic particles by the mucociliary clearance mechanism. Contact between cells and fibers may be only indirect and brief. Soluble carcinogens like PAH have a better chance of reaching the epithelial cells than "insoluble" ones, whose elimination by mucociliary clearance normally takes only hours or a few days. By contrast, the long-term clearance of insoluble, nontoxic particles retained in the deep lung has a half-life of about 70 days in rats and 500 days in humans.

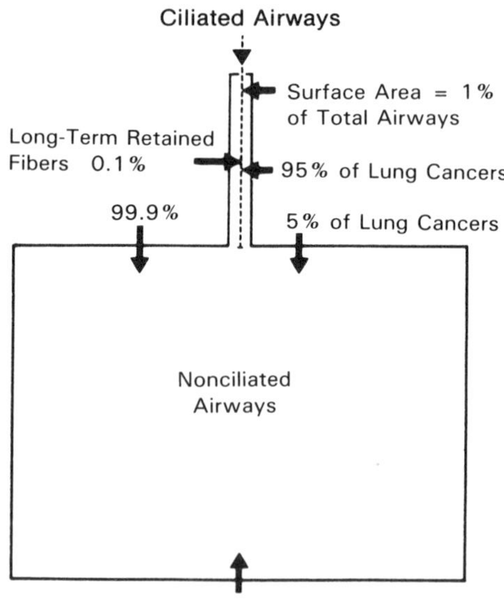

Figure 1. Comparison of surface area (Yu and Xu, 1987), lung-cancer incidence (Greenberg, 1987), and long-term asbestos fiber retention (percentages estimated) in ciliated and nonciliated human airways.

In explaining the induction of a bronchial carcinoma by fibers, it is reasonable to assume that the fibers stop prematurely on their way to the esophagus, and that they penetrate the epithelium and become implanted in the basal layer of the bronchial wall. Moreover, they must remain intact and persist in this location until, by an unknown mechanism, they convert the target cells into precursors of tumor cells. Many years can elapse between this stage and death by cancer. In the meantime, the fibers may disappear, so that the cause of the cancer is not detectable in the tissue after death. As yet there are no data on the percentage of fibers that are implanted and persist in the basal layer of the ciliated airways; most chronically retained mineral fibers (possibly 99.9%; Figure 1) are found in the nonciliated airways and in the interstitium (Brody and Hill, 1982), although they seem to have only a very weak carcinogenic effect there. Conversely, the small number of fibers that are chronically retained in the ciliated airways may be responsible for most of the asbestos-induced lung cancers in humans.

If these hypotheses are true, the effective fiber masses in both inhalation and injection experiments may be similar. After exposing rats to UICC crocidolite for 1 year (10 mg/m^3, 5 x 7 hours/week), about 8 mg of crocidolite was detected in the lungs (Wagner et al., 1974). This may have deposited an effective mass of 5 to 10 μg of fibers in the walls of the ciliated airways, but because of the animals' short remaining life span, only a low tumor incidence could be expected.

DAMAGE OF BRONCHIAL WALLS INDUCED BY CIGARETTE SMOKE

It can be hypothesized that cigarette-smoke-induced lesions of the bronchial walls are an important factor in increasing the effective fiber dose to target cells in that tissue.

Under physiological conditions, it is probably rare for bronchial clearance of fibers to be interrupted and for fibers to be embedded in the basal layer of the epithelium. This may explain the relatively low lung-cancer incidence observed in rats and hamsters (0 to 8%) after exposure to very high concentrations of crocidolite, even when the lungs were overloaded (Reeves et al., 1974; Davis et al., 1978; Wagner et al., 1985; Smith et al., 1987; Muhle et al., 1987). Therefore, inhalation experiments in healthy rats are not a realistic model for detecting the carcinogenicity of fibers, because they will result in only (false) negative findings when extrapolated to humans.

The bronchial epithelium and the clearance mechanism in rats can, however, be damaged by inflammation caused by infections, air pollutants, and, last but not least, long-term exposure to cigarette smoke. Under these conditions, many fibers can be expected to become implanted in the basal layer of the epithelium on the way from the alveoli to the esophagus. Figure 2 demonstrates a model of these conditions, under which fibers are trapped and persist in the bronchial wall. This can therefore be called the "fiber-implantation hypothesis." The greater the number of fibers that become implanted in the bronchial wall and persist for a long time, the greater the carcinogenic risk.

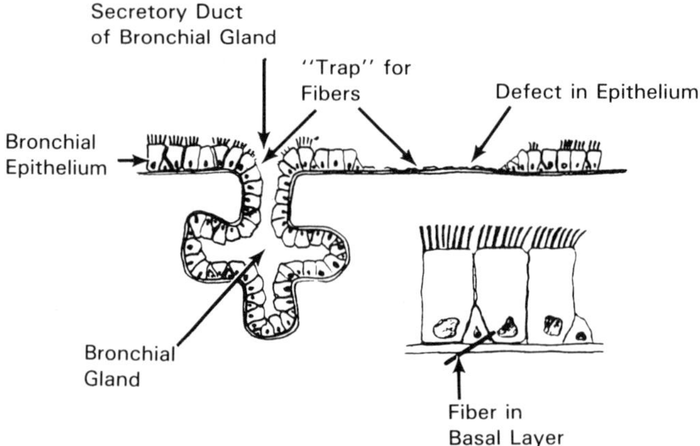

Figure 2. Model showing preconditions for implantation of fibers in basal layer of bronchial epithelium or bronchial gland (Pott et al., 1984).

DISCUSSION

To examine the validity of the fiber-implantation hypothesis, one must determine whether it is consistent with most epidemiological observations in smoking asbestos workers, compared with those in their nonsmoking counterparts. The two most frequent observations are:

(1) the synergistic (multiplicative) effect of active smoking and asbestos exposure with regard to lung-cancer incidence; and

(2) the absence of an effect of smoking on the incidence of mesotheliomas.

The hypothesis can explain the multiplicative effect on the lung-cancer incidence, because it is plausible that impairment of the bronchial clearance mechanism greatly increases the very small number of fibers that usually persist in the bronchial wall. It can be assumed that, even in smokers, only a small percentage of the fibers retained in the lung are located in the wall of the epithelium. Without impairment of alveolar clearance and the resulting increase in the number of fibers retained in alveoli, a difference is not likely to be detectable between the number of fibers in the lungs of smokers and nonsmokers. The consequences are discussed later.

In contrast to lung-cancer incidence, mesothelioma incidence depends on the number of fibers that migrate from the alveoli to the pleura and peritoneum. When cigarette smoke damages the ciliated epithelium and impairs bronchial clearance of particles, it does not necessarily also significantly impair the mechanism of long-term alveolar clearance, which differs greatly from bronchial clearance. In an inhalation experiment, Muhle et al. (1983) found that the number of crocidolite fibers in rat lungs was about twice as high in "smokers" as in "nonsmokers"; no effect was detected with chrysotile (see also Muhle et al., this volume). It is not known whether these results also apply to humans, but if so, they would agree with epidemiological results, because asbestos workers were exposed mainly to chrysotile.

Because most retained fibers are located in the nonciliated airways and in the interstitium, diffuse asbestosis can be observed in the interstitial tissue of animals (Wehner et al., 1975; Davis et al., 1986; Wagner et al., 1974) and of humans (Selikoff and Lee, 1978). It is therefore reasonable to assume that the multiplicative effect of smoking on fiber numbers retained in bronchial walls does not increase the total fiber numbers within the lung and the degree of fibrosis. Fibrosis and cancer induced by fibers are end points of two unknown mechanisms that may work independently of one another. After prolonged asbestos exposure, cancer does not occur without asbestosis. But after a short exposure, cancer can be expected, albeit at a low incidence, without clinically detectable asbestosis. In older humans, slight fibrotic reactions are normal findings in the lung; therefore, many asbestos-induced lung-cancer cases cannot be confirmed with sufficient certainty to justify compensation.

If this fiber-implantation hypothesis is correct, it leads to further conclusions:

- The number of asbestos fibers found in the lung is related to the severity of asbestosis rather than to the lung-cancer risk.
- It is theoretically possible that a single persistent fiber can induce malignant growth after a long period of cell irritation. But it is also important to avoid the reciprocal misunderstanding: that inhalation of a few fibers leads inevitably to unacceptable cancer risk. This may be explained with an example from reproduction: There is no doubt that only a single sperm is necessary to fertilize an ovum, but an ejaculation containing less than 20 million sperm is a condition termed oligospermia, which may be a cause of infertility.

- Asbestos fibers may also be a complete carcinogen in the lung as well as in the abdominal cavity when inducing mesothelioma.

- Although cigarette smoke contains several carcinogens and promoters that have produced lung cancer in millions of humans, these substances are not necessarily responsible for the multiplicative cancer risk caused by their combination with asbestos. Instead, the irritants in cigarette smoke may act as very effective cocarcinogens by impairing bronchial clearance of carcinogenic asbestos fibers.

- The syncarcinogenic effect of intratracheal administration of a combination of benzo[a]pyrene (BaP) and asbestos in rats and hamsters appears to support the PAH carrier hypothesis. However, in these animal experiments, similar large amounts of asbestos and of PAH (in the milligram range) have been instilled (Smith et al., 1970; Pylev and Shabad, 1973; Bogovski et al., 1982). This may have led to inflammation of the bronchi that enhanced implantation of fibers. In contrast, asbestos workers now usually inhale only about 1 mg asbestos in 10 m^3 air per day and only 0.5 μg BaP when smoking 30 cigarettes. (In earlier times, asbestos exposure may have been somewhat higher.) In a recent study, long-term inhalation of highly concentrated pyrolyzed pitch (90 μg BaP/m^3) and crocidolite instilled intratracheally resulted in a syncarcinogenic effect (Heinrich et al., 1986). However, the multiplicative carcinogenic effect of BaP and asbestos has been observed only in the lung; it was not detected after intraperitoneal or intrapleural injection (Pott et al., 1972; Pylev, 1980).

- The conclusion from several animal experiments that the carcinogenicity of ingested asbestos is not proven may be erroneous because it is based on an unrealistic model: healthy rats. So far as is known, the treated rats and hamsters had no chronic inflammation in the gastrointestinal tract. Such lesions would be more comparable to those that occur in many humans and would provide better conditions for the implantation of fibers in the mucosa.

If the fiber-implantation hypothesis is incorrect, and the PAH carrier hypothesis is true, then the durability and persistence of fibers are of lesser importance, and the surface properties are more relevant. This means that fibers with short durability also contribute to the carcinogenic effect if their surfaces can serve as suitable carriers for organic carcinogens, if these substances are present.

Evaluation of the carcinogenic potency of inhaled fibers is likely to remain a complex issue because more and more types of respirable natural and man-made fibers have been introduced in recent years.

DAMAGE TO BRONCHIAL WALLS BY FORMALDEHYDE AND INFLUENCE ON FIBER NUMBER—A FIRST EXPERIMENT

To test the hypothesis of fiber implantation after damage to the bronchial mucosa, an animal experiment was carried out, which will be described here very briefly (Althaus and Pott, unpublished).

Ten-week-old female Wistar rats were treated several times by intratracheal instillations. First, they were pretreated with 30 μl of a 1% formaldehyde solution to induce inflammation of the trachea and the upper bronchi. Four to twelve days after pretreatment, the rats were instilled six times with 10 μg crocidolite or glass microfibers suspended in 30 μl of saline solution. Control groups were pretreated with saline instead of formaldehyde. Another control group was treated seven times with saline only. Four weeks after the last instillation, the animals were sacrificed, and tissues of interest collected and ashed. The fibers in the ash of the trachea, including the main bronchi and those in the lung were counted. So far, no clear effect is evident regarding the number of fibers retained after pretreatment with formaldehyde (Table 1). However, this first experiment does not prove conclusively whether or not the hypothesis is correct because, with modifications in the experimental design, long-term effects may be demonstrable.

Table 1. Preliminary results of six intratracheal instillations of 10 μg crocidolite (UICC) or glass microfibers (M 104/475) in rats pretreated with 30 μl formaldehyde and in controls. Numbers of fibers longer than 5 μm that were visible by light microscopy were counted in part of ashed tissue; total fiber numbers per organ were calculated (Althaus and Pott, unpublished).

	Pretreated with 30 μl Saline (Control)			Pretreated with 30 μl Formaldehyde (1%)			P-Value (Mann-Whitney U-Test)
	N	No. Fibers, Median ± SD (x 10^3)	% of Instilled Fibers	N	No. Fibers, Median ± SD (x 10^3)	% of Instilled Fibers	
Crocidolite							
Trachea + main bronchi	7	8.0 ± 2.7	0.12	7	5.5 ± 4.8	0.08	0.31
Lung	12	456 ± 224	6.61	12	405 ± 342	5.87	0.67
Glass microfibers							
Trachea + main bronchi	9	3.9 ± 2.1	0.07	10	2.4 ± 1.9	0.04	0.05
Lung	12	222 ± 112	3.7	10	129 ± 74	2.17	0.22
Control (saline)							
Trachea + main bronchi	10	0 ± 0	0	10	0 ± 0	0	—
Lung	3	0 ± 0.5	0	3	0 ± 1.2	0	—

REFERENCES

Bastie-Sigeac, I, M Hubert-Habart, MC Jaurand, and J Bignon. **1983.** Action des fibres diamante sur le métabolisme du benzo(a)pyrene par les cellules pleurales en culture, pp. 283-288. In: *Faserige Stäube—Messung,* Wirkung, Abhilfe, VDI-Berichte, 475. VDI-Verlag, Düsseldorf; Federal Republic of Germany.

Bellmann, B, H Muhle, F Pott, H König, H Klöppel, and K Spurny. **1987.** Persistence of man-made mineral fibres (MMMF) and asbestos in rat lungs. Ann Occup Hyg 31: 493-709.

Bogovski, P, A Küng, and F Winkmann. **1982.** Phenole, andere Bestandteile des Brennschieferteers und Asbest als modifizierende Faktoren der karzinogenen Wirkung von Benzo(a)pyren. Arch Geschwulstforsch 52:49-55.

Brody, AR and LH Hill. **1982.** Interstitial accumulation of inhaled chrysotile asbestos fibers and consequent formation of microcalcifications. Am J Pathol 109:107-114.

Davis, JMG. **1986.** A review of experimental evidence for the carcinogenicity of man-made vitreous fibers. Scand J Work Environ Health 12 (Suppl.1):12-17.

Davis, JMG, ST Beckett, RE Bolton, P Collings, and AP Middleton. **1978.** Mass and number of fibres in the pathogenesis of asbestos-related lung disease in rats. Br J Cancer 37:673-688.

Davis, JMG, RE Bolton, D Brown, and HE Tully. **1986.** Experimental lesions in rats corresponding to advanced human asbestosis. Exp Mol Pathol 44:207-221.

Doll, R. Summing-up. In: *Mineral Fibres in the Non-Occupational Environment,* Proceedings of a joint symposium held at IARC, September 8-10, 1987, Lyon, France, IARC Scientific Publication. International Agency for Research on Cancer, Lyon, France (in press).

Gerde, P. **1987.** *A Model for the Uptake of Polycyclic Aromatic Hydrocarbons by the Human Lung—Influence of Inhaled Mineral Fibres,* Thesis. Department of Chemical Engineering, Royal Institute of Technology, Stockholm, Sweden.

Greenberg, SD. **1987.** Carcinomas of the peripheral airways, pp. 286-309. In: *Lung Carcinomas,* EM McDowell (ed.). Churchill Livingston, Edinburgh, London, Melbourne, New York.

Heinrich, U, F Pott, and S Rittinghausen. **1986.** Comparison of chronic inhalation effects in rodents after long-term exposure to either coal oven flue gas mixed with pyrolyzed pitch or diesel engine exhaust, pp. 441-457. In: *Carcinogenic and Mutagenic Effects of Diesel Engine Exhaust,* N Ishinishi, A Koizumi RO McClellan, and W Stöber (eds.), Developments in Toxicology and Environmental Science, Vol. 13. Elsevier (Biomedical Div.), Amsterdam, The Netherlands.

Jaurand, MC. A particulate state carcinogenesis: Recent data on the mechanisms of action of fibres. In: *Mineral Fibres in the Non-Occupational Environment,* Proceedings of a joint symposium held at IARC, September 8-10, 1987, Lyon, France, IARC Scientific Publication. International Agency for Research on Cancer, Lyon, France (**in press**).

Linzbach, AJ and HW Wedler. **1941.** Beitrag zum Berufskrebs der Asbestarbeiter. Virchows Arch 307:387-409.

Mossman, BT. **1983.** In vitro approaches for determining mechanisms of toxicity and carcinogenicity by asbestos in the gastrointestinal and respiratory tracts. Environ Health Perspect 53:155-161.

Muhle, H, K Spurny, and F Pott. **1983.** Inhalationsexperimente zur Retention, Lungenreinigung und Wanderungsfähigkeit von Asbest und Glasfasern unter Einfluβ von Zigarettenrauch, pp. 247-251. In: *Faserige Stäube—Messung, Wirkung,* Abhilfe, VDI-Berichte, 475. VDI-Verlag, Düsseldorf, Federal Republic of Germany.

Muhle, H, F Pott, B Bellmann, S Takenaka, and U Ziem. **1987.** Inhalation and injection experiments in rats for testing man-made mineral fibres in the working environment. Ann Occup Hyg 31:755-764.

Nordmann, M. **1938.** Der Berufskrebs der Asbestarbeiter. Z Krebsforsch 47:288-302.

Pott, F. **1978.** Some aspects on the dosimetry of the carcinogenic potency of asbestos and other fibrous dusts. Staub-Reinhalt Luft 38:486-490.

Pott, F. **1984.** On the problems of experimental carcinogenicity studies with fibrous dusts administered intraperitoneally, intratracheally, and by inhalation, pp. 211-220. In: *Problems of Inhalatory Toxicity Studies,* P Grosdanoff et al. (eds.), BGA-Schriften 5/1984. MMV Medizin Verlag, München, Federal Republic of Germany.

Pott, F and KH Friedrichs. **1972.** Tumoren der Ratte nach i.p.-Injektion faserförmiger Stäube. Naturwissenschaften 59:318.

Pott, F, F Huth, and KH Friedrichs. **1972.** Tumoren der Ratte nach i.p.-Injektion von gemahlenem Chrysotil und Benzo(a)pyren. Zentralbl Bakteriol Abt Orig B Hyg Krankenhausyg Betriebshyg Praev Med 155:463-469.

Pott, F, U Ziem, and U Mohr. **1984.** Lung carcinomas and mesotheliomas following intratracheal instillation of glass fibres and asbestos, pp. 746-756. In: *VIth International Pneumoconiosis Conference 1983,* Vol. 2, September 20-23, 1983, Bergbau-Berufsgenossenschaft, Bochum, Federal Republic of Germany. Wirtschaftsverlag, Verlag für neue Wissenschaft, Bremerhaven, Federal Republic of Germany.

Pott, F, U Ziem, F-J Reiffer, F Huth, H Ernst, and U Mohr. **1987.** Carcinogenicity studies on fibres, metal compounds, and some other dusts in rats. Exp Pathol (Jena) 32: 129-152.

Pott, F, M Roller, U Ziem, F-J Reiffer, B Bellmann, M Rosenbruch, and F Huth. Carcinogenicity studies on natural and man-made fibres with the intraperitoneal test in rats. In: *Mineral Fibres in the Non-Occupational Environment,* Proceedings of a joint symposium held at IARC, September 8-10, 1987, Lyon, France, IARC Scientific Publication. International Agency for Research on Cancer, Lyon, France (**in press**).

Pylev, LN. **1980.** Pretumorous lesions and lung and pleural tumours induced by asbestos in rats, Syrian golden hamsters and *Macaca mulatta* (Rhesus) monkeys, pp. 343-355. In: *Biological Effects of Asbestos,* Vol. 1, GC Wagner (ed.), IARC Scientific Publication No 30. International Agency for Research on Cancer, Lyon, France.

Pylev, LN and LM Shabad. **1973.** Some results of experimental studies in asbestos carcinogenesis, pp. 99-105. In: *Biological Aspects of Asbestos,* P Bogovski, JC Gilson, V Timbrell, and JC Wagner (eds.), IARC Scientific Publication No. 8. International Agency for Research on Cancer, Lyon, France.

Reeves, AL, HE Puro, and RG Smith. **1974.** Inhalation carcinogenesis from various forms of asbestos. Environ Res 8:178-202.

Selikoff, IJ, EC Hammond, and J Churg. **1968.** Asbestos exposure, smoking, and neoplasia. J Am Med Assoc 204:104-110.

Selikoff, IJ and DHK Lee. **1978.** *Asbestos and Disease. Environmental Sciences.* Academic Press, New York, NY.

Smith, WE, L Miller, and J Churg. **1970.** An experimental model for study of carcinogenesis in the respiratory tract, pp. 299-316. In: *Morphology of Experimental Respiratory Carcinogenesis.* CONF-700501, NTIS, Springfield, VA.

Smith, DM, LW Ortiz, RF Archuleta, and NF Johnson. **1987.** Health effects in Osborne-Mendel rats and Syrian golden hamsters chronically exposed to man-made vitreous fibres. Ann Occup Hyg 31:731-754.

Stanton, MF and M Layard. **1978.** The carcinogenicity of fibrous minerals, pp. 143-151. In: *Proceedings of the Workshop on Asbestos: Definitions and Measurement Methods,* CC Gravatt, PD LaFleur, and KFJ Heinrich (eds.). U.S. Department of Commerce, National Bureau of Standards, Washington, DC.

Stanton, MF and C Wrench. **1972.** Mechanisms of mesothelioma induction with asbestos and fibrous glass. J Natl Cancer Inst 48:797-821.

Wagner, JC, G Berry, and V Timbrell. **1973.** Mesotheliomata in rats after inoculation with asbestos and other materials. Br J Cancer 28:175-185.

Wagner, JC, G Berry, W Skidmore, and V Timbrell. **1974.** The effect of the inhalation of asbestos in rats. Br J Cancer 29:252-269.

Wagner, JC, JW Skidmore, RJ Hill, and DM Griffiths. **1985.** Erionite exposure and mesotheliomas in rats. Br J Cancer 51:727-730.

Wehner, AP, RH Busch, RJ Olson, and DK Craig. **1975.** Chronic inhalation of asbestos and cigarette smoke by hamsters. Environ Res 10:368-383.

Yu, CP and GB Xu. **1987.** *Predictive Models for Deposition of Inhaled Diesel Exhaust Particles in Humans and Laboratory Species,* Research Report No. 10. Health Effects Institute, Cambridge, MA.

How Smoking and Asbestos Exposure Interact to Increase the Risk of Pulmonary Carcinoma: A Mechanistic Hypothesis

Juraj Ferin

University of Rochester, Department of Biophysics, School of Medicine & Dentistry, University of Rochester, Rochester, NY 14642

KEY WORDS: asbestos, cigarette smoke, carcinoma, interaction, mechanism

---

ABSTRACT

Cigarette-smoking increases the incidence of bronchogenic carcinoma in those who are exposed to asbestos; however, smoking is not a known risk factor for malignant mesothelioma in humans. Differences in particle clearance mechanisms related to the airways, in the case of pulmonary cancer, or the pleura, in the case of mesothelioma, and the effects of smoking on the clearance pathways may be essential for the seeming discrepancy. Asbestos fibers can be translocated from the airways to the pleura. Once in the pleural tissue, fibers are not cleared via the airways. In view of the sensitivity of the pleural tissue to fibers, and considering structural factors that prevent cigarette smoke from reaching the pleural sites directly, potentiation of carcinogenicity by asbestos and cigarette smoke would be surprising. On the other hand, clearance via the airways is impaired by both cigarette smoke and asbestos fibers compared to the clearance of particles with low toxicity; this increases the exposure of airway cells to the two carcinogens. The first essential step required for the synergistic effect of two factors to occur is thus established.

INTRODUCTION

It is generally accepted that the exposure to asbestos dust and to cigarette-smoking multiplies the risk of each factor in regard to the incidence of bronchogenic carcinoma. It has been reported that asbestos exposure increases the risk of bronchogenic carcinoma by a factor of about 5, cigarette-smoking by a factor of about 10, and combined exposure to cigarette smoke and asbestos by a factor of about 50. Cigarette-smoking also seems to shorten the latency interval preceding bronchogenic carcinoma in asbestos workers. However, smoking is not a known risk factor for mesothelioma, another death-causing tumor related to asbestos exposure (Fontana et al., 1981). Why this discrepancy? Obviously, different tissues are involved in these two distinct malignancies. However, the differences in particle clearance mechanisms related to the airways, in the case of pulmonary cancer, or to the pleura, in the case of mesothelioma, may be essential for the apparent discrepancy. The relation of pulmonary lesions to asbestos and/or smoking can be summarized as follows: There is synergism in the case of lung cancer, possible synergism in fibrosis, and no known synergism between pleural disease and chronic obstructive pulmonary disease.

In response to encouragement by the organizers of this meeting to speculate on interactions of mineral fibers and cigarette smoke, I am suggesting that the synergistic interaction between cigarette smoke and asbestos fibers in the respiratory tract is the result of an increased dose to airway cells, resulting mainly from impaired pulmonary clearance.

PLEURAL PROCESSES

It is not well known how mineral particles reach the pleural tissue. However, there is no doubt that asbestos fibers move from the site of initial deposition. The inhaled fibers may pass through or between the cells, enter the interstitial space and the lymphatic system, and may reach the pleura by a combination of these pathways. Once in the pleural tissue, the fibers are no longer cleared via the airways. Polycyclic aromatic hydrocarbons (PAH) from the cigarette smoke that have been adsorbed to the surface of the fibers are released quite readily in the pulmonary tissue (Mossman, 1983). After a single exposure to particles of various materials coated with benzo[a]pyrene (BaP), the clearance time of BaP from the lungs of hamsters was on the order of hours (Henry and Kaufman, 1973). In addition, asbestos fibers are more effective in facilitating rapid uptake of PAH by membranes than nonfibrous materials (Lakowicz and Bevan, 1980). It is therefore probable that during the translocation from airways to the pleural tissues, the fibers lose the adsorbed PAH. The asbestos fibers in the pleural tissue may, of course, become exposed to PAH and other constituents of cigarette smoke after being lodged there. However, this exposure apparently does not increase the risk of mesothelioma. Thus, the adsorption of PAH to the fiber may not be the primary factor in the synergism between asbestos and cigarette smoke.

In view of the sensitivity of the pleural tissue per se to fibers and considering anatomical factors that prevent constituents of cigarette smoke from reaching the pleural sites directly, potentiation of the tumorigenicity of asbestos by cigarette smoke to produce mesotheliomas would be surprising.

AIRWAY PROCESSES

The processes occurring in the airways are different from those in pleural sites. Inhaled particles deposited in the airways are cleared by mechanisms that have evolved in the respiratory system to keep the alveolar surfaces clean. Generally, pulmonary clearance of particles is quite effective, although clearance mechanisms can be overwhelmed, and some particles are cleared less efficiently than others. The lung clearance of particles has recently been reviewed by Oberdörster (in press).

Is pulmonary clearance affected by cigarette smoke or by asbestos? In two very early papers, Bair and Dilley (1967) reported little effect of smoking on the clearance of $^{59}Fe_2O_3$ or $^{51}Cr_2O_3$. However, we found that smoking depressed clearance of SiO_2 particles in rats (Ferin et al., 1965). The different methods used in these two studies may explain the inconsistency. Park et al. (1977) reported that 6-month and 1-year periods of mild to moderate smoking impaired tracheal mucociliary transport and the bacteriosuppressive activity of alveolar macrophages in dogs. It was also reported (Green, 1985) that components of cigarette smoke produced various cellular deficiencies in alveolar macrophages, a finding which may explain, at least in part, the altered host resistance to respiratory infections in smokers. In a study on guinea pigs, Tron et al. (1987) showed that smoking potentiated fibrosis induced by asbestos, possibly because of increased fiber retention. Among men exposed to asbestos for less than 20 years, only cigarette smokers had roentgenographic evidence of pulmonary fibrosis; among those exposed to asbestos for 20 years or more, smokers had a high frequency of asbestosis (Weiss, 1971). Lung clearance of amosite asbestos fibers was dramatically decreased in guinea pigs by cigarette smoke exposure (McFadden et al., 1986). Changes in alveolar macrophage functions after asbestos exposure have been observed in rats (Warheit et al., 1984). We have reported that rats clear TiO_2 test particles more slowly if the animals have been pre-exposed for a short time to asbestos dust (Ferin and Leach, 1976). In addition, experimental studies on particle clearance and cigarette smoke that are listed in the program of this meeting apparently led to the conclusion that cigarette-smoke exposure increased pulmonary retention of inhaled particles in animals (see, for example, Churg et al., Mauderly et al., Muhle et al., this volume).

Clearance studies in humans require a harmless probe that can be monitored externally in living subjects. Because of the inherent problems, only a few long- term clearance studies on smokers have been reported. Cohen et al. (1979) used magnetite (Fe_3O_4) particles as the probe. During a single session, the subjects inhaled about 1 mg of magnetite dust. Periodically, the amount of dust remaining in the lung was measured with a sensitive magnetic detector. The individual clearance curves indicated that, in heavy smokers, clearance of magnetite particles was considerably slower than in nonsmokers. After about a year, approximately 50% of the originally deposited dust remained in the lungs of the smokers, whereas only about 10% was retained in the lungs of the nonsmokers.

Bohning et al. (1982) used polystyrene particles tagged with ^{85}Sr as their probe. The long-term particle clearance had two phases in healthy nonsmokers, with half-times of 30 and 296 days, respectively. Cigarette-smoking suppressed the first phase and increased the half-time of the second phase by 14.7 days per pack-year of smoking.

The available data strongly suggest that both cigarette smoke and/or asbestos fibers impair pulmonary clearance mechanisms. It seems that both the mucociliary system and alveolar macrophages are affected. How cigarette smoke or asbestos fibers affect the cells involved in clearance is not known. It has been suggested that, in addition to the toxic effects on cells, asbestos fibers physically affect alveolar macrophages by their size, which is sometimes larger than that of the macrophage. In addition, an apparently nonspecific overload effect must also be considered. Bolton et al. (1983) reported that, at lung burdens exceeding about 1.5 mg amosite fibers per rat lung, clearance mechanisms break down. The phenomenon of overloading was also observed with other dust particles, e.g., TiO_2, diesel particles, photocopier toner particles, and quartz (Ferin, 1972; Chan et al., 1984; Wolff et al., 1987; Bellmann et al., 1986; Muhle et al., 1988). It seems that overloading occurs at a lung burden of 1 to 2 mg of dust/g lung tissue. This phenomenon has been observed with many different kinds of particles, including those with low toxicity. Following pulmonary overload, we have observed impaired lung clearance and redistribution of particles into the interstitium (e.g., for TiO_2; Ferin and Feldstein, 1978) in addition to inflammation, macrophage recruitment, and cell proliferation. Although the mechanisms leading to pulmonary overloading are not clear, the involvement of alveolar macrophages in this process seems to be certain, as stressed by Morrow (1986).

LOCALIZED PROCESSES IN AIRWAYS

Inhaled fibers are preferentially deposited at bifurcations of bronchi and bronchioles by impaction and interception. Brody et al. (1981) showed that small inhaled chrysotile asbestos fibers were also deposited mainly at bifurcations of alveolar ducts. Warheit et al. (1984) studied the changes triggered by asbestos fiber deposition at alveolar duct bifurcations and described asbestos-induced lesions at these sites. The authors suggested that early lesions of asbestos-related fibrotic lung disease occur at anatomic sites where asbestos-laden macrophages initially accumulate. Lung carcinomas associated with smoking or asbestos exposure are almost always bronchogenic. It can be assumed that in the bronchi or bronchioles, asbestos will also exert toxic effects, mainly on the airway cells that are in contact with the fiber. In cases of pulmonary carcinoma, changes in the mucosa of bronchi are commonly found at sites some distance from the tumor. These changes, which range from basal cell hyperplasia to squamous metaplasia, have been found in almost all those who died with pulmonary carcinoma. Furthermore, most smokers who died from diseases other than pulmonary carcinoma also had these changes. Metaplasia occurs readily with smoke alone; however, exacerbation of epithelial proliferation and metaplasia following exposure to both asbestos and cigarette smoke suggests that the contribution made by asbestos fibers is an additional stimulus to epithelial proliferation (Selikoff and Lee, 1978). Morphological and functional changes in the bronchial mucosa exacerbate local impairment of particle clearance. The normally uneven distribution of the total lung dose over the airways can also be increased by local changes, and increased total dose to the airways enhances the potential for this focal exacerbation.

PULMONARY CLEARANCE AND DOSE

At least three factors that lead to clearance impairment by cigarette smoke and asbestos should be considered: toxic effects on cells, physical characteristics of the fibers, and pulmonary overload. The main result of impaired clearance is, of course, an increased dose of both asbestos and cigarette smoke to airway cells. Even after cessation of asbestos exposure, particles accumulate in lung tissue and may become a source of airway cell exposure after they are mobilized from sequestered sites. The extent of this mobilization is not known, but asbestos bodies in the sputum of humans indicate such a possibility. The synergism of asbestos and cigarette smoke may be the result of increased dose to airway cells, resulting from impairment of pulmonary clearance mechanisms.

CONCLUSIONS

Epidemiological studies and clinical experience indicate that cigarette smoke increases the asbestos-associated risk of bronchogenic carcinoma in man, but smoking is not a known risk factor for developing mesothelioma.

The differences between the tissues involved and the effect of asbestos and/or cigarette smoke on particle clearance from the airways may account for this apparent discrepancy.

Evidence strongly suggests that pulmonary particle clearance is impaired by asbestos or by cigarette-smoke exposure. Toxic effects on cells, the physical characteristics of the fibers, and pulmonary overload appear to be the main factors that account for this phenomenon.

Impaired clearance increases pulmonary retention, which, in turn, increases the dose of asbestos and cigarette-smoke constituents to airway cells. Focal exacerbation of biological effects may be expected from localized morphological and functional changes in the bronchial mucosa. This increased dose may be the basis for the synergism between mineral fibers and cigarette smoke.

REFERENCES

Bair, WJ and JV Dilley. **1967.** Pulmonary clearance of $^{59}Fe_2O_3$ and $^{51}Cr_2O_3$ in rat and dogs exposed to cigarette smoke, pp. 251-268. In: *Inhaled Particles and Vapours, II,* CN Davies (ed.). Pergamon Press, New York, NY.

Bellmann, B, H Muhle, and O Crentzenberg O. **1986.** The effect of a "nuisance" dust inhalation on lung clearance, pp. 209-211. In: *Aerosols: Formation and Reactivity,* Second International Conference, Berlin. Pergamon Journals, Ltd., Oxford, Great Britain.

Bohning, DE, HL Atkins, and SH Cohn. **1982.** Long-term particle clearance in man: Normal and impaired. Ann Occup Hyg 26:259-271.

Bolton, RE, JH Vincent, AD Jones, J Addison, and ST Beckett. **1983.** An overload hypothesis for pulmonary clearance of UICC amosite fibres inhaled by rats. Br J Ind Med 40:264-272.

Brody, AR, LH Hill, B Adkins, and RW O'Connor. **1981.** Chrysotile asbestos inhalation: Deposition pattern and reaction of alveolar epithelium and pulmonary macrophages. Am Rev Respir Dis 123:670-679.

Chan, TL, PS Lee, and WE Hering. **1984.** Pulmonary retention of inhaled diesel particles after prolonged exposures to diesel exhaust. Fundam Appl Toxicol 4:624-631.

Cohen, D, SF Arai, and JD Brain. **1979.** Smoking impairs long-term dust clearance from the lung. Science 204:514-517.

Ferin, J. **1972.** Observations concerning alveolar dust clearance. Ann NY Acad Sci 200:66-72.

Ferin, J and LJ Leach. **1976.** The effect of amosite and chrysotile asbestos on the clearance of TiO_2 particles from the lung. Environ Res 12:250-254.

Ferin, J and M Feldstein. **1978.** Pulmonary clearance and hilar lymph node content in rats after particle exposure. Environ Res 16:342-352.

Ferin, J, G Urbankova, and A Vlckova. **1965.** Influence of tobacco smoke on the elimination of particles from the lungs. Nature 206:515-516.

Fontana, RS, et al. **1981.** *Lung Cancer and Asbestos Related Pulmonary Disease,* pp 1-40. The American College of Chest Physicians, Chicago, IL.

Green, GM. **1985.** Mechanisms of tobacco smoke toxicity on pulmonary macrophage cells. Eur J Respir Dis 66:82-85.

Henry, MC and DG Kaufman. **1973.** Clearance of benzo(a)pyrene from hamster lungs after administration on coated particles. J Natl Cancer Inst 51:1961-1964.

Lakowicz, JR and DR Bevan. **1980.** Benzo(a)pyrene uptake into rat liver microsomes: Effects of adsorption of benzo(a)pyrene to asbestos and nonfibrous mineral particulates. Chem Biol Interact 29:129-138.

McFadden, J, L Wright, B Wiggs, and A Churg. **1986.** Smoking inhibits asbestos clearance. Am Rev Respir Dis 133:372-374.

Morrow, PE. **1986.** The setting of particulate exposure levels for chronic inhalation toxicity studies. J Am Coll Toxicol 5:533-544.

Mossman, B. **1983.** Asbestos: Mechanisms of toxicity and carcinogenicity in the respiratory tract. Ann Rev Pharmacol Toxicol 23:595-615.

Muhle, H, B Bellmann, O Crentzenberg, W Stober, R Kilpper, J MacKenzie, PE Morrow, and R Mermelstein. **1988.** Pulmonary deposition, clearance and retention of test toner, TiO_2 and quartz during a long-term inhalation study in rats. The Toxicologist 8:272 (abstract).

Oberdörster, G. Lung clearance of inhaled insoluble and soluble particles. J Aerosol Med 1 (**in press**).

Park, SS, Y Kikkawa, IP Goldring, MM Daly, M Zeletsky, C-H Shim, M Spierer, and T Morita. **1977.** An animal model of cigarette smoking in beagle dogs: Correlative evaluation of effects on pulmonary function, defense, and morphology. Am Rev Respir Dis 115:971-979.

Selikoff, IJ and DHK Lee. **1978.** *Asbestos and Disease.* Academic Press, Inc., New York, NY, 422 p.

Tron, V, JL Wright, N Harrison, B Wiggs, and A Churg. **1987.** Cigarette smoke makes airway and early parenchymal asbestos-induced lung disease worse in the guinea pig. Am Rev Respir Dis 136:271-275.

Warheit, DB, LY Chang, LH Hill, GER Hook, JD Crapo, and AR Brody. **1984.** Pulmonary macrophage accumulation and asbestos induced lesions at sites of fiber deposition. Am Rev Respir Dis 129:301-310.

Weiss, W. **1971.** Cigarette smoking, asbestos and pulmonary fibrosis. Am Rev Respir Dis 104:223-227.

Wolff, RK, RF Henderson, MB Snipes, WC Griffith, JL Mauderly, RG Cuddihy, and RO McClellan. **1987.** Alterations in particle accumulation and clearance in lungs of rats chronically exposed to diesel exhaust. Fundam Appl Toxicol 9:154-166.

Factors Affecting the Carcinogenicity of Mineral Fibers and Their Relationship to the Synergistic Effects of Tobacco Smoke

John M. G. Davis

Institute of Occupational Medicine, Roxburgh Place, Edinburgh EH8 95U, Great Britain

KEY WORDS: carcinogenesis, chrysotile, amphiboles, tobacco smoke, synergism

---

ABSTRACT

Experimental studies by several workers have demonstrated that whether administered by inhalation, or by intraperitoneal or intrapleural injection, the carcinogenic effects of any asbestos sample are related to the mass dose. With injection studies, the dose response appears to be linear, although the results from inhalation studies published so far are insufficiently detailed to be certain that the response follows exactly the same pattern. Differences in fiber length between different dust samples of the same mineral type are important factors in carcinogenicity. Many detailed injection studies with carefully sized dusts have indicated that the most carcinogenic fibers are long and thin; maximum carcinogenicity was reached at lengths of >8 μm and diameters of <0.25 μm. The results from inhalation exposure are less detailed, but recent studies suggest that short fibers (<5 μm in length) have little or no carcinogenic potential. Even with fibers in the most dangerous size range, their durability in lung tissue varies considerably, probably affecting carcinogenicity. Fibers that dissolve within a relatively few months seem much less likely to accumulate in lung tissue to levels at which tumor production is likely. This factor most probably explains the different carcinogenic effects seen with chrysotile and the amphibole asbestos types in humans and experimental animals. In experimental animals, chrysotile appears to survive for the 1 to 2 years needed for it to be as carcinogenic as the amphiboles. In humans, where tumor induction takes many years, the same rate of chrysotile dissolution appears to reduce its carcinogenic effect considerably, while the durable amphiboles remain almost unchanged.

While it has been clearly demonstrated that there is a synergistic effect between asbestos and tobacco-smoke inhalation for the production of pulmonary tumors, little is known about the mechanisms involved. For a full understanding of this process, it is necessary to know how the combined effects of tobacco smoke and asbestos relate to the fiber mass inhaled, the dimensions of the fibers inhaled, and the durability of these fibers in lung tissue.

INTRODUCTION

Selikoff et al. (1968) first demonstrated that a synergistic relationship existed between asbestos exposure and cigarette smoking for the production of bronchial carcinomas. While the risk for asbestos workers who smoked heavily was increased more than 90 times that of the general population, nonsmoking asbestos workers showed a relatively small increase in tumor incidence compared to nonsmokers in the general population. Since cigarette smoke contains a number of well-known chemical carcinogens, particularly polycyclic aromatic hydrocarbons (PAH), which are readily adsorbed onto asbestos fibers, it has been assumed that synergism in some way relates to this adsorption. Indeed, it was originally suggested that the carcinogenicity of asbestos fibers might be entirely caused by the adsorption of hydrocarbons during processing and particularly from packaging materials, such as hessian bags. This was disproved by Harington et al. (1974), who showed that asbestos carcinogenicity in experimental animals was not affected by the complete removal of adsorbed hydrocarbons by benzene.

Using a variety of *in vitro* techniques, Kandaswami and O'Brien (1980), Lakowicz and Bevan (1980), Reiss et al. (1983), and Poole et al. (1983) all reported changes in the biological activity of asbestos fibers in the presence of chemical carcinogens. In some mutagenicity studies, asbestos alone had no effect, while the combined effect of the two materials was much greater than that of the chemical carcinogen on its own.

Similar results have been obtained from animal experimental studies. Pylev (1972), Pylev and Shabad (1973), and Shabad et al. (1974) reported on work involving the intratracheal injection of Russian chrysotile asbestos into rats with and without the addition of benzo[a]pyrene (BaP). The injected chrysotile dose was 2 mg, and the BaP was either adsorbed onto chrysotile before injection or, in another experiment, given as a separate injection of 5 mg. No tumors developed with either chrysotile or BaP alone, but in both experiments using these materials together, substantial numbers of pulmonary tumors or mesotheliomas developed. Inhalation studies using chrysotile asbestos, BaP and cigarette smoke (Shabad et al., 1974) did not cause pulmonary tumors with any combination of materials, although precancerous lesions were found more frequently in animals treated with asbestos and BaP than in the other groups. The mass dose of chrysotile administered by inhalation seems very large (230 mg/m^3), and it was continued for over 1 year. However, this was not a measure of respirable dust, and exposure was conducted for only 10 hours each week. Exposure to cigarette smoke, administered between periods of asbestos inhalation, was trivial (1.5 cigarettes/rat/month), and exposure to BaP was by means of a single intratracheal injection of 1 mg. Wehner et al. (1975) and Wehner (1980) reported on more detailed inhalation studies with asbestos and cigarette smoke. Exposure of hamsters to chrysotile asbestos at a respirable mass concentration of 23 mg/m^3 resulted in severe pulmonary asbestosis by 11 months and an increase in the incidence of benign pulmonary tumors. Concurrent exposure to cigarette smoke (10 minutes, three times a day, 5 days a week) produced no additional carcinogenic effect.

Harrison* reported a study in which the synergistic effects of chrysotile (administered as a single intratracheal injection of 2 mg) and a number of potential carcinogens were examined. These included cadmium and BaP, which were mixed with the chrysotile before intratracheal injection into rats and N-nitroso-heptamethyleneimine (NHMI), which was administered by subcutaneous injection. While the development of "precancerous" lesions was common, neither chrysotile alone or in conjunction with most of the other materials tested caused an increase in definitive pulmonary tumors. The only group of animals with a significantly increased incidence of pulmonary tumors was that treated with chrysotile and NHMI.

Topping and Nettesheim (1980) used a novel technique to examine the combined effects of chrysotile and dimethylbenz[a]anthracene (DMBA). Tracheal explants from rats were treated with these materials and implanted subcutaneously into syngeneic rats. In these studies, a combination of supposedly nontumorigenic doses of the two materials produced carcinomas in 15 to 25% of animals.

---

*Harrison, PTC. Some Histopathological Changes in Rat Lung Induced by Chrysotile Asbestos, Powdered Metallic Cadmium and a Nitrosamine. Presented at the British Association for Lung Research Meeting, 1987, Guildford, Surrey, U.K.

FACTORS AFFECTING THE CARCINOGENICITY OF ASBESTOS AND OTHER MINERAL FIBERS

In many early experimental studies with asbestos, little attention was paid to the content of the asbestos sample used. In some cases, only the generic term "asbestos" was given, with no indication whether it was chrysotile or amphibole. The production of standard reference samples by the International Union Against Cancer (UICC) eliminated some of these problems. However, it rapidly became apparent that the carcinogenicity of different samples of one asbestos type could vary greatly, and a large amount of experimental work has been undertaken in an attempt to learn exactly which dust parameters affect tumor production. It now appears that the mass of dust administered, the fiber size distribution of the dust, and the length of time the dust remains in lung tissues are all important. The carcinogenicity of a dust sample depends on a combination of these factors.

The importance of the mass dose of any asbestos type was examined by Wagner et al. (1974), who reported long-term inhalation studies using rats that had been exposed to dust clouds of the main asbestos varieties. While the mass concentration of respirable dust aerosol remained constant at approximately 10 mg/m^3 of air, exposure time was varied between 1 day and 24 months, so that the total dose received by the animals varied greatly. For all asbestos types, the degree of pulmonary fibrosis (asbestosis) that was produced varied proportionally with the duration of exposure. The values for rats exposed for 1 day only were similar to those of unexposed control animals. The production of pulmonary tumors was less clearly related to exposure duration than asbestosis but, in general, more tumors occurred in animals exposed for long periods. Some animals exposed for a single day developed pulmonary neoplasms, but similar numbers of tumors were found in control animals.

In 1978, Davis et al. reported inhalation studies using rats exposed to UICC chrysotile A for 1 year at a respirable mass concentration of either 10 or 2 mg/m^3. Both pulmonary fibrosis and the occurrence of pulmonary tumors were functions of the aerosol concentrations, with the 10-mg concentration producing significantly more tumors than the 2-mg dose.

Pleural mesotheliomas following dust inhalation were rare in both these inhalation studies, and no relationship with dose could be demonstrated. Dose-related production of mesotheliomas has, however, been demonstrated on several occasions following intrapleural or intraperitoneal implantation of asbestos. Smith et al. (1968) reported a progressive reduction in tumor incidence with a reduced dose of both chrysotile or amosite injected into the pleural cavity of hamsters, although tumors still developed following injection of as little as 1 mg of dust. Stanton and Wrench (1972) confirmed this dose-response effect with crocidolite implanted in the pleural cavities of rats. Similar results were reported by Wagner et al. (1973): mesothelioma production by both chrysotile and crocidolite following the injection of as little as 0.6 mg of dust into rats.

In 1985, Davis reported more extensive studies, in which the UICC reference samples of crocidolite, amosite and chrysotile A had been injected into the peritoneal cavities of rats at doses from 25 to 0.01 mg. A clear dose response was found for all three asbestos varieties (Figure 1). Although crocidolite and amosite did not produce tumors at the lowest dose level, chrysotile did, and the dose response in each case was linear when plotted on a log scale. This pattern of response could imply that there is no threshold below which tumors will not occur if the number of animals injected is large enough. However, evidence for a safety threshold comes from examination of the tumor induction period at very low dose levels. For all three asbestos types, both the time to first tumor and the mean induction period of all tumors increased progressively with decreasing dose (Figure 2). Tumors produced by the lowest doses occurred, in general, during the last few months of the rat's life, indicating that even lower doses would have had insufficient time to produce tumors. The numbers of fibers in the lowest doses injected in this study were approximately 25 x 10^6 for chrysotile, 10 x 10^6 for crocidolite, and 4 x 10^6 for amosite.

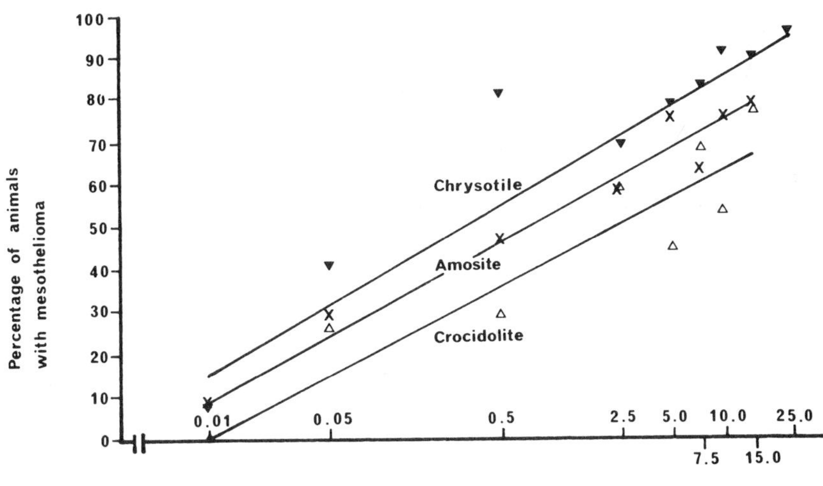

Figure 1. The percentage of animals developing mesotheliomas following the intraperiteoneal injection of varying doses of the UICC reference samples of chrysotile A, crocidolite and amosite.

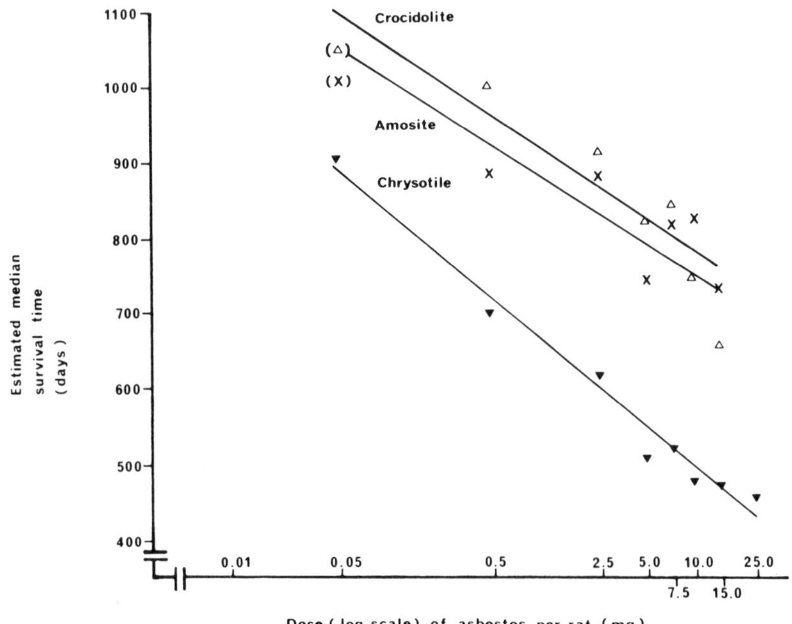

Figure 2. The median tumor induction period for rats developing mesothelioma following the intraperitoneal injection of varying doses of IUCC chrysotile A, crocidolite and amosite.

The studies described above provide good evidence that asbestos carcinogenicity is closely related to the mass of dust administered. However, it appears that not all fibers included in any exposure are equally harmful, and evidence is accumulating that very short fibers may be innocuous. Both Stanton and Wrench (1972) and Pott and Friedrichs (1972) reported that dust samples that produced the most mesotheliomas in rats following implantation were those that contained the highest number of long thin fibers. This work was progressively refined (Stanton et al., 1977; Stanton and Layard, 1978; Pott, 1978, 1983), and it now appears that the most dangerous fibers are those with a length >8 μm and a diameter >0.25 μm. For many years, it was not possible to confirm that long fibers are necessary to cause pulmonary damage following dust inhalation because of the difficulties in preparing sufficiently large quantities of suitably sized dust. Recently, however, long-term inhalation studies have been conducted using short-fiber preparations of amosite and chrysotile (Davis et al., 1986a; Davis and Jones, in press). In these experiments, the effects of short-fiber dust were compared with a dust cloud of the same batch of asbestos containing many long fibers. The short-fiber amosite preparation available had almost no fibers >5 μm in length. The short-fiber chrysotile had some long fibers. The short-fiber preparation had only six times fewer fibers >5 μm long than the long, although for fibers >20 μm in length the ratio increased to approximately 30:1. Tables 1, 2 and 3 show the levels of pulmonary disease produced in rats following a 1-year inhalation of these dust preparations and the number of mesotheliomas produced following intraperitoneal injection. Inhalation of the short-fiber amosite preparation produced no detectable pulmonary disease in rats, although large amounts of dust were visible in pulmonary macrophages in even the oldest animals. Inhalation of short-fiber chrysotile produced pulmonary fibrosis and neoplasia roughly in proportion to the number of 5-μm-long fibers present. Following dust injection at two dose levels, the short-fiber amosite preparation produced only a single mesothelioma at the highest dose (25 mg). When injected at three dose levels, short-fiber chrysotile readily produced mesotheliomas at the two highest dose levels (25 and 2.5 mg), although no mesotheliomas developed following injection of 0.25 mg of dust. A comparison of both tumor numbers and tumor induction period between long- and short-fiber chrysotile, however, indicates that response was proportional at each dose level to the number of relatively long fibers present in the two materials.

In addition to dust mass and the number of long, thin fibers present in the dust, it is becoming apparent that a hypothesis regarding the dose effect of asbestos needs to be considered; that is, the concept that to cause disease, asbestos fibers need to be

Table 1. Mean areas of lung tissue occupied by interstitial fibrosis in rats of advanced age treated with long- and short-fiber samples of amosite and chrysotile asbestos[a]

	Percentage of Lung Containing Interstitial Fibrosis	
	Amosite	Chrysotile
Long fiber (Range of length, μm)	11.0 (0.4-34.6)	12.6 (6.4-23.9)
Short fiber (Range of length, μm)	0.15 (0-2.8)	2.4 (0.3-6.7)

[a]All rats that survived to within 2 months of the end of their respective studies were included in the estimates of interstitial fibrosis. They were, therefore, aged between 30 and 33 months, and the group numbers varied between 10 and 23 animals.

Table 2. Numbers of pulmonary tumors and pleural mesotheliomas produced in rats by inhalation of long- and short-fiber samples of amosite and chrysotile[a]

	Pulmonary Tumors and Pleural Mesotheliomas	
	Amosite	Chrysotile
Long fiber	13	22
Short fiber	0	7

[a]Number of animals in each group available for examination ranged between 40 and 42.

Table 3. Percentage of mesotheliomas produced following intraperitoneal injection of varying doses of long- and short-fiber preparations of amosite and chrysotile

	Amosite		Chrysotile	
Injected Dose (mg)	Long Fiber	Short Fiber	Long Fiber	Short Fiber
25	95	4	95	91
10	88	0	—	—
2.5	—	—	91	33
0.25	—	—	67	0

retained in the lung tissues for long periods and that a low retained dose will produce little disease regardless of the number of fibers inhaled. In the matter of retained dose, chrysotile asbestos differs from amphibole varieties. This has been demonstrated by a number of workers, including Wagner et al. (1974), Middleton et al. (1977) and Davis et al. (1978). Following varying inhalation periods at high concentrations, rats have been shown to retain up to 10 times more amphibole than chrysotile. The recent studies of Davis et al. (1986a) for amosite and Davis and Jones (in press) for chrysotile have extended these findings to involve the importance of fiber length. The combined findings for lung dust retention from both these studies are given in Table 4. The differing retention of chrysotile and amosite is clearly demonstrated, but fiber length appears important in pulmonary deposition and retention of both asbestos types. Less long-fiber amosite than short was present at the end of exposure for both chrysotile and amosite, indicating that the longer fibers tended to impact higher up in the bronchial tree, where clearance was rapid. Following the end of exposure, the clearance of short fibers was faster, but the amount of all sizes of chrysotile was reduced in the lung tissue much faster than amosite. While 14% of long-fiber amosite and 20% of short-fiber amosite was cleared during the 6 months following the end of exposure, the comparable figures for long- and short-fiber chrysotile were 55 and 90%.

Table 4. Lung burdens of asbestos for rats exposed for 12 months to a respirable mass concentration of long- or short-fiber preparations of 10 mg/m^3 of amosite or chrysotile

	Lung Asbestos Burdens (μg)			
Time After End of Exposure (Months)	Long-Fiber Amosite	Short-Fiber Amosite	Long-Fiber Chrysotile	Short-Fiber Chrysotile
0	3570	5640	350	1020
6	3080	4470	161	109

Amphibole fibers are extremely durable, even in aggressive chemical environments, but chrysotile undergoes decomposition much more readily. Even in water, magnesium is progressively leached from chrysotile, and mild acids can cause rapid dissolution of chrysotile fibers (Hodgson, 1986). It appears likely, therefore, that observed differences in pulmonary clearance between chrysotile and the amphiboles are due mainly to the solubility of chrysotile in the lung tissues. Davis et al. (1986b) reported that in old rats, 18 months after a 1-year inhalation period of chrysotile at a concentration of 10 mg/m^3, no chrysotile fibers remained in pulmonary macrophages or in direct contact with any other pulmonary cells. Only very small amounts of chrysotile were detected, either among the collagen fibrils in old acellular fibrous tissue or in the thickened basement membranes of the air spaces. Both these sites may be considered chemical backwaters, where fiber dissolution is retarded. The rapid removal of chrysotile from human lung tissues and the durability of amphibole fibers have been confirmed by several studies (Pooley, 1976; Gylseth et al., 1983).

The rapid dissolution of chrysotile in lung tissues implies a much lower hazard following dust inhalation than that for the durable amphiboles. Human epidemiological evidence appears to confirm this, certainly as far as tumor production is concerned. With rats, however, chrysotile appears equally as pathogenic as amphiboles of similar fiber length. This apparent anomaly is probably due to the fact that in order to produce disease, asbestos fibers need to remain in tissue for a large proportion of the life span of any species, while chemical dissolution of chrysotile fibers occurs at similar rates in all lung tissues. Using a 1-year inhalation period, large quantities of chrysotile can be retained in the rat lung for at least half of the animal's life span. In humans, the same dissolution rate would clear fibers inhaled during industrial or, particularly, environmental exposures before they were able to build up to a dangerous level.

The dissolution of fibers in lung tissue is particularly important for many types of man-made mineral fibers, and rapid dissolution of glass fibers has been reported from *in vitro* and *in vivo* studies (Forster, 1984; Klingholz and Steinkopf, 1984; Leinweber, 1984). Probably as a result of this short retention in lung tissue, fine glass fibers appear to produce very few lesions in rat lungs following long-term inhalation (Wagner et al., 1984; McConnell et al., 1984). Lungs heavily burdened with visible glass fibers at the end of the exposure period appeared to contain none within a few months after exposure (McConnell, personal communication). Man-made fibers that are able to remain in lung tissue for many years may be as dangerous as asbestos for the same number and size of fibers. For instance, pulmonary tumors have been reported in rats following the inhalation of ceramic fibers (Davis et al., 1984) and aramid fiber (Reinhardt).*

DISCUSSION

The mechanisms by which asbestos and chemical carcinogens such as PAH react synergistically to produce tumors are not known. However, the factors affecting the carcinogenicity of asbestos fibers suggest that different dust parameters might well conflict in this synergism. Perhaps the synergism results from the adsorption of PAH onto the fiber surface, although in one respect this would conflict with the carcinogenic effects of fiber size. For any asbestos type, carcinogenicity has been shown to depend on the presence of relatively long thin fibers. At the same time, adsorption of carcinogenic hydrocarbons depends on fiber surface area (Fournier and Pezerat, 1986). Reducing the fiber length in a dust sample would reduce the carcinogenicity of the pure material but would provide greater surface area for adsorption, so that the potential for carrying hydrocarbons would be increased. It is obviously important to determine whether or not these conflicting factors would cancel each other. In addition, while both chrysotile and the amphiboles can adsorb PAH readily, chrysotile retention in tissue is much lower than for the amphiboles. It seems likely that chrysotile undergoes dissolution in tissue fluids, which would release

*Reinhardt, CF. Letter circulated to customers by the Du Pont Company, Wilmington, DE on 4/4/85.

adsorbed carcinogens. If synergism only occurs when fibers and chemical carcinogens are in physical contact, then one would expect it to be eliminated by this dissolution. In this context, it would be important to know whether the carcinogenic synergism reported by Harrison (1987) for chrysotile and NHMI resulted from the NHMI, which was injected subcutaneously, traveling in the circulation, and adsorbing onto chrysotile fibers already deposited in lung tissue. This factor could be important in relation to the use of artificially modified asbestos fibers. Menard et al. (1986) have demonstrated that treating chrysotile fibers with phosphate largely eliminates the adsorption of PAH, so that little of these materials could be carried into the tissues following contact with cigarette smoke. However, the residence time of phosphate-coated chrysotile in lung tissues has not been investigated as yet. If it was removed before dissolution of the chrysotile fibers, then the potential for adsorption onto these fibers of PAH that were deposited in the tissue directly from tobacco smoke might be as great as for untreated chrysotile.

Although these factors obviously need careful examination, it seems possible that the synergism between asbestos and cigarette smoke might result from the two carcinogens acting separately. It is suggested that increased lung cancer in asbestos workers does not occur without a significant level of asbestosis (Browne, 1986). It may be that the effect of the fibrotic inflammation of asbestosis on lung tissue is to produce a population of epithelial cells that are unusually sensitive to the additional effects of chemical carcinogens. One finding that may support the idea that the synergism between asbestos and cigarette smoke results from separate action by the two carcinogens is that there is no evidence for this synergism in relation to mesothelioma production. If carcinogens from cigarette smoke remain firmly bound to asbestos fibers, then it would be expected that they would be carried to the pleural cavity along with the fibers. It would be very surprising if mesothelial cells reacted differently to fibers coated with carcinogen than do pulmonary epithelial cells. If, however, chemical carcinogens and asbestos fibers merely act in the same sites in lung tissue, there is no reason why fiber transport to the pleura should not take place on its own.

REFERENCES

Browne, K. 1986. Is asbestos or asbestosis the cause of increased risk of lung cancer in asbestos workers? Br J Ind Med 43:145-149.

Davis, JMG. 1985. A review of recent experiments on the mechanisms of asbestos pathogenicity, pp. 25-35. In: *Proceedings of the*

Vth International Colloquium on Dust Measuring Technique and Strategy. Asbestos International Association, Johannesburg, Republic of South Africa.

Davis, JMG, SR Beckett, RE Bolton, P Collings, and AP Middleton. **1978.** Mass and number of fibres in the pathogenesis of asbestos-related lung disease in rats. Br J Cancer 37:673-688.

Davis, JMG, J Addison, RE Bolton, K Donaldson, AD Jones, and A Wright. **1984.** The pathogenic effects of fibrous ceramic aluminum silicate glass administered to rats by inhalation or peritoneal injection, pp. 303-322. In: *Biological Effects of Man-Made Mineral Fibres,* Proceedings of the World Health Organization Symposium. World Health Organization, Copenhagen, Denmark.

Davis, JMG, J Addison, RE Bolton, K Donaldson, AD Jones, and T Smith. **1986a.** The pathogenicity of long versus short fibre samples of amosite asbestos administered to rats by inhalation and intraperitoneal injection. Br J Exp Pathol 67:415-430.

Davis, JMG, RE Bolton, D Brown, and HE Tully. **1986b.** Experimental lesions in rats corresponding to advanced human asbestosis. Exp Mol Pathol 44:207-221.

Davis, JMG and AD Jones. Comparisons of the pathogenicity of long and short fibre samples of chrysotile asbestos in rats. Br J Exp Pathol (**in press**).

Forster, H. **1984.** The behavior of mineral fibres in physiological solutions, pp.27-60. In: *Biological Effects of Man-Made Mineral Fibres,* Proceedings of the World Health Organization Symposium. World Health Organization, Copenhagen, Denmark.

Fournier, J and H Pezerat. **1986.** Interactions between asbestos and polynuclear aromatic hydrocarbons. Environ Res 41:276-295.

Gylseth, B, G Mowe, and A Wannag. **1983.** Fibre type and concentration in the lungs of workers in an asbestos cement factory. Br J Ind Med 40:375-379.

Harington, JS, AC Allison, and DV Badami. **1974.** Mineral fibers: Chemical, physicochemical and biological properties. Adv Pharmacol Chemotherap 12:291-302.

Hodgson, AA. **1986.** *Scientific Advances in Asbestos 1967-1985,* Anjalena Publications. Jupiter Press, Croydon, UK.

Kandaswami, C and PJ O'Brien. **1980.** Effects of asbestos on membrane transport and metabolism of benzo[a]pyrene. Biochem Biophys Res Commun 97:794-801.

Klingholz, R and B Steinkopf. **1984.** The reactions of MMMF in a physiological model fluid and in water, pp. 60-87. In: *Biological Effects of Man-Made Mineral Fibres,* Proceedings of the World Health Organization Symposium. World Health Organization, Copenhagen, Denmark.

Lakowicz, JR and DR Bevan. **1980.** Benzo[a]pyrene uptake into rat liver microsomes: Effects of adsorption of benzo[a]pyrene to asbestos and non-fibrous mineral particulates. Chem Biol Interact 29:129-138.

Leinweber, JP. **1984.** Solubility of fibres *in vitro* and *in vivo,* pp. 87-102. In: *Biological Effects of Man-Made Mineral Fibres,* Proceedings of the World Health Organization Symposium. World Health Organization, Copenhagen, Denmark.

McConnell, EE, JC Wagner, JW Skidmore, and JA Moore. **1984.** A comparative study of the fibrogenic and carcinogenic effects of UICC Canadian chrysotile B asbestos and glass microfibre (JM100), pp. 234-252. In: *Biological Effects of Man-Made Mineral Fibres,* Proceedings of the World Health Organization Symposium. World Health Organization, Copenhagen, Denmark.

Menard, H, L Noel, J Khorami, J Jouve, and J Dunningan. **1986.** The adsorption of polyaromatic hydrocarbons on natural and chemically modified asbestos fibers. Environ Res 40:84-91.

Middleton, AP, ST Beckett, and JMG Davis. **1977.** A study of the short-term retention and clearance of inhaled asbestos using UICC standard reference samples, pp. 247-259. In: *Inhaled Particles, IV,* WH Walton (ed.). Pergamon Press, Oxford.

Poole, A, RC Brown, and GTA Fleming. **1983.** Study of the cell transforming ability of amosite and crocidolite asbestos and the ability to induce changes in the metabolism and macromolecular binding of benzo[a]pyrene in C3H10T cells. Environ Health Perspect 51:319-324.

Pooley, FD. **1976.** An examination of the fibrous mineral content of asbestos lung tissue from the Canadian chrysotile mining industry. Environ Res 12:281-298.

Pott, F. **1978.** Some aspects on the dosimetry of the carcinogenic potency of asbestos and other fibrous dusts. Staub-Reinhalt Luft 38:486-490.

Pott, F. **1983.** Animal experiments with mineral fibres, pp. 133-161. In: *Short and Thin Mineral Fibres,* Proceedings of the Arbete Och Halsa Symposium. Arbete Och Halsa, Stockholm.

Pott, F and KH Friedrichs. **1972.** Tumours in rats after intraperitoneal injection of asbestos dusts. Naturwissenschaften 59:318-332.

Pylev, LN. **1972.** Morphological changes in rat lungs caused by intratracheal injection of chrysotile alone and with a mixture of benzo[a]pyrene. Vopr Onkol 18:40-55

Pylev, LN and LM Shabad. **1973.** Some results of experimental studies in asbestos carcinogenesis, pp. 99-106. In: *Biological Effects of Asbestos,* P Bogovski (ed.). IARC, Lyon.

Reiss, B, C Tong, S Telang, and GM Williams. **1983.** Enhancement of benzo[a]pyrene mutagenicity of chrysotile asbestos in rat liver epithelial cells. Environ Res 31:100-104.

Selikoff, IJ, EC Hammond, and J Churg. **1968.** Asbestos exposure, smoking and neoplasia. J Am Med Assoc 204:106-112.

Shabad, LM, LN Pyler, LV Krivosheeva, TF Kulagina, and BA Nemenko. **1974.** Experimental studies on asbestos carcinogenicity. J Natl Cancer Inst 52:1175-1180.

Smith, WE, DD Hubert, L Miller, MS Badollet, and J Churg. **1968.** Tests for threshold levels of carcinogenicity of asbestos, pp. 240-242. In: *Biologische Wirkungen des Asbestos.* Deutches Zentralinstitut für Arbeitsmedizin, Berlin, Federal Republic of Germany.

Stanton, MF and C Wrench, C. **1972.** Mechanisms of mesothelioma induction with asbestos and fibrous glass. J Natl Cancer Inst 48:797-821.

Stanton, MF, M Layard, A Tegeris, M Miller, M May, and E Kent. **1977.** Carcinogenicity of fibrous glass: Pleural response in the rat in relation to fibre dimension. J Natl Cancer Inst 58:587-603.

Stanton, MF and M Layard. **1978.** The carcinogenicity of fibrous minerals, pp. 143-157. In: Proceedings of the Workshop on Asbestos, Special Publication #506. National Bureau of Standards, Gaithersburg, MD.

Topping, DC and P Nettesheim. **1980.** Two stage carcinogenesis studies with asbestos in Fisher 344 rats. J Natl Cancer Inst 65:627-630.

Wagner, JC, G Berry, and V Timbrell. **1973.** Mesotheliomata in rats after inoculation with asbestos and other materials. Br J Cancer 28:173-185.

Wagner, JC, G Berry, JW Skidmore, and V Timbrell. **1974.** The effects of the inhalation of asbestos in rats. Br J Cancer 29:252-269.

Wagner, JC, GB Berry, RJ Hill, DE Munday, and JW Skidmore. **1984.** Animal experiments with MMM(V)F—effects of inhalation and intrapleural inoculation in rats, pp. 207-233. In: *Biological Effects of Man-Made Mineral Fibres,* Proceedings of the World Health Organization Symposium. World Health Organization, Copenhagen, Denmark.

Wehner, AP. **1980.** Effects of inhaled asbestos, asbestos plus cigarette smoke, asbestos-cement and talc baby powder in hamsters, pp. 373-376. In: **Biological Effects of Mineral Fibres,** JC Wagner (ed.), IARC Scientific Publication No. 30. IARC, Lyon, France.

Wehner, AP, RH Busch, RJ Olson, and DK Craig. **1975.** Chronic inhalation of asbestos and cigarette smoke by hamsters. Environ Res 10:368-383.

An Animal Model of Co-Exposure to Cigarette Smoke and Mineral Dust*

Andrew Churg and Joanne L Wright

Department of Pathology and University of British Columbia Health Sciences Centre Hospital, University of British Columbia, Vancouver, B.C., Canada

KEY WORDS: cigarette smoke, asbestos, iron oxide, intratracheal instillation, guinea pig

---

ABSTRACT

Co-exposure to mineral dusts and cigarette smoke is extremely common for many workers. In man, the combination of smoke and asbestos produces synergistic increases in incidence rates for carcinoma of the lung and, probably, for asbestosis as well. It is possible that similar effects occur with other dusts. The mechanisms of these processes are unknown. We have begun to examine this problem using a guinea-pig model and have thus far considered the effects of asbestos, a dust of known pathogenicity, as well as those of iron oxide, a dust generally considered inert.

In our system, dusts are administered as a single intratracheal instillation. In our smoke-exposure apparatus, a very simple one originally described by Hogg and colleagues, air is drawn once per minute through a cigarette by a syringe. The whole smoke is then expelled into a 1-L, head-only exposure chamber. This apparatus produces a blood carboxyhemoglobin level in the range of 5% after a 2-hour exposure to 10 cigarettes (the usual dose), a value similar to that seen in chronic human smokers.

Using this system, we have shown that clearance of asbestos from the lung is markedly inhibited. Whereas non-smoke-exposed animals clear more than 80% of a 1-mg dose of UICC amosite in 1 month,

*Supported by grants MA8051 and MA7820 from the Medical Research Council of Canada.

smoke-exposed animals have only about a 20% clearance. Histologically, penetration of asbestos fibers into the walls of small airways can be seen by light microscopy in both smoke-exposed and unexposed animals, but the number of penetrating fibers is statistically much greater with smoke exposure.

Examination of fiber sizes in lavaged macrophages, and of fiber sizes and concentrations in lavaged tissues, indicates that in both smoke-exposed and unexposed animals, macrophages phagocytize primarily short fibers, while long fibers are associated with tissue. However, in smoke-exposed animals, retention of tissue-associated short fibers is greatly increased by 1 month after exposure, in unexposed animals, short fibers are cleared. These observations may imply that smoke exposure interferes with macrophage function, with subsequent release of phagocytized short fibers back into the medium and, ultimately, into tissue. This raises the possibility that short fibers may be of more pathogenetic importance in those who smoke than in those who do not.

Using slightly higher doses of asbestos and longer-term (6-month) animal exposures, it is apparent that smoke increases the disease-producing potential of asbestos. Such animals had poorer pulmonary function, increased tissue collagen, and morphometric evidence of more severe disease than was seen with exposure to asbestos alone. Moreover, the two agents tended to interact in a synergistic fashion.

In our system, exposure to iron oxide plus smoke reduced particle clearance and increased particle penetration into tissue in a fashion very similar to that of combined asbestos and smoke. However, in contrast to asbestos, iron oxide that reached the interstitium in either smoke-exposed or unexposed animals was rapidly removed. These observations suggest that a primary effect of cigarette smoke is to increase particle penetration into tissue, but that smoke does not interfere with removal of particles from the interstitium.

INTRODUCTION

Although there are extensive investigations on the effects of cigarette smoke in man and animals, relatively little information exists on co-exposure to cigarette smoke and mineral dust. This is a problem of considerable significance, because many workers who are exposed to dust also smoke. Smoking affects the way in which dust is cleared from the lungs, as shown by experiments in which volunteers were exposed to inert particles. The long-term clearance times for dust particles were greatly increased in smokers compared to those for nonsmokers (Cohen et al., 1979). In fact, the clearance times were proportional to the amount of smoking (Bohning et al., 1982). This observation applies not only to inert particles in experimental situations but also to the numerous particles deposited in the lungs from the environment. In the general population, those who smoke and have no occupational dust exposure have a pulmonary mineral-particle concentration that is proportional to their pack-years of smoking (Churg and Wiggs, 1987).

Because many toxic dusts act in a dose-response fashion, any effect that leads to greater retention of such particles should produce greater incidences of disease. Virtually the only information in this regard comes from studies of asbestos-exposed workers. Asbestos workers who smoke have markedly greater increases in lung cancer rates than those who do not smoke. The interaction between asbestos exposure and smoking appears to be more than additive and, in some studies, multiplicative (Hammond et al., 1979). It has been suggested that exposure to silica also increases the risk of lung cancer, and it is possible that a synergistic relationship with smoking, similar to that for asbestos, may exist. However, at present the issue of silica and lung cancer is hotly disputed (Goldsmith et al., 1986).

Other data imply that smoking may increase the incidence of fibrotic, asbestos-induced, parenchymal disease. Weiss (1984), in reviewing a large number of radiographic surveys, found that most showed a greater incidence of new cases of asbestosis and/or a more rapid progression rate for established cases of asbestosis in those who smoke compared to those who did not, although this conclusion is not universally accepted (Weiss, 1984; Blanc et al., 1988). Parenchymal fibrosis induced by asbestos is known to be proportional to retained asbestos dose, hence any agent that increases retention should increase the attack rate for asbestosis. On the other hand, pleural disease, which in many respects seems to be more a function of time from first exposure than of dose, generally does not appear to be affected by smoking.

EXPOSURE SYSTEM

To examine how smoking may affect dust retention and what the mechanisms of these effects may be, we have established the guinea pig as a model for co-exposure to smoke and mineral dust. For this purpose, we have used a single intratracheal instillation of dust, a procedure that is far from ideal in terms of physiologic distribution of dust (Pritchard et al., 1985). However, it permits delivery of a very large dose, avoids the necessity for interpreting clearance patterns caused by repeated or continuous exposure over extended periods, and it is very economical.

The smoking apparatus that we use was first described by Simani et al. (1974). It consists of a syringe that draws air through a cigarette once per minute, then injects the whole smoke into a 1-L, head-only, exposure chamber. The standard smoke volume is

20 ml/puff, and our standard exposure has been 10 cigarettes per day, 5 days a week (about 2 hours of smoke exposure each day). We have used a standard commercial, nonfiltered cigarette. This system produces a carboxyhemoglobin level of about 5% in guinea pigs at the end of a 2-hour exposure, a value comparable to that found in chronic cigarette smokers.

Our investigations to date have used UICC amosite asbestos and a finely divided iron oxide (Pfizer R2999-R). Amosite was chosen because its fiber content in lung and lavage fluid can easily be quantitated by electron microscopic techniques, as opposed to chrysotile asbestos, which tends to aggregate and may also dissolve. The UICC preparation has a wide size distribution, with a geometric mean length of about 4 μm and 20% of fibers greater than 10 μm. Using this material allows us to observe the differential clearance of both short and long fibers in one preparation. Iron oxide serves as a comparison dust because it is generally considered inert, in contrast to asbestos, which is highly toxic. For the short-term experiments described below we used a dose of 0.5 to 1 mg of UICC amosite or a dose of 25 mg of iron oxide. For the longer experiments with amosite, the dose was 5 mg.

EFFECTS OF SMOKING ON PARTICLE CLEARANCE

In our initial experiments, we examined the effects of smoking on amosite clearance at 1 week and at 1 month after exposure. As shown in Figure 1, in nonsmoking animals, the concentration (as determined by bleach digestion of tissue, and fiber collection and analysis by electron microscopy) of retained asbestos per gram of dry lung decreased about sixfold between 1 week and 1 month. By contrast, in animals exposed to smoke, the decrease in concentration averaged only about 20%, a statistically nonsignificant value (McFadden et al., 1986a). When a larger dose of asbestos was used and the observation period continued for 6 months, smoke-exposed animals retained about three times the fiber burden of the animals not exposed to smoke (Tron et al., 1987).

As shown in Figure 2, the increase in particle retention with iron oxide at 1 day and 1 week after exposure is similar to that for asbestos (Gilks et al., in press). The iron concentrations were determined chemically, by atomic absorption spectrometry. In contrast to results with asbestos, by 1 month iron concentration was the same in both smoke-exposed and unexposed animals. This point is discusssed in more detail later in this report.

Smoking affects lung clearance of different sizes of fiber in different ways; this difference was obvious both immediately after exposure (McFadden et al., 1986a; Churg et al., 1987) and at 6 months

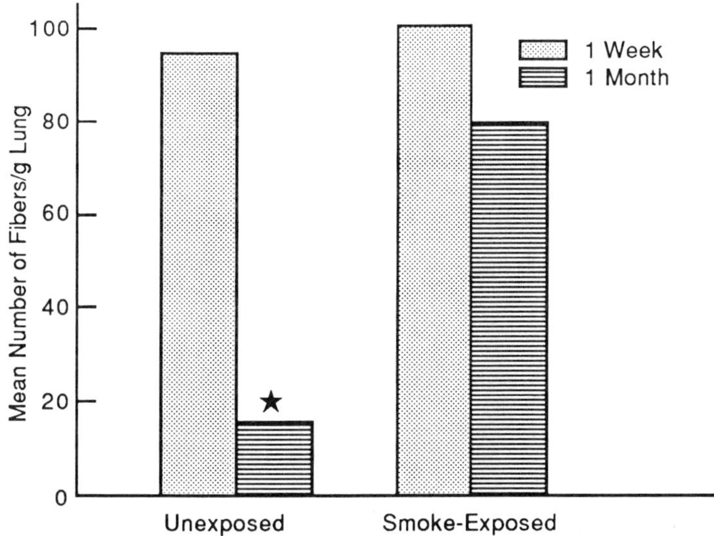

Figure 1. Mean asbestos fiber concentrations in cigarette-smoke-exposed and unexposed guinea pigs at 1 week and 1 month after intratracheal asbestos instillation. Star indicates significant difference; statistics were performed using non-parametric methods, hence no error bars. (Modified from McFadden et al., 1986a.)

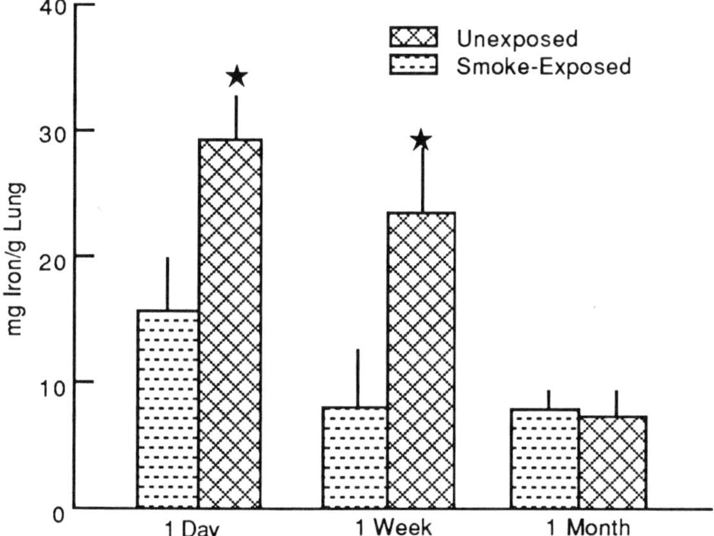

Figure 2. Chemically determined iron concentrations in lung tissue of cigarette-smoke-exposed and unexposed guinea pigs. Stars indicate significant differences between smoke-exposed animals and animals not exposed to smoke. Values are mean ± standard error (from Gilks et al., in press).

after exposure (Tron et al., 1987). Figure 3 shows mean lengths, by time and tissue compartment, of fibers found in lavaged macrophages, cell-free lavage fluid, and residual tissue in a short-term experiment. Macrophages always contained the shortest fibers; those associated with tissue were generally longest; and those that were free in lavage fluid were intermediate in length (Churg et al., 1987). In animals not exposed to cigarette smoke, tissue fiber length increased by 1 month after exposure; in smoke-exposed animals, tissue fiber length decreased by 1 month.

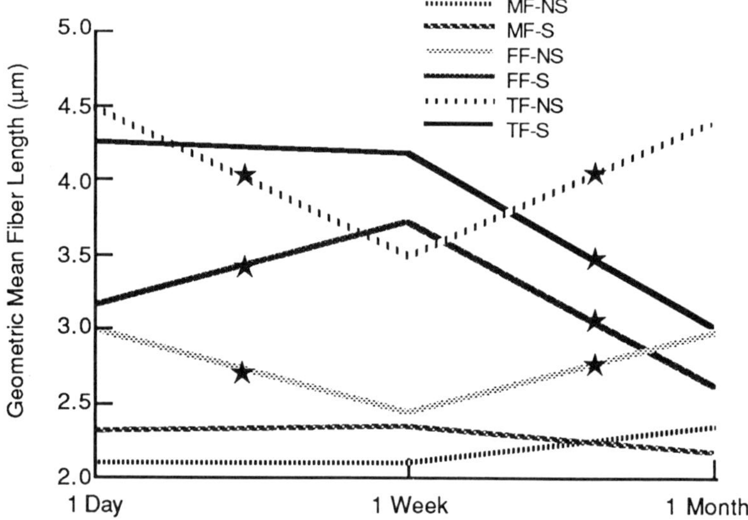

Figure 3. Geometric mean fiber lengths found in lungs of cigarette-smoke-exposed and unexposed guinea pigs as a function of time and treatment. MF = fiber in microphages; FF = fibers free in lavage fluid; TF = fibers associated with tissue; NS = nonsmokers; S = smokers. (From Churg et al., 1987.)

The mean length of fibers in macrophages did not appear to change with either time or smoke exposure; however, the lengths of fibers in tissues and of those free in lavage fluid were greatly affected. In the animals not exposed to cigarette smoke, length of retained fibers initially decreased, but by 1 month it had increased beyond its original length. In smoke-exposed animals, retained tissue fiber length was initially stable, then decreased, so that by 1 month the tissue from smoke-exposed animals contained much shorter fibers than that of the animals not exposed to smoke. From these data it appears that clearance of short fibers was impeded to a much greater extent than that of long fibers, although clearance of all fibers was impaired to some extent. A possible explanation is that one effect of cigarette smoke is to interfere with the macrophage clearance of fibers. As shown in Figure 4, the absolute number of fibers contained in macrophages appeared to increase over the course of 1 month in the smoke-exposed animals, whereas it was essentially stable in animals not exposed to smoke. Whether this process reflects interference with macrophage motility, or failure of the mucociliary escalator, or both, is not known. However, it is generally accepted that particles that are free in air spaces are very likely to cross epithelia. Therefore, if particles were stored in macrophages, then re-released into the medium (possibly as a result of the cytotoxic effects of the asbestos), more short fibers would be available to cross the epithelium and deposit in tissue. This schema postulates that interference with macrophage clearance is a major effect of cigarette smoke; however, it is only one possible explanation of the data, and other smoke effects are likely.

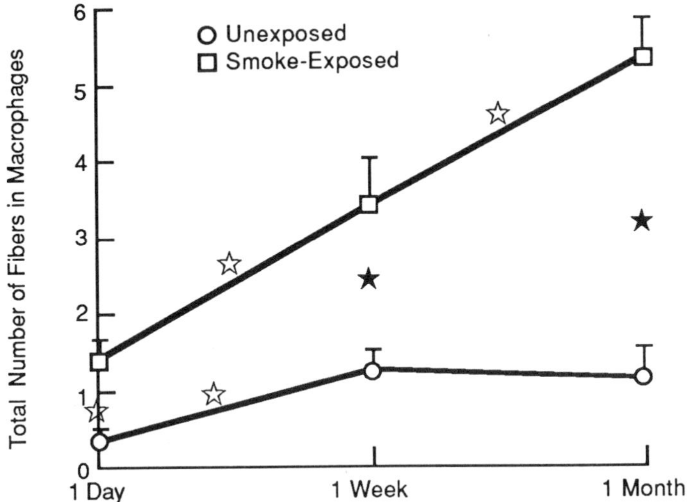

Figure 4. Total fiber burden retained in macrophages (as determined from lavaged macrophages) in cigarette-smoke-exposed guinea pigs and guinea pigs not exposed to smoke. Stars indicate significant differences over time and between groups. Values are mean ± standard error. (From Church et al., 1987.)

EFFECTS ON TISSUE

It is very clear from our experimental data that particles and fibers do, in fact, cross epithelia and deposit in tissue in great numbers, by some mechanism. As shown in Figure 5, administration of a single dose of asbestos led to increased numbers of fibers that were visible by light microscopy in the walls of the respiratory bronchioles between 1 week and 1 month after exposure. This observation suggests that asbestos was progressively transported into tissues even in the absence of smoke. However, in smoke-exposed animals, the number of bronchioles that contained such fibers was considerably greater than in animals not exposed to smoke at both 1 week and 1 month. When the data are broken down by fibers per square millimeter of airway wall, the differences are even more dramatic and highly significant (McFadden et al., 1986b). Somewhat similar observations were made for iron oxide particles in the walls and epithelia of respiratory bronchioles. The one notable difference was that by 1 month, particle counts were the same in both smoke-exposed groups and groups not exposed to smoke (Gilks et al., in press; Figures 6 and 7). These observations suggest that the effect of smoking was to increase particle transport into tissues, but that smoking did not affect the "normal" mechanisms for removing particles from the interstitium.

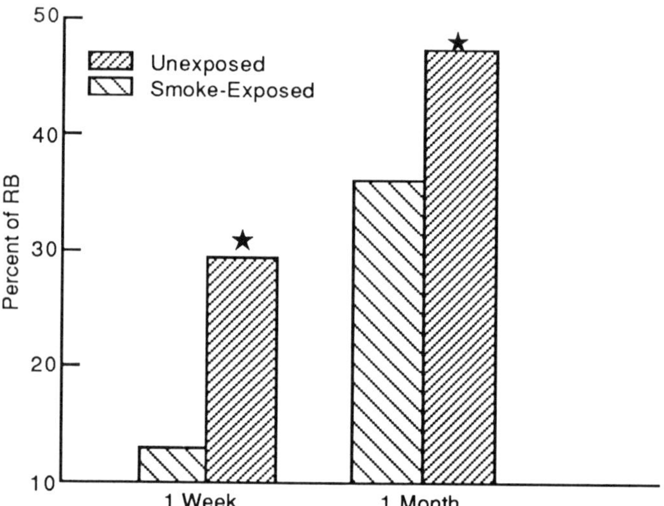

Figure 5. Percentage of respiratory bronchiolar (RB) walls with fibers longer than 5 μm, visualized by light microscopy. Guinea pigs received a single dose of asbestos and were divided into cigarette-smoke-exposed and unexposed groups. At both 1 week and 1 month after exposure, smoke-exposed animals had significantly more fibers than animals not exposed to smoke. Numbers of fibers in walls increased significantly as a function of time. Figure is representational; statistics were obtained by nonparametric methods, using fibers/mm^2 of airway wall (McFadden et al., 1986b).

The way in which particles cross epithelia is, in general, obscure, and the effects of cigarette smoke on particle penetration are not known. It has been suggested that amphibole asbestos fibers tend to ulcerate epithelia (Adamson and Bowden, 1986), and that

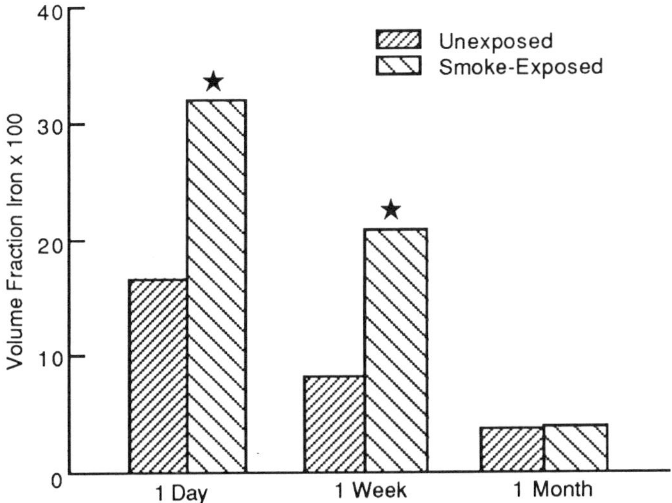

Figure 6. Volume fraction of iron in respiratory bronchiolar epithelia, as determined by light microscopic morphometry. Stars indicate significant differences between guinea pigs treated with iron oxide and exposed to cigarette smoke, or not exposed to smoke. Analysis was by nonparametric methods, hence no error bars are shown. (From Gilks et al., in press.)

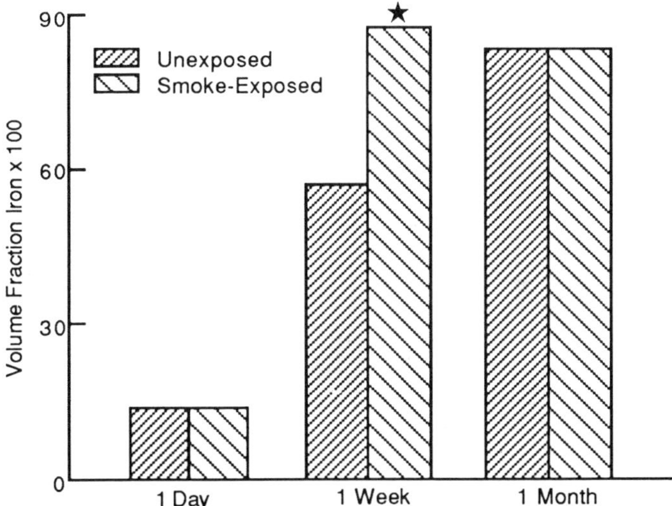

Figure 7. Volume fraction of iron in respiratory bronchiolar walls, as determined by light microscopic morphometry. Star indicates significant differences between guinea pigs treated with iron oxide and exposed to cigarette smoke, or unexposed. Analysis was by nonparametric methods, hence no error bars are shown. (From Gilks et al., in press.)

particle penetration is, in large measure, a reflection of the amount of ulceration. On the other hand, asbestos fibers have been shown to penetrate bronchial epithelial cells directly in a variety of systems (Brody et al., 1981). It is possible that in the smoke-exposed animals both ulceration and transepithelial transport of asbestos are greater than normal.

For iron oxide, the route of transport is quite clear because, although we did not observe ulceration, we found greater numbers of particles in the respiratory bronchiolar epithelium of smoke-exposed animals compared to those in animals not exposed to smoke, at 1 day and 1 week after exposure (Gilks et al., in press). This observation leaves no doubt that in cigarette-smoke-exposed animals, transepithelial transport of particles is greater than normal.

We are currently exploring the possibility that smoke-mediated increases in particle transport result from the direct effects of smoke on epithelia. There is a precedent for such effects, because smoke is known to directly affect the epithelial transport of small molecules (Simani et al., 1974). It is interesting that, for both asbestos and iron oxide, light microscopic counting of particles in airway walls and epithelium showed an increase in transport only for respiratory bronchioles. In fibers and particles observed in the walls of the more proximal membranous bronchioles, no differences in numbers of particles were apparent, by light microscopy, between smoke-exposed animals and animals not exposed to smoke. Because numbers of particles in alveolar epithelium cannot be counted by light microscopy, no data are available on this parameter. If electron microscopic techniques were used, all three types of epithelia and the underlying interstitium might show increased numbers of particles and fibers, but it is also possible that cigarette-smoke effects are selective, primarily disturbing only the respiratory bronchioles.

Whatever the route of transport into the airway walls may be, the effects of smoke-induced increases in fiber concentration can be clearly demonstrated (Tron et al., 1987). As shown in Figure 8, cigarette smoke increased the hydroxyproline content of the lung as well as the thickness of airway walls and the volume fraction of tissue surrounding airways. We have performed the latter measurement in an attempt to determine whether true asbestosis (diffuse interstitial fibrosis) is exacerbated by cigarette smoking, because asbestosis is thought to begin in the parenchyma around the respiratory bronchioles. The data suggest that our hypothesis is correct and, furthermore, that the effects of cigarette smoke and asbestos are largely synergistic in this regard. These effects are not confined to morphologic measurements: when pulmonary function was assessed, cigarette-smoking also exacerbated asbestos-induced changes in those measurements (Wright et al., in press).

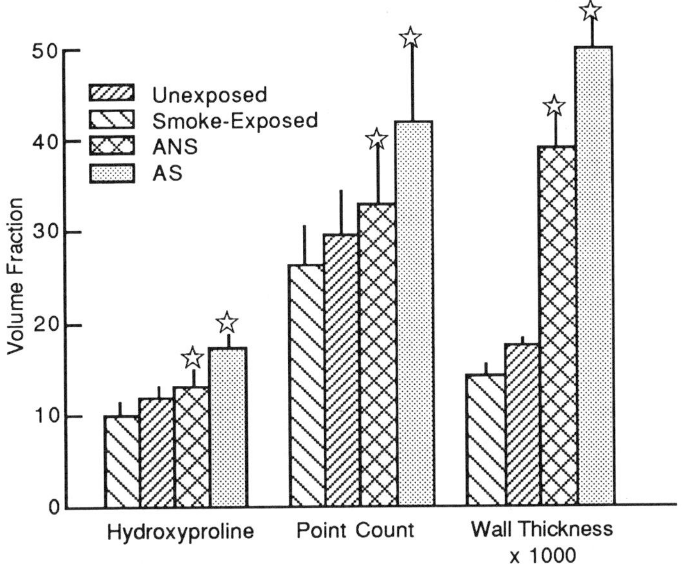

Figure 8. Effects of asbestos plus cigarette-smoke exposure in guinea pigs 6 months after a single instillation of 5 mg UICC amosite. Volume fraction of alveolar walls surrounding respiratory bronchioles, point count (a measure of early asbestosis), and thickness of respiratory bronchiolar walls were significantly increased by a combination of smoke plus asbestos. Note that interactions appear to be synergistic. ANS = amosite only; AS = amosite plus smoke. (Data from Tron et al., 1987.)

In summary, exposure of guinea pigs to cigarette smoke after instillation of either asbestos or iron oxide increased retention of both dusts as well as their penetration into tissue. Clearance of short fibers appeared to be impaired more than clearance of long fibers. Initial data suggest that one mechanism for this process may be that cigarette smoke interfered with removal of asbestos-bearing macrophages from the lung. With both asbestos and iron oxide, the number of particles that crossed the epithelium to reach the airway walls increased. As measured by collagen content or morphometric evidence of fibrosis, the combination of asbestos and smoke synergistically exacerbated the disease compared with the results of exposure to asbestos alone. As judged by pulmonary-function tests, smoking also potentiated the functional consequences of asbestos exposure. This model showed that smoking aggravates mineral-dust-induced disease and provides a means of exploring the mechanism of this phenomenon.

REFERENCES

Adamson, IYR and DH Bowden. **1986.** Crocidolite-induced pulmonary fibrosis in mice. Am J Pathol 122:261-267.

Blanc, PD, JA Golden, GG Gamsu, DR Aberle, and WR Gold. **1988.** Asbestos exposure-cigarette smoking interactions among shipyard workers. J Am Med Assoc 259:370-373.

Bohning, DE, HL Atkins, and SH Cohn. **1982.** Long-term particle clearance in man: Normal and impaired. Ann Occup Hyg 26:259-271.

Brody, AR, LH Hill, B Adkins, and RW O'Connor. **1981.** Chrysotile asbestos inhalation in rats: Deposition pattern and reaction of alveolar epithelium and pulmonary macrophages. Am Rev Respir Dis 123:670-679.

Churg, A and B Wiggs. **1987.** Types, numbers, sizes, and distribution of mineral particles in the lungs of urban male cigarette smokers. Environ Res 42:121-129.

Churg, A, V Tron, and JL Wright. **1987.** Effects of cigarette smoke on retention of asbestos from various morphologic compartments of the guinea pig lung. Am J Pathol 129:385-393.

Cohen, D, SF Arai, and JD Brain. **1979.** Smoking impairs long-term clearance from the lung. Science 204:514-516.

Gilks, B, J Wright, and A Churg. Effects of cigarette smoke on uptake and retention of iron oxide in the guinea pig. Am Rev Respir Dis (**in press**).

Goldsmith, DF, DM Winn, and CM Shy. **1986.** *Silica, Silicosis, and Cancer.* Praeger Publishers, New York, NY.

Hammond, EC, IJ Selikoff, and H Seidman. **1979.** Asbestos exposure, smoking, and death rates. Ann NY Acad Sci 330:473-492.

McFadden, D, JL Wright, B Wiggs, and A Churg. **1986a.** Smoking inhibits asbestos clearance. Am Rev Respir Dis 133:372-374.

McFadden, D, JL Wright, B Wiggs, and A Churg. **1986b.** Cigarette smoke increases the penetration of asbestos fibers into airway walls. Am J Pathol 123:95-99.

Pritchard, JN, A Knudson, JC Evans, et al. **1985.** The distribution of dust in the rat lung following administration by inhalation and by single intratracheal instillation. Environ Res 36:268.

Simani, AS, S Inoue, and JC Hogg. **1974.** Penetration of respiratory epithelium of guinea pigs following exposure to cigarette smoke. Lab Invest 31:75-87.

Tron, V, JL Wright, N Harrison, B Wiggs, and A Churg. **1987.** Cigarette smoke makes airway and early parenchymal asbestos-induced lung disease worse in the guinea pig. Am Rev Respir Dis 136:271-275.

Weiss, W. **1984.** Cigarette smoke, asbestos, and small irregular opacities. Am Rev Respir Dis 130:293-301.

Wright, JL, V Tron, B Wiggs, and A Churg. Cigarette smoke potentiates asbestos-induced airflow obstruction. Exp Lung Res (**in press**).

A Model for the Influence of Inhaled Mineral Fibers on the Pulmonary Uptake of Polycyclic Aromatic Hydrocarbons (PAH) from Cigarette Smoke

Per Gerde and Peter Scholander

Department of Chemical Engineering, Royal Institute of Technology, S-100 44, Stockholm, Sweden

KEY WORDS: adsorption, fibers, cigarette smoke, polycyclic aromatic hydrocarbons, pulmonary deposition

---

ABSTRACT

A model has been developed for the way physiochemical mechanisms, such as molecular diffusion, convection, adsorption onto solids and partition among various phases, can influence the uptake of particle-associated polycyclic aromatic hydrocarbons (PAH) by the human lung. Particular attention has been paid to the possible effects of inhaled mineral fibers on this transport process. The main reason for such a study is the strong synergistic effect observed between tobacco-smoking and asbestos exposure for the induction of bronchial cancer. In this case, a direct adsorption of PAH from the smoke onto the fiber surfaces has been a frequently studied starting point for such an interaction. Both nonbiological laboratory experiments and theoretical models of the transport phenomena involved have been utilized. Results show that the uptake of PAH by the human lung is probably governed much more by properties of the bronchial lining layer (BLL) that covers the airways of the lung than by properties of the carrier particles of PAH. This implies that the direct adsorption of PAH onto the fibers is probably a parameter of little relevance for the synergistic interaction between tobacco smoke and inhaled mineral fibers. Instead, the BLL seems to be a dense barrier not only to impinging particles but also to diffusing lipophilic substances in the ambient air. The mechanism behind this effect is the high degree of lipid-aqueous heterogeneity of the BLL, created by its surfactant lipid content. These lipids have a great capacity to solubilize PAH, in which state these hydrocarbons are very reluctant to diffuse into the neighboring aqueous phase of the BLL. However, the denser the aqueous-lipid barrier, the greater the effect of any leak in it. Mineral fibers, particularly those of asbestos, adsorb layers of phospholipids from lung surfactant. If such fibers traverse the BLL, a lipid connection can be created between contaminated surfactant lipids at the air interface and the epithelial cellular membranes. Thus, lipophilic substances (e.g., PAH) can be transported across the otherwise highly impermeable aqueous regions of the BLL. One would expect this "lipid-link" mechanism to result in very localized but extremely high cellular doses of PAH in the lung when tobacco smoke and lipid-adsorbing fibers are inhaled.

INTRODUCTION

Two lines of research concerning the health hazards of mineral fibers, on the one hand, and of polycyclic aromatic hydrocarbons (PAH) on the other, proceeded independently until about 2 decades ago, when they interconnected at one important point. It was then discovered that the previously observed enhanced incidence of bronchial cancer in workers exposed to asbestos (Doll, 1955) exhibited a strong synergistic interaction with tobacco-smoking (Selikoff et al., 1968). Since then, several attempts have been made to find a plausible mechanism for this interaction. One proposed hypothesis has been that asbestos fibers can increase pulmonary deposition of carcinogenic compounds, such as PAH in tobacco smoke. During the last decade or so, man-made mineral fibers (MMMF), which have replaced asbestos in many applications, have also been of concern. This paper describes a model for the uptake of PAH by the human lung and our efforts to assess the influence of inhaled mineral fibers on this uptake. Emphasis is on the initial and essentially physiochemical processes that lead to the introduction of PAH in target tissues in the lung. These transport phenomena, including mechanisms such as molecular diffusion, convection, adsorption onto solids and partition among various phases, probably govern, to some extent, the subsequent and far more complex biological action of PAH.

Suggested Mechanisms for an Interaction Between PAH and Mineral Fibers

Several mechanisms have been suggested to explain the synergistic effect between tobacco-smoking and asbestos exposure for the induction of bronchial cancer. On the basis of the known preferential bronchial location of these tumors (Selikoff et al., 1968), a simple sketch can be drawn to outline the possible positions for an interaction (Figure 1). This is a schematic illustration of the routes of fibers and PAH from inhaled air, across the extracellular lining layer of the lung, and into the epithelial cells below. Hypothetical locations for interaction between the agents are: (I) in the air, before inhalation, as a gas-phase process; (II) in the liquid phase of the bronchial lining layer (BLL); or (III) within the cellular membrane. A fourth possibility is, of course, that there is no interaction. At the first two locations, before the cellular membrane is reached, physical transport phenomena are thought to play an important role, whereas biomedical processes are more important for uptake in cellular membranes.

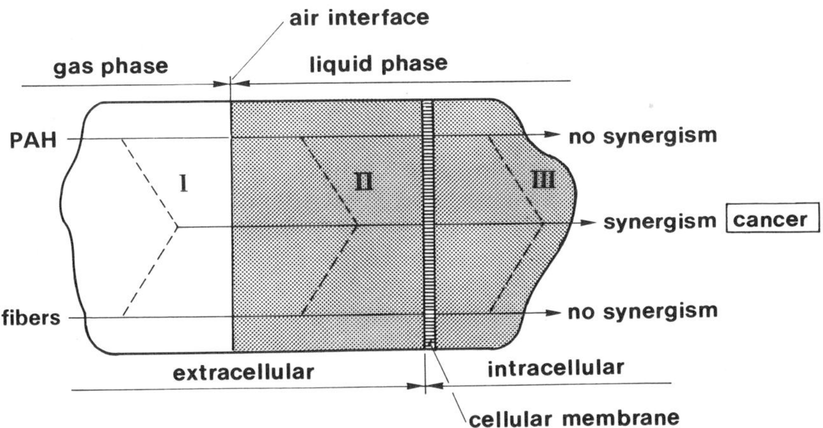

Figure 1. Schematic illustration of the possible positions for a synergistic interaction between mineral fibers and polycyclic aromatic hydrocarbons (PAH) in the bronchial lining layer (BLL). Positions along the routes of PAH and fibers from the ambient air, across the lining layer, and into the epithelial cells below are: I, in the air before inhalation as a gas-phase process; II, the liquid phase of the BLL; or III, within the cellular membrane.

The mechanisms suggested for the first interaction described above can be considered part of the "physical carrier concept" (Mossman and Craighead, 1981). This concept hypothesizes that the fiber somehow acts as a vehicle for PAH, thereby increasing the uptake of these carcinogens by their target tissues. Harington (1973) suggested that the mechanism for this carrier function is direct adsorption of PAH onto the fiber surfaces. Several investigators have studied the adsorption of various PAH onto asbestos fibers, mostly in organic solvents (Harington and Smith, 1964; Shabad et al., 1974). The surface charge of the asbestos fibers proved to be an important parameter in the adsorption of PAH (Fournier and Pezerat, 1986), and modifying this charge by phosphorylation drastically reduced the adsorptivity of chrysotile asbestos for PAH (Menard et al., 1986). These mechanisms are addressed in this paper, and the epithelial cellular membrane shown in Figure 1 represents the ultimate boundary in this model.

The other principal theory for mechanisms to induce bronchial cancer is that asbestos fibers somehow alter the metabolic activation of PAH, thereby increasing their carcinogenic potency. The negligible metabolic activity of PAH outside the cells (Thust and Gräbner, 1984) make it more likely that this interaction would take place within the cell. We will not deal here with these possible indirect effects of mineral fibers on the carcinogenicity of PAH, but they cannot be excluded as a possibility. A number of experiments have been performed to demonstrate the influence of mineral fibers on the uptake of PAH by target tissue. Both *in vivo* animal experiments and *in vitro* experiments with cellular cultures or noncellular model fluids have been used. The modes of administration of fibers and PAH determine in which location (Figure 1) interaction is simulated. Location I is simulated if the PAH is adsorbed or precoated on the fiber before being introduced into the test system. This is an adsorption in the gas phase of PAH onto the fibers before inhalation. However, this does not rule out the other mechanisms. Introduction of PAH and fibers separately into the test system would be expected to result in interaction in locations II or III. If synergism is detected with PAH precoated on fibers and not with PAH added separately, type I interaction is indicated. A positive response in location II but not in location I is not plausible and apparently has not happened.

Parameters measured to indicate the response of the test system include tumors in experimental animals, number of revertants or amounts of PAH/PAH metabolites/PAH bound to cellular DNA in cell cultures, and transfer rates of PAH from the fiber to a surrounding medium. All of the mechanisms suggested for interaction between asbestos fibers and PAH, including an absence of interaction, have been observed in experiments. Response in location I, where interaction occurred only when PAH were precoated onto fibers, was demonstrated using cell cultures (Mossman et al., 1983; Szyba and Lange, 1983). The rate of mass transfer of PAH precipitated onto various particles, to microsomes, or to phospholipid vesicles in suspension has also been measured (Lakowicz et al., 1980; Kandaswami and O'Brien, 1980; Brown et al., 1983). Asbestos fibers were found to mediate a rapid transfer of PAH to vesicles and microsomes. This apparent characteristic of asbestos fibers was presumed to be important in the etiology of bronchial cancer. This view has been criticized, because precipitation of PAH onto fibers before administration is not normally found in nature (Chang et al., 1981). Furthermore, critics have said that the rate of mass transfer should mirror the total interfacial area of the hydrocarbon exposed to the surroundings rather than being a characteristic parameter of the carrier particles (Light, 1979). A synergistic interaction occurred between asbestos and PAH not only when it was pre-adsorbed but also when it was administered separately, both in animal experiments (Shabad et al., 1974) and in cell cultures (DiPaolo et al., 1983; Poole et al., 1983; Reiss et al., 1983; Brown et al., 1984). Where agents were separately administered, both an enhanced uptake of PAH and changes in the metabolism of PAH, caused by asbestos fiber, have been suggested as mechanisms for this interaction. Several investigations have also been conducted with aromatic hydrocarbons and fibers administered separately, where only a very weak interaction, or none, could be detected (Jaurand et al., 1983a; Kandaswami and O'Brien, 1983; Stephens et al., 1983; Paterour et al., 1985). This suggested a mechanism for the asbestos/smoking synergism that did not involve an interaction between fibers and PAH. The ambiguity of these results indicates that asbestos may have an influence on the *in vivo* transformation of PAH, but no clear mechanism has been demonstrated for this.

Transport Phenomena

Modeling of transport phenomena has been used in chemical engineering for decades; with the development of advanced computers, great progress has been made in techniques. One of the main objectives of such modeling is to gain a better insight into the underlying physiochemical mechanisms for various chemical processes and to understand how different parameters affect these processes. A vast body of literature exists in this field, especially regarding the numerous special applications. The mathematics of fundamental transport phenomena have been described, for example, by Carslaw and Jaeger (1959), Crank (1975), and Bird et al. (1960). Lightfoot (1974) published work on transport phenomena in biological systems in general. In this study, great attention is paid to the physiochemical behavior of PAH in a biological system. As such a system constitutes a highly heterogeneous lipid-aqueous medium for diffusing PAH, further information could be useful in the studies we are concerned with. Higuchi and Higuchi (1960) developed theories on the penetration of a diffusant through a heterogeneous barrier, with one phase distributed as droplets in a continuous phase. Similarly, Ash et al. (1963) presented a model describing a heterogeneous barrier consisting of laminar layers.

When particles contaminated with PAH are inhaled, physical transport phenomena are likely to be dominant temporarily. They could thus be suitable for modeling, using the same fundamental equations as in chemical engineering. This is the phase that occurs from the time when PAH and particles are emitted into the air until the released hydrocarbons are first absorbed by cellular membranes in the lung (Figure 1). We need to know more about the duration of these processes, particularly those that involve mechanisms such as molecular diffusion, convection, adsorption onto solids and partition into various phases. Because many of the parameters probably have ranges of several orders of magnitude, results obtained from simplified models of these processes cannot be more than approximations. Still, models can be of considerable value for understanding subsequent biological actions of these mostly unknown phenomena. This is particularly true because mechanisms involving very low concentrations and a micron-size scale are extremely difficult to discover experimentally without any *a priori* knowledge of what is expected. Results from using models must, of course, be tested in appropriate biological systems.

METHODS

This study involves an interactive use of both experiments and theoretical models of transport phenomena. Experiments were performed to provide data for the theoretical models and to verify results obtained in the model simulations. The considerable complexity of the problem, even at this physiochemical level, makes simplification important, but difficult. The most important general simplification was to replace the multitude of PAH occurring in the environment with one model PAH. This PAH has been ascribed properties similar to that of benzo[a]pyrene (BaP), which is one of the most often studied substances in this group.

In designing the theoretical models, we devoted great effort to choosing limited systems with a few important parameters to be modeled and to fitting these models to biological facts, typical dimensions and realistic concentrations, rather than refining complex models with many parameters. Because of this, we often found solutions to our problems in published solutions for standard problems of transport phenomena. One way of doing this is to use one-dimensional geometries and simple initial and boundary conditions for the transport equations. This is facilitated by assuming that all expressions for equilibria of the model PAH among the various phases involved are linear.

Important input data were obtained by measuring the adsorption of aromatic hydrocarbons onto mineral fibers in both the gas phase and in liquid phases relevant to the composition of the BLL of the lung. The solubility of BaP in models of the principal liquid phases of the lung has also been measured.

Adsorption as a Possible Mechanism for an Interaction Between PAH and Mineral Fibers in the Lung

The earliest possible interaction between PAH and mineral fibers would be in the ambient air before inhalation, in the gas phase, in the form of adsorption of the hydrocarbons onto the fiber surfaces. This has been the case in most experiments where an enhanced biological effect of PAH has been detected after administering the hydrocarbons together with mineral fibers. The hydrocarbon is most often adsorbed (or, rather, precipitated) onto the fibers before being introduced in the biological test system.

We have studied adsorption in the gas phase of naphthalene and phenanthrene onto various asbestos types and onto MMMF. We also investigated the influence of moisture content of the gas on this adsorption (Gerde and Scholander, 1987a). When dry gas phase was used, the experimental results appear to support the adsorption hypothesis. Chrysotile asbestos readily adsorbed aromatic hydrocarbons in dry gas. The amphibolic asbestos types adsorbed less, and the MMMF adsorbed far less PAH than chrysotile. At lower concentrations of hydrocarbons in the gas phase, adsorptivity varies by a factor of about 100,000 between chrysotile (greatest capacity) and glass wool (lowest capacity). However, if the gas phase is humidified to typical ambient air values, adsorptivity dramatically decreases in the highly adsorbent materials. At ambient humidities, adsorption of PAH was rather weak: about the same order of magnitude for all fibrous materials tested, asbestos types as well as MMMF. This adsorption by mineral fibers appears to be rather less than that by other ambient air particles. On the other hand, increased humidity in the gas phase immediately caused a release of PAH from fibers, indicating a dynamic equilibrium of PAH adsorption on mineral fibers as a function of ambient relative humidity. This permits certain conclusions as to the fate of such hydrocarbons when they are inhaled and deposited in the lung. Therefore, when PAH adsorbed on fibers are inhaled, an enhanced biological effect may be related to properties other than just the degree to which fibers adsorb PAH.

A second possible period during which PAH is substantially adsorbed onto mineral fibers is after inhalation, probably in the BLL of the lung (Gerde, 1987). The adsorption of BaP onto various mineral fibers was measured both in aqueous solution and in an aqueous solution containing phosphatidylcholine, which is a principal constituent of lung surfactant. Measurements of the adsorption of BaP on the fibers in the pure aqueous solution confirmed the results from experiments with a highly humid gas phase. All mineral fibers tested exhibited weak adsorption of BaP of roughly the same order of magnitude. Experiments to measure adsorption using a pure aqueous phase, to simulate the principal solvent of the lung, were supplemented by experiments in which lipids, the other important liquid phase of the lining layer of the lung, were added. Phospholipids in water form a separate lipid phase, consisting of micellar liposomes or planar bilayers. As might be expected, the highly lipophilic BaP dissolved or solubilized rapidly in phosphatidylcholine, leaving an extremely low concentration of BaP in the aqueous phase. However, the mineral fibers adsorbed phosphatidylcholine, the solubilized BaP accompanying the adsorbed phospholipids onto the fibers. The adsorbed phosphatidylcholine constituted a continuous bilayer, at least along the surfaces of the asbestos fibers, into which BaP was solubilized. The lipid bilayer merely rested against the solid surface, and there may be a layer of water, only one or a few molecules thick, between the lipid layer and the fiber surface. In this environment, direct adsorption of PAH onto the fiber surfaces is not likely. Therefore, one would not expect mineral fibers to enhance the uptake of PAH by the lung through direct adsorption of such hydrocarbons on surfaces of the mineral fibers in the lung. Any aromatic hydrocarbons adsorbed onto the fibers before inhalation should be rapidly desorbed from the fibers when deposited on the lining layer of the lung. After this desorption, PAH are likely to be found solubilized in lipid phases in the vicinity of the fibers. The fundamental difference between adsorption of PAH onto fibers in a homogeneous aqueous solution and in a lipid-aqueous heterogeneous solution is depicted in Figure 2.

At this stage, it is of interest to know the probable length of time required both for adsorption of PAH onto fibers in ambient air and for their desorption from the fibers in a liquid such as the lining layer of the lung. This will show how specific the carrier function of the fibers can be with regard to adsorption of PAH in ambient air and subsequent desorption from them in the lung. We have made theoretical estimates of mass transfer rates of PAH between micron-size particles and their environment (Gerde, 1987). Two types of surfaces are treated: the outer surface of a smooth sphere and the surface of the walls of a straight cylindrical pore. Simulations were made of both the adsorption by these surfaces of a model PAH at typical ambient air conditions and the subsequent desorption of the model PAH from these surfaces in water, which is the principal solvent of the BLL of the lung. Because the medium surrounding a free-settling micron-size particle can be regarded as stagnant, theoretical solutions to the problem in question can be obtained from standard models of diffusion without convection.

From results in these models we have concluded that, in general, adsorption of PAH in the gas phase under typical ambient air conditions is much slower than the rate at which these hydrocarbons are likely to be desorbed in the lung. The main reason is that the concentrations of PAH in the gas phase are considerably lower than the solubility of these hydrocarbons in any type of aqueous solution. The time required for solid micron-size particles to reach near-equilibrium with PAH under typical ambient air conditions ranges from 1 minute to 1 hour; in the case of the porous surfaces of, say, a chrysotile fiber, it may take up to several days. From this, it must be concluded that the amount of PAH carried into the lung adsorbed on an asbestos fiber is probably not appreciably altered if it is inhaled with the smoke from a cigarette. If the synergistic effect between tobacco-smoking and asbestos exposure were caused by an adsorption of PAH onto the fibers before inhalation, this effect would be more or less the same, whether the fiber is inhaled by a smoker or a nonsmoker.

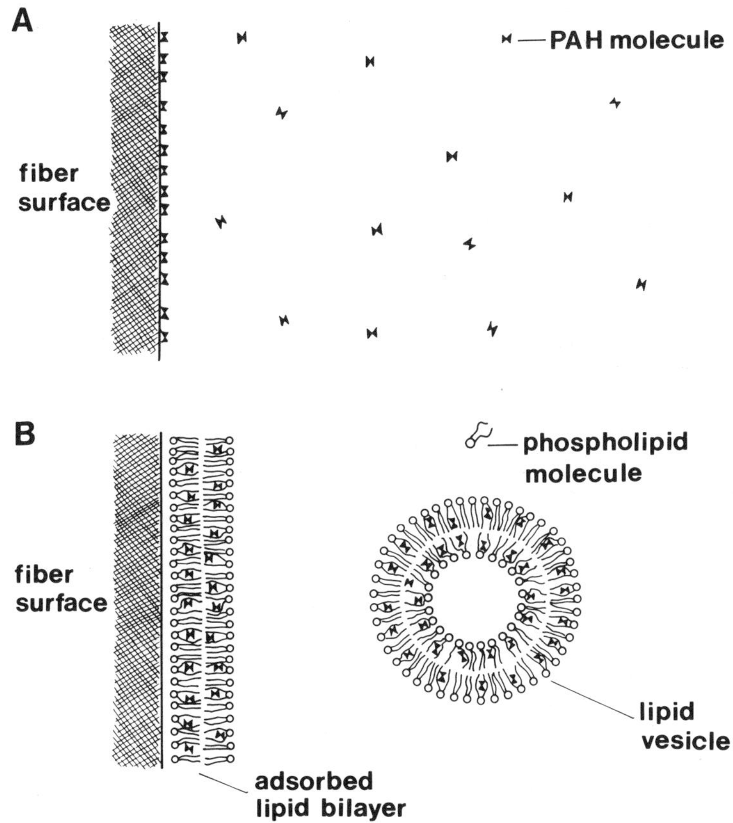

Figure 2. A, Schematic description of the equilibrium between a mineral fiber surface and a polycyclic aromatic hydrocarbon (PAH) in a homogeneous aqueous solution. A certain fraction of the hydrocarbon is adsorbed onto the fiber surface. B, A schematic description of the equilibrium between a mineral fiber surface and a PAH in a heterogeneous phospholipid-water suspension. The phospholipid adsorbs onto the fiber surface, but there may be a thin layer of water, perhaps one or a few molecules thick, between the lipid bilayer and the fiber surface. The PAH is readily solubilized into both adsorbed and free lipid phases.

Desorption of reversibly adsorbed PAH from micron-size particles in the lining layer is much more rapid than the adsorption, previously described, in ambient air. Nonporous particles deposited in the lung will probably release their more reversibly adsorbed PAH within a fraction of a second. The majority of more-or-less nonporous particles in ambient air as well as solid mineral fibers such as MMMF and the amphibolic asbestos types probably release PAH at this rate. The PAH adsorbed onto surfaces of pores in the particles are likely to add an extended asymptotic tail to the release curve of PAH. There will be a further tailing-off of the release curve, particularly on carbonaceous particles, through the desorption of PAH of high binding energies. Under these circumstances, the surface reaction is very slow (Rivin and Atkins, 1987). Nevertheless, for most of the more reversibly adsorbed PAH on the porous interiors of particles this release will occur within a matter of minutes.

It can therefore be concluded that PAH are adsorbed onto respirable particles before inhalation and that this process is comparatively slow if it occurs at typical ambient air conditions. These adsorbed PAH will be released from particles after deposition in the lung, probably within seconds for most PAH deposited on nonporous mineral particles. The only mineral fiber likely to retain its adsorbed PAH for a slightly longer time in the lung is the porous chrysotile fiber. Thin chrysotile fibers can penetrate living cells, thereby permitting direct delivery of desorbed PAH into tissues. Except for this direct delivery, the small amount of PAH adsorbed on mineral fibers and thus available for deposition in tissues is less than that adsorbed on most other particle types. In addition, probably only a small fraction of these PAH comes from the smoker's own smoke. The direct adsorption of PAH onto asbestos fibers, either before inhalation in the ambient air or in the BLL of the lung, does not seem to explain the strong synergism observed between tobacco-smoking and asbestos exposure in the induction of bronchial cancer.

An Alternative Mechanism by Means of Which Mineral Fibers may Increase Uptake of PAH by the Lung

There are two reasons for studying in detail the physiochemical behavior of PAH in the BLL. First, if there is another, primarily physiochemical, mechanism for the interaction between PAH and mineral fibers besides a direct adsorption affecting the uptake of PAH by the lung, it can be expected to occur before the hydrocarbons are absorbed by the epithelial cellular membranes; in other words, in the BLL. It is here that both agents have their highest deposition following inhalation, and most lung cancers connected with smoking and asbestos exposure are of bronchial origin. Another reason for such a study is an interesting "misfit" between reasonable release rates of PAH from their carrier particles, estimated from modeling transport phenomena, and the release rate of PAH ascribed to such particles based on results of various biological experiments. In general, the true release rate of PAH from solitary, micron-size particles appears to be considerably more rapid than is required to explain some aspects of particle and PAH behavior in biological systems. One aspect is the role of the carrier particle itself. An enhanced biological activity of PAH bound to particles has been explained by assuming that the carrier particles cause increased retention of the hydrocarbons in the target tissue because of the slow release of their adsorbed PAH (Henry et al., 1975). Another situation in which the release rate is considered important is the rapid redistribution of PAH from the lung to the gastrointestinal tract, apparently through mucociliary action, observed in animals during perhaps the first half-hour after inhalation of these substances (Sun et al., 1982).

Our model, which focuses on the physiochemical properties of the BLL (Gerde and Scholander, 1987b), has a thin layer that, because of its high viscosity, constitutes a fairly rigid barrier that should retain its identity during any period under consideration. The dominant fraction of the BLL is an aqueous phase, containing surfactant lipids, a few per mill. This causes the lining layer to act as a very heterogeneous barrier towards diffusing lipophilic substances like PAH that have a very low solubility in the aqueous phase. Also, most micron-size carrier particles of PAH are likely to be deposited at the air interface in the outer part of this barrier. In the simplest model, all of the lipids are assumed to be concentrated as a continuous layer at the air interface, resembling a morphology of the lining layer established by Ueda et al. (1984). This model is depicted in Figure 3.

The very high lipid-aqueous partition coefficient of PAH makes the penetration of PAH through a lipid-aqueous barrier with several lipid layers fairly simple to simulate. The slow rate of penetration presents a pseudo-steady-state situation, with a straight concentration profile through the barrier.

If realistic dimensions and concentrations of PAH are assumed, lipids in the barrier reduce the penetration of lipophilic substances by orders of magnitude compared with a purely aqueous barrier. This is a more plausible explanation than is the release rate of PAH from their carrier particles for the residence times required to redistribute particles and hydrocarbons from the upper bronchial tree to the gastrointestinal tract, as observed in animal experiments. Thus it seems that the rate-determining step in the overall transport of PAH from carrier particles to the bronchial epithelium often lies not within the particles but, rather, within the BLL. This implies that the BLL acts not only as a mechanical shield against inhaled particles but also as a physiochemical barrier against diffusing lipophilic substances in ambient air. In the case of a laminated barrier, this protective function is exerted not only through a reduction in the rate of penetration of PAH. It may also cause a redistribution of the quantity of PAH on a single carrier particle from a localized and therefore high dose, affecting perhaps one or a few cells close to this particle, to a more dispersed and therefore much lower dose, shared by a larger number of cells. This important protective mechanism of the lung thus shifts from being controlled by an exogenous agent, the carrier particle, to being a parameter of the biological system.

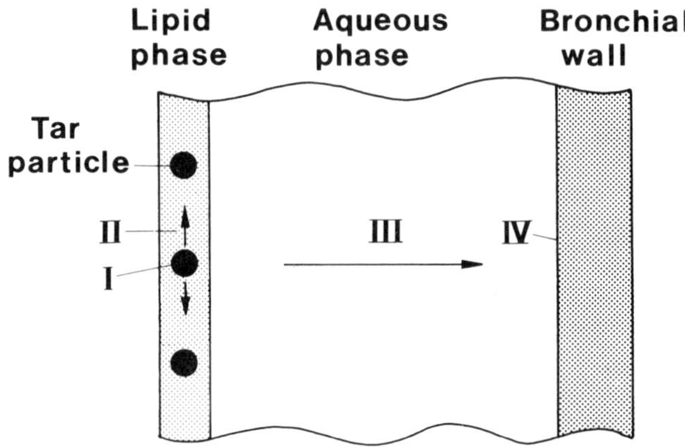

Figure 3. Simplified model of the bronchial lining layer with tar particles deposited from tobacco smoke. Roman numerals represent consecutive steps in the penetration of polycyclic aromatic hydrocarbons (PAH) through the lining layer. (I) Release of PAH from tar particles; (II) dispersion of PAH within top lipid layer; (III) penetration of PAH through the aqueous phase; and (IV) uptake of PAH by cellular membranes.

As these results contradict the quite common view that the carrier particles of PAH control the rate of uptake of these hydrocarbons by the lung, it was necessary to test the influence of the lipid-aqueous structure of the BLL on the rate of PAH penetration. A simple model of the lining layer was built up in a petri dish to simulate the physiochemical characteristics of the theoretical model. With paraffin at the bottom and an aqueous starch gel on top, and, finally, a thin layer of phosphatidylcholine at the air interface, the penetration of the diffusing BaP from the top layer into the paraffin simulates the penetration of PAH through the BLL and into the epithelium. We verified that a thin layer of phosphatidylcholine dramatically reduced the rate of PAH penetration.

The aqueous phase of the BLL, if intact, is a strong barrier. It is therefore of interest to investigate mechanisms that might short-circuit the aqueous phase (Gerde and Scholander, 1987c). Fibers are important in this contest because they are the only respirable particles long enough to bridge the BLL. Asbestos fibers, with their documented ability to adsorb phospholipids from lung surfactant (Light and Wei, 1977), are particularly interesting. The phospholipids are adsorbed in continuous bilayers along the surface of the fibers. Thin fibers have been demonstrated to penetrate cellular membranes without causing lysis of these cells. Thus, an adsorbed layer of surfactant phospholipids may form on such a fiber penetrating the BLL, constituting a continuous lipid link between the outer, contaminated lipid phase of the BLL and the lipid environment of the epithelial cellular membranes (Figure 4). A formidable short-circuit for lipophilic compounds across the BLL is thus created. Assuming realistic figures, the huge transport capacity of such a hypothetical lipid connection can be readily estimated. It may well be that a cell penetrated by phospholipid-adsorbing fibers receives on the order of 100 times more PAH through such a lipid corridor than it would have received as a result of PAH diffusion through the aqueous phase.

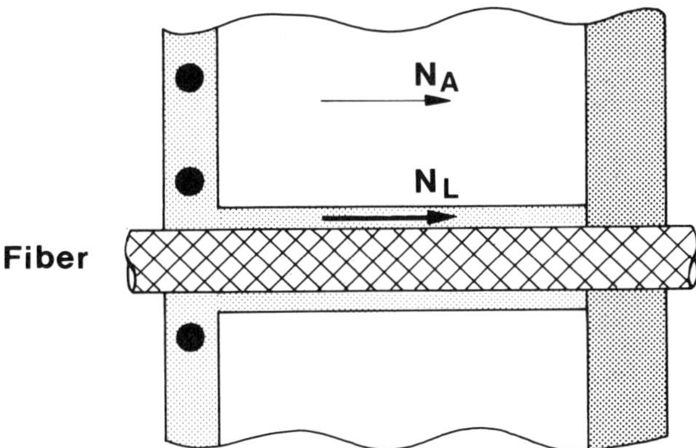

Figure 4. An inhaled fiber traversing the bronchial lining layer; this fiber has an adsorbed layer of phospholipids. N_A is the mass flux (G/m²/s) of the polycyclic aromatic hydrocarbon (PAH) in the aqueous phase; N_L is the mass flux of PAH in the adsorbed lipid layer.

The proposed "lipid-link" mechanism predicts a strong synergism between lipid-adsorbing fibers and the average concentration of PAH in the BLL for the deposition of very high cellular doses of PAH in the lung. Because tobacco smoke is a primary source of PAH in the human lung, and because focally concentrated high doses of tumor initiators can be assumed to increase the risk of cancer, the proposed mechanism may shed some light on the synergism between smoking and asbestos exposure for the induction of bronchial cancer.

This mechanistic model for a synergistic interaction between mineral fibers and PAH in the lung presupposes certain parameters of a hypothetical "high-risk" fiber. Such a fiber has to have surface properties conducive to selective adsorption of phospholipids in the lung, whereas the direct adsorption of PAH onto the fiber will be of little relevance. Dimensions are important: the fiber must be long enough to traverse the BLL and must probably retain this position for a fairly long period of time. This suggests a fiber length of at least 5 μm but, preferably, much longer, as the chance of a fiber bridging the BLL in a random position increases with its length. The fiber must also be thin enough to reach into the tracheobronchial region. However, it should not be so thin that it can easily be swept away by movements of the mucus blanket. Furthermore, a thin fiber may cause less physical damage when penetrating a cellular membrane than a thicker one.

The epithelial cellular membrane constitutes the ultimate boundary for modeling physical transport phenomena likely to be associated with the introduction of particle-associated PAH to the human lung. This model is, of course, only a crude simulation of the *in vivo* situation, and, as such, it must be tested in an appropriate biological system. We hope, however, that even a crude mechanistic model will prove valuable in better understanding these initial transport phenomena in biological test systems.

DISCUSSION

Physical transport phenomena seem to have a great influence on the introduction of particle-associated PAH to the lungs through inhalation. Processes like molecular diffusion, convection, adsorption onto solid surfaces, and partition between various phases are likely to influence the subsequent biological action of these hydrocarbon carcinogens.

We paid particular attention to the BLL when modeling the uptake of particle-associated PAH by the lung because of a series of circumstances. Some concern the properties of the exogenous agents; others concern the properties of the biological system itself. Owing to its viscosity, the BLL acts as a fairly rigid barrier, consisting of a minor lipid phase dispersed in a major aqueous one.

Inhalable particles deposited on this viscous layer are immediately swept toward the trachea by ciliary action, a process that requires the outer, viscous part of the lining layer to retain its identity. The deposition of airborne particles on this barrier therefore entails a change from a three-dimensional volume of air to the nearly two-dimensional, outer part of the lining layer. This causes a considerable accumulation of particles, including PAH bound to these particles. The low vapor pressures of these compounds, in combination with their comparatively high aqueous solubility, will prevent the escape of PAH into the air. Furthermore, the tiny fraction of lipids dispersed in the aqueous phase will trap the highly lipophilic hydrocarbons with the thin lining layer. The PAH will then slowly leak through the aqueous phase of the lining layer into the bronchial epithelium below. Exposure to PAH-contaminated particles, i.e., through tobacco-smoking, should therefore lead to a very high concentration of PAH in the surfactant lipids of the BLL during the first hour or so after deposition. The resulting steep concentration gradient through the aqueous region of the lining layer accentuates the importance of diffusional mass transfer at this early stage in the biological action of PAH. This also justifies the search for a mechanism, in this particular region of the lung, through which mineral fibers may increase the pulmonary uptake of PAH.

The very slow rate of transport into an adjacent aqueous phase of PAH that have been solubilized in a phospholipid membrane underscores the problem of lipid accumulation that challenges all organisms exposed to highly lipophilic exogenous compounds. The inhalation of smoke from fires must have confronted many species of land-living animals with the problem of accumulated, highly lipophilic substances, such as PAH, in the epithelial cellular membranes of their airways. This, in turn, should have provided a strong pressure for the evolution of various metabolizing enzymes designed to transform the lipophilic properties of exogenous compounds into more easily excretable, hydrophilic ones. To function in the lipid membranes of the cell, these enzymes must have initial substrate concentrations that may be millions of times higher than that of the extra- or intracellular aqueous fluids.

Nevertheless, it seems that nature has exploited the mechanism of prolonged retention of lipophilic substances in lipid phases to protect the very same tissues in the respiratory tract that are likely to be exposed to this adverse effect. The suggested protective function of surfactant lipids in the BLL causes a very slow penetration of lipophilic substances through aqueous regions of the lining layer. This increases clearance of these substances via the gastrointestinal tract, through mucociliary action. Thus, the lipids in lung surfactant also have another important function in the central airways: to provide the lipid phase in the otherwise aqueous BLL.

There are at least two advantages in redistributing PAH from the lung to the gastrointestinal tract. The first is simply to dilute the lipophilic substances that must be dealt with by the organism. The volume of the BLL excreted from the lung to the esophagus is estimated at 10 to 100 ml/24 hours (Pavia et al., 1980), whereas the volume passing through the gastrointestinal tract during that time can be measured in liters. The other advantage is that metabolic transformation of PAH is transferred from the bronchial epithelium to the liver, with its specialized function for such detoxification.

In this model, the role of the carrier particle for PAH is somewhat changed from that described above. Instead of providing a slow release of PAH in the lung, the carrier seems to release a significant quantity of adsorbed PAH at the moment of deposition in the BLL, followed by an extended asymptotic tailing-off of the PAH release curve. This indicates that the behavior of the carrier particle is most important during the first second or so after its deposition in the lung. This draws attention to what could be called the ballistic properties of the particle. A steep angle of impact on the mucous membrane and high speed should increase the probability for a particle to penetrate through the gel phase into the underlying epithelium. Reducing the fraction of the initially released quantity of PAH absorbed by the superficial layer of surfactant lipids should increase the risk of more localized and considerably higher cellular doses of PAH. Particles at the upper end of the respirable size range may therefore be of greater interest than previously thought. Although they have a lower weight ratio of PAH, these particles may carry more PAH per particle than the smaller ones, and, in combination with a greater tendency for inertial impact, larger particles may give much higher cellular doses of PAH at their preferential sites of deposition in the lung. This should further increase the quantities of PAH deposited at the bifurcations of the upper bronchial tree. These locations have long been suspected as the points of origin for bronchial cancer (Auerbach et al., 1961; Schlesinger and Lippmann, 1978).

Coughing is another clearance mechanism of the lung that may be affected by the characteristic behavior of a lipophilic diffusant in a lipid-aqueous heterogeneous medium. The cough reflex involves deep inspiration, followed by a forceful expiratory effort against the closed glottis, resulting in a considerable pressure increase in the lungs (Richardson and Peatfield, 1981). The subsequent explosive opening of the glottis allows air to rush out of the trachea, causing a decrease in static pressure that collapses the upper part of the bronchial tree. The high pressure and greatly reduced cross-sectional area in the collapsed bronchi force out the air at high velocity. If the mucous layer is thick enough, it will be sheared off the bronchial wall and follow the airstream toward the pharynx as sputum. This defensive reflex mechanism of the lung can be very effective in removing inhaled particles or excess mucus. The violent treatment of the sputum during this reflex may cause further dispersal of its surfactant lipids. As under normal conditions in the BLL, the lipid-aqueous heterogeneous nature of the sputum may prove effective in reducing the mobility of lipophilic substances within these liquid elements, thereby reducing the risk of their escape before the sputum reaches the pharynx and is swallowed.

This suggested protective mechanism in the BLL appears to work well with smaller granular particles that have diameters considerably less than the thickness of the lining layer. The thickness and the viscosity of the lining layer at a given depth in the airways appears to be related to the maximal diameter of granular particles likely to reach this region of the lung. The lining layer becomes thinner and less viscous with increasing depth in the lung. A major fraction of the inhaled particles is therefore rapidly cleared from the lung on the mucociliary escalator. In contrast, this system works poorly with long fibers that threaten the lipid-aqueous structure of the lining layer. The hypothetical formation of a continuous lipid link along a fiber between the contaminated surfactant lipids and the epithelial cellular membranes suddenly turns the advantage of the lipid-aqueous structure into a disadvantage. Instead of reducing the penetration rate and providing a more even distribution of the cellular doses of PAH, the lipids adsorbed onto a traversing fiber may deliver to one penetrated cell considerably higher doses of PAH than doses received by unpenetrated cells, in what seems to be a failure of nature. On the other hand, being largely a cultural phenomenon, massive exposure to mineral fibers was probably very rare during the eons when the human respiratory system was evolving.

Of course, there may be other protective mechanisms of the lung that counteract the suggested lipid-link phenomenon, such as coughing, phagocytosis by macrophages, and protein coating. The expulsion of the BLL in the upper part of the bronchial tree by coughing will most likely remove any fibers traversing the lining layer, together with the mucus. This should reduce the amount of fibers traversing the lining layer within the range of this clearance mechanism. The wrapping of pulmonary macrophages around long asbestos fibers (Miller, 1978) probably breaks the lipid corridor and sends diffusing PAH into the cellular membrane of the macrophage instead. Adsorption of various proteins onto the fibers in competition with the surfactant phospholipids may also lead to inactivation of the lipid-link mechanism. Albumin partly removes a bilayer of phosphatidylcholine previously adsorbed on the surface of chrysotile asbestos (Jaurand et al., 1983b). The heterogeneous surface of a continuous layer of proteins on the fiber probably cannot provide suitable support for an adsorbed bilayer of phospholipids. The bulkier protein molecules, however, have lower diffusivities than phospholipids. Albumin has a diffusivity in water at 20°C of about $6 \cdot 10^{-11}$ m^2/s (Shaw, 1980), compared with a diffusivity of phospholipid monomers on the order of 10^{-9} m^2/s. This, in combination with their probably greater steric restrictions in the adsorption of proteins, should make adsorption of phospholipids a precursor of the former process. As suggested for other biological effects of asbestos, the fully protein-coated fiber probably represents an inactivated form of the material (Morgan and Holmes, 1980).

Of course this has to be investigated more thoroughly, but, taken together, these effects indicate that asbestos-related lung cancers do not necessarily have to occur at the same positions as lung cancers induced solely by smoking. It might be postulated that the more peripheral positions of asbestos-related lung cancers that have been suggested (Whitwell et al., 1974) may be consistent with the proposed lipid-link mechanism. If coughing is such a radical clearance mechanism, fibers traversing the BLL may be found more frequently at positions more peripheral than, and beyond, the reach of this clearance mechanism. Two other factors may favor the hypothetical lipid-link mechanism at a more peripheral position: a decreasing viscosity, and decreasing thickness of the lining layer with increasing depth in the lung. The latter may decrease the viscous drag exerted by the lining layer on the fiber and shorten lipid corridors that must be passed by diffusing PAH. This, together with the probably increasing concentration of phospholipids with greater depth in the lung, may offset the reduced pulmonary deposition of both PAH and fibers, which decreases with increasing depth in the lung.

Caution must be exercised when ranking various fibrous materials with respect to their hazard to health. The results of the model described here merely estimate the influence of fibers on the uptake of PAH. If the weak adsorption of PAH onto mineral fibers that is likely to occur under typical ambient air conditions is of any significance, adsorbed PAH should be retained for at least a slightly longer period of time than the almost instantaneous release of PAH from MMMF and the amphibolic asbestos types. If, on the other hand, the suggested lipid-link mechanism is a significant factor *in vivo,* attention will have to focus on other parameters of the fibers. Rapid adsorption of phospholipids from lung surfactant, forming dense and continuous lipid layers along the fibers, will be of crucial importance, whereas direct adsorption of PAH onto fibers will be of little relevance. Too few measurements of the adsorption of phospholipids onto mineral fibers have been made to rank the materials according to this parameter with any certainty. It is evident, however, that both the common types of asbestos and

MMMF adsorb phospholipids. This adsorption occurs in the form of lipid bilayers on asbestos fibers. These layers are particularly dense and stable on the amphibolic asbestos types crocidolite and amosite (Light and Wei, 1977). To qualify for the hypothetical lipid-link mechanism, fibers must also be long and thin; must resist transverse cleavage; and must have a large total surface area. Taken together, these parameters point toward a smaller influence of MMMF on the uptake of PAH by the lung through this hypothetical mechanism than that of the asbestos types.

One obvious and important objection to both the suggested very slow penetration of PAH through the lining layer and the proposed lipid-link mechanism is that these hypothesized effects have not yet been demonstrated experimentally. The most important reason for this probably involves the doses of PAH used. The comparatively low sensitivity of both the analytical instruments used and the biological systems studied has necessitated large doses of carcinogens that often exceed realistic *in vivo* concentrations by several orders of magnitude. This changes the role of the carrier particle from that of an adsorbent of a highly scattered monomolecular layer of PAH to (at worst) constituting a core within a crystalline shell of PAH. The transport phenomena studied are not likely to behave linearly at these unrealistically increased concentrations that cause localized PAH saturation in the medium around the carrier particle. The PAH concentration in the medium, in turn, probably determines the rate of release of PAH from the particle. There is a possibility, however, that this limited solubility in the surrounding medium, in combination with large amounts of PAH on the particle, causes a rather artificial retention of the PAH, which is erroneously regarded as characteristic of the carrier particle. Another problem could be the disruption of the highly structured geometry of the original model, with deposition of particles and PAH in the BLL. This is likely caused by agitation of an experimental vessel, or by administering a liquid suspension of the agents into the lungs of experimental animals. Medium in the near vicinity of a micron-size particle in the lung is, most probably, stagnant.

The use of mechanistic models of transport phenomena associated with biological processes should be helpful for understanding such processes, but great care must be taken when integrating the nonbiological with biological models. Inhalation of particle-associated PAH represents, perhaps, a somewhat unusual situation in that drastic physical transport phenomena are involved. In this case, the nonbiological and the biological/biochemical parts of the problem can be fairly well separated both in time and space. The clear indications for the nonbiological model should increase its chances of surviving the necessary integration with the biological model. In most cases, it is probably not possible to make this separation. Integration of physiochemical mass transfer processes with enzyme kinetics, in particular, will probably be required right from the start under less well-defined initial and boundary conditions, and with much lower driving forces.

A parallel to this study can be seen in the significance of phospholipids in the gastric mucosa for protecting the gastric epithelium against the action of hydrochloric acid in gastric juices (Lichtenberger et al., 1983). According to those authors, this is probably the inverse of the problem described in this paper. The lipid-aqueous barrier to lipophilic substances has been exchanged for an aqueous-lipid barrier to hydrophilic diffusants.

CONCLUSIONS

The results of our investigations indicate that transport phenomena such as molecular diffusion, convection, adsorption onto solids, and partition between various phases greatly influence the uptake of PAH by the human lung. Most probably, they also influence the subsequent biological action of these compounds.

The composition of the BLL is such that this important means of clearance for the lung probably also has a significant moderating influence on the rate of penetration of lipophilic substances such as PAH. This is the result of its surfactant lipid content, which creates a lipid-aqueous heterogeneic barrier. This barrier causes a drastic reduction in the rate of penetration of lipophilic substances such as PAH compared with the rate in an aqueous barrier. The faster the mucociliary transport toward the esophagus, the greater the fraction of PAH that will be cleared from the lung via the gastrointestinal tract.

Although asbestos fibers, particularly those of chrysotile, are very good adsorbents of PAH in dry gas, only a weak adsorption of PAH occurs on asbestos and MMMF at typical ambient air humidities. These adsorbed PAH are likely to be released rapidly when the fiber is inhaled and deposited in the BLL of the lung. It is probably only the porous chrysotile fiber that retains a limited amount of PAH as long as it takes the fiber to penetrate an epithelial cell. The fiber thereby serves as a carrier for adsorbed PAH into the target tissue. Because adsorption of these PAH in ambient air is slow, the amount of PAH adsorbed is probably not influenced by whether or not the fiber is inhaled together with tobacco smoke. Thus, ascribing a carrier function to mineral fibers for PAH into target tissues through direct adsorption of hydrocarbons on the fibers does not seem to be a good explanation for the synergistic interaction between asbestos exposure and tobacco-smoking in the induction of bronchial cancer.

However, PAH are readily solubilized in phospholipids from lung surfactant and remain solubilized in layers of phospholipids when these layers are adsorbed onto mineral fibers. Asbestos fibers, in particular, have a strong affinity for phospholipids, which are adsorbed in bilayers on the surface. This may create a continuous lipid layer along the fiber, within which solubilized PAH are likely to have high mobility. This may create lipid connections across aqueous regions otherwise highly impermeable to lipophilic substances, particularly in the BLL, with its highly structured lipid-aqueous phases. Thin, phospholipid-adsorbing fibers that are long enough to both penetrate an epithelial cell and to traverse the BLL may create a formidable short circuit for lipophilic substances between the contaminated surfactant lipids in the lining layer and the epithelial cellular membranes. Inhalation of such fibers in combination with tobacco-smoking probably delivers focalized, very high doses of PAH to target cells in the lung.

REFERENCES

Ash, R, RM Barrer, and JH Petropoulos. **1963.** Diffusion in heterogeneous media: Properties of a laminated slab. Br J Appl Phys 14:854-862.

Auerbach, O, AP Stout, EC Hammond, and L Garfinkel. **1961.** Changes in bronchial epithelium in relation to cigarette smoking and in relation to lung cancer. N Engl J Med 265:253-267.

Bird, RB, WE Stewart, and EN Lightfoot. **1960.** *Transport Phenomena.* John Wiley & Sons, New York, NY.

Brown, RC, GTA Fleming, and AI Knight. **1983.** Asbestos affects the *in vitro* uptake and detoxification of aromatic compounds. Environ Health Perspect 51:315-318.

Brown, RC, A Poole, and GTA Fleming. **1984.** The metabolism of benzo(a)pyrene by the lungs of asbestos exposed rats. Exp Pathol 26:101-105.

Carslaw, HS and JC Jaeger. **1959.** *Conduction of Heat in Solids.* Clarendon Press, Oxford, England.

Chang, MJW, NP Singh, A Turturro, and RW Hart. **1981.** Interaction of benzo(a)pyrene and chrysotile, pp. 167-176. In: *International Symposium on Polynuclear Aromatic Hydrocarbons,* Vol. 6. Battelle Press, Columbus, OH.

Crank, J. **1975.** *The Mathematics of Diffusion.* Clarendon Press, Oxford, England.

DiPaolo, JA, AJ DeMarinis, and J Doniger. **1983.** Asbestos and benzo(a)pyrene synergism in the transformation of Syrian hamster embryo cells. Pharmacology 27:65-73.

Doll, R. **1955.** Mortality from lung cancer in asbestos workers. Br J Ind Med 12:81-86.

Fournier, J and H Pezerat. **1986.** Studies on surface properties of asbestos. III. Interactions between asbestos and polynuclear aromatic hydrocarbons. Environ Res 41: 276-295.

Gerde, P. **1987.** *A Model for Uptake of Polycyclic Aromatic Hydrocarbons by the Human Lung—Influence of Inhaled Mineral Fibres,* Thesis, Department of Chemical Engineering, Royal Institute of Technology, Stockholm, Sweden.

Gerde, P and P Scholander. **1987a.** Adsorption of polycyclic aromatic hydrocarbons onto asbestos and man-made mineral fibers in the gas phase. In: *Mineral Fibres in the Non-Occupational Environment,* IARC Conference, September 8-10, 1987. International Agency for Research on Cancer, Lyon, France.

Gerde, P and P Scholander. **1987b.** A mathematical model of the penetration of polycyclic hydrocarbons through the bronchial lining layer. Environ Res 44:321-334.

Gerde, P and P Scholander. **1987c.** A hypothesis concerning asbestos carcinogenicity: The migration of lipophilic carcinogens in adsorbed lipid bilayers. Ann Occup Hyg 31:395-400.

Harington, JA. **1973.** Chemical factors (including trace elements) as etiological mechanisms, pp. 304-311. In: *Biological Effects of Asbestos,* P Bogovski, JC Gilson, V Timbrell, and JC Wagner (eds.), IARC, Scientific Publications No. 8. International Agency for Research on Cancer, Lyon, France.

Harington, JS and M Smith. **1964.** Studies of hydrocarbons on mineral dusts. Arch Environ Health 8:453-458.

Henry, MC, CD Port, and DG Kaufman. **1975.** Importance of physical properties of benzo(a)pyrene-ferric oxide mixtures in lung tumor induction. Cancer Res 35:207-217.

Higuchi, W and T Higuchi. **1960.** Theoretical analysis of diffusional movement through heterogeneous barriers. J Am Pharmacol Assoc 49:598-606.

Jaurand, M-C, I Bastie-Sigeac, L Magne, M Hubert-Habart, and J Bignon. **1983a.** Studies on *in vitro* chrysotile-pleural mesothelial cell interaction: Morphological aspects and metabolism of benzo-3,4-pyrene. Environ Health Perspect 51:159-165.

Jaurand, M-C, P Baillif, J-H Thomassin, L Magne, and J-C Touray. **1983b.** X-ray photoelectron spectroscopy and chemical study of the adsorption of biological molecules on chrysotile asbestos surface. J Colloid Interface Sci 95:1-9.

Kandaswami, C and PJ O'Brien. **1980.** Effects of asbestos on membrane transport and metabolism of benzo(a)pyrene. Biochem Biophys Res Commun 97:794-801.

Kandaswami, C and PJ O'Brien. **1983.** Effects of chrysotile asbestos and silica on the microsomal metabolism of benzo(a)pyrene. Environ Health Perspect 51:311-314.

Lakowicz, JR, DR Bevan, and SC Riemer. **1980.** Transport of a carcinogen, benzo(a)pyrene from particulates to lipid bilayers. A model for the fate of particle-adsorbed polynuclear aromatic hydrocarbons which are retained in the lung. Biochim Biophys Acta 629:243-258.

Lichtenberger, LM, LA Graziani, EJ Dial, BD Butler, and BA Hills. **1983.** Role of surface-active phospholipids in gastric cytoprotection. Science 219:1327-1329.

Light, WG. **1979.** Asbestos-enhanced uptake of carcinogens. Nature 279:349-350.

Light, WG and ET Wei. **1977.** Surface charge and hemolytic activity of asbestos. Environ Res 13:135-145.

Lightfoot, EN. **1974.** *Transport Phenomena and Living Systems.* John Wiley & Sons, New York, NY.

Menard, H, L Noel, J Khorami, J-L Jouve, and J Dunnigan. **1986.** The adsorption of polyaromatic hydrocarbons on natural and chemically modified asbestos fibers. Environ Res 40:84-91.

Miller, K. **1978.** The effects of asbestos on macrophages, pp. 319-354. In: *Critical Reviews of Toxicology.* CRC Press, Boca Raton, FL.

Morgan, A and A Holmes. **1980.** Concentrations and dimensions of coated and uncoated asbestos fibres in the human lung. Br J Ind Med 37:25-32.

Mossman, BT and JE Craighead. **1981.** Mechanisms of asbestos carcinogenesis. Environ Res 25:269-280.

Mossman, BT, A Eastman, JM Landesman, and E Bresnick. **1983.** Effects of crocidolite and chrysotile asbestos on cellular uptake and metabolism of benzo(a)pyrene in hamster tracheal epithelial cells. Environ Health Perspect 51:331-335.

Paterour, MJ, J Bignon, and MC Jaurand. **1985.** *In vitro* transformation of rat pleural mesothelial cells by chrysotile fibres and/or benzo(a)pyrene. Carcinogenesis 6:523-529.

Pavia, D, JRM Bateman, NF Sheahan, JE Agnew, SP Newman, and SW Clarke. **1980.** Techniques for measuring lung mucociliary clearance. Eur J Respir Dis 61 (Suppl. 110):157-177.

Poole, A, RC Brown, GTA Fleming. **1983.** Study of the cell-transforming ability of amosite and crocidolite asbestos and the ability to induce changes in the metabolism and macromolecular binding of benzo(a)pyrene in C3H10T½ cells. Environ Health Perspect 51:319-324.

Reiss, B, C Tong, S Telang, and GM Williams. **1983.** Enhancement of benzo(a)pyrene mutagenicity by chrysotile asbestos in rat liver epithelial cells. Environ Res 31:100-104.

Richardson, PS and AC Peatfield. **1981.** Reflexes concerned in the defence of the lungs. Bull Eur Physiopathol Respir 17:979-1012.

Rivin, D and JH Atkins. **1987.** Sorption of bioactive materials on carbon. Carbon 25: 135-145.

Schlesinger, RB and M Lippmann. **1978.** Selective particle deposition and bronchogenic carcinoma. Environ Res 15:424-431.

Selikoff, IJ, EC Hammond, and J Churg. **1968.** Asbestos exposure, smoking and neoplasia. J Am Med Assoc 204:106-112.

Shabad, LM, LN Pylev, LV Krivosheeva, TF Kulagina, and BA Nemenko. **1974.** Experimental studies on asbestos carcinogenicity. J Natl Cancer Inst 52:1175-1180.

Shaw, DJ. **1980.** *Introduction to Colloid and Surface Chemistry.* Butterworths, London, England, 35 p.

Stephens, RE, LB Joseph, FB Daniel, KM Schenck, HAI Newman, PD Lipetz, and JR Milette. **1983.** Interactions of chrysotile and benzo(a)pyrene in a human cell culture systems. Environ Health Perspect 51:257-265.

Sun, JD, RK Wolff, and GM Kanapilly. **1982.** Deposition, retention and biological fate of inhaled benzo(a)pyrene adsorbed onto ultrafine particles and as a pure aerosol. Toxicol Appl Pharmacol 65:231-244.

Szyba, K and A Lange. **1983.** Presentation of benzo(a)pyrene to microsomal enzymes by asbestos fibers in the *Salmonella*/mammalian microsome mutagenicity test. Environ Health Perspect 51:337-341.

Thust, R and R Gräbner. **1984.** Incorporation in liposomes as a method for the application of genotoxins of low water solubility in the SCE assay. Mutat Res 139:207-210.

Ueda, S, K Kawamura, N Ishii, S Matsumoto, K Hayashi, M Okayasu, M Saito, and I Sakurai. **1984.** Ultrastructural studies on surface lining layer (SLL) of the lungs: Part III. J Jpn Med Soc Biol Interface 15:67-88.

Whitwell, F, ML Newhouse, and DR Bennett. **1974.** A study of the histological types of lung cancer in workers suffering from asbestos in the United Kingdom. Br J Ind Med 31:298-303.

CLINICAL STUDIES

Chemoprevention of Lung Cancer with Beta-Carotene and Retinol in Persons at High Risk Due to Asbestos Occupational Exposures and/or Cigarette Smoking, a Double-Blind Randomized Trial

Gilbert S Omenn, GE Goodman, M Thornquist, L Rosenstock, S Barnhart, and P Feigl

University of Washington School of Public Health and Community Medicine and Fred Hutchinson Cancer Research Center, Seattle, WA

KEY WORDS: beta-carotene, retinol, asbestos, cigarette smoke, lung cancer, chemoprevention

---

ABSTRACT

This chemoprevention trial tests the efficacy of retinol and β-carotene in preventing lung cancer in two related high-risk populations: (1) heavy smokers recruited from insurance-based sources, and (2) current and former workers with heavy occupational asbestos exposure, recruited from Workers' Compensation and employment-based sources. The double-blind, two-arm, randomized trial compares the apparent effects of placebos with those of a daily combination of 30 mg β-carotene plus 25,000 IU retinol. Successful recruitment, excellent compliance, and minimal side effects are evident thus far in over 1700 subjects enrolled in our two current chemoprevention projects using these agents. We have decided to integrate the two high-risk populations in a cost-effective, multiclinic strategy, with a Seattle coordinating center for project management and data analysis. Current assumptions and projections are that the full-scale study will be capable of detecting significant reductions in lung-cancer incidence in the high-risk groups combined, and in either subgroup alone, with 13,000 smokers and 4000 asbestos-exposed subjects.

INTRODUCTION AND BACKGROUND

Lung cancer is the leading cause of death from cancer among both men and women in the United States, accounting for approximately 25% of cancer deaths and 5% of all deaths. More than 130,000 Americans died of this disease in 1986. Despite aggressive therapy, 5-year survival remains poor: approximately 10% (Silverberg and Lubera, 1986). Thus, the National Cancer Institute (NCI) Cancer Control Program goals for lung cancer are focused almost entirely on prevention (Greenwald and Sondik, 1986).

Primary prevention of lung cancers is eminently feasible. The two leading risk factors are well established; namely, cigarette-smoking and exposures to respirable fibers of asbestos, which interact synergistically (Hammond and Horn, 1958a,b; Doll and Hill, 1956; Hammond et al., 1979; Doll and Peto, 1985; Berry et al., 1985). Doses, dose rates, years from first exposure to asbestos, individual susceptibility factors, and other variables influence the absolute rates and individual risks. The latency period is at least 10 years and, often, 30 to 40 years.

Smoking cessation and prevention of relapse to smoking have a deservedly prominent place in the National Cancer Control Program plans to reduce age-adjusted cancer death rates by 25 to 50% by the year 2000 (Greenwald and Sondik, 1986). In parallel, occupational exposure standards, protective equipment, and efforts to substitute other materials for asbestos are aimed at primary prevention of asbestos-related lung cancer. However, in concert with those efforts, cancer control strategies aimed at preventing the development and/or progression of tumors in persons who already have histories of cigarette smoking and/or occupational exposures to asbestos are essential. Some 79% of men and 50% of women in the 55 to 64 age group are current or former smokers (Havlik, 1986), and an estimated 4 million workers were significantly exposed to asbestos in shipyards and related activities during the period of World War II alone (Nicholson et al., 1982). Nicholson et al. have predicted that those already exposed to asbestos will suffer asbestos-related cancer deaths at an excess rate of 8000 to 10,000 per year at least to the end of the century; a consensus figure is 4000 to 6000 lung-cancer deaths per year (Omenn et al., 1986). The latency period offers a major opportunity to intervene in preventing cancers in these high-risk persons.

The chemopreventive activity of vitamin A and its synthetic and naturally occurring analogues, the retinoids, as well as that of β-carotene, a major dietary source of vitamin A, has attracted wide interest (Peto et al., 1981; Sestili and Dell, 1984; Bertram et al., 1987). Many animal studies have shown that these compounds can prevent and reverse chemically induced pulmonary neoplasia (Saffiotti et al., 1967; Port et al., 1975; Lasnitzki and Bollag, 1982).

Most importantly, some studies have demonstrated that substantial reductions in tumor incidence and size can be obtained when the retinoids are administered long after the exposures to inducing carcinogens. For example, retinyl acetate decreased the incidence of breast cancers at 20 weeks by about 50% when given to rats for a 6-week period starting 2 weeks prior to dimethylbenzanthracene (DMBA); starting 12 weeks after exposure to DMBA, there was still a 40% decrease in incidence of breast tumors at 20 weeks (McCormick et al., 1980). In cultures of hamster tracheal cells, retinyl methyl ether inhibited the metaplastic transformation induced by crocidolite or amosite asbestos (Mossman et al., 1980). In mice, β-carotene treatment resulted in a 3.1% incidence of adenocarcinoma of the colon in dimethylhydrazine-treated mice, as opposed to a 32.3% incidence in controls (Temple and Basu, 1987).

In humans, retinoids have reversed cigarette-smoking-induced, preneoplastic bronchial lesions and reduced the incidence of micronuclei in buccal smear cells. Mathe et al. (1982) administered etretinate for 6 months at 30 mg/day to 67 heavy cigarette smokers, who underwent serial bronchoscopies with biopsies. In the 34 subjects with severe metaplasia at the start of the study, treatment significantly decreased the degree of metaplasia ($P < 0.01$). In studies with betel nut chewers by Stich et al. (1984), the proportion of buccal mucosal cells with micronuclei (an indicator of nuclear chromatin damage) decreased to normal during 3 months of treatment with the combination of retinol and β-carotene. Bollag and Matter (1981) have reviewed the beneficial effects of retinoids on other precancerous lesions in man.

Epidemiologic investigations generally have shown a striking inverse relationship between intake of β-carotene and/or vitamin A-rich foods and lung-cancer risk (Bjelke, 1975; Shekele et al., 1977; Zeigler et al., 1984; Hinds et al., 1984), and between serum concentrations of β-carotene and lung-cancer risk (Nomura et al., 1986; Kark et al., 1981; Wald et al., 1980; Willett et al., 1984; Byers et al.*). To estimate the potential effect of dietary supplementation with β-carotene/retinol, Byers and co-workers (Byers et al., 1987; Byers, 1987) reviewed seven epidemiologic studies evaluating β-carotene/retinol and lung cancer. The relative risk (RR) for lung cancer was standardized to 1.0 for those subjects in the lowest category (quintile/quartile) of intake. In these seven trials, subjects in the highest category of intake had an average lung-cancer risk of 0.59. These findings are potentially compatible with our objective to detect a maximal potential chemopreventive effect that yields a risk

*Diet and Cancer: Any Progress in the Interim?, presented at the Second National Conference on Cancer Prevention and Detection, Seattle, WA, 1987.

of 0.67. Such epidemiologic associations, of course, cannot establish that increasing the intake or blood concentrations of vitamin A and β-carotene would actually decrease the incidence of lung cancers. Only the intervention studies being supported under the NCI Cancer Control Program can address that crucial question. In addition to our studies, the NCI portfolio includes the Harvard trial of β-carotene in physicians and the Finnish trial of β-carotene and vitamin E in 20,000 smokers (Sestili and Dell, 1984).

The combination of β-carotene and retinol employed in this study has the dual attraction of avoiding possible dose-related toxicity from higher doses of either agent, especially retinol, and of gaining the potential complementary antitumor actions of the two agents. We have demonstrated that the doses chosen are capable of substantially increasing serum β-carotene and serum retinyl palmitate concentrations without any early signs of liver toxicity or marked increases in triglycerides. The β-carotene is thought to function as an electron-scavenging anti-oxidant (Peto et al., 1981; Goodman, 1984) as well as a precursor of retinol. Retinol functions to maintain or enhance the differentiated state of epithelial cells, including those in bronchial epithelium (Peto et al., 1981; Goodman, 1984). Retinol *in vitro* inhibits cell growth, possibly via changes in cell surface glycolipids and glycoproteins (Patt et al.,1978; Lotan et al., 1987). We recognize that these mechanisms and their chemopreventive significance in humans are currently speculative.

Establishing the safety of any chemopreventive agent is essential, especially since subjects in chemoprevention trials are healthy volunteers without cancers, not patients (Omenn et al., 1988a). Even high-risk participants have less than one chance of lung cancer per 100/year. Thus, it is important to avoid significant side effects, both subjective and objective. Our ongoing studies address directly the potential of cumulative side effects. If our expanded trials provide evidence for the chemopreventive efficacy of β-carotene and retinol, further work to develop safe and efficacious agents will be stimulated.

The costs of full-scale chemoprevention trials, even for common cancers, are very high. We have devised a strategic plan to pool the two high-risk populations in ways that make project management more efficient, that moderate costs, that permit pooled as well as separate analyses of efficacy, and that generate side effects and observations on adherence of subjects to instructions from identical protocols.

It is likely that the underlying carcinogenic mechanisms for these two high-risk populations have much in common. Asbestos fibers retained in the pulmonary parenchyma are thought to act as cocarcinogens with the carcinogens in cigarette smoke (and other inhaled pollutants; Nicholson et al., 1982; Omenn et al., 1986). The distribution of histologic types of lung cancers is comparable between asbestos-exposed and non-asbestos-exposed smokers (Churg, 1985; Kannerstein and Churg, 1972). There is little or no basis to exclude adenocarcinomas in either population (Omenn et al., 1986); furthermore, the retinoids and β-carotene have chemopreventive activity in animals against adenocarcinomas of breast and colon (McCormick et al., 1980; Temple and Basu, 1987). It is likely that the chemoprevention of bronchogenic carcinoma in smokers and in asbestos-exposed workers would be acting on similar tumor promotion and tumor progression steps.

CURRENT TRIALS: PROGRESS TO DATE

Smokers Pilot Study

Goodman and associates (Goodman et al., 1985) have conducted a 2 x 2 factorial, four-group, Phase II pilot trial of β-carotene and retinol as potential cancer prevention agents in high-risk smokers (Figure 1). The objectives were to address the feasibility of a larger intervention trial, subject adherence, and potential side effects.

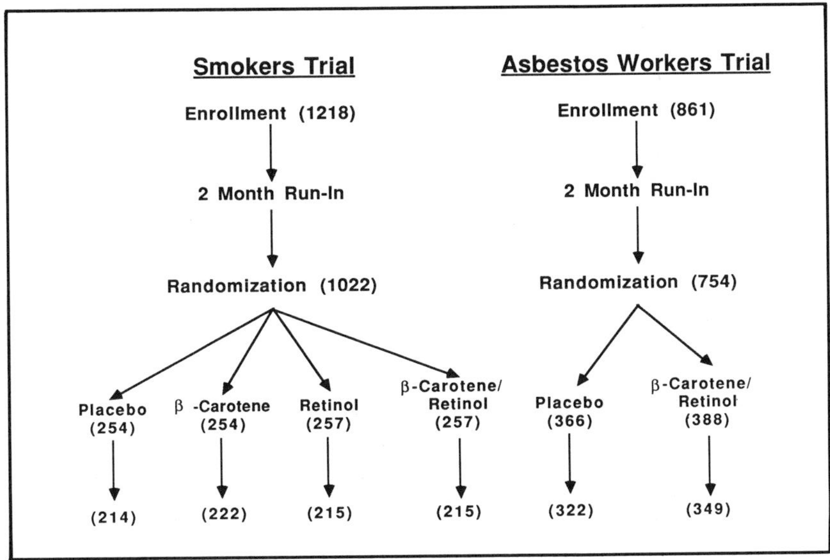

Figure 1. Schematic array of four-group trial of smokers and two-group trial of asbestos-exposed workers for safety and efficacy of β-carotene and retinol, with numbers of active randomized subjects as of 31 December 1987. Numbers of subjects in each group are given in parentheses.

Subjects were recruited from a local health insurer, King County Medical Blue Shield. A mailing to 29,927 subscribers described the trial and elicited responses about eligibility and interests in participating. Potentially eligible subjects (men and women, aged 50 to 67, with smoking history of at least 20 pack-years, either current smokers or those who had quit less than 6 years previously) were contacted, and an initial clinic visit was scheduled. At this first appointment, subjects' informed consent was obtained, a food frequency questionnaire was administered, a baseline side-effect evaluation was made, a limited physical examination was done, and blood samples were obtained. At the end of a 2-month placebo run-in, subjects returned for randomization to: (1) β-carotene placebo and retinol placebo; (2) β-carotene (30 mg) and retinol placebo; (3) β-carotene placebo and retinol (25,000 IU); or (4) β-carotene (30 mg) and retinol (25,000 IU). Subsequently, phone contacts were alternated with clinic visits at 2-month intervals to evaluate side effects and adherence. As of January 1988, 1296 subjects had completed their initial clinic visit, and 1022 had been randomized. We have exceeded our goal of 920 randomized subjects. The cohort comprises 69% current smokers and 31% former smokers, with 45.5 and 48.6 mean pack-years of smoking, respectively.

Subjective and objective side effects were measured with a standardized symptom questionnaire and symptom-grading scale, and a standardized physical examination. Scores for 15 different symptoms were grouped into eight categories: skin dryness or nosebleeds; yellowing of the skin; headaches; weight loss or appetite loss; psychological symptoms; bone pain; nausea or vomiting; change of bowel habits. Threshold symptoms were defined on our standardized grading scale as moderate or severe symptoms compatible with retinol or β-carotene excess. Threshold-grade symptoms triggered our side-effect management protocol.

The only significant objective finding was yellow coloration of the skin in 28% of subjects in the β-carotene-containing groups. No one has reported distress about the yellowing, and no subject has gone off study because of it. There were no differences across the treatment groups for subjective symptoms as of December 31, 1987, corresponding to mean follow-up of 12 months and total follow-up of 1003 person-years. Subjective symptom grades in all groups were higher on the initial visits, decreasing as the subjects became more familiar with the study nurses and the questionnaire, and as anxiety about taking the daily medication lessened. There were no changes in serum glutamic oxalic transaminase (SGOT) or alkaline phosphatase over time or across the four treatment groups.

Among 1218 subjects started on placebo, 187 subjects dropped out during the 2-month run-in period, including 29 found to be ineligible. The leading reasons were symptoms defined as side effects by our protocol (N = 44) and the fear of side effects (N = 34). Subjects reported being greatly influenced by the detailed, explicit consent form. After randomization, 7% of subjects dropped out during the first 4 months, then 3 to 5% during each subsequent 4-month interval through 16 months. Many of those who dropped out, both on the placebo run-in and after randomization, did so because of nonspecific side effects. The current side-effect monitoring protocol presumes all symptoms to be related to the drugs. At the 12-month follow-up of the first 415 smoker subjects, 304 were continuing on the pilot study; 111 (27%) had dropped out after randomization, and 62 were attributed to various symptoms and signs; of these 62, only 14 dropped out due to the development of symptoms graded as threshold on our grading scale. Based on these findings, the efficacy trial protocol has been designed to minimize these dropouts. As of 12/31/87, there have been 12 deaths (two due to cancer, one to lung cancer) and 14 additional cancer cases (six in the lung), with no excess in any treatment groups (total, 1003 person-years follow-up).

Medication rates were identical by pill counts and by subject reports and were stable over time: 87 to 92% of the subjects missed 5 or fewer days of treatment during six successive 4-month periods after randomization. A quarterly newsletter is mailed to all subjects to buttress compliance. No subject has refused to complete the side-effects questionnaire or fill out other forms.

There was no significant change in the serum concentrations of retinol, but retinyl palmitate concentrations increased in both groups receiving retinol. Mean β-carotene concentrations in groups that received β-carotene increased from 200 to 2600 ng/ml by 4 months (and to 2700 ng/ml at 12 months).

Asbestos-Exposed Workers

Omenn and associates (Omenn et al., 1988a,b) have enrolled men aged 45 to 74 who were occupationally exposed to asbestos in a Phase IV two-arm trial of 15 mg β-carotene plus 25,000 IU retinol versus placebos. Recruitment involved federal and state Workers' Compensation programs, selected occupational-medicine and pulmonary physicians, plaintiffs' attorneys, the Navy Asbestos Medical Surveillance Program at Bremerton, WA, and major unions in the Puget Sound area. The enrollment strategy included a 2-month placebo run-in, with follow-up every 2 months that alternated between phone calls and clinic visits. As of January 1988, 1007 subjects had completed the evaluation visit, and 754 were randomized.

The first 500 subjects recruited included 36% shipyard boilermakers, 30% plumbers and pipefitters, and 9% insulators, with the rest from high-risk shipyard trades (including ship scalers, electricians, and sheet-metal workers). In this cohort the prevalence of asbestos-related radiographic abnormalities (fibrosis and/or pleural changes) is 66%. In previous studies by others, prevalence was 52% for shipyard insulators and 46% for all crafts (Selikoff et al., 1979). The RR of asbestos exposure was 3.9 for mortality from lung cancer in the shipyard insulators. It is reasonable to conclude that the study cohort has significant asbestos exposure and lung-cancer risks similar to those of the asbestos insulators (Selikoff et al., 1979). Doll and Peto (1985) and Nicholson et al. (1982) have used an RR model in which lung-cancer risk is independent of age and smoking status and increases with duration and intensity of exposure. For those with 15 to 19 years from first exposure, RR was from 3.4, rising to 6.0 for those with 30 to 34 years, and declining to 3.9 for those who had more than 45 years since first exposure. The mean latency of our first 500 subjects was 34 years from first exposure, with a mean of 24 years cumulative duration of exposure in the respective high-risk trades.

Subjective and objective symptoms and signs were evaluated exactly as in the smokers study. There were no differences in subjective symptom grade or in objective physical findings between the two treatment groups. At 12 months there was no difference in the incidence of slight yellowing of the skin in the placebo group (8%) or the treatment group (6.5%). As of 12/31/87, 30 of the 754 randomized subjects had reported symptoms defined as threshold grade, requiring dosage reduction according to the protocol. There were no differences in biochemical indicators, deaths (four versus six), or cancer cases (eight versus four) between the two groups. In 1983 the Food and Drug Administration had decided that the "upper limit of normal" for SGOT and alkaline phosphatase be used to exclude subjects or to define toxicity once they were enrolled, rather than the usual 2.5 times the upper limit of normal used in other studies and in the Tyler, TX study (directed by J. McLarty; based on our protocol). As a result, 22 subjects were excluded, and 19 randomized subjects were treated as toxic, of whom 9 were dropped from the study before our originally proposed limits were approved in July 1987.

Among the 861 subjects who completed the initial clinic visit and began on placebos, 83 dropped out during the 2-month run-in period, including 20 who were found to be ineligible, and 83 more have gone off medication after randomization. During the 2-month run-in, 95% of subjects missed 5 or fewer days of medication. Subsequently, 87 to 93% missed 5 or fewer days of medication during six successive 4-month periods following randomization.

DESIGN FEATURES FOR THE FULL-SCALE EFFICACY TRIAL

The single most important design consideration, sample size, is discussed in detail here (Figure 2). Sample size requirements have been computed taking explicit account of seven parameters which will affect the magnitude of detectable decrease in lung-cancer incidence resulting from any chemopreventive effects (Figure 3). Values for these parameters have been chosen based on review of relevant literature and various specific assumptions. For some of these parameters, further field experience will refine the assumptions and projections.

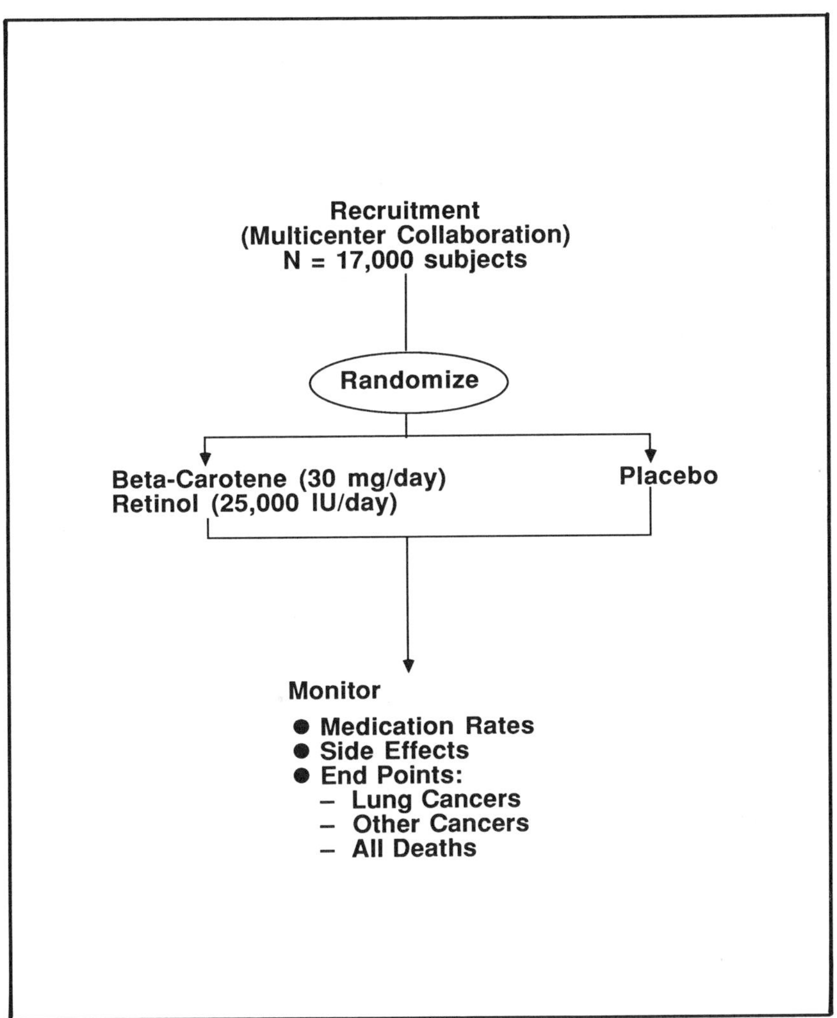

Figure 2. Study design for two-group chemoprevention efficacy trial of β-carotene plus retinol in heavy smokers and asbestos-exposed workers (multicenter collaboration).

Parameters	Assumptions
Incidence of Lung Cancer in Placebo Groups	
Smokers	0.5/100 Person-Years
Asbestos-Exposed Subjects	1.2/100 Person Years
Maximal Potential Chemoprevention Effect	33% Reduction of Lung Cancer Incidence
Accrual Period	3 Years
Time Lag for Full Effect	2 Years
Medication Rate (%)	
Treatment Group	100 Initially 70% at 3 Years 65% at 8 Years
Placebo Group	50% at 3 Years
Loss to Competing Risks	2% per Year
Loss to Follow-Up	2%
Test Statistic: Stratified, Weighted Log-Rank Test	Two-Sided Power: $\chi = 0.05$ $\beta = 0.80$

Figure 3. Parameters affecting sample size in study design for full-scale efficacy trial.

Incidence of Lung Cancer in Placebo Groups

This parameter has been estimated separately for the two high-risk populations of subjects. The overall incidence of lung cancer has been computed as the weighted mean of the estimates for the two groups in proportion to their numbers.

The lung-cancer incidence for heavy smokers is estimated to be 0.50 cases per 100 person-years, based upon: (1) the 1984 age- and sex-specific statistical epidemiology and end results (SEER) lung-cancer incidence rates of 0.24 per 100 per year for males 50 to 69 and 0.11 per 100 per year for females 50 to 69 (National Cancer Institute, 1986); (2) relative risks of 1 for never-smokers, 10 for all smokers, and 20 for heavy smokers (more than 20 pack-years or more than 25 cigarettes per day; Smoking and Health, 1964); (3) prevalence of smoking history, based upon the 1985 Health Promotion/Disease Prevention supplement to the National Health Interview Study (National Center for Health Statistics, 1986) for ages 45 to 64: 29% never, 40% ex-smoker, 20% light (less than 25 cigarettes per day), and 11% heavy smokers among males, and 46, 24, 21, and 8%, respectively, for the same categories in women; (4) uniform distribution by age through the eligible range; and (5) equal proportions of men and women. Based on the report of Lubin et al. (1984), we have made an adjustment of 0.9 for ex-smokers 0 to 6 years since cessation at enrollment and 3 to 9 years since cessation at study midpoint.

The lung-cancer incidence rate for asbestos-exposed subjects is estimated to be 1.2 per 100 person-years, based on: (1) the 1984 SEER lung-cancer incidence of about 0.23 per 100 per year for males 45 to 69; (2) relative risks for asbestos exposure in our highly exposed subjects of not less than 3 (Doll and Peto, 1985; Nicholson et al., 1982; Breslow, 1984); and (3) estimated RR of 15 for average smoking history in current and former smokers (based on observed proportion of light and heavy [20-plus pack-years] smokers in Seattle recruitment of 81/19% compared with 65/35% ratio for national data above), adjusted to 0.9 for ex-smokers 0 to 6 years since cessation and 0.6 for ex-smokers 6 to 15 years since cessation (Lubin et al., 1984). Support for this estimate comes from review of the Selikoff-Hammond studies of United States insulators, in which the observed lung-cancer incidence rate among workers with 20-plus years since first exposure to asbestos was 1.1 per 100 per year (Selikoff et al., 1979b). Mean age in the Seattle recruitment is 59, while the insulator subgroup's mean age was only 49, an age difference associated with a threefold higher risk, according to SEER data. Conversely, the insulators probably had higher asbestos exposures and higher current smoking incidence.

Analysis of this parameter must be a composite of rates for the smokers, for the higher-risk asbestos subjects to be enrolled at new sites, and for the already-enrolled asbestos subjects in Seattle. For the recruitment to date in Seattle of 22% current smokers, 62% ex-smokers, and 16% never-smokers, aged 45 to 74, the N of 754 may correspond to about 550 subjects recruited under the proposed, more stringent criteria of smoking history.

Maximal Potential Chemopreventive Effect

For public-health purposes, a sizable reduction in lung-cancer risk is needed to justify a general intervention program. Efficacy corresponding to 33% reduction in a fully compliant population of the two high-risk groups combined and, secondarily, to 50% reductions in each subgroup alone has been postulated. Such major effects may be feasible, based upon reductions of that magnitude observed in animals, the prompt effects on micronucleus formation and on bronchial biopsies in humans, and the two- to fivefold variation in lung-cancer risk between extreme quintiles or quartiles of β-carotene/vitamin A intake or blood levels. Other parameters (see below) diminish the actual reductions that can be observed.

Time Lag for Full Effect on Reduction of Cancer Risk

We have used a time lag of 2 years to full effect that is linear from zero effect to full effect. There is no experimental basis at present that would clarify this matter. We know from studies of serial chest radiographs that lung cancers grow very rapidly once they are detectable radiographically (Weiss et al., 1982; Fontana and Taylor, 1985). Specifically, 3-month intervals were too long for clinically useful detection for treatment. We begin with direct pharmacologic intervention, and we know from animal studies, *in vitro* studies, and human intermediate-endpoint studies that vitamin A and β-carotene achieve chemopreventive effects within weeks.

Accrual Period and Length of Followup

We are using 3 years for accrual and a total of 8 years for the study, hence an average follow-up of 6.5 years. Obviously, extension of the follow-up (if attrition is low and medication rate is high) would be valuable. In Seattle, we have exceeded the target of 920 subjects for the smokers study and accrued over 600 subjects in the asbestos study within 2 years from the actual start in May 1985 (when drugs were made available). Three years for accrual seems reasonable. Our sources for the collaborating sites are well identified and seem ready to make rapid initial-recruitment efforts.

Loss to Competing Risks

We have used 0.02 per year for deaths unrelated to lung cancer in these high-risk populations, based on actuarial estimates (U.S. Department of Commerce, 1980; National Center for Health Statistics, 1985) and experience from other long-term intervention trials (Lipid Research Clinics [LRC] Program, 1984; Aspirin Myocardial Infarction Study Research Group, 1980; Beta-Blocker Heart Attack Trial Research Group, 1982). A detailed calculation shows that this factor for smokers increases from 0.015 to 0.024 from ages 45-49 to ages 65-69.

Medication Rate

This parameter, the average fraction of full dose taken, may involve both placebo subjects taking significant doses of active drug from nonstudy sources and subjects on an active drug taking less than the assigned dose of drug. Users of more than one MultiVit tablet (Barre, Baltimore, MD) or 5500 IU retinol per day are excluded from randomization. Only extremely positive publicity about the chemopreventive value of vitamin A compounds is likely to induce crossover in the placebo group. We allow for 5% medication rate after 3 years in the placebo group.

We have reviewed data from the three large-scale, cardiovascular-intervention studies cited above. Our calculations use a medication rate that declines from 100 to 70% over 3 years and then to 65% at 8 years after randomization. These assumptions are consistent with a 7-year 0.63 medication rate and 0.73 adherence rate in the LRC trial, a 0.80 medication rate over 3 years in the aspirin trial, and 0.85 adherence at 27 months in the beta-blocker trial.

Loss to Follow Up

We estimate 2% among all randomized individuals as the fraction for whom the lung-cancer end point cannot be ascertained despite both active and passive follow-up methods.

In sum, with these parameters, a two-sided alpha 0.05 test using a modified log-rank test statistic down-weighted over 2 years, and power of 0.80, about 13,000 heavy smokers and about 4000 asbestos-exposed subjects are needed. Specifically, with a maximal potential chemopreventive effect of 33% reduction in lung-cancer incidence, the projected actual reduction would be 22% from the placebo group to the β-carotene/retinol group. After down-weighting for cases occurring during the first 2 years, the distribution of analyzable cases would be as follows:

Population	Number of Lung Cancer Cases	Group	Percent Change	Odds Ratio
Combined	269	Placebo		
	210	β-carotene/retinol	-22	0.78
Heavy smokers	158	Placebo		
	123	β-carotene/retinol	-22	0.78
Asbestos workers	111	Placebo		
	87	β-carotene/retinol	-22	0.78

DISCUSSION

Design Features

The eligibility criteria define two high-risk populations: (1) smokers, men and women, aged 50 to 69, with a history of at least 20 pack-years, currently smoking cigarettes or stopped within 6 years; and (2) men, aged 45 to 69, with evidence of extensive occupational exposure to asbestos beginning at least 15 years earlier and based on chest radiograph findings and/or employment in one of seven defined high-risk trades, currently smoking or stopped smoking within 15 years. These eligibility criteria represent certain refinements of the criteria used in the preceding Seattle studies. Since minimal exposure to the potent cocarcinogenic action of asbestos fibers in this study is 15 years, we have chosen to accept ex-smokers up to 15 years in this subpopulation of the trial. According to Lubin et al. (1984), after 10 to 14 years, the relative risk of lung cancer is still 0.56 compared with current smokers with similar duration; also, the risk declines much less rapidly in those with longer smoking histories. An additional RR of 3 for asbestos history would place these individuals at higher risk than current smokers and should be cost-effective. From data about effects of smoking cessation on lung-cancer risk in asbestos-exposed cohorts, the time course roughly parallels the decline in risk among unexposed smokers (Hammond et al., 1979; Berry et al., 1985). There is no apparent decline in duration-adjusted risk from ending asbestos exposure (Seidman et al., 1979).

The design of this trial is based on our experience with the Seattle populations of 1022 smokers and 754 asbestos-exposed subjects already randomized (as of 12/31/87, see Figure 1). The placebo run-in will be extended from 2 to 3 months. A uniform dosage intervention has been chosen: 30 mg per day β-carotene and 25,000 IU per day retinol. After randomization, subjects will be followed at a participating clinic at 3-month intervals for the first year after randomization, and at 4-month intervals thereafter (annual clinic visit and two phone contacts).

In the efficacy trial protocol, the inquiry about and management of side effects is streamlined. Subjects will receive an abbreviated symptom questionnaire and a more limited physical examination initially; follow-up evaluations by telephone and in the clinic will elicit self-report of symptoms. Any responses representing a threshold symptom as defined in the grading scale will trigger side-effect management with administration of the full, standardized questionnaire and side-effect management protocol. These protocol changes recognize that most symptoms are unrelated to the study agents and are predicated upon our expectation that any significant side effects will be identified first in the group of the 1700 subjects already enrolled; they will continue much closer monitoring of symptoms and signs. We are aware that uncommon side effects might appear only in the larger population, and the clinic staffs will be alerted to that fact. The Fred Hutchinson Cancer Research Center (FHCRC) Institutional Safety and Endpoints Monitoring Committee for the Cancer Prevention Research Program (CPRP) will make periodic reviews of the comparative frequency of symptoms in the placebo and treatment groups of the Vanguard group and in a 10% sample of the efficacy trial and will recommend changes in the protocol, should any be indicated.

The chest radiograph and spirometry results have been included, as before, as independent variables in the asbestos cohort. The high prevalence of parenchymal fibrosis (37%) and pleural changes (55%), comprising 11% with parenchymal changes only, 29% with pleural changes only, and 26% with both, and of restrictive abnormalities on spirometry (17%) are consistent with enrollment of a population with high asbestos exposure and high risk for asbestos-associated cancers. These functions will be monitored at the new clinics to ensure enrollment of similar high-risk subjects. In addition, there is some evidence that parenchymal and/or pleural abnormalities may be a predictor of lung-cancer risk independent of exposure dose (Breslow, 1984; Cullen, 1987; Liddell and McDonald, 1980; Finkelstein and Vingilis, 1984; Becklake et al., 1970; Bader et al., 1970; Weill et al., 1975; Harber et al., 1987).

During our current studies, subjects who are still smoking are encouraged to stop and to seek assistance if they wish. Henceforth, our protocol will include more explicit guidance, based upon the extensive experience in our CPRP with smoking cessation strategies, including the Hanford studies for which Omenn was Principal Investigator (Omenn et al., in press; Schwartz, 1987), and the National Heart, Lung, and Blood Institute Smoking Education Program (NHLBI, 1986) report. Smokers will be offered the manual *Freedom from Smoking in 20 Days* produced by the American Lung Association specifically for blue-collar workers. The manual emphasizes the benefits of a nonsmoking lifestyle, recommends a day-by-day technique to quit, recordkeeping, identification of smoking triggers, personal contracts, and techniques to resist relapse. For those participants interested and willing to be assisted, clinic staff will help them set a target date for smoking cessation and will contact them for reinforcement at that time. Smoking cessation will have little effect on lung-cancer risk for at least the first few years of follow-up (Lubin et al., 1984).

Management Structure

The Data Management Center already established at the FHCRC is being reorganized and expanded to meet substantially increased responsibilities. The Coordinating Center will consist of a medical core and a statistical center. The medical core will be responsible for close communication with clinic sites on all clinical questions, as well as staffing; procurement and distribution of drugs; analysis of blood samples and periodic review of chest radiographs; human subjects matters; arrangements for evaluation of pathology reports and occasional reviews of slides or specimens critical to endpoint decisions; and communications with Steering and Policy Committees, including agenda-setting and convening functions. The statistical center will comprise an administrative support unit and three technical units: a field unit, a data processing unit, and a data analysis unit.

Randomization of eligible subjects will be performed centrally. The clinics will remain blind to the sampling scheme. The Center will maintain selected administrative data on all enrolled subjects for use in generating status reports to the clinics and others and for follow-up tracking activities. As needed, the Coordinating Center will assist the clinics in preparing mass mailings for recruiting efforts.

Data Analysis

Data analysis will be organized around the case-cohort method. The primary end point is the incidence of lung cancer in the two high-risk populations treated with a combination of β-carotene and retinol versus placebos. Explanatory variables computerized for all subjects include age, sex, smoking history, threshold toxicity and toxicity management reports, and endpoint data, plus summaries of asbestos occupational exposure history, chest radiograph ILO interpretation, and annual spirometry test for the asbestos population. Variables computerized only for lung-cancer cases and a 10% subcohort include blood serum measures, dietary-intake analyses, clinic attendance records, compliance data, and side-effects reports.

The primary analysis will test for differences between the groups in the incidence of lung cancer. Let t_i denote the detection time of the i'th lung-cancer case, O_i the number of lung-cancer cases in the intervention group occurring at time t_i, and E_i the conditionally expected number of such cases under the null hypothesis of no risk reduction due to β-carotene and retinol. The weighted log-rank statistic, $T = \Sigma\, w_i\,(O_i - E_i)$, where

$$w_i = \begin{cases} t_i \tfrac{1}{2} \; if\, t_i < 2 \\ 1 \quad if\, t_i \geq 2 \end{cases}$$

will be used as the primary test of the null hypothesis. This weighted log-rank statistic down-weights cases occurring in the first 2 years, before the full effect is predicted to occur. In addition, the analysis will be stratified to deal with the 1700 subjects included in the group, allowing for differences in eligibility criteria, initial assignment to treatment groups, and initial dosages.

Secondary analyses will test for differences in the lung-cancer rates between the groups with adjustment for known and suspected factors that may influence the rates. Any such differences will be subjected to explanatory analyses. Variables include detailed smoking and occupational-exposure histories; presence and extent of asbestos-induced radiographic changes (for asbestos subjects); age and sex; dietary and supplementary intake of vitamin A and β-carotene; time and cumulative dose on study; and smoking cessation success and interval. When all potential covariates are computerized for all subjects, the analysis will use the Cox model (Kalbfleisch and Prentice, 1973) applied to prospectively collected data. When some potential covariates are available only for cases and the subcohort, the case-cohort method (Prentice, 1986) will be used for the analysis.

Ancillary analyses will be carried out as well, including potential efficacy against mesothelioma or other cancer sites, competing causes of death, roles of smoking in fibrosis and of fibrosis as an independent risk factor in lung cancer, variation in β-carotene from different sources and suppliers, and behavioral aspects of participation and compliance. We have already completed significant methods development for the analysis of β-carotene, α-carotene, retinol, and retinyl palmitate (Kalman et al., 1987); analyses of food-frequency questionnaires for β-carotene and vitamin A intake versus serum values (Roidt et al., in press); and initial correlations among smoking history, asbestos exposure history, radiographic and spirometric abnormalities (Barnhart et al.*). Psychological, sociological, and economic analyses of the trial results will be made especially to characterize their general applicability.

Each year, a sample size calculation will be performed. Instead of using the assumptions made above about accrual patterns, distribution of risk factors among study participants, and medication rates among participants, the values for these factors actually observed in the trial or projections for these values based on trial data will be used. The technique of stochastic curtailed testing (Halperin et al., 1982; Lan et al., 1985) will be used in monitoring recruitment of subjects and the medication rate in the two groups. In addition, the assumptions about lung-cancer incidence rate in the placebo group and rate of loss of subjects to competing risks will be assessed in light of the trial experience and changed accordingly. The resultant power calculation for detection of the desired chemopreventive effect of retinoids will serve as a guide for modifying the proportions of asbestos-exposed and smoker subjects and clinics as enrollment is completed. If necessary, we will initiate remedial actions to improve recruitment or compliance, changing some of the

*Barnhart, SL et al. Does Smoking Behavior Affect Fibrosis Among an Asbestos-Exposed Cohort? Presented at the 22nd International Congress on Occupational Health, September 27-October 2, 1987, Sydney, Australia.

fundamental parameters of the trial (such as length of follow-up), or abandoning the trial. Decision rules for abandoning the trial or drastically changing its parameters will be developed in concert with a National Policy Advisory Committee or an alternative mechanism established by the NCI and the FHCRC/University of Washington Cancer Prevention Research Program. We expect the full efficacy trial to run through 1996.

This trial should yield information crucial to our efforts to reduce lung cancer, especially in the high-risk smoker and asbestos-exposed populations in this country and throughout the world.

ACKNOWLEDGMENTS

We gratefully acknowledge the work of our excellent clinical and statistical center staff for this trial. Work was supported by Grant CA 34704 from the National Cancer Institute.

REFERENCES

Aspirin Myocardial Infarction Study Research Group. 1980. A randomized, controlled trial of aspirin in persons recovered from myocardial infarction. J Am Med Assoc 243:661-669.

Bader, ME, RA Mader, AS Tierstein, A Miller, and IJ Selikoff. **1970.** Pulmonary function and radiographic changes in 598 workers with varying duration of asbestos exposure. Mt Sinai J Med 37:492-500.

Becklake, MR, G Fournier-Massey, JC McDonald, et al. **1970.** Lung function in relation to chest radiographic changes in Quebec asbestos workers. Bull Physiopathol Respir 6:637-59.

Berry, G, ML Newhouse, and P Antonis. **1985.** Combined effect of asbestos and smoking on mortality from lung cancer and mesothelioma in factory workers. Br J Ind Med 42:12-18.

Bertram, JS, LN Kolonel, and F Meyskens. **1987.** Rationale and strategies for chemoprevention of cancer in humans. Cancer Res 47:3012-3031.

Beta-Blocker Heart Attack Trial Research Group. 1982. A randomized trial of propranolol in patients with acute myocardial infarction. J Am Med Assoc 247:1707-1714.

Bjelke, E. **1975.** Dietary vitamin A and human lung cancer. Int J Cancer 15:561-565.

Bollag, W and A Matter. **1981.** From vitamin A to retinoids in experimental and clinical oncology: Achievements, failures and outlook. Ann NY Acad Sci 351:9-23.

Breslow, L (ed.). **1984.** *Asbestiform Fibers, Nonoccupational Health Risks.* National Academy Press, Washington, DC.

Byers, TE, S Graham, BP Haughey, JR Marshall, and MK Swanson. **1987.** Diet and lung cancer risk: Findings from the Western New York Diet Study. Am J Epidemiol 125:351-363.

Churg, J. **1985.** Lung cancer cell type and asbestos exposure. J Am Med Assoc 253:2984-2985.

Cullen, MR. **1987.** Controversies in asbestos-related lung cancer. In: *Occupational Medicine State of the Art Reviews: Occupational Pulmonary Disease,* L Rosenstock (ed.). Hanley & Belfus, Philadelphia, PA.

Doll, R and AB Hill. **1956.** Lung cancer and other causes of death in relation to smoking. Second report on mortality of British doctors. Br Med J 2:1071-1081.

Doll, R and J Peto. **1985.** *Effects on Health of Exposure to Asbestos,* Health and Safety Commission Report. Her Majesty's Stationery Office, London, England.

Finkelstein, MM and JJ Vingilis. **1984.** Radiologic abnormalities among asbestos-cement workers: An exposure-response study. Am Rev Respir Dis 129:17-22.

Fontana, RS and WF Taylor. **1985.** Screening for lung cancer: the Mayo Lung Project, pp. 161-174. In: *Lung Cancer: Causes and Prevention,* M Mizel and P Correa (eds.). Verlag Chemie Int., Deerfield Beach, FL.

Goodman, DS. **1984.** Vitamin A and retinoids in health and disease. N Engl J Med 310:1023-1031.

Goodman, GE, GS Omenn, P Feigl, GD Kleinman, B Lund, DD Thomas, MM Henderson and R Prentice. **1985.** Chemoprevention of lung cancer with retinol/beta-carotene, pp. 341-350. In: *Vitamins and Cancer—Human Cancer Prevention by Vitamins and Micronutrients,* FL Meyskens and KN Prasad (eds.). Humana Press, Clifton, NJ.

Greenwald, P and EJ Sondik (eds.). **1986.** Cancer Control Objectives for the Nation 1985-2000, NCI Monograph #2, National Cancer Institute, Bethesda, MD, pp. 1-105; Appendix B, Tables B-2,3,4,5.

Halperin, M, KKG Lan, JH Ware, NJ Johnson, and DL DeMets. **1982.** An aid to data monitoring in long-term clinical trials. Controlled Clinic Trials 3:311-323.

Hammond, EC and D Horn. **1958a.** Smoking and death rates—Report on 44 months of following 187,783 men. I—Total mortality. J Am Med Assoc 166:1159-1172.

Hammond, EC and D Horn. **1958b.** Smoking and death rates—Report on 44 months of follow-up of 187,783 men. II—Death rates by cancer. J Am Med Assoc 166:1294-1308.

Hammond, EC, IJ Selikoff, and H Seidman. **1979.** Asbestos exposure, cigarette smoking, and death rates. Ann NY Acad Sci 330:473-490.

Harber, P, Z Mohsenifar, and M Lew. **1987.** Pleural plaques and asbestos associated malignancy. J Occup Med 29:641-644.

Havlik, RJ. **1986.** Determinants of health—Cardiovascular risk factors, p. 40. In: *Health Statistics on Older Persons, United States 1986,* DHHS Publication No. (PHS) 87-1409. Department of Health and Human Services, Washington, DC.

Hinds, MW, LN Kolonel, JN Hankin, and J Lee. **1984.** Dietary vitamin A, carotene, vitamin C and risk of lung cancer in Hawaii. Am J Epidemiol 119:227-237.

Kalbfleisch, JD and RL Prentice. **1973.** Marginal likelihoods based on Cox's regression and life model. Biometrika 60:267-278.

Kalman, DA, GE Goodman, GS Omenn, G Bellamy, and B Rollins. **1987.** Micronutrient assay for cancer prevention clinical trials: Serum retinol, retinyl palmitate, alpha-carotene, and beta-carotene with the use of high-performance liquid chromatography. J Natl Cancer Inst 79:975-982.

Kannerstein, M and J Churg. **1972.** Pathology of carcinoma of the lung associated with asbestos exposure. Cancer 30:14-21.

Kark, JD, AH Smith, BR Switzer, CG Hames. **1981.** Serum vitamin A (retinol) and cancer incidence in Evans County, Georgia. J Natl Cancer Inst 66:7-16.

Lan, KKG, R Simon, and M Halperin. **1985.** Stochastically curtailed tests in long-term clinical trials. Commun Stat Seq Anal 1(3):207-219.

Lasnitzki, I and W Bollag. **1982.** Prevention and reversal of 3,4-benzpyrene and cigarette smoke condensate induced hyperplasia and metaplasia of rodent respiratory epithelia in organ culture. Cancer Treat Rep 66:1375-1380.

Liddell, FDK and JC McDonald. **1980.** Radiologic findings as predictors of mortality in Quebec asbestos workers. Br J Ind Med 37:257-267.

Lipid Research Clinics Program. 1984. The lipid research clinics coronary primary prevention trial results. I. Reduction in incidence of coronary heart disease. J Am Med Assoc 251:351-364.

Lotan, R, D Lotan D, and V Deutsch. **1987.** Growth inhibition of murine melanoma cells by antibodies to a cell surface glycoprotein implicated in retinoic acid action. Cancer Res 47:3152-3158.

Lubin, JH, WJ Blot, F Berrino, R Famant, CR Gillis, M Kunze, D Schmahl, and G Visco. **1984.** Modifying risk of developing lung cancer by changing habits of cigarette smoking. Br Med J 288:1953-1956.

Mathe, G, J Gouveia, et al. **1982.** Detection of precancerous bronchus metaplasia in heavy smokers and its regression following retinoid treatment. Proceedings, First International Conference on Modulation and Mediation of Cancer by Vitamins, February 23-26, 1982, Tucson, AZ.

McCormick, DL, FJ Burns, and RE Albert. **1980.** Inhibition of rat mammary carcinogenesis by short dietary exposure to retinyl acetate. Cancer Res 40:1140-1143.

Mossman, BT, JE Craighead, and BV MacPherson. **1980.** Asbestos induced epithelial changes in organ cultures of hamster trachea: Inhibition by retinyl methyl ether. Science 207:311-313.

National Cancer Institute (NCI). 1986. *1986 Annual Cancer Statistics Review,* p. II.B.39, NCI, Division of Cancer Prevention and Controls, NIH Publication No. 87-2789. National Institutes of Health, Washington, DC.

National Center for Health Statistics. 1985. *Vital Statistics of the United States, 1980, Volume II. Mortality, Part B,* p. 131, DHHA Publication No. (PHS) 85-1102. U.S. Public Health Service, Washington, DC.

National Center for Health Statistics. 1986. *National Health Interview Survey: United States, January-March, 1985,* Provisional Data from the Health Promotion and Disease Prevention Supplement. Vital and Health Statistics, No. 113, advance data, DHHS Pub. No. (PHS) 86-1250. National Center for Health Statistics, Hyattsville, MD.

National Heart, Lung, and Blood Institute Smoking Education Program. 1986. Clinical Opportunities for Smoking Intervention: A Guide for the Busy Physician, NIH Publication No. 86-2718. National Institutes of Health, Washington, DC.

Nicholson, WJ, G Perkel, and IJ Selikoff. **1982.** Occupational exposure to asbestos: Population at risk and projected mortality. Am J Ind Med 3:259-311.

Nomura, AM, GN Stemmermann, LK Heilbrun, RM Salkeld, and JP Vuilleumier. **1986.** Serum vitamin levels and the risk of cancer in specific sites in men of Japanese ancestry in Hawaii. Cancer Res 45:2369-2372.

Omenn, GS, J Merchant, E Boatman, JM Dement, M Kuschner, W Nicholson, J Peto, and L Rosenstock. **1986.** Contribution of environmental fibers to respiratory cancer. Environ Health Perspect 70:51-56.

Omenn, GS, GE Goodman, GD Kleinman, L Rosenstock, S Barnhart, P Feigl, DB Thomas, D Kalman, B Lund, RL Prentice, and MM Henderson. **1988a.** The role of intervention studies in ascertaining the contribution of dietary factors in lung cancer: The Seattle chemoprevention trial of retinoids in asbestos-exposed workers. Ann NY Acad Sci 534:575-583.

Omenn, GS, GE Goodman, L Rosenstock, S Barnhart, B Lund, M Thornquist, P Feigl. **1988b.** Cancer chemoprevention with vitamin A and beta-carotene in populations at high risk for lung cancer, pp. 279-283. In: *Anticarcinogenesis and Radiation Protection,* OF Nygaard, M Simic, and P Cerutti (eds.). Plenum Press, New York, NY.

Omenn, GS, B Thompson, M Sexton, N Hessol, B Breitenstein, S Curry, M Michnich, and A Peterson. A randomized comparison of worksite-sponsored smoking cessation programs. Am J Prevent Med **(in press)**.

Patt, LM, K Itaya, S-I Hakomori. **1978.** Retinol induces density-dependent growth inhibition and changes in glycolipids and LETS. Nature 273:379-381.

Peto, R, R Doll, JD Buckley, and MB Sporn. **1981.** Can dietary beta-carotene materially reduce human cancer rates? Nature 290:201-209.

Port, C, M Sporn, and D Kaufman. **1975.** Prevention of lung cancers in hamsters by 13-cis-retinoic acid. Proc Am Assoc Cancer Res 16:21.

Prentice, RL. **1986.** A case-cohort design for epidemiologic cohort studies and disease prevention trials. Biometrika 73:1-11

Roidt, L, EM White, GE Goodman, PW Wahl, GS Omenn, B Rollins, JM Karkeck. Association of food frequency questionnaire estimates of vitamin A intake with serum vitamin A levels. Am J Epidemiol **(in press)**.

Saffiotti, U, R Montesano, AR Sellakumar, and SA Borg. **1967.** Experimental cancer of the lung: Inhibition by vitamin A of the induction of tracheobronchial squamous metaplasia and squamous cell tumors. Cancer 20:857-864.

Schwartz, JL. **1987.** *Review and Evaluation of Smoking Cessation Methods: The United States and Canada, 1978-1985,* NIH Publication No. 87-2940, April 1987. National Institutes of Health, Bethesda, MD.

Seidman, H, IJ Selikoff, EC Hammond. **1979.** Short-term asbestos work exposure and long-term observations. Ann NY Acad Sci 330:61-79.

Selikoff, I, R Lilis, and W Nicholson. **1979a.** Asbestos disease in United States shipyards. Ann NY Acad Sci 330:295-312.

Selikoff, IJ, EC Hammond, and H Seidman. **1979b.** Mortality experience of insulation workers in the United States and Canada, 1943-1976. Ann NY Acad Sci 330:91-116.

Sestili, MA and JG Dell (eds.). **1984.** *Chemoprevention Clinical Trials. Problems and Solutions,* Proceedings of a Workshop, May 17-18, 1984, NIH Publication No. 85-2715. National Cancer Institute, Bethesda, MD.

Shekele, RB, L Shuguey, WJ William, M Lepper, C Maliza, and AH Rossof. **1977.** Dietary vitamin A and risk of cancer in the Western Electric study. Lancet 2:1185-1190.

Silverberg, E and J Lubera. **1986.** Cancer statistics, 1986. Cancer 36:9-25.

Smoking and Health. 1964. *Report of the Advisory Committee to the Surgeon General of the Public Health Service.* U.S. Department of Health, Education, and Welfare, Washington, DC, 164 p.

Stich, H, M Rosin, and M Vallejera. **1984.** Reduction with Vitamin A and beta-carotene administration of proportion of micronucleated buccal mucosal cells in Asian betel nut and tobacco chewers. Lancet 1:1204-1206.

Temple, NJ and TK Basu. **1987.** Protective effect of β-carotene against colon tumors in mice. J Natl Cancer Inst 78:1211-1214.

U.S. Department of Commerce. 1980. *General Population Characteristics,* pp. 1-127, Table 140, Vol. I. U.S. Department of Commerce, Bureau of the Census, Washington, DC.

U.S. Surgeon General's Advisory Committee on Smoking and Health. 1964. Smoking and Health: Report of the Advisory Committee to the Surgeon General of the Public Health Service. U.S. Department of Health, Education and Welfare, Washington, DC.

Wald, N, M Idle, J Boreham, and A Bailey. **1980.** Low serum-vitamin-A and subsequent risk of cancer. Lancet 2:813-815.

Weill, H, MM Ziskind, C Waggenspack, and CE Rossiter. **1975.** Lung function consequences of dust exposure in asbestos cement manufacturing plants. Arch Environ Health 30:88-96.

Weiss, W, KR Boucot, and H Seidman. **1982.** The Philadelphia pulmonary neoplasm research project. Clin Chest Med 3:243-256.

Willett, WC, BF Polk, BA Underwood, MJ Stampfer, S Pressel, B Rosner, JO Taylor, K Schneider, and CG Hames. **1984.** Relation of serum vitamins A and E and carotenoids to the risk of cancer. N Engl J Med 310:430-434.

Zeigler, RG, RJ Mason, A Stemhagen, R Hoover, JB Schoenberg, G Gridley, PW Virgo, R Altman, and JF Fraumeni, Jr. **1984.** Dietary carotene and vitamin A and risk of lung cancer among white males in New Jersey. J Natl Cancer Inst 73:1429-1434.

Evaluation of Breathlessness by Exercise Testing in Cigarette-Smoking and Nonsmoking Asbestos Workers

Piergiuseppe Agostoni,[1] Dorsett Smith,[2] Robert B. Schoene,[2] H. Thomas Robertson,[2] and John Butler[2]

[1]Istituto di Cardiologia, Universita di Milano, Milan, Italy

[2]Division of Pulmonary and Critical Care Medicine, University of Washington School of Medicine, Seattle, WA 98195

KEY WORDS: asbestos, smoking, pulmonary function, exercise, rest, restrictive disease, obstructive disease, cardiac limitation

---

ABSTRACT

We endeavored to identify objective criteria for functional impairment in 120 male asbestos-exposed workers, most of whom were smokers or ex-smokers. They were consecutively referred patients claiming compensation for asbestos inhalation injury that was allegedly causing disability because of breathlessness. We assumed that the presence and severity of asbestosis were reflected by radiographic changes (International Labour Office [ILO] score), and that cigarette-smoking had caused any chronic obstructive pulmonary disease (COPD), identified by reduced expiratory flow rates. However, because radiographic changes are not necessarily correlated with functional impairment, we assessed whether their severity (ILO score) was matched by the abnormal gas transfer [alveolar-to-arterial oxygen pressure differential, $P(A\text{-}a)O_2$] characteristic of the diseases that cause pulmonary fibrosis. We used a progressive exercise test (increments in load each minute) and scored the data to identify the organ system (ventilatory, cardiac, pulmonary vascular or peripheral circulatory) which was mainly responsible for limiting performance. The $P(A\text{-}a)O_2/\dot{V}O_2$ on exercise correlated well with the radiographic ILO score, suggesting that the latter could be used to assess the presence of asbestosis and its severity. A $P(A\text{-}a)O_2/\dot{V}O_2$ of 35 mm Hg/L or above was specific for individuals with asbestosis, although sensitivity of this parameter was poor. Groups of workers with asbestosis, or with asbestosis and COPD, had higher $P(A\text{-}a)O_2/\dot{V}O_2$ than groups of normal workers or those who had COPD without asbestosis. Half (49.2%) of the claimants had no abnormal limitation to exercise, based on our criteria. Of those who were limited, more had a cardiac (37%) than a ventilatory (26%) cause. Ventilatory limitations were usually due to COPD and occurred in smokers (32%) and ex-smokers (22%). The only two nonsmokers with ventilatory limitations also had obstructive abnormalities, and it seemed likely that they had asthma. Thus, objective evidence of ventilatory limitation due to asbestos-related disease was uncommon in this group of asbestos-exposed workers.

INTRODUCTION

The assessment of the cause of breathlessness is particularly difficult in patients who are claiming compensation (Adams et al., 1985; Lindgren et al., 1965; Morgan, 1979). Thus, objective criteria for functional impairment are very important (American Medical Association, 1984). We studied asbestos-exposed workers who were claiming compensation for disability because of breathlessness on exercise, which was allegedly caused by asbestos-related disease. Because such problems become apparent only 30 or more years after the initial exposure to asbestos, the patients are usually elderly cigarette-smokers and thus likely to have other diseases (Becklake, 1976).

Cigarette-smoking causes chronic obstructive pulmonary disease (COPD) in some people. This is characterized by reduced expiratory flow rates (forced expiratory volume in 1 second, FEV_1) and maximum voluntary ventilation (MVV). Asbestosis is a form of pulmonary fibrosis that causes a restrictive pulmonary-function defect (low total lung capacity, TLC), with clinically insignificant airflow obstruction. It also reduces maximum ventilation, because lung expansion is impaired. Thus, both COPD and asbestosis may cause a ventilatory limitation which impairs exercise abilities. However, pulmonary fibrosis causes a characteristic, marked increase in the alveolar-to-arterial oxygen pressure differential on exercise, whereas moderate obstructive pulmonary disease usually does not. We assumed that the presence and severity of asbestosis was reflected by the amount of radiographic opacity (ILO score; ILO, 1980). We used the radiographic ILO score as a measure of asbestosis, and we needed to show that this was associated with the functional impairment of asbestosis. Therefore, we tested the patients' exercise performance to ascertain whether the alveolar-to-arterial oxygen pressure differential related to the ILO score for asbestosis.

Our study was aimed at finding objective criteria for evaluating the cause of the breathlessness which limited exercise by asbestos workers.

SUBJECTS

We surveyed all asbestos workers referred over a 4-year period for assessment of the breathlessness that they attributed to asbestos exposure. Subjects were excluded if they were unable or unwilling to exercise, if they had evidence of past or present lung disease other than that attributable to asbestos exposure or cigarette-smoking, and if they had clinical or electrocardiographically visible signs of drug intoxication (digitalis, quinidine, etc.), or if they were receiving beta-blocker therapy. Of the 120 subjects surveyed, 94 had arterial blood-gas values during exercise that were adequate for measuring alveolar-to-arterial oxygen pressure differentials. All subjects were men; 116 were Caucasian; 63% were smokers, 19% ex-smokers, and 18% were nonsmokers (Table 1).

Table 1. History of asbestos exposure and cigarette-smoking in dyspneic asbestos workers (total number of subjects, 120).

	Range	Mean	SD
Age:	36 to 81	60	9.5
History of Asbestos Exposure			
Years of exposure	0.5 to 45	23	11
Years since exposure	9 to 52	34	10
History of Cigarette-Smoking	Number in Study		Percent of Total
Smokers	75		63
Ex-smokers	23		19
Nonsmokers	22		18

METHODS

Pulmonary Function at Rest

Total lung capacity was measured by helium dilution. Spirometry included MVV, usually at a rate of 70 breaths per minute. In assessing exercise limitation, we used the greater of the measured MVV and that calculated from FEV_1 x 40 (American Thoracic Society, 1979). The prediction equation of Kory and co-workers (Kory et al., 1961) was used for the MVV, that of Goldman and Becklake (1959) for TLC, and that of Morris and associates for FEV_1 and forced vital capacity (FVC; Morris et al., 1971). We reduced the predicted values for lung volumes of the four non-Caucasian men by 15% (U.S. Department of Labor, 1974).

Exercise Test

Subjects were exercised on a bicycle ergometer (19 subjects) or a treadmill (101 subjects, including all those for whom we measured alveolar-to-arterial oxygen differentials). Electrocardiographs were recorded throughout the test and for 10 minutes afterwards. Blood pressure was measured with a cuff manometer. Arterial blood was withdrawn from a percutaneously catheterized radial artery. In the bicycle ergometer test, we used the standard 15-watt increment each minute (Hansen et al., 1984). A modified Bruce protocol was used for the treadmill subjects (Bruce et al., 1973, 1979). All subjects were encouraged to continue exercising as long as they could. Because oxygen consumption was measured as an indicator of workload, it was not necessary to attempt to match the external mechanical stresses of bicycle and treadmill. We judged when maximal exercise had been achieved from a heart rate greater than 90% of that predicted for at least 20 seconds and/or a stable oxygen uptake during at least two 1-minute increments of workload. Oxygen pulse was calculated from oxygen uptake divided by heart rate. Alveolar-to-arterial oxygen differential and physiological dead space were calculated from blood and expired-gas measurements, using standard formulas (Furuike et al., 1982). Maximum values were defined as the highest values reached by the subject during any 30-second period of measurement.

Predicted Values

The following predicted values were proposed by Hansen et al. (1984):

Weight (kg) = 0.79 x [height (cm) - 60.7]
Maximal heart rate = 210 - 0.65 x age

Predicted maximum oxygen consumption = observed weight x (50.75 - 0.372 x age)

Predicted maximum oxygen pulse = predicted maximum oxygen uptake divided by predicted maximal heart rate.

The predicted maximum values were corrected on the basis of the subject's observed-to-predicted weight relationship. For this, we separated our population into five groups, selected from the relationship of their actual to their predicted weight, using the criteria of Hansen et al. (1984). For treadmill data, we used 100% of these values; for bicycle ergometer data, 90%.

INTERPRETATION

Radiography

Posteroanterior, lateral and oblique radiographs, taken at full inspiration within 1 month after the exercise test, were interpreted by at least three observers who did not know the exercise data. One was an experienced ILO category "B" reader. Observations were reported as normal, pleural disease, or parenchymal disease with profusion of 1/0 or greater, using ILO criteria (ILO, 1980). Some patients had combined pleuroparenchymal disease.

Pulmonary-Function Tests

Obstructive abnormalities were defined as those that had an FEV_1/FVC relationship of more than 1.6 SD below predicted values. A restrictive abnormality was defined as one that resulted from a TLC decrement of more than 1.6 SD below that predicted. If the latter was combined with obstructive dysfunction, restriction was usually not evident (Barnhart et al., 1988).

Alveolar-to-Arterial Oxygen Pressure Differential [$P(A\text{-}a)O_2$]

The 94 asbestos-exposed workers in whom blood-gas measurements were made were divided into four groups (Table 2) to study the alveolar-to-arterial oxygen differential during exercise in relation to the extent of the changes shown by radiography (ILO score). We also wished to determine whether that differential discriminated between asbestosis and COPD. We assumed that pleural plaques were indicative of asbestos exposure, but that they were without functional significance. No diffuse pleural thickening was found in these subjects.

Because ventilation/perfusion abnormalities are exacerbated as blood flow increases (Jones and Campbell, 1982), we attempted to standardize the $P(A\text{-}a)O_2$ for this effect. We did not measure cardiac output, so we used the oxygen consumption ($\dot{V}O_2$) at each level of exercise as a reflection of pulmonary blood flow and divided the $P(A\text{-}a)O_2$ by the $\dot{V}O_2$.

Table 2. Radiographic and ventilatory criteria for 94 subjects who had blood gas measurements made during exercise.

Group	Number	ILO Profusion[a]	Pulmonary Function
Normal	40	<1/1	Normal pulmonary function at rest
Chronic obstructive pulmonary disease (COPD) without asbestosis	29	<1/1	FEV_1/FVC[b] = 1.6 SD or more below predicted
Asbestosis alone	22	>1/0	Normal FEV_1/FVC
COPD with asbestosis	3	>1/0	FEV_1/FVC = 1.6 SD or more below predicted

[a]Radiographic score (ILO = International Labour Office; see ILO, 1980)
[b]Forced expiratory volume in 1 second/forced vital capacity

Exercise Tests

Using arbitrary criteria (Table 3), we evaluated whether exercise limitation was primarily caused by a ventilatory, cardiac, pulmonary vascular or peripheral circulatory abnormality. A single patient may sometimes have a limitation in more than one system.

STATISTICS

Data were analyzed by analysis of variance and Student's *t*-tests. A value of $P < 0.05$ was considered significant. When comparing one group with another of the test groups, a P value of <0.0125 was considered significant (Remington and Schork, 1970).

RESULTS

The alveolar-to-arterial oxygen pressure differential widened with increasing ILO score (Figure 1). This parameter discriminated between asbestosis and COPD ($P < 0.01$) and also differentiated ($P < 0.05$) between those with asbestosis and normal subjects (Figure 2). The $P(A\text{-}a)O_2/\dot{V}O_2$ was specific when values were greater than 35 mm Hg/L (Figure 3); however, its sensitivity was poor, in that it identified only 8 of 26 patients presumed to have asbestosis.

Table 3. Ventilatory and cardiac limitation criteria and scores of subjects while performing exercise.

Limitations	Positive	Score
VENTILATORY LIMITATION at exercise maximum	≥4	
Positive MVV[a] impaired (i.e., greater of MVV measured or FEV_1[b] x 40 ≤ 80% of predicted value) *and* $\dot{V}E_{max}$[c] ≥ 80% of impaired MVV *or* $\dot{V}E_{max}$ ≥ 70 to 79% of impaired MVV		4
When maximum exercise not achieved (because of poor effort or other causes). Positive MVV impaired *and* $\dot{V}E_{max}$ estimated from $\dot{V}E/\dot{V}O_2$ and predicted $\dot{V}O_{2max}$ (corrected for weight; Goldman and Becklake, 1959) ≥ 80% of impaired MVV.[c]		2
$\Delta P_{a_{CO_2}}$ from start of exercise to limit ≥ 3 mm Hg, with pH unchanged or decreasing		4
or $P_{a_{CO_2}}$ ≥ 45 mm Hg, with pH unchanged or decreasing		2
CARDIAC LIMITATION	≥4	
Blood pressure falls with heart rate over 120 beats per minute; $P_{systolic}$ and $P_{diastolic}$ fall ≥ 10 mm Hg		3
If only $P_{systolic}$ available, fall ≥ 10 mm Hg *but* $P_{systolic}$ fall constant with $P_{diastolic}$		2
O_2 pulse (O_2P) with hemoglobin ≥ 10 g/100 ml. O_2P below prediction for age, sex, height and weight by 1 SD or more.		4
Angina, severe enough to limit the test, *with* electrocardiograph ST-wave change ≥ 1 mm		4
or angina, severe during test and continuing for at least 3 minutes after exercise		1
ST-wave depression ≥ 3 mm (not a curved depression), persisting for at least 2 minutes		3
or ST-wave elevation ≥ 1 mm (plateau elevation		3
Lesser ST-wave depression (3 to 2 mm)		1
Sustained atrial or ventricular tachycardiac arrhythmia		4
or premature ventricular contraction, doubling in rate or occurring more than 20 times/min		1
PULMONARY VASCULAR LIMITATION	≥4	
$P(A\text{-}a)O_2$ more than 35 mm Hg during exercise		1
or $P(A\text{-}a)O_2$ increasing during exercise to between 35 and 45 mm Hg		2
or increasing during exercise to 45 mm Hg or more		3
or oximeter desaturation ≥ 3% without $P_{a_{CO_2}}$ elevation		2
Volume of dead space/tidal volume (VD/VT) not decreasing during exercise		1
or VD/VT increasing to 30 to 59% during exercise		3
or VD/VT increasing to ≥ 60% during exercise		4
PERIPHERAL CIRCULATORY LIMITATION	≥4	
Intermittent claudication, severe enough to stop test, with other (i.e., Doppler) confirmation of peripheral vascular disease		4

[a]Maximum voluntary ventilation
[b]Forced expiratory volume in 1 second
[c]Maximum expiratory volume; predicted from $\dot{V}E/\dot{V}O_2$ (expiratory volume/oxygen consumption) in 9% of subjects)
[d]Alveolar-to-arterial oxygen pressure differential

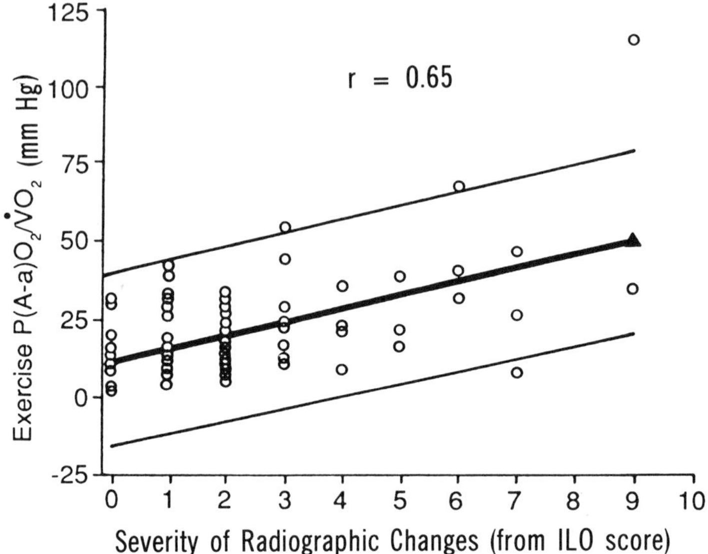

Figure 1. Relationship between alveolar-to-arterial oxygen pressure differential/ oxygen consumption [$P(A\text{-}a)O_2/\dot{V}O_2$ (functional impairment)] and severity of radiographic changes (ILO score). Significant at r = 0.65.

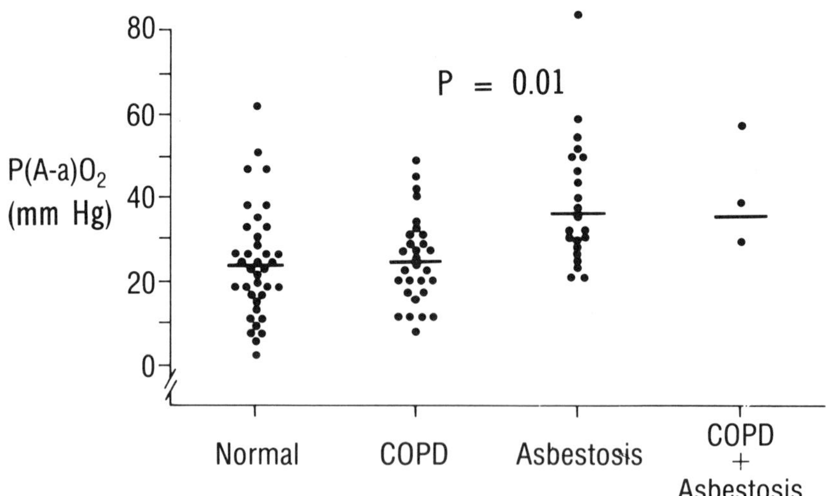

Figure 2. Alveolar-to-arterial oxygen pressure differential on exercise in asbesetos-exposed subjects in four groups: normal; with chronic obstructive pulmonary disease (COPD); with asbestosis; with COPD and asbestosis.

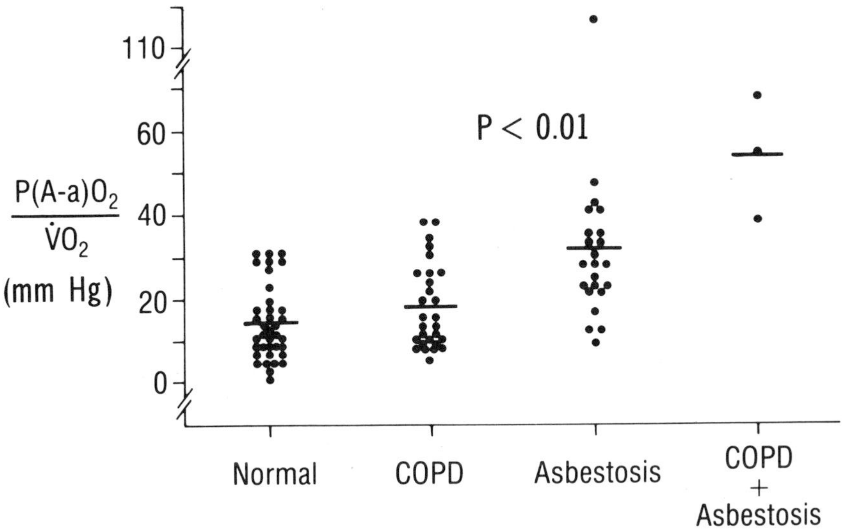

Figure 3. Data from subjects described in Figure 2, after correcting for increased blood flow. See text for details.

Half (49.2%) of the subjects had only normal limitation to exercise. Of those who had abnormal limitation, more were caused by a cardiac (37%) than a ventilatory (26%) abnormality. Combined cardiac and ventilatory limitations were slightly more frequent than a ventilatory limitation alone (14 versus 12%). Ventilatory limitations were more frequent with obstructive than with restrictive abnormalities, and they were more frequent in smokers and ex-smokers than in nonsmokers.

DISCUSSION

The radiographic changes which, we assumed, reflected the presence and severity of asbestosis proved to be related to the functional $P(A\text{-}a)O_2$ impairment shown by these asbestos-exposed workers.

Although the mechanical problem of asbestos-related lung disease is generally thought to be caused largely by restrictive lung disease, the percentage of subjects in our study with such a restrictive abnormality was low (25%). However, if COPD was present, a restriction might not have been apparent (Barnhart et al., 1988). When asbestosis was established according to ILO criteria, the alveolar-to-oxygen pressure differential divided by the oxygen consumption was highly specific when above 35, as demonstrated by the observation that only 2 of the 65 patients without asbestosis would have been considered abnormal. Thus, an alveolar-to-arterial oxygen pressure differential (normalized for blood flow) of 35 or above on exercise strongly suggested asbestosis, although some increase in that measurement occurred in patients with COPD. However, our categorization of these subjects was inexact, and it is likely that subjects with mild and radiographically unrecognizable degrees of asbestosis were included in both the normal and COPD groups.

Only 31 (26%) of the subjects appeared to have a ventilatory limitation, and 24 of the 31 were cigarette smokers. By contrast, 45 of our subjects (37%) had a cardiac limitation; and 17 (14%) had a combined cardiac and ventilatory limitation. These results must be interpreted with caution, because this was a retrospective study, and our scoring system for exercise limitation was arbitrary and incomplete.

Our results are similar to those of Howard and co-workers (1982) who also reported that half of their subjects with dyspnea did not show objective criteria of exercise limitation. Our results were also remarkably similar to those of Sue et al. (1985) and Pearle (1981) in relation to smoking. In our subjects whose exercise performance was limited, more were limited by cardiovascular problems than by ventilatory defects. Only 9% of the nonsmokers had ventilatory limitations, in contrast with 32% of smokers and 22% of ex-smokers. (The two nonsmokers with ventilatory limitation also had obstructive abnormalities, probably asthma.) Thus, objectively documented exercise limitation from restrictive ventilatory abnormalities was an uncommon finding in these workers who were claiming compensation for asbestos-induced breathlessness.

REFERENCES

Adams, L, N Chronos, R Lane, and A Guz. **1985.** The measurement of breathlessness induced in normal subjects: Validity of two scaling techniques. Clin Sci 69:7-16.

American Medical Association. 1984. *Guides to Evaluation of Permanent Impairment,* Vol. 85, 2nd Edition. American Medical Association, Council on Scientific Affairs, Chicago, IL, 101 p.

American Thoracic Society. 1979. Snowbird Workshop on Standardization of Spirometry. Am Rev Respir Dis 119:831-838.

Barnhart, S, LD Hudson, SE Mason, DJ Pierson, and L Rosenstock. **1988.** Total lung capacity. An insensitive measure of impairment in patients with asbestosis and chronic obstructive pulmonary disease Chest 93:299-302.

Becklake, MR. **1976.** Asbestos related diseases of the lung and other organs. Their epidemiology and implications for clinical practice. Am Rev Respir Dis 114:187-226.

Bruce, RA, F Kusimi, and D Mosmer. **1973.** Maximal oxygen intake and monographic assessment of functional aerobic impairment in cardiovascular disease. Am Heart J 85:546-562.

Bruce, RA, K Mossak, F Kusimi, and J Clark. **1979.** Acute effect of oral propranolol on hemodynamic response to upright exercise. Am J Cardiol 44:132-140.

Furuike, A, DY Sue, J Hansen, and K Wasserman. **1982.** Comparison of physiologic dead space/tidal volume ratio and alveolar arterial PO_2 difference during incremental and constant work exercise. Am Rev Respir Dis 126:578-583.

Goldman, H and MR Becklake. **1959.** Respiratory function test: Normal values at medium altitudes and the prediction of normal results. Am Rev Tuberc 79:457-467.

Hansen, JE, DY Sue, and K Wasserman. **1984.** Predicted values for clinical exercise test. Am Rev Respir Dis 129 (Suppl):549-555.

Howard, J, Z Mohsenifar, HV Brown, and SK Koerner. **1982.** Role of exercise testing in assessing functional respiratory impairment due to asbestos exposure. J Occup Med 24:685-689.

ILO (International Labour Office). **1980.** Guidelines for the use of ILO international classification of radiographs of pneumoconiosis. In: *Occupational Safety and Health Series,* Number 22. International Labour Office, Geneva, Switzerland.

Jones, ML and EM Campbell. **1982.** *Clinical Exercise Testing,* 2nd Edition. WB Saunders, Philadelphia, PA.

Kory, RC, R Callahan, HG Boren, and JC Syner. **1961.** The Veterans Administration cooperative study of pulmonary function. 1. Clinical spirometry in normal man. Am J Med 30:243-258.

Lindgren, I, B Mueller, and EA Gaensler. **1965.** Pulmonary impairment and disability claims. J Am Med Assoc 194:499-506.

Morgan, WK. **1979.** Clinical significance of pulmonary function test. Disability or disinclination—impairment or importuning? Chest 75:6.

Morris, JF, A Kosky, and LC Johnson. **1971.** Spirometric standards for healthy non-smoking adults. Am Rev Respir Dis 103:57-67.

Pearle, J. **1981.** Exercise performance and functional impairment in asbestos-exposed workers. Chest 80:701-705.

Remington, RD and MA Schork. **1970.** *Statistics with Application to the Biological and Health Sciences.* Prentice Hall, New York, NY.

Sue, DY, A Oren, JE Hansen, and K Wasserman. **1985.** Lung function and exercise performance in smoking and nonsmoking asbestos-exposed workers. Am Rev Respir Dis 132:612-618.

U. S. Department of Labor. 1974. Occupational exposure to cotton dust. Final mandatory occupational safety and health standard. Appendix D: Pulmonary function standards. Fed Reg 43:122.

Effect of Cigarette-Smoking on the Cardio-respiratory Reponses to Exercise in Young Men and Middle-Aged Asbestos Workers

Karlman Wasserman, Darryl Y. Sue, Ami Oren, Gregory L. Hirsch, Terry E. Robinson, and James E. Hansen

Division of Respiratory and Critical Physiology and Medicine, Department of Medicine, Harbor-UCLA Medical Center, 1000 W. Carson St., Torrance, CA 90509

---

*Dr. Wasserman's presentation at the symposium is summarized in the following abstract. The information has been published previously.**

ABSTRACT

To determine the acute action of cigarette-smoking on cardiorespiratory function under stress, the immediate effects of cigarette-smoking on the ventilatory, gas exchange, and cardiovascular responses to exercise were studied in nine healthy male subjects. Each subject performed an incremental exercise test to exhaustion on two separate days, one without smoking (control) and one after smoking 3 cigarettes/hour for 5 hours. The order of the two tests was randomized. Arterial blood gases and pH were measured during rest and all levels of exercise; CO blood levels confirmed the absorption of cigarette smoke. In addition, minute ventilation (V_E), end-tidal P_{CO_2} and P_{O_2}, O_2 uptake (V_{O_2}), CO_2 production, directly measured blood pressure, electrocardiogram, and heart rate (HR) were recorded every 30 seconds. The dead space-to-tidal volume ratio V_D/V_T), maximal aerobic capacity ($V_{O_{2max}}$), and the anaerobic threshold (*AT*) were determined from the gas exchange data. Cigarette-smoking resulted in a significantly lower $V_{O_{2max}}$, *AT*, and (V_{O2}/HR, (O_2 pulse) and a

---

*Sue et al., Am. Rev. Respir. Dis. *132:*612-618 (1985); Hirsch et al., J. Appl. Physiol. *58:*1975-1981 (1985).

significantly higher HR, pulse-pressure product, and pulse pressure ($P < 0.05$) compared with the control. Additionally, a trend toward a higher V_D/V_T and arterial-end-tidal P_{CO_2} difference was found during exercise after smoking. We conclude that cigarette-smoking causes immediate detrimental effects on cardiovascular function during exercise, including tachycardia, increased pulse-pressure product, and impaired O_2 delivery to the exercising muscles. The acute effects on respiratory function were less striking and were primarily limited to abnormalities reflecting ventilation-perfusion mismatching. Because the cardiovascular effects of smoking seen during exercise are similar to those seen in subjects exposed to CO and nicotine, we believe that the adverse acute effects of cigarette smoke on exercise performance are likely due to the effects of these two substances.

Because cigarette-smoking can complicate the evaluation of impairment caused by exposure of aerosolized occupational toxins, and because cigarette-smoking is common and cigarettes are implicated in obstructive lung disease and cardiovascular diseases, we assessed the contribution of smoking to functional abnormalities in a group of asbestos-exposed shipyard workers. Seventy-three workers who never smoked were paired with 73 current smokers, by age and asbestos exposure. Pulmonary function and performance during cycle incremental exercise were compared between the two groups. Nonsmokers had significantly higher VC, FEV_1, FEV_1/VC, and diffusing capacity for CO than did smokers. Only 3 of the 73 nonsmokers, but 23 of the 73 smokers, had a FEV_1/VC below the 95% confidence limit of predicted value. During exercise, despite the fact that there was no difference in maximal heart rate, the maximal O_2 uptake ($V_{O_{2max}}$) and oxygen-pulse were lower among smokers than among nonsmokers. In addition, smokers more frequently had an abnormal alveolar-arterial O_2 differential at maximal exercise. Of 33 smokers who had a $V_{O_{2max}} < 80\%$ of predicted, 16 were judged to have cardiac disease, whereas only 2 appeared to be limited by obstruction. Only 15 of the 73 nonsmokers had a $V_{O_{2max}} < 80\%$. We conclude that cigarette-smoking was the major contributing factor to the obstructive lung disease observed in asbestos workers, and it also had a strong influence on the occurrence, nature, and magnitude of exercise limitation. An asbestos worker's history of cigarette-smoking has an important effect on the assessment of impairment from asbestos.

DEPOSITION AND CLEARANCE OF INHALED PARTICLES: MACROPHAGES

Physical Factors Affecting Lung Deposition of Cigarette Smoke (with Syncarcinogenic Radon Progeny Effects) and Mineral Fibers*

Ted B. Martonen,[1] Werner Hofmann,[2] and Imre Balásházy[3]

[1]Toxicology Branch, Inhalation Toxicology Division, Health Effects Research Laboratory, U.S. Environmental Protection Agency, Research Triangle Park, NC 27711

[2]Center for Extrapolation Modeling, Duke University Medical Center, Durham, NC 27710 (Permanent Address: Abteilung für Biophysik, Universität Salzburg, Hellbrunnerstr. 34, A-5020 Salzburg, Austria)

[3]International Atomic Energy Agency Postdoctoral Fellowship, U. S. Environmental Protection Agency, Research Triangle Park, NC 27711 (Permanent Address: Radiation Protection Department, Central Research Institute for Physics, H-1525 Budapest, Hungary)

KEY WORDS: pulmonary deposition, cigarette smoke, cloud settling, radon progeny, mineral fibers, syncarcinogenesis

---

ABSTRACT

We will address the unusual dynamic factors affecting the behavior and fate of inhaled cigarette-smoke particles and mineral fibers within the human lung. The actions of interception for fiber particles, and cloud-settling for concentrated cigarette smoke, can enhance focal deposition in locations that would not have been anticipated for dilute aerosols or for the more regularly shaped, sphere-like particles. It is important to quantitate the efficiencies of these deposition

*The research described in this article has been reviewed by the Health Effects Research Laboratory, U.S. EPA, and approved for publication. Approval does not signify that the contents necessarily reflect the views and policies of the Agency nor does mention of trade names or commercial products constitute endorsement or recommendation for use.

mechanisms because it is *after* deposition that deleterious biological effects can occur. Here, we present theoretical deposition models that simulate the actions of the interception and cloud-settling processes, which are validated by comparison with *in vitro* and *in vivo* data. The sites of preferential deposition are regions whose cells receive increased doses of hazardous substances associated with smokes and fibers. They must, therefore, be considered in risk-assessment analyses of human inhalation exposures to airborne toxicants. Incorporation of these mechanisms in aerosol therapy protocols—the reverse of the usual inhalation toxicology concerns—could conceivably lead to improved therapeutic procedures, by which medication would be preferentially deposited at desired target locations within the lung so as to achieve optimal effects.

INTRODUCTION

The primary physical mechanisms that influence the deposition of inhaled particulate matter are inertial impaction, sedimentation, and diffusion. In our contribution to this international symposium, we shall focus on rather rare physical processes that influence the regional dispersion patterns of cigarette-smoke particles and mineral fibers.

The geometric shape of a fiber results in the introduction of another effective deposition mechanism, interception. Deposition may occur when a rod-shaped particle's center of mass remains on a fluid streamline, because a portion of it can still come in contact with an airway's surface. Interception is relatively insignificant for more regularly shaped particles. Here, we compare the efficacy of theoretical equations predicting the efficiency of the interception mechanism with experimental observations.

A cigarette-smoke aerosol also has a relatively uncommon feature that affects its motion. Deposition studies performed using a surrogate tracheobronchial airway system have indicated that the smoke particles, predominantly submicron-size, are preferentially deposited at upper airway branching sites, or bifurcations. Furthermore, deposition studies conducted with human test subjects have suggested enhanced deposition of cigarette smoke *in vivo*. In this work we present a mathematical theory describing the occurrence of cloud-settling, which promotes cigarette-smoke deposition in agreement with laboratory findings. Since cigarette-smoke particles contain chemical carcinogens and radionuclides, cells located within bifurcations receive increased exposure. This, together with possible synergistic effects of ambient radon progeny, may explain the increase in clinical observations of bronchogenic tumors in uranium miners who smoke relative to those observed in the general population.

The simultaneous physical interaction of the phenomenon of cloud-settling and interception may lead to preferential deposition of an inhaled aerosol mass of mixed (i.e., mineral fibers and cigarette-smoke particles) composition, resulting in delivery of a relatively increased dose to airway cells located within bifurcations. This increased dose may be of significance and is a subject worthy of further investigation regarding potential biological interactions.

BASIC PARTICLE MOTION AND INTERACTIONS

Single-Particle Kinetics

For airborne particles that have relatively regular geometric forms (i.e., not agglomerate or fiber-like in dimensions), the most efficient deposition mechanisms are inertial impaction, sedimentation, and diffusion (Figure 1). Inertial impaction [denoted (A)] is predominant when particles carried by the airstream have sufficient momentum to deviate from fluid streamlines and impact on airway surfaces. Sedimentation (B) predominates in the lower, more peripheral airways of the lung, where airflow velocities have been sufficiently reduced—for a given inspiratory flow rate—so that particle residence times in airways permit gravity to exert its effect. For submicron-size particles, the dominant mechanism of deposition is diffusion (C), or random Brownian motion. Other mechanisms of deposition, depending on the physical, physicochemical and electrical properties of the inhaled particles and the exposure conditions, include electrophoresis, etc., thermophoresis, etc. (Mercer, 1973) and, as we will discuss, interception and cloud-settling.

The motion of assemblages of particles has been studied extensively by Happel and Brenner (1973). Here, we will address only the topics most relevant to our proposed simulation of the phenomenon of cloud-settling.

The terminal settling velocity of an isolated solid spherical particle in a motionless fluid under viscous flow conditions may be expressed by Stokes' Law (Stokes, 1845, 1846) as:

$$U_p = \frac{g \rho_p D_p^2}{18 \mu} , \tag{1}$$

where ρ_p and D_p are the particle's density and geometric diameter, respectively; g is the gravitational constant; and μ is the fluid's absolute viscosity. The conditions necessary for equation (1) to be applicable to the size range of particles relevant to inhalation toxicology have been detailed by Fuchs (1964). The numerator of equation (1) may, if necessary, be modified by a slip correction factor, as originally proposed by Cunningham (1910), in this form: $1 + 1.63/\lambda/r_p$, where λ is the mean free path of air molecules and r_p "... the effective radius of the particle, inasmuch as it is assumed to be large compared with the molecule" (Cunningham, 1910).

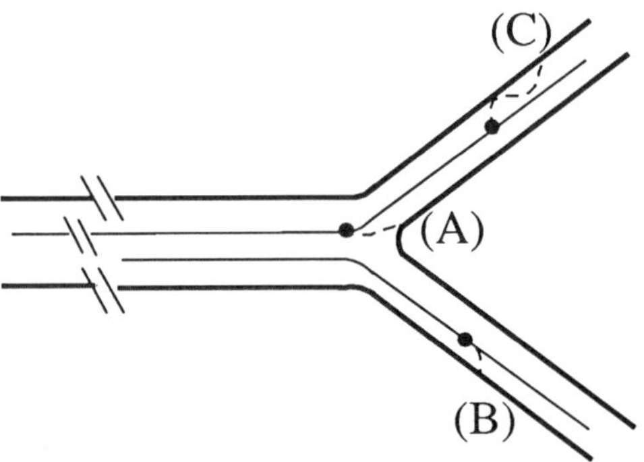

Figure 1. Primary deposition mechanisms for regularly shaped particles in a respiratory tract passage: (A) inertial impaction; (B) sedimentation; and (C) Brownian motion.

For a liquid droplet of viscosity μ' that settles in the fluid, equation (1) now becomes:

$$U_p = \frac{g\rho_p D_p^2}{18\,\mu}\left\{\frac{3\mu' + 3\mu}{3\mu' + 2\mu}\right\} . \tag{2}$$

The velocity of the droplet is greater than that of a similarly sized solid particle because the resistive drag force acting on it is lessened by the internal currents induced by tangential friction forces (Figure 2). Equation (2) was derived independently by two investigators: Rybczynski and Hadamard, both of whom published in 1911; but these publications are difficult to obtain, so we have included in our references the citation for von Smoluchowski (1912) where the derivation of the equation is also given.

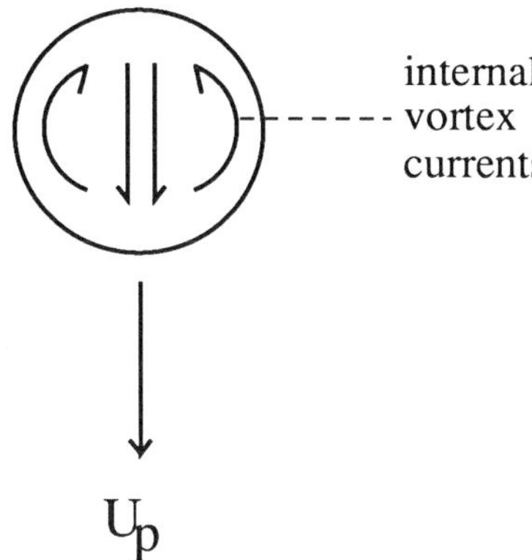

Figure 2. Circulating currents within a liquid droplet that are caused by external drag forces.

Transitional Particle/Fluid Motion

The introduction of another particle, solid or droplet, in the vicinity of the first has the effect of enhancing the rate of sedimentation (U_p') of both particles via mutual hydrodynamic interactions (Figure 3), of the form:

$$\frac{U'_p}{U_p} = 1 + \frac{3D_p}{8d}\left\{1 + cos^2\theta + \left(\frac{D_p}{2d}\right)^2\left(\frac{1}{3} - cos^2\theta\right)\right\}, \qquad (3)$$

where θ is the angle between the line-of-centers between the particles and the vertical, and d is the distance between the centers. Other terms are as defined previously. Consideration of additional particles results in increasingly complex equations describing individual motion.

Whether particles are solid or liquid, their presence alters the physical properties of the fluid entraining them. For example, Einstein,* in 1906 and 1911, showed that the viscosity, μ_s, of a

*See citation for Einstein (1956), where the subject is discussed in English.

dilute, uniform suspension of spherical particles may be expressed as:

$$\mu_s = \mu \left\{ 1 + \frac{5}{2} \phi \right\} \tag{4}$$

where μ, as before, is the viscosity of the fluid, and ϕ is the volume fraction of particles present.

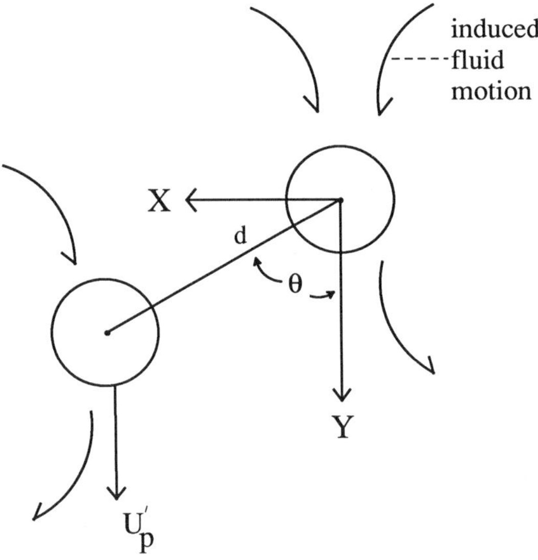

Figure 3. Hydrodynamic interactions between two moving particles.

Aerosol Dynamics

Particle kinetics and related fluid dynamics are described in numerous publications. Even a cursory review of the subject is beyond the focus of our work. We therefore refer the reader interested in more information to Lamb (1932), Fuchs (1964), and Reist (1984).

When we investigate the settling of an array of particles within a "bounded" medium such as the air occupying the lung, it is important to distinguish between particles that are distributed throughout the fluid and particles that are not. Although the settling particles create fields that tend to increase the velocities of neighboring particles, mass conservation within the closed system requires that a fluid flow field exist (in an opposite sense to the particulate matter) to compensate for the settling particles and dragged fluid. If particles are dispersed, then settling will be slower because the compensating flow must penetrate, rather than bypass, the particle array. This may be termed hindered settling. If the particles are not dispersed, this compensating flow occurs mainly in particle-free regions and will not effectively retard particle settling. The resistance to a fluid flowing through a spatial arrangement of particles increases with the number of particles in a given volume. As long as flow continues, individual particle settling, even when modified by mutual hydrodynamic interactions, can exist. Soon, however, the path of least resistance for the fluid will be to flow partially around the space occupied by the particles rather than to completely penetrate the particle array (Fuchs, 1964). At this point, the particle array starts to become an entity and attains a certain velocity that is superimposed on the settling velocities of the individual particles. This effect continues to increase with the addition of particles in the space. Finally, as the concentration is further increased, individual particle settling is completely masked as fluid no longer penetrates the array but, rather, flows around it. At this stage, cloud-settling occurs, and its motion may be considered that of a fluid sphere settling through a surrounding fluid of different material properties [equations (2) and (4); Figure 4].

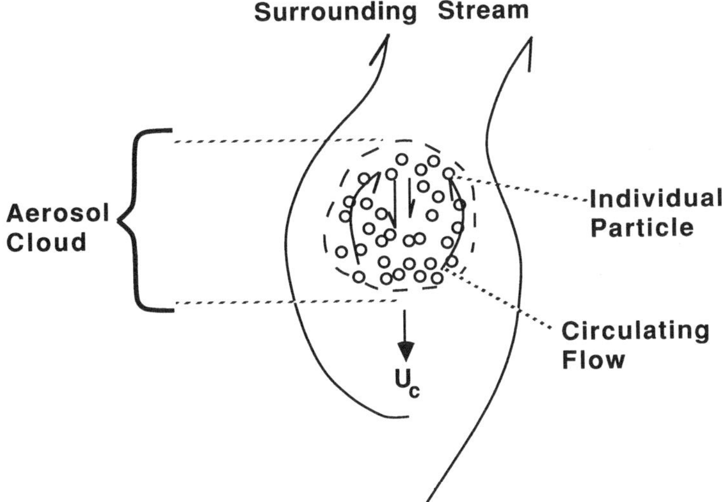

Figure 4. Aerosol cloud-settling at sufficient particle concentration to exhibit aerodynamic properties that are relatively independent of component particles.

Von Smoluchowski (1912) expressed the settling velocity of a spherical cloud, U_c, in an "unbounded" (for mathematical simplicity) medium as:

$$U_c = \frac{2g\rho_c R_c^2}{9\mu}\left\{\frac{3\mu_c + 3\mu}{3\mu_c + 2\mu}\right\} , \tag{5}$$

where μ_c is the viscosity of the cloud in the bracketed correction term, equation (2); and, ρ_c and R_c are the density and geometric radius of the cloud, respectively. (The concepts of bounded versus unbounded fluid dynamics problems are definite, important distinctions, from engineering perspectives.) He assumed that the cloud was dilute and, therefore, that the fractional solid volume, ϕ, was negligible, and $\mu_c = \mu$ [equation (4)]. The cloud's density, or particulate mass concentration (relative to the surrounding medium), could be expressed as:

$$\rho_c = N_p\rho_p\left(\frac{r_p}{R_c}\right)^3 \tag{6}$$

where N_p is the total number of particles in the cloud. Equation (5) could then be rewritten as:

$$U_c = \frac{4gN_p\rho_p r_p^3}{15\mu R_c} \tag{7}$$

emphasizing the constituent particulate properties. Von Smoluchowski (1912) pointed out that Stokes' Law (Stokes, 1845, 1846) is not an accurate description of particle motion unless cloud-settling is *not* significant, a condition formulated as $U_c << U_p$, or, from equations (1) and (7):

$$\frac{6N_p r_p}{5R_c} << 1 \tag{8}$$

for particle-settling. At the time of his derivation, there were no experimental data to validate the theoretical findings.

Apparently unaware of von Smoluchowski's (1912) theoretical work (i.e., it was not cited), Slack (1963a,b) conducted tests which, we believe, demonstrated the existence of cloud-settling experimentally, although he did not use that terminology. He examined the sedimentation under gravity of spherically shaped suspensions of spherical Diakon® particles in still air. The investigations revealed that 50-cm-diameter monodisperse suspensions, which contained as little as 2 g of particulate matter of geometric diameter $< 64\ \mu m$, developed and sustained internal circulations. These currents were directed upward at the periphery of the suspensions and downward at their center, as illustrated in Figure 2 for a liquid droplet. We surmise that the existence of these circulatory flow patterns indicated that air was flowing around rather than penetrating the arrays of settling particulate matter. For 10-μm particles that settled in the experiments, with $\rho_p = 1.18$ g cm^{-3}, the total number of particles in the suspension was approximately $N_p = 3 \times 10^9$, so that the condition of equation (8) is not satisfied. Von Smoluchowski's (1912) earlier theoretical model, now substantiated, thus predicted the interactive particle motion and cloud-settling effects observed later by Slack (1963a,b) in the laboratory.

To express the influence of particulate mass concentration, ρ_c, on the transition from single-particle motion to hydrodynamic interactions, the onset of cloud-settling [equation (8)] may be put in the form:

$$\frac{6\,\rho_c}{5\,\rho_p}\left(\frac{R_c}{r_p}\right)^2 << 1 \quad . \qquad (9)$$

In the previously mentioned tests of Slack (1963a,b) the value of ρ_c was 3.1×10^{-5} g/cm^3, at cloud-settling conditions.

Interception

There is, of course, a wide range of potentially hazardous fibers, ranging from naturally occurring mineral fibers, such as forms of asbestos, to man-made glass fibers (Joint ACGIH-AIHA Aerosol Hazards Evaluation Committee, 1975; HEW, 1976; Spurny, 1983).

For airborne mineral fiber particles, a significant deposition mechanism is termed interception. Interception is important when a particle can contact an airway wall even though its center of mass remains on a fluid streamline. Of course, particle orientation is a most relevant factor to consider in computing the deposition efficiency of mineral fibers. In Figure 5 we illustrate three specific instances of rod-shaped particle motion relative to fluid flow patterns. For (A), we assume the fiber is arranged longitudinally to the entraining fluid motion. For (B), the particle is in an assigned spatial fix, perpendicular to a streamline transporting it. We consider (C) a randomly moving fiber. (A) and (B) may be considered limiting conditions, but a tumbling fiber may be a more probable, realistic case.

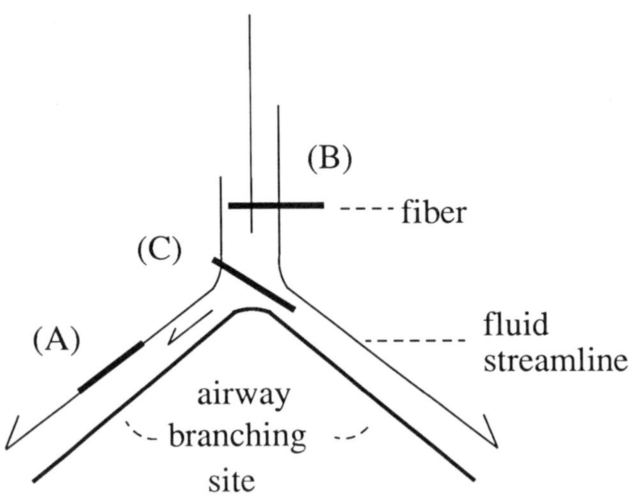

Figure 5. Fiber deposition at an airway branching site.

Timbrell (1965) demonstrated experimentally that there is no preferential orientation for fibers with an aspect ratio (i.e., a length-to-diameter ratio) of less than 5, while rod-like fibers tend to align themselves with the streamlines if their aspect ratio is larger than 5. For aligned rod-like inhaled fibers, the key deposition parameter of the interception mechanism is the fiber's diameter rather than its length, and the depth that the fibers penetrate within the airway system is determined by their aerodynamic equivalent diameter (defined as the geometric diameter of a unit density sphere having the same terminal settling velocity [see equation (1)] as the particle considered). The aerodynamic equivalent diameter and the terminal settling velocity obviously depend on the orientation of a fiber relative to the fluid within which it is moving.

Harris and Fraser (1976) have proposed mathematical expressions for the probability of the interception deposition mechanism of straight, cylindrical fibers at airway bifurcations and at the entrance of alveoli as functions of airway geometry and fiber characteristics for different airflow profiles and fiber orientations. Later, Harris and Timbrell (1977) extended this mathematical concept to incorporate irregularly shaped or aggregated fibers. While Harris and Fraser (1976) assumed that all deposition mechanisms that act on fibers are independent from one other, Harris and Timbrell (1977) considered the simultaneous actions of impaction and interception. In a recent theoretical effort, we have developed a model for the simultaneous action of impaction, sedimentation, and interception deposition of fibers in a single-bend tube of circular cross-section that simulates an airway bifurcation (Balásházy et al., submitted).

Recently, Myojo (1987) measured the deposition of glass fibers in a single bifurcation (branching angle, 45°) of a machined brass model, which corresponded approximately to the junction between generations 3 and 4 of Weibel's (1963) lung Model A. In Myojo's (1987) tests considered here, the length of the fibers was 20 to 40 μm, with an average diameter of 0.52 μm. Although the density of the fibers was not reported in the manuscript, we derived a value of 1.28 g/cm^3 from the published aerodynamic equivalent diameter for random orientation of fibers within the bifurcation. In our mathematical simulations of these experimental data, we assumed that interception occurs only within a distance $D_d/4$ of the downstream airway, with diameter D_d, from the airflow dividing point, or carinal ridge.

In Figure 6, our model predictions are compared to Myojo's (1987) experimental results, presenting the deposition velocity as a function of the distance from the carina along the inner part of a downstream airway. The measured deposition velocity lies between the calculated values for the deposition of fibers moving parallel to the streamlines [(A), Figure 5] and those for randomly oriented fibers [(C), Figure 5]. This finding is supported by the experimental results of Timbrell (1965) for symmetrical fibrous particles and by the scanning electron microscope illustrations made by Myojo (1987). It is important that the maximum deposition velocity occurs at the carinal ridge, suggesting that potential deleterious effects of inhaled fibers arise preferentially at bifurcation sites.

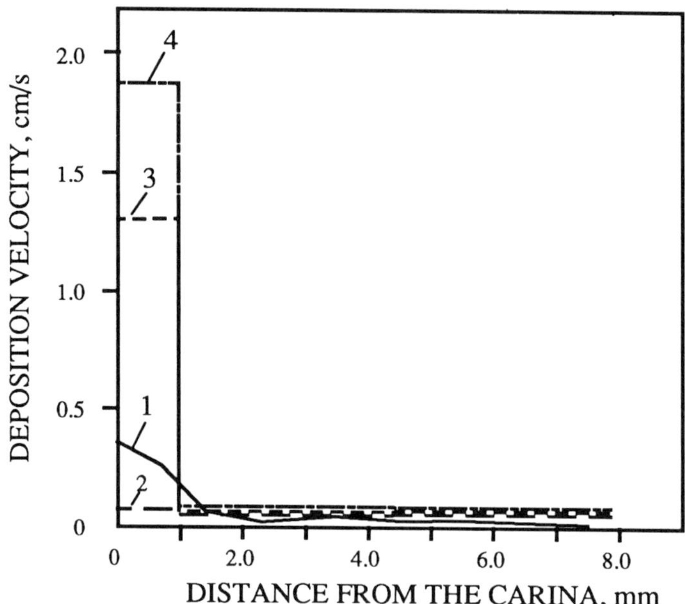

Figure 6. Predicted and measured (plot 1) fiber deposition within a surrogate bifurcation. (Computations are for fiber orientations, relative to fluid streamlines [see Figure 5], of longitudinal, or parallel [plot 2], random [plot 3], and perpendicular [plot 4] alignment.)

CIGARETTE-SMOKE DEPOSITION

The heterogeneous patterns in which inhaled particles are deposited within lung airways are of importance to our text. We must therefore define a few morphological terms for subsequent applications and refer to certain particle-size parameters of cigarette smoke for deposition considerations.

Following Weibel's (1963) symmetrical, dichotomously dividing lung Model A, we will assume that an airway branching site consists of a "parent" that divides into two "daughters." The daughters will consist of two tubular segments with a common bifurcation zone (Figure 7). The carinal ridge is the airstream divider at the junction of the daughter airways, within the bifurcation zone.

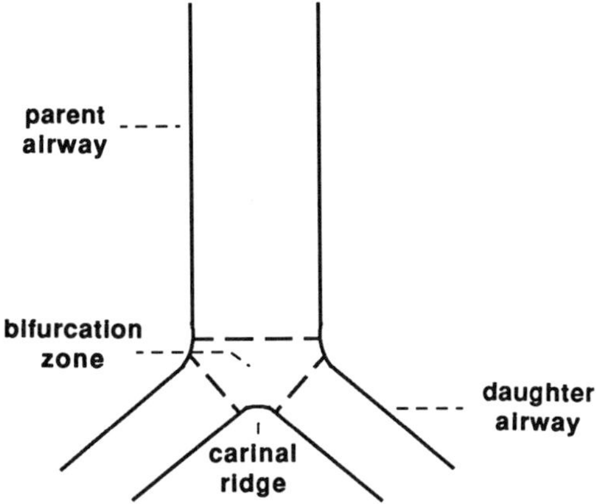

Figure 7. Branching region between airways of succeeding generations.

The work of Sam (1956) and Keith and Derrick (1960) suggests that cigarette smoke has aerodynamic equivalent diameters in the 0.1- to 1.0-μm range, the most prevalent (based on number frequency) being 0.2 to 0.25 μm. One may expect that aerosols of this size may penetrate the oro- and nasopharyngeal, laryngeal and large, upper bronchial airway regions of the human respiratory tract before being deposited in the more peripheral airways of the tracheobronchial tree and distal pulmonary passages (Task Group on Lung Dynamics, 1966; Lippmann and Albert, 1969; Heyder et al., 1986).

In Vitro Experiments

Ermala and Holsti (1955) studied the deposition of tobacco smoke in full-scale plaster models of the human respiratory tract. Locations of enhanced deposition were detected in the mouth and throat, the larynx, and at airway bifurcation zones (Figure 7) in large bronchi.

Complementary studies, using Silastic® silicone rubber surrogates of human oropharyngeal/laryngeal/upper tracheobronchial regions have been performed by Martonen and Hofmann (1986) and Martonen et al. (1987). (The oropharyngeal unit, a new component to systems used in previous experiments [Martonen, 1983; Martonen and Lowe, 1983], was incorporated to simulate smoke-mixing before entering the lung proper.) Aerosol dispersion through a surrogate during a test was controlled by an integrated system of rotameters and vacuum pumps (see Figure 1; Martonen et al., 1987). The findings confirmed the earlier Ermala and Holsti (1955) data and revealed two additional sites of preferential deposition for cigarette smoke. Highly localized particle deposition occurred at carinal ridges within upper bronchial bifurcation zones and on the posterior surfaces of the tubular segments of daughter airways. These elements of a deposition pattern were visible within the tracheobronchial tree of a surrogate (see Figure 2; Martonen and Hofmann, 1986).

Deposition experiments conducted with surrogate airway models (Martin and Jacobi, 1972) and laryngeal/tracheobronchial replica casts (Schlesinger et al., 1974) have investigated the extent to which submicron-sized aerosols are concentrated within the bifurcation zones (relative to neighboring airway locations) of several generations of upper bronchi. Although the tests were not conducted with cigarette smoke, some particle size diameters were comparable to the major constituents of smoke: 0.2 to 0.4 μm (see Figure 7; Martin and Jacobi, 1972), and 0.26 to 0.28 μm (see Table 1 and Figure 3; Schlesinger et al., 1974).

In Vivo Experiments

There is clinical evidence that carcinogenic tumors occur primarily in the main, lobar and segmental airways of the human lung (Bryson and Spencer, 1951; Herman and Crittenden, 1961; Garland, 1961; Garland et al., 1962). Additional findings (Kotin and Falk, 1959; Auerbach et al., 1961) are consistent with the theory that such cancers may originate within bifurcations. However, it is impossible to establish with certainty the preferential morphological sites of cancer, as most tumors are detected only in advanced stages.

In the Ermala and Holsti (1955) studies, and in the Martonen and Hofmann (1986) and Martonen et al. (1987) experiments, the upper surrogate bronchial airways, where deposition was enhanced, corresponded to *in vivo* main, lobar, segmental, and first-generation subsegmental bronchi. This may relate to the predilection of lung carcinomas for certain locations, as noted above. Indeed, Ermala and Holsti (1955) wrote that "... a striking parallelism becomes apparent ..." when the distribution of tobacco tar in their surrogate model was compared with the frequency of cancer noted clinically. Moreover, Schlesinger and Lippmann (1978) have referred to the strong correlation between the clinically observed incidence of tumors among the five lobar bronchi of the human lung and the aerosol patterns they measured within laryngeal/tracheobronchial replica casts (see their Figure 1). Although their deposition tests were not conducted with cigarette smoke, some experiments were done using particles ranging in diameter from 0.26 to 1.2 μm, that is, diameters similar to those of cigarette-smoke particles.

Hicks et al. (1986) conducted inhalation exposure experiments with human volunteers to investigate the influence of hygroscopicity on the dynamics of aerosol deposition. The possible effect of hygroscopic particle growth on the deposition of cigarette smoke in human lungs was noted earlier by Davies (1974). The results of their investigation of two aerosols, mainstream cigarette smoke, and sodium chloride, are presented in Figure 8. Aerosol sizes were measured directly with a quartz-crystal microbalance cascade impactor before inhalation and after exhalation. The authors calculated a growth factor of approximately 1.7 for inhaled cigarette-smoke particles, whereas sodium chloride aerosols grew by a factor of about 4.5. Nevertheless, the deposition of comparably sized inhaled smoke particles was much greater.

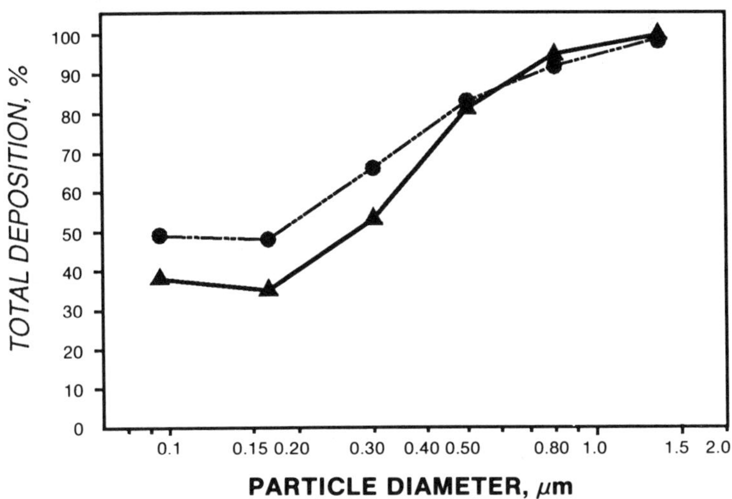

Figure 8. Comparison of hygroscopic aerosol deposition in human subjects: ● = cigarette smoke inhalation exposures, and ▲ = sodium chloride.

Because of the difference in growth factors, Hicks et al. (1986) expected the two aerosols to have different deposition patterns. However, the minimal total deposition for both aerosols occurred with particle sizes of about 0.15 μm. This suggested to the authors that, "... there are other mechanisms contributing to the deposition pattern of cigarette smoke," although no explanations were given.

Cloud-Settling in the Lung and in Surrogate Models

Martonen (1977) showed that the particulate number [for use in equation (8)] and mass [for use in equation (9)] concentrations of cigarette smoke are $N_p \simeq 3 \times 10^9$ particles/cm^3 and $\rho_c \simeq 10^{-4}$ g/cm^3, respectively. Those determinations were based on the cigarette-smoke characterization studies of Sam (1956), Keith and Derrick (1960), and Keith and Tesh (1966; see also Stöber et al., 1978). Smoke, therefore, has sufficient constituent particles, in terms of number and/or mass, for the cloud-settling effect to occur; see Slack, 1963a,b for magnitudes of relevant comparable physical parameters. It is possible that cloud-settling within the lungs of the human subjects of Hicks et al. (1986) may partially explain their findings, especially because we shall introduce a mechanistic and mathematical basis for cloud-settling motion of dense aerosols. Similarly, the enhanced deposition of cigarette smoke in the simulated respiratory tracts of Ermala and Holsti (1955), Martonen and Hofmann (1986), and Martonen et al. (1987) is consistent with the proposed action of cloud-settling.

We surmise that the onset of cloud-settling within a bounded medium like that within the lung and the surrogate models depends on a physical situation which permits fluid to flow around a spatial array of particles. This is possible when a free surface exists at an interface between a particle array and its entraining medium. The formation, size, and shape of a cloud will depend primarily on the given fluid dynamics and geometry of a specific problem. The magnitude of the cloud-settling effect will depend on the particle concentration of the aerosol. Parenthetically, Martonen (1977) demonstrated the existence of cylindrical clouds in aerosol spectrometers (instruments used to aerodynamically characterize airborne particles).

Flow separation, which occurs when an airstream is disjoined from a bounding surface, takes place as inhaled air passes through the narrow glottic aperture of the larynx and enters the trachea in the form of a laryngeal jet (Chan et al., 1980; Martonen, 1986). Flow separation has been observed by Schroter and Sudlow (1969) in idealized laboratory models and replica casts of bifurcations of the human lung and reported by Pedley et al. (1977) in other investigations performed at the Physiological Flow Studies Unit of Cambridge University. The respective authors used a variety of airway geometries and flow patterns to simulate physiological conditions. A mathematical basis for flow separation was theorized by Lakin and Fox (1974), who analyzed fluid dynamics at airway branching sites in the tracheobronchial network. We hypothesize that, within the lung, replica casts, and surrogate models, the onset of flow separation may initiate cloud-settling.

SYNCARCINOGENIC EFFECTS: CIGARETTE SMOKE AND RADON PROGENY

For cigarette-smokers, the etiology of lung cancer may be affected by synergistic carcinogenic interactions following exposure to naturally occurring ambient radon progeny. We speak of "synergism" if the combined effect of two toxic agents is given by the product of the two individual responses.

A recent analysis (Whittemore and McMillan, 1983) of lung-cancer mortality among a cohort of Caucasian uranium miners in the Colorado plateau demonstrates the synergism between concurrent exposure to cigarette smoke and radon progeny. The relative risk factor, R, is expressed as a multiplicative function:

$$R = (1 + 0.31 \times 10^{-2}\, WLM)(1 + 0.51 \times 10^{-3}\, Pk) \quad , \quad (10)$$

where a miner's total exposure to radon decay products (daughters) is given in units of working level months (WLM), and packages of cigarettes (Pk) are counted from the start of exposure until 10 years before the subject's current age.

Cigarette smoke may, however, have a paradoxical effect on concurrent exposure to radon progeny. Experimental data on beagle dogs (Cross et al., 1982) indicate a possible protective role of cigarette smoke, which could be ascribed to a stimulatory effect on the mucociliary clearance process, although the opposite effect has been observed in heavy, long-term human smokers. The protective effect may arise from increased mucus production, which provides a thicker protective barrier, thereby limiting exposure of underlying sensitive cells. Possibly, such factors may slightly reduce the lung-cancer risk from radiation kinetics alone, but it seems unlikely that they compensate for the synergistic mechanism of cigarette smoke and radon daughters.

Experiments with rodents have shown that the sequence in which cigarette smoke and radon exposures are administered is important (Cross, 1984). It appears that the absorbed energy of deposited radon progeny is the initiating event and that cigarette smoke has a promotional effect. This would explain the earlier occurrence of lung cancer by stimulated proliferation of cells that have already been transformed by ionizing radiation and/or other carcinogens, including chemical substances.

Earlier histological studies have noted highly localized preneoplastic and neoplastic lesions at airway bifurcations following inhalation exposures to cigarette smoke and other environmental pollutants (Kotin and Falk, 1959; Auerbach et al., 1961). In a study of lung-tissue specimens from deceased smokers, highly concentrated deposits of ^{210}Po were found in the bifurcation-zone epithelium of large bronchial airways (Little et al., 1965). The authors concluded that alpha-radiation emitted from ^{210}Po may be an important factor in the initiation of bronchial cancers in smokers. Martell (1983) attributed the high incidence of malignant transformations at airway bifurcations in cigarette smokers to the cumulative alpha-radiation dose resulting from enhanced deposition of insoluble ^{210}Po-enriched particles produced in burning cigarettes, as well as to ambient radon progeny inhaled between cigarettes or that contained in mainstream cigarette smoke. The latter idea has been developed and is presented in more detail by Martonen and Hofmann (1986), Martonen et al. (1987), and Hofmann and Martonen (in press).

Mucociliary clearance may be significantly slowed, or reduced in efficiency, at airway branching sites. A reduced rate of mucociliary clearance at the first tracheobronchial bifurcation with marked accumulations of deposited particles at the carina has been observed in laboratory test animals (Gore and Patrick, 1978; Svartengren et al., 1981). In man, the rate of mucociliary clearance is slower within bronchial bifurcations, at least down to the level of segmental and subsegmental bronchi (Macklin, 1956; Hilding, 1957).

Based on the deposition and clearance patterns at airway bifurcations described above, we have developed a dosimetry model in which each airway generation is divided into three distinct compartments: (1) two tubular airway segments with normal clearance rates, (2) a bifurcation zone (excluding the contiguous carina) with reduced clearance efficiency, and (3) a carinal ridge without clearance (Hofmann and Martonen, in press). Our calculations suggest that the combined effect of enhanced radionuclide deposition and reduced clearance at bronchial bifurcations (relative to tubular airway segments) may lead to highly localized accumulations of radon progeny within bifurcation zones and, subsequently, to concentrated radiation doses being delivered to sensitive progenitor cells located at such sites.

It is important, we believe, that both inhaled radon progeny and cigarette smoke exhibit, qualitatively, the same nonuniform dose patterns. Assuming that cigarette smoke acts mainly as a promoting agent, the effect of cigarette smoke on lung-cancer induction by inhaled radon progeny in the three compartments of an airway generation (lobar bronchi) is illustrated in Table 1. The lung-cancer risk for each exposure regimen is normalized to the integer 1, assuming: (1) that risk is proportional to the annual radiation dose for environmental radon-progeny exposure and also proportional to the local retention pattern for cigarette-smoke inhalation, and

(2) that radiation and cigarette smoke interact in a synergistic, i.e., multiplicative, fashion. These calculations clearly demonstrate that the predicted nonuniformity of radiation-induced lung-cancer risk is aggravated by the interaction with cigarette smoke.

Table 1. Lung-cancer risk from radon progeny and cigarette smoke as a function of aerosol exposure and airway morphology.

	Lung Cancer Risk (%)		
Exposure Protocol	Tubular Airway Segments	Bifurcation Zone	Carinal Ridge
Radon progeny	7.34	18.80	73.85
Cigarette smoke	0.56	8.69	90.76
Radon progeny and cigarette smoke	0.06	2.38	97.56

SUMMARY AND CONCLUSIONS

Cloud-settling is a physical phenomenon in which a finite population of particles that occupy a discrete region of space settles at a rate exceeding the terminal settling speed (Stokes, 1845, 1846) of a constituent particle of the cloud, even when modified by hydrodynamic interaction from surrounding particles. Cloud-settling, and the extent to which it influences individual particle trajectories, has been discussed by von Smoluchowski (1912) and demonstrated by Martonen (1977) in aerosol particle-sizing instruments and, we believe, by the engineering particle physics laboratory tests of Slack (1963a,b). Moreover, we propose that cloud-settling may explain the previously mentioned data anomalies observed by Hicks et al. (1986) in human subjects and the enhanced cigarette-smoke deposition observed in surrogate lungs by Ermala and Holsti (1955), Martonen and Hofmann (1986), and Martonen et al. (1987). The separation of flow at bifurcations within the bronchial tree, as observed *in vitro,* may permit the formation of aerosol clouds within the human lung. Such upper airway sites are known to have enhanced deposition *in vitro* and increased incidence of cancer *in vivo.* It seems reasonable to recommend, therefore, that further efforts be made to establish the significance of the cloud-settling mechanism on the distribution of inhaled particulate matter. Assuming that such formation does occur, our simple analytical model has been developed, which predicts that cloud-settling will take place unless equations (8) and (10) are valid. The theoretical model predicts that cigarette smoke may have to be significantly diluted before the influence of cloud-settling on the deposition of cigarette-smoke particles in the lung can be ignored.

Because of the correlation between clinically observed bronchial carcinomas and enhanced deposition at these sites that was detected *in vitro,* we propose that the tumors develop there because cigarette smoke is *initially* deposited at corresponding bronchial locations *in vivo.* This is in contrast to the most popular current school of thought: that the submicron-sized cigarette-smoke particles are originally deposited in more distal regions of the lung and are subsequently transported to and accumulate at upper bronchial bifurcations, primarily because of reduced mucociliary clearance at those sites.

Regarding simultaneous exposure to radon progeny and cigarette smoke, we surmise that interactions may increase the absolute number of lung-cancer cases [see equation (10)] and affect the relative distribution within a given generation of the respiratory tree (Table 1). Considering the role of mucociliary clearance, perhaps the significance of cloud-settling is greater for short-lived radionuclides than for chemical carcinogens. This may be the case for ^{210}Po, a naturally occurring component of cigarette smoke, or for syncarcinogenic effects of interactions between cigarette smoke and ambient radon progeny, which occur within residences and workplaces.

Exposure to mineral fibers may act in a manner similar to that discussed above for cigarette smoke. Thus, concurrent inhalation of fibers, by smokers and nonsmokers alike, may also synergistically increase the probability of lung-cancer induction from naturally occurring radon progeny.

REFERENCES

Auerbach, O, AP Stout, EC Hammond, and L Garfinkel. **1961.** Changes in bronchial epithelium in relation to cigarette smoking and in relation to cancer. N Engl J Med 265:253-267.

Balásházy, I, W Hofmann, and TB Martonen. Fiber deposition in an airway bifurcation: Simultaneous action of interception, impaction and sedimentation deposition mechanisms. Submitted to J Aerosol Sci.

Bryson, CC, and H Spencer. **1951.** Carcinoma of the bronchus. Q J Med 20:173-186.

Chan, TL, RM Shreck, and M Lippmann. **1980.** Effect of the laryngeal jet on particle deposition in the human trachea and upper bronchial airways. J Aerosol Sci 11:447-459.

Cross, FT. **1984.** Radioactivity and cigarette smoke. Health Phys 46:205-208.

Cross, FT, RF Palmer, RE Filipy, GE Dagle, and BO Stuart. **1982.** Carcinogenic effects of radon daughters, uranium ore dust and cigarette smoke in beagle dogs. Health Phys 42:33-52.

Cunningham, E. **1910.** On the velocity of steady fall of spherical particles through fluid medium. Proc R Soc London 83:357-365.

Davies, CN. **1974.** Deposition of inhaled particles in man. Chem Ind 1:441-444.

Einstein, A. **1956.** *The Theory of Brownian Movement.* Dover, New York, NY.

Ermala, P and LR Holsti. **1955.** Distribution and absorption of tobacco tar in the organs of the respiratory tract. Cancer 8:673-678.

Fuchs, NA. **1964.** *The Mechanics of Aerosols.* Pergamon Press, Oxford, England.

Garland, LH. **1961.** Bronchial carcinoma. Lobar distribution of lesions in 250 cases. Calif Med 940:7-8.

Garland, LH, RL Beier, W Coulson, JH Heald, and RL Stein. **1962.** The apparent sites of origin of carcinomas of the lung. Radiology 78:1-11.

Gore, DJ and G Patrick. **1978.** The distribution and clearance of inhaled UO_2 particles on the first bifurcation and trachea of rats. Phys Med Biol 23:730-737.

Happel, J and H Brenner. **1973.** *Low Reynolds Number Hydrodynamics.* Noordhoff International Publishing, Leyden, The Netherlands.

Harris, RL, Jr and DA Fraser. **1976.** A model for deposition of fibres in the human respiratory tract. Am Ind Hyg Assoc J 37:73-89.

Harris, RL, Jr and V Timbrell. **1977.** The influence of fibre shape in lung deposition—Mathematical estimates, pp. 75-89. In: *Inhaled Particles IV,* WH Walton (ed.). Pergamon Press, Oxford, England.

Herman, DL and M Crittenden. **1961.** Distribution of primary lung carcinomas in relation to time as determined by histochemical techniques. J Natl Cancer Inst 27: 1227-1271.

HEW Publication No. (NIOSH) 76-151. **1976.** Occupational exposure to fibrous glass, Proceedings of a Symposium. Superintendent of Documents, U.S. Government Printing Office, Washington, D.C.

Heyder, J, J Gebhart, G Rudolf, CF Schiller, and W Stahlhofen. **1986.** Deposition of particles in the human respiratory tract in the size range 0.005-15 μm. J Aerosol Sci 17:811-825.

Hicks, JF, JN Pritchard, A Black, and WJ Megaw. **1986.** Experimental evaluation of aerosol growth in the human respiratory tract, pp. 244-247. In: *Aerosols: Formation and Reactivity.* Pergamon Press, Oxford, England.

Hilding, AC. **1957.** Ciliary streaming in the bronchial tree and the time element in carcinogenesis. N Engl J Med 256:634-640.

Hofmann, W. and TB Martonen. The significance of enhanced radionuclide deposition at bronchial bifurcations. Ann Occup Hyg **(in press)**.

Joint ACGIH-AIHA Aerosol Hazards Evaluation Committee. **1975.** Background documentation on evaluation of occupational exposure to airborne asbestos. Am Ind Hyg Assoc J 36:91-103.

Keith, CH and JC Derrick. **1960.** Measurement of the particle size distribution and concentration of cigarette smoke by the "Conifuge." J Colloid Interface Sci 15:340-356.

Keith, CH and PG Tesh. **1966.** Measurement of the total smoke issuing from a burning cigarette. Tob Sci 61-64.

Kotin, P and HL Falk. **1959.** The role and action of environmental agents in the pathogenesis of lung cancer. I. Air pollutants. Cancer 12:147-163.

Lakin, MB and VG Fox. **1974.** Transient flow characteristics in an idealized bronchial bifurcation. Respir Physiol 21:101-117.

Lamb, H. **1932.** *Hydrodynamics* (Sixth Edition). Dover, New York, NY.

Lippmann, M and RE Albert. **1969.** The effect of particle size on the regional deposition of inhaled aerosols in the human respiratory tract. Am Ind Hyg Assoc J 30: 257-275.

Little, JB, EP Radford, Jr, HL McCombs, and VR Hunt. **1965.** Distribution of polonium 210 in pulmonary tissues of cigarette smokers. N Engl J Med 273:1343-1351.

Macklin, CC. **1956.** Induction of bronchial cancer by local massing of carcinogen in outdrifting mucus. J Thorac Surg 31:238-244.

Martell, EA. **1983.** Alpha-radiation dose at bronchial bifurcations of smokers from indoor exposure to radon progeny. Proc Natl Acad Sci USA 80:1285-1289.

Martin, D and W Jacobi. **1972.** Diffusion deposition of small-sized particles in the bronchial tree. Health Phys 23:23-29.

Martonen, TB. **1977.** *Aerosol Characterization in a Spinning Spiral Duct Centrifuge,* Ph.D. Thesis. University of Rochester, Rochester, NY.

Martonen, TB. **1983.** Measurements of particle dose distribution in a model of a human larynx and tracheobronchial tree. J Aerosol Sci 14:11-22.

Martonen, TB. **1986.** Surrogate experimental models for studying particle deposition in the human respiratory tract: An overview, pp. 547-568. In: *Aerosols: Research, Risk Assessment and Control Strategies,* SD Lee, T Schneider, LD Grant, and PJ Verkerk (eds.). Lewis Publishers, Inc., Chelsea, MI.

Martonen, T and W Hofmann. **1986.** Factors to be considered in a dosimetry model for risk assessment of inhaled particles. Radiat Protect Dosim 15:225-232.

Martonen, TB, W Hofmann, and JF Lowe. **1987.** Cigarette smoke and lung cancer. Health Phys 52:213-217.

Martonen, TB and J Lowe. **1983.** Assessment of aerosol deposition patterns in human respiratory tract casts, pp. 151-164. In: *International Symposium on Aerosols in the Mining and Industrial Work Environment,* B Liu and V Marple (eds.). Ann Arbor Science, Ann Arbor, MI.

Mercer, TT. **1973.** *Aerosol Technology in Hazard Evaluation,* pp. 159-185. Academic Press, New York, NY.

Myojo, T. **1987.** Deposition of fibrous aerosols in model bifurcations. J Aerosol Sci 18:338-347.

Pedley, TJ, RC Schroter, and MF Sudlow. **1977.** Gas flow and mixing in the airways, pp. 163-265. In: *Lung Biology in Health and Disease.* Marcel Dekker, Inc., New York, NY.

Reist, PC. **1984.** *Introduction to Aerosol Science.* McGraw-Hill Book Co, New York, NY. [Russian edition, Mir Publishers; Moscow, 1987.]

Sam, A. **1956.** *A Study of Particle Size Distribution and Dilution of Cigarette Smoke,* Ph.D. Thesis. Duke University, Durham, NC.

Schlesinger, RB, VR Cohen, and M Lippmann. **1974.** Studies of intrabronchial particle deposition using hollow bronchial casts, pp. 116-127. In: *Experimental Lung Cancer: Carcinogenesis and Bioassays,* E Karbe and JF Park (eds.). Springer-Verlag, New York, NY.

Schlesinger, RB and M Lippmann. **1978.** Selective particle deposition and bronchogenic carcinoma. Environ Res 15:424-431.

Schroter, RC and MF Sudlow. **1969.** Flow patterns in models of human bronchial airways. Respir Physiol 7:341-355.

Slack, GW. **1963a.** Sedimentation of compact clusters of uniform spheres. Nature 200:466-467.

Slack, GW. **1963b.** Sedimentation of a large number of particles as a cluster in air. Nature 200:1306.

Spurny, KR. **1983.** Measurement and analysis of chemically changed mineral fibers after experiments *in vitro* and *in vivo.* Environ Health Perspect 51:343-355.

Stöber, W, TB Martonen, and S Osborne, Jr. **1978.** On the limitations of aerodynamical size separation of dense aerosols with the spiral duct centrifuge, pp. 263-278. In: *Recent Developments in Aerosol Science.* J. Wiley and Sons, New York, NY.

Stokes, GG. **1845.** On the theories of the internal friction of fluids in motion and of the equilibrium and motion of elastic solids. Cambridge Philosoph Trans IX, Pt II: 8-106.

Stokes, GG. **1846.** On the effect of the internal friction of fluids on the motion of pendulum. Cambridge Philosoph Trans IX, Pt II: 287-305.

Svartengren, M, K Widtskiöld-Olsson, K Philipson, and P Camner. **1981.** Retention of particles on the first bifurcation and trachea of rabbits. Bull Eur Physiopathol Respir 17:87-91.

Task Group on Lung Dynamics. 1966. Deposition and retention models for internal dosimetry of the human respiratory tract. Health Phys 12:173-207.

Timbrell, V. **1965.** The inhalation of fibrous dusts. Ann NY Acad Sci 132:255-273.

von Smoluchowski, MS. **1912.** On the practical applicability of Stokes' Law of resistance and modifications of it required in certain cases, pp. 192-201. In: *Fifth International Conference of Mathematics,* Vol. 2. Cambridge University, England.

Weibel, ER. **1963.** *Morphometry of the Lung.* Springer-Verlag, West Berlin, Federal Republic of Germany.

Whittemore, AS and A McMillan. **1983.** Lung cancer mortality among U.S. uranium miners: A reappraisal. J Natl Cancer Inst 71:489-499.

Inhalation Experiments on Retention and Lung Clearance of Asbestos in Combination with Cigarette-Smoking

Hartwig Muhle,[1] Bernd Bellmann,[1] Kvetoslav R. Spurny,[2] and Friedrich Pott[3]

[1]Fraunhofer-Institut für Toxikologie und Aerosolforschung, Hannover, Federal Republic of Germany

[2]Fraunhofer-Institut für Umweltchemie und Ökotoxikologie, Schmallenberg, Federal Republic of Germany

[3]Medizinisches Institut für Umwelthygiene, Düsseldorf, Federal Republic of Germany

KEY WORDS: asbestos, crocidolite, cigarette-smoking, inhalation, exposure, pulmonary retention, lung clearance, rat

---

ABSTRACT

Rats received nose-only exposure to 11.4 mg/m^3 UICC crocidolite and 2.5 mg/m^3 UICC chrysotile A for 2 hours a week for a period of up to 1 year. One-half of the animals also inhaled cigarette smoke, diluted 1:5 with filtered air, twice daily for 34 minutes at a time, 5 days a week.

Long-term lung clearance of a radioactively labeled aerosol was determined after 2 and 9 months of exposure. Cigarette-smoking decreased lung clearance of inhaled labeled particles. After 2, 6 and 12 months of exposure, the animals were sacrificed, and organs were ashed in a low-temperature ashing furnace. The number of fibers, and their length and diameter distribution, were examined in both tissue samples and in samples of exposure-chamber air, using a scanning electron microscope.

Results showed a factor-of-two increase of crocidolite fibers in the lungs of groups also exposed to cigarette smoke, compared to the animals that did not inhale cigarette smoke. No such effect of cigarette-smoking was found on chrysotile fiber retention. The difference between these results may be due to the different deposition patterns of the two fiber types.

The slowing of alveolar clearance is probably of minor importance for the synergistic effect of smoking and asbestos inhalation in humans, because the majority of lung cancers develop in the ciliated airways.

INTRODUCTION

The combination of cigarette-smoking and asbestos inhalation leads to a synergistic effect of bronchogenic tumor induction but not to an increased incidence of mesothelioma (Selikoff et al., 1968; Hammond et al., 1979). Why do these differences exist in epidemiologic findings

There are various hypotheses to explain these observations. Three of them are:

- Fiber retention in lungs is increased by cigarette-smoking. This effect could be caused by the reduced clearance reported for smokers (Cohen et al., 1979; Bohning et al., 1982).
- Cigarette smoke and asbestos react on lung cells by a special mechanism, e.g., by adsorption of carcinogenic substances onto the fibers and enhanced transport to target molecules.
- Penetration of fibers into the basal layer of the epithelium of the upper airways is increased after impairment of clearance by cigarette-smoking.

The objective of this study was to test the first hypothesis.

Some of the data presented here were reported at a Congress of the Verein Deutscher Ingenieure (Muhle et al., 1983).

MATERIALS AND METHODS

Fiber Exposure

Standard UICC samples of chrysotile A, originating from Zimbabwe, and crocidolite, from South Africa, were used. A vibrating-bed aerosol generator was used to produce the fiber aerosol (Spurny et al., 1975). The core of this device is a vibrating tube that is filled with fibers; air is blown from underneath and carries out the fibers. The frequency and amplitude of the vibrations can be changed to optimize aerosol production. The fiber aerosol concentration in the study is shown in Table 1. The process of aerosol generation resulted in a higher concentration for crocidolite than for chrysotile.

Table 1. Characterization of fiber exposure.

Fiber Type	Aerosol Concentration (mg/m³)	Fiber Concentration (Number of Fibers/ml)	Concentration of Fibers Longer than 5 μm	Calculated Median Aerodynamic Diameter (μm)
Crocidolite	11.1 ± 4.3	15,900 ± 5200	1500 ± 600	0.85
Chrysotile	2.5 ± 1.2	5,000 ± 1200	1600 ± 500	1.08

The aerodynamic diameter was calculated according to Harris and Fraser (1976), based on length and diameter of the fibers. The aerosol was discharged by a ^{85}Kr source before entering a nose-only exposure chamber that could house up to 24 rats.

Exposures to fibers were for 1 hour a day, twice a week for up to 12 months. After exposure, rats were kept in Makrolon® cages containing softwood chips as bedding. The animals had free access to feed and water except when being exposed to asbestos or cigarette smoke.

Analysis of Fibers

The number of fibers and their size distribution were determined monthly by collecting samples from the exposure chamber on Nuclepore® filters.

Rats were sacrificed by anesthesia with 50 mg/kg body weight pentobarbital and subsequent exsanguination. The lungs were isolated, weighed, dried, and ashed in oxygen plasma. The lung ash was weighed, suspended in 5% HCl and filtered on a Nuclepore® filter (pore size, 0.2 μm). The filter was sputtered with gold and analyzed for fibers at a magnification of 3000 to 5000X. One hundred fifty fibers per sample were analyzed.

Analysis of chrysotile is difficult because the fibers can split into fibrils while in the lungs and/or during sample preparation. The size of the fibrils is sometimes smaller than the detection limit of the scanning electron microscope.

Cigarette Smoke

Special research cigarettes (Type E 76) were smoked according to the German standard DIN 10240 in a Hamburg-type smoking machine (H. Burghart, Hamburg). The smoke was diluted 1:5 by filtered air before being inhaled by the animals. The concentration of CO in the exposure chamber was about 1500 ppm. Animals were exposed via nose-only tubes twice a day for 34 minutes, at a time interval of about 5 hours, 5 days a week, up to 12 months. At 6 minutes after exposure, the CO-hemoglobin level was about 40%. The value had decreased to 5% by 2 hours after exposure. The animals were not exposed simultaneously to cigarette smoke and fibers. Control animals were sham-exposed to clean air.

Minute Volume

The animals were anesthetized with 40 mg/kg pentobarbital, and the tidal volume was determined in a whole-body plethysmograph.

Labeled Particles

The effect of fiber and cigarette-smoke exposure on deep lung clearance was investigated by using a labeled test aerosol of iron oxide ($^{59}Fe_2O_3$). This test aerosol was inhaled by nose-only exposure for 1 hour at 2 and 9 months after the start of the study.

Particles of iron oxide can be used for this purpose because they show negligible secondary biological effects in lungs and their solubility is relatively low. Their mass median aerodynamic diameter was about 0.25 μm. Over a period of up to 75 days after inhalation of the labeled iron oxide, lung clearance was measured by the decrease of gamma-activity in the thoracic area with a sodium iodide scintillation detector. Results were corrected for physical decay. Exposure continued throughout this period of 75 days. The spatial dissolution of the measuring geometry was not sufficient to distinguish between tracheobronchial and alveolar clearance. Quantitative evaluation of the data was limited to 15 to 75 days after exposure to the labeled particles. In this time period, the fast clearance processes of the upper respiratory tract can be ignored. Because alveolar clearance of iron oxide particles is considered a macrophage-mediated activity, it was used to determine the impairment of macrophage-mediated clearance. The method is described by Gibb and Morrow (1962) and by Bellmann et al. (1983).

Study Design

The study was designed to investigate retention and clearance but not carcinogenicity. Only limited histopathology was performed.

Female Wistar rats, weighing 180 to 200 g each at the beginning of the experiment, were purchased from Winkelmann, West Germany. Besides the unexposed control group, there were five groups. They were exposed, respectively, to (1) cigarette smoke,

(2) crocidolite, (3) crocidolite plus cigarette smoke, (4) chrysotile, or (5) chrysotile plus cigarette smoke. Usually, six rats per group were exposed for 2, 6 or 12 months, respectively. The total number of rats in the control group was 42.

Statistical Analysis

Data for body weights, clearance rates, and retained fibers were evaluated by Student's *t*-test. Results were considered statistically significant if the P value of the test statistic was <0.05.

For determining the alveolar clearance rate, k, an exponential curve ($y = a \cdot e^{-kt}$) was applied to the data for each animal from day 15 to about day 75 after exposure to the labeled particles. The statistical analysis was performed on the resulting k-values. For clarity, the corresponding half-times are given, using the following approximations:

$$t_{\frac{1}{2}}\,(mean) = \frac{ln\,2}{k\,(mean)} \tag{1}$$

$$t_{\frac{1}{2}}\,(SD) = \frac{k\,(SD)}{k\;mean} \cdot t_{\frac{1}{2}}\,mean\;. \tag{2}$$

RESULTS

Body Weight and Minute Volume

Body weights of rats after 2, 6, and 12 months of the study are presented in Table 2. Cigarette-smoking significantly reduced body weights by 5 to 15% compared to those of sham-exposed animals. Minute volumes in anesthetized animals were consistently lower in all smoke-exposed groups than in the sham-exposed control group (Table 3). This reduction was not statistically significant because of the relatively large standard deviation, which may have been influenced by individual differences in the effect of the anesthetic. Reduced minute volume is important because it leads to fewer inhaled fibers.

Alveolar Clearance

Figure 1 shows alveolar clearance in rats as a function of time and cigarette-smoke exposure. Table 4 shows half-times of alveolar clearance, demonstrating reduced alveolar clearance after 9 months of exposure to cigarette smoke.

Table 2. Body weight (mean ± SD) of rats exposed by inhalation to mineral fibers and/or cigarette smoke.

	Body Weight (g)					
Exposure	At 2 Months	Number of Animals	At 6 Months	Number of Animals	At 12 Months	Number of Animals
Control	224 ± 16	42	262 ± 27	20	265 ± 25	14
Cigarette smoke	212 ± 17[a]	12	207 ± 19[a]	6	238 ± 17[a]	6
Crocidolite	232 ± 18	12	230 ± 17	6	264 ± 21	6
Crocidolite plus cigarette smoke	208 ± 13[a]	12	209 ± 12[a]	6	229 ± 12[a]	6
Chrysotile	225 ± 20	12	232 ± 17	6	257 ± 25	6
Chrysotile plus cigarette smoke	210 ± 16[a]	12	212 ± 22[a]	6	215 ± 17[a]	6

*Statistically significantly different from controls, $P < 0.05$.

Table 3. Minute volume (mean ± SD) during the same study as in Table 2.

	Minute Volume (ml/min)					
Exposure	At 2 Months	Number of Animals	At 6 Months	Number of Animals	At 12 Months	Number of Animals
Control	129 ± 33	42	116 ± 30	20	104 ± 22	14
Cigarette smoke	119 ± 12	11	105 ± 25	6	87 ± 25	6
Crocidolite	ND[a]	ND	98 ± 16	6	123 ± 18	6
Crocidolite plus cigarette smoke	ND	ND	91 ± 12	6	103 ± 17	6
Chrysotile	88 ± 14	12	74 ± 23	5	119 ± 23	6
Chrysotile plus cigarette smoke	94 ± 19	12	64 ± 20	6	106 ± 22	6

[a]Not determined.

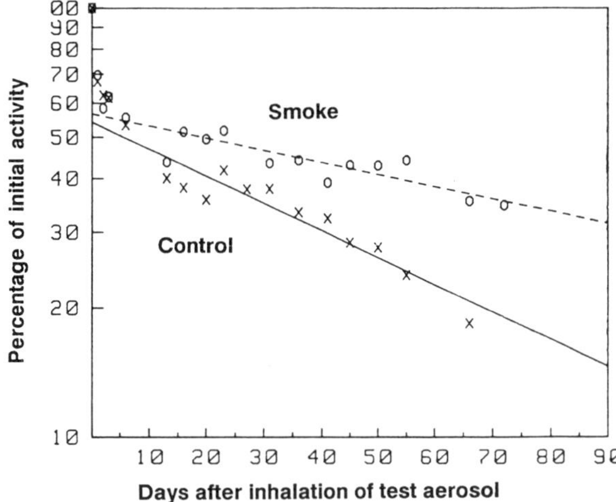

Figure 1. Reduced alveolar clearance of labeled iron oxide in rats after exposure to cigarette smoke for 9 months.

Table 4. Half-times (mean ± SD) for alveolar clearance of $^{59}Fe_2O_3$-labeled particles.

Exposure Group[a]	Half-Time (Days) of Alveolar Clearance after Stated Exposure Time	
	2 Months	9 Months
Control	47 ± 14	42 ± 8
Smoke	ND[b]	77 ± 26[c]
Crocidolite	53 ± 9	53 ± 12
Crocidolite plus cigarette smoke	92 ± 44	99 ± 25[c,d]
Chrysotile	51 ± 24	ND
Chrysotile plus cigarette smoke	114 ± 75	ND

[a]Six animals per group
[b]Not determined
[c]Significantly different from controls, $P < 0.05$
[d]Significantly different from comparable group exposed only to fibers

Retention of Fibers

The number of fibers retained in lungs is presented in Table 5. In groups exposed to cigarette smoke and crocidolite, the number of fibers retained increased significantly after both 6- and 12-month exposures. In contrast, the number of chrysotile fibers retained was not altered by cigarette-smoking.

Table 5. Number (mean ± SD) of fibers retained in the lungs.

Exposure	Number of Retained Fibers/Lung (x 10^6)					
	At 2 Months	N[a]	At 6 Months	N	At 12 Months	N
Crocidolite	197 ± 47	6	160 ± 31	6	441 ± 85	6
Crocidolite plus cigarette smoke	236 ± 81	6	340 ± 111[b]	6	808 ± 170[b]	5
Chrysotile	22 ± 4	3	100 ± 15	6	85 ± 23	5
Chrysotile plus cigarette smoke	25 ± 2	3	92 ± 37	6	80 ± 75	5

[a]Number of lungs investigated
[b]Statistically significant difference from groups exposed to fibers only, $P < 0.05$

The length and diameter distribution of the retained fibers was determined by scanning electron microscopy. Data on fibers retained in lungs after 12 months are presented in Table 6 and are compared with the size distribution of fibers in the exposure chamber. In general, the fibers retained in lungs were shorter and thinner than the ones to which the animals were exposed. In particular, the diameter of the chrysotile fibers in the lungs was considerably smaller.

Table 6. Mean fiber length and GSD (τ_g).

			Median Values			
			Fiber Length		Fiber Diameter	
Fiber Type	Sample From	Exposure Group	μm	τ_g	μm	τ_g
Crocidolite	Exposure chamber		1.7	2.0	0.28	1.5
	Lung	Fiber	1.4	2.2	0.28	1.5
	Lung	Fiber plus cigarette smoke	1.3	2.1	0.25	1.5
Chrysotile	Exposure chamber		3.7	1.8	0.33	1.5
	Lung	Fiber	3.6	2.1	0.16	1.7
	Lung	Fiber plus cigarette smoke	3.5	2.0	0.20	1.6

Histopathology

An increased incidence of macrophage aggregates in lungs was found in all exposed groups. In smoke-exposed animals, focal hyperplasia was observed in the larynx.

DISCUSSION

The clearance rate of the inhaled iron-oxide-labeled particles differs from that for fiber clearance because of variations in size and solubility (Bellmann et al., 1987; Muhle et al., 1987).

Measuring impairment of long-term lung clearance by using labeled marker aerosols during exposure is of special value for assessing the effect of toxic particles with low solubility that are inhaled in addition to other airborne dusts. After cigarette-smoking, long-term clearance was slowed in the rats in this study. Cohen et al. (1979) and Bohning et al. (1982) have also reported reduced deep lung clearance in smokers.

Fiber retention in the lungs showed different patterns for crocidolite and chrysotile, not only with respect to the effect of smoking in combination with fiber exposure, but also for fiber inhalation alone. Numbers of fibers retained increased with increasing exposure time to crocidolite; this was not true of chrysotile. Similar differences in the retention of chrysotile and crocidolite were described by Wagner et al. (1974). After a 3-month exposure period, a plateau was reached for chrysotile fibers retained in lungs. For crocidolite, the mass of fibers retained in the lungs increased during the 2-year exposure period.

Timbrell (1972) reported that the curved shape of chrysotile particles causes greater deposition of this fiber type in the upper airways compared with that of crocidolite. This difference in the deposition site may be one reason for the steady state of chrysotile retention after 6 months of exposure found in the study reported here. Another reason for the steady state of chrysotile retention may be the tendency of chrysotile to split into fibrils while in the lungs. This leads to a larger surface area and, therefore, to a higher dissolution rate. Furthermore, the disintegration of fibers may lead to their more rapid translocation from lung tissue (Bellmann et al., 1987). The smaller diameter of the chrysotile fibers in lungs, compared to that of the fibers in the exposure chamber, is indicative of such a process.

In our study, cigarette-smoking affected clearance rates of each fiber type differently. In the case of crocidolite, for which a higher alveolar deposition could be expected because of its shape and its smaller aerodynamic diameter, cigarette-smoking increased fiber retention. This can be explained by the reduced alveolar clearance, which was also seen for labeled particles.

In contrast, no such effect was detected for chrysotile; the dynamic equilibrium of deposition and clearance of chrysotile fibers was not influenced by cigarette smoke. Studies by Albert et al. (1974), Camner et al. (1971), and Lippmann et al. (1980) on the effect of cigarette-smoking on clearance of the ciliated airways indicated no effects or only a slight increase, in contrast to the reduced alveolar clearance observed. Furthermore, cigarette-smoking may lead to bronchoconstriction, which could also influence the deposition pattern.

Fibers retained in lungs can retard alveolar clearance (Bolton et al., 1983; Vincent et al., 1985). According to the calculations of these investigators, a lung burden of 1.5 mg amosite leads to reduced lung clearance in rats. Retained fiber mass at 12 months, calculated on the basis of measurements of numbers and shape of fibers, was 0.58 ± 0.14 mg/lung after crocidolite plus cigarette-smoke inhalation, and 0.051 ± 0.024 mg/lung after chrysotile plus cigarette-smoke inhalation. These data show that the value for the retained crocidolite mass is lower than the value believed to impair alveolar clearance.

In our opinion, the impaired long-term lung clearance is not a sufficient explanation for the synergistic carcinogenic effect of cigarette smoke and asbestos that has been reported for humans because the majority of lung cancers develop in the ciliated airways (Greenberg, 1987). It is suggested that the penetration and settling of fibers into the basal layer of the bronchial epithelium, already damaged by cigarette smoke, may be the reason for the increased tumor rate (see Pott, this volume). The settling rate in nonsmokers is likely to be much lower. The fraction of settled fibers in the upper airways may be relatively small compared to the total mass of fibers retained in the entire lung. Therefore, analysis of the total number of fibers retained in the lung will not show whether such an effect occurs.

REFERENCES

Albert, RE, J Berger, K Sanborn, and M Lippmann. **1974.** Effects of cigarette smoke components on bronchial clearance in the donkey. Arch Environ Health 29:96-101.

Bellmann, B, H Muhle, and U Heinrich. **1983.** Lung clearance after long time exposure of rats to airborne pollutants. J Aerosol Sci 14:194-196.

Bellmann, B, H Muhle, F Pott, H König, H Klöppel, and K Spurny. **1987.** Persistence of man-made mineral fibers (MMMF) and asbestos in rat lungs. Ann Occup Hyg 4B:693-709.

Bohning, DE, HL Atkins, and SH Cohn. **1982.** Long-term particle clearance in man: Normal and impaired. Ann Occup Hyg 26:259-271.

Bolton, RE, JH Vincent, AD Jones, J Addison, and ST Becket. **1983.** An overload hypothesis for pulmonary clearance of UICC amosite fibers inhaled by rats. Br J Ind Med 40:264-272.

Camner, P, K Philipson, and T Arvidsson. **1971.** Cigarette smoking in man. Environ Health 23:421-426.

Cohen, D, S Arai, and JD Brain. **1979.** Smoking impairs long-term dust clearance from the lung. Science 204:514-517.

Gibb, FR and PE Morrow. **1962.** Alveolar clearance in dogs following inhalation of an iron-59 oxide aerosol. J Appl Physiol 17:429-432.

Greenberg, SD. **1987.** Carcinomas of the peripheral airways, pp. 286-309. In: *Lung Carcinomas,* EM McDowell (ed.). Churchill Livingstone, New York.

Hammond, EC, IJ Selikoff, and H Seidman. **1979.** Asbestos exposure, cigarette smoking and death rates. Ann NY Acad Sci 330:473-492.

Harris, RL and AA Fraser. **1976.** A model for deposition of fibres in the human respiratory system. Am Ind Hyg Assoc J 37:73-89.

Lippmann, M, DB Yeates, and RE Albert. **1980.** Deposition, retention, and clearance of inhaled particles. Br J Ind Med 37:337-362.

Muhle, H, K Spurny, and F Pott. **1983.** Inhalationsexperimente zur Retention, Lungenreinigung und Wanderungsfähigkeit von Asbest und Glasfasern unter Einfluss von Zigarettenrauch. VDI-Berichte 475:247-251.

Muhle, H, F Pott, B Bellmann, S Takenaka, and U Ziem. **1987.** Inhalation and injection experiments in rats for testing man-made mineral fibres on carcinogenicity. Ann Occup Hyg 4B:755-764.

Selikoff, IJ, EC Hammond, and J Churg. **1968.** Asbestos exposure, smoking and neoplasia. J Am Med Assoc 204:106-110.

Spurny, KR, C Boose, and D Hochrainer. **1975.** Zur Zerstäubung von Asbestfasern in einem Fliessbett-Aerosolgenerator. Staub-Reinhalt Luft 35:440-445.

Timbrell, V. **1972.** Inhalation and biological effects of asbestos, pp. 429-445. In: *Assessment of Airborne Particles,* TT Mercer, et al. (eds.). CC Thomas, Springfield, MA.

Vincent, JH, AM Johnston, AD Jones, RE Bolton, and J Addison. **1985.** Kinetics of deposition and clearance of inhaled mineral dusts during chronic exposure. Br J Ind Med 42:707-715.

Wagner, JC, G Berry, JW Skidmore, and V Timbrell. **1974.** The effect of the inhalation of asbestos in rats. Br J Cancer 29:252-269.

Combined Effects of Tobacco Smoke and Asbestos Fibers in the Lung: Synergism or Increased Dose to Target Sites?*

Günter Oberdörster

Environmental Health Sciences Center and Department of Biophysics, University of Rochester, Rochester, NY 14642

KEY WORDS: asbestos, tobacco smoke, synergism, lung dosimetry

---

ABSTRACT

The following hypothesis is proposed with regard to lung cancer: that the observed synergistic effect of exposure to asbestos and cigarette smoke is caused by an increase in dose of carcinogens to target tissues, and that this results in additive rather than synergistic effects. This hypothesis is supported by studies indicating that the interaction of several factors could indeed increase the dose of toxic agents to critical target sites. Such interactive factors may also contribute to the development of diseases other than lung cancer, which are known to arise from chronic exposure to asbestos (i.e., lung fibrosis, pleural diseases) and from active smoking alone, when it results in chronic obstructive pulmonary disease. Among those factors are impaired mucociliary clearance, induced by long-term smoking, which leads to increased retention of fibers in the tracheobronchial region; chronic bronchitis, which results in increased deposition of inhaled asbestos fibers in the conducting airways; and the effects of mediators released from inflammatory cells in this region. For the alveolar/interstitial lung region, impairment of the alveolar-macrophage-mediated clearance function for particles can lead to increased fiber retention and greater access of fibers to the interstitium, where they can affect interstitial macrophages. In addition, the release of mediators from activated

*This paper is partially based on work supported by grants ES01247 and ES01248 from the National Institutes of Health. Paper presented by Dr. Ferin.

alveolar macrophages and their effects on the integrity of the alveolar epithelium may enhance the access of other mediators to the interstitium, where they can interact with fibroblasts. Last but not least, fibers may be transported, via interstitial and pleural lymphatics, to the pleural space. This concept may at least partly explain the observed "synergism" for lung cancer. However, it is not possible, at present, to estimate the magnitude of a dose increase at different target sites that results from combined exposure to mainstream cigarette smoke and asbestos.

INTRODUCTION

It is known from epidemiologic studies that combined exposure to asbestos and smoking can have a greater effect on the development of lung cancer than would be expected from simply adding the pulmonary carcinogenic response to both agents (Hammond et al., 1979). Consequently, this effect has been termed "synergistic." Both chronic exposure to asbestos and active cigarette-smoking can cause other effects in the respiratory system, some of which are shown in Table 1. Chronic asbestos inhalation can lead to induction of lung tumors, lung fibrosis (asbestosis), and pleural diseases, including plaques and mesothelioma. Cigarette-smoking does not cause pleural disease, but it can lead to chronic obstructive pulmonary disease (COPD). Combined exposures lead to synergistic effects with regard to lung cancer, and a possible additive effect on the development of lung fibrosis is also suggested (Weiss, 1984; Tron et al., 1987). However, additive or potentiating effects have not been confirmed with regard to pleural diseases or to COPD, although such effects cannot be ruled out (Weiss and Theodos, 1978).

Table 1. Epidemiologic findings relative to asbestos and smoking.

Exposure	Lung Cancer	Lung Fibrosis	Pleural Disease	Chronic Obstructive Pulmonary Disease
Asbestos	yes	yes	yes	no
Smoking	yes	(yes)	no	yes
Asbestos plus smoking	yes (synergistic)	(yes) (additive?)	? (potentiating?)	? (potentiating?)

Obviously, the dose of inhaled asbestos and cigarette-smoke particles deposited and retained in different parts of the respiratory tract has a significant impact on the response, i.e., lung cancer, lung fibrosis, pleural disease, and COPD. Therefore, dosimetric aspects which are related to the development of these lung diseases will be addressed in this paper: the role of lung dosimetry in the lung for the synergism of effects.

SYNERGISM AND LUNG DOSIMETRY

The following hypothesis is proposed: the interactive effect of smoking cigarettes and asbestos exposure is not the result of synergism or potentiation but is due to an increase in dose, i.e., they are additive. Figure 1 illustrates this hypothesis. Unfortunately, the definition of the term synergism is not always the same in various pharmacology or toxicology textbooks (e.g., Klaassen et al., 1986; Hodgson and Levi, 1987). Therefore, the term synergism will be used here as it is defined in *Casarett and Doull's Toxicology* (Klaassen et al., 1986): the simultaneous action of separate substances which, together, have greater total effect than the sum of their individual effects; i.e., synergism refers to a more than additive effect when individual doses of two substances act together. Likewise, potentiation occurs when one substance has no effect but potentiates the effect of a given dose of another substance.

Synergism has been observed for lung cancer between asbestos exposure and mainstream cigarette-smoke exposure, as shown in the upper left panel of Figure 1. The dashed line refers to a purely additive effect, i.e., reduction in exposure to one compound requires an increase in exposure to the other compound to achieve the same effect. In contrast, the solid line illustrates synergism, i.e., reducing exposure to both compounds results in the same effect. Specifically, combined exposure to lower concentrations of asbestos plus mainstream smoke yields the same response as does exposure to higher concentrations of asbestos or smoking alone, as reflected by the hyperbolic function in this graph. Or, translated into an exposure-response curve, as shown in the lower left panel of Figure 1, the same exposure concentration leads to a greater response when exposure to both compounds (asbestos and tobacco smoke) occurs in combination (solid curve) compared to the response to one compound alone (dashed curve). The exposure-response curve has shifted to the left. For simplicity, the slope and the location of the exposure-response curves for both compounds are assumed to be the same (dashed curve). It does not change the basic concept that the two exposure-response curves could be quite different from one another in reality. Daily exposure may be expressed as μg asbestos/m^3 air or μg particulate mass/m^3 air (for cigarette smoke). However, *exposure* to a compound, expressed as a given concentration in the air, is not equivalent to *dose*. Thus, if one considers the doses of asbestos and mainstream smoke reaching the target tissue (upper right panel of Figure 1), we propose that the two compounds act together in a simple additive fashion, and the observed synergism during combined asbestos and mainstream smoke *exposure* results from an increase in *dose* at the target site. This means that the *dose-response* curve (lower right panel of Figure 1) does not shift, but the increase in dose leads to an increase in response on the same dose-response curve (arrows on x- and y-axes). Obviously, the outcome (increased response) is the same, but it is the conceptual difference that should be emphasized in the proposed hypothesis.

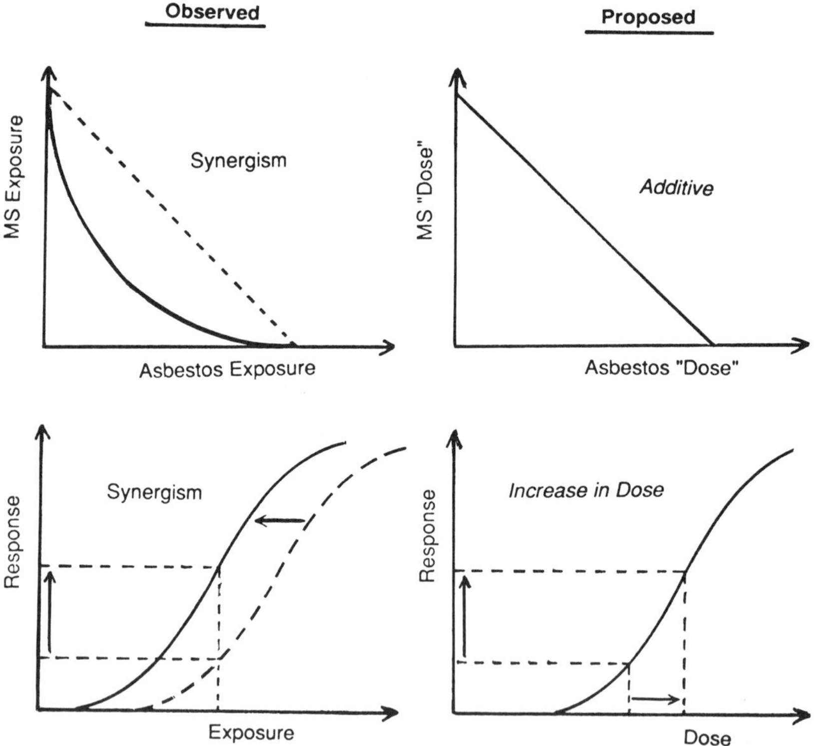

Figure 1. Schematic of synergistic effects of combined exposure to cigarette mainstream smoke (MS) and asbestos (left panels) and of additive effects of the respective doses to target tissues (right panels). See text for details.

The additive interaction between doses of asbestos and cigarette-smoke particles with regard to lung cancer proposed here is plausible also because the two carcinogenic agents are different in nature. One is a physical carcinogen (asbestos), and the other contains chemical carcinogens (cigarette-smoke constituents), which very likely act by means of different mechanisms. Similarly, potentiating effects between the two compounds, if observed (e.g., with regard to pleural diseases or COPD), could also be explained by increases in dose. Both synergistic and additive effects are most obvious at doses that lead to a relatively low response to the individual agent, i.e., in the low dose range (flat part of the dose-response curve), as is the case for asbestos exposure and smoking.

A few examples may serve to illustrate the possibilities for increased doses to regions of the respiratory tract and may clarify the proposed concept. Figure 2 shows the influence of smoking on the lung clearance of both solid and soluble particles. Smokers retain inhaled test particles (magnetite or polystyrene) for a much longer period of time and to a greater degree than nonsmokers (Cohen et al., 1979; Bohning et al., 1982). Obviously, if those test particles were toxic (as is asbestos, for example), it would increase the dose of the toxic agent to the lung. Although the measured particle retention, in this case, is in the alveolar region of the lung (i.e., it involves long-term clearance of particles), it is known from other experiments that, in a chronic smoker, tracheobronchial clearance is also retarded (Weiss et al., 1983; Vastag et al., 1986). Thus, doses of inhaled insoluble particles to the conducting airways will also increase. On the other hand, solute particles, such as the nonreactive hydrophilic chelator ^{99m}Tc-DTPA, are cleared more rapidly in smokers than in nonsmokers (Jones et al., 1980; Figure 2). This reflects an effect of smoking on the integrity of the alveolar epithelium, i.e., it has become more permeable, and hydrophilic solutes reach the interstitium more easily and at higher doses than in a healthy lung. This could also mean an increase in the dose to the interstitium of reactive biological mediators, e.g., growth factors, which are generated by inflammatory cells in the alveolar space of smokers' lungs, or of other toxic hydrophilic solutes. For both situations shown in Figure 2, the alveolar macrophages of smokers play a central role in increasing dose. The mechanical clearance function of the macrophage for solid particles is impaired; inflammatory mediators, such as oxidants, are released and affect the integrity of the alveolar epithelium (Mossman and Landesman, 1983; Mossman et al., 1986), resulting in an increased access of solutes to the interstitium.

Another example of increased dose is the increased retention of inhaled carcinogens that are adsorbed onto particles. Bond et al. (1985) found that when benzo[a]pyrene (BaP) was adsorbed onto diesel particles, BaP was retained much longer than when it was inhaled alone, and therefore its dose to the lung was increased. With other particles tested, this increased retention was not as obvious, or it may have been absent (Bond et al., 1985). Thus, both the type of particle as well as the chemical nature of the adsorbed compound are important. These studies show that polycyclic aromatic hydrocarbons (PAH) are retained longer in the lung and may also reach different target tissues (e.g., interstitial sites) when they interact with inhaled particles. Such an effect was also found by Pylev et al. (1969) for asbestos and BaP when they were instilled together into the lung, resulting in an increase in retained dose.

A third example is from the results of a study by Harrison and Heath (1986), in which combined exposure to cadmium and nitrosamine, both constituents of mainstream cigarette smoke, plus asbestos, increased lung-cancer incidence in rats. Because particle clearance was slowed by exposure to cadmium (Oberdörster and Hochrainer, 1980), it can be assumed that the asbestos particles also administered in that study were probably retained longer, thereby increasing their dose.

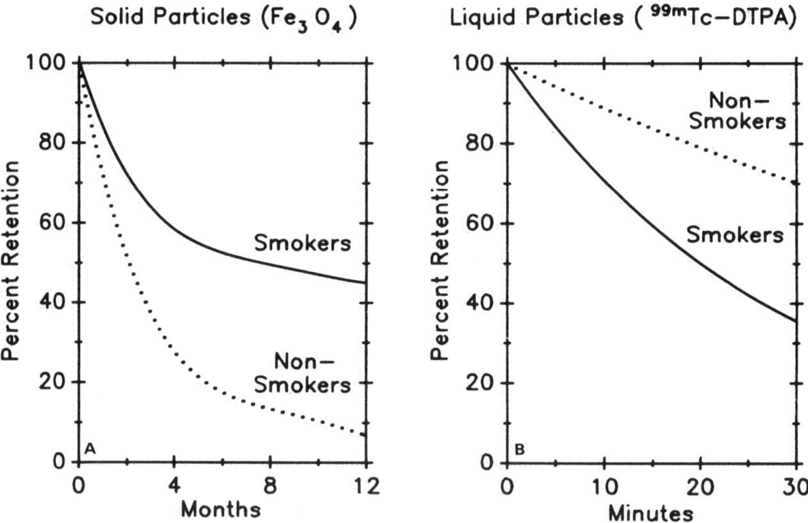

Figure 2. Effect of smoking on lung clearance of solid particles and of an inhaled hydrophilic solute, demonstrating the adverse effect of chronic smoking on alveolar-macrophage-mediated particle clearance and on the barrier function of the alveolar epithelium. [Modified from: Cohen et al., 1979 (A) and Jones et al., 1980 (B).]

To evaluate the concept of dose increase versus synergism of action, our objectives will be twofold: firstly, to evaluate lung-model prediction of doses of inhaled mainstream smoke particles and inhaled asbestos deposited in the respiratory tract; secondly, to discuss possible interactive mechanisms that increase doses at target sites, i.e., to address the importance of tissue dose versus synergism of effects.

LUNG DOSIMETRY OF INHALED CIGARETTE SMOKE AND ASBESTOS

Figure 3 lists several factors that can modify doses to target sites and the resulting effects. This figure shows the respiratory tract dosimetry following exposure to airborne asbestos or mainstream cigarette smoke. Inhalation of both compounds results in an inhaled dose, part of which is deposited, resulting in the deposited dose. Part of the deposited dose is cleared relatively quickly, whereas the rest is cleared more slowly. If the clearance rate is lower than the deposition rate, the compound accumulates, resulting in a retained dose, which eventually will cause an effect.

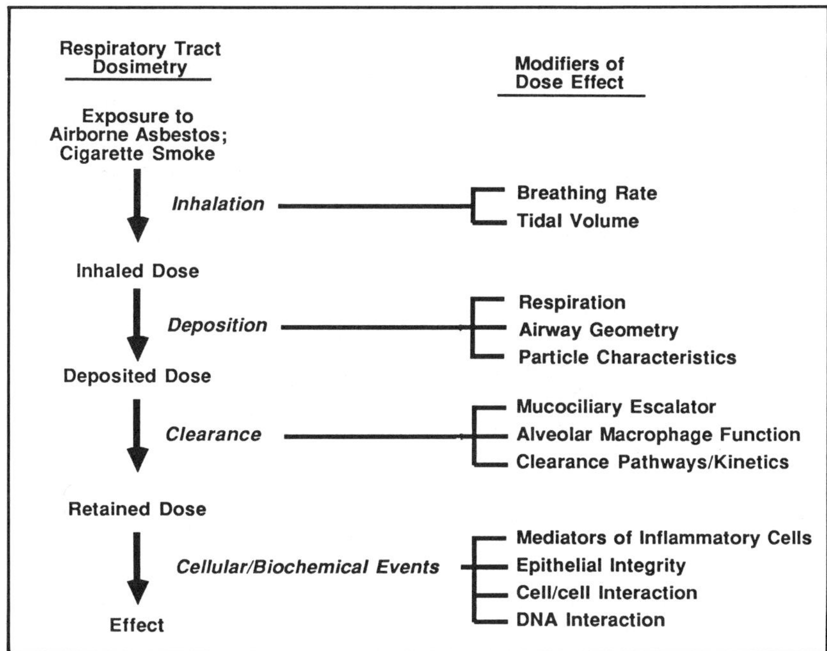

Figure 3. Influence of modifiers on respiratory tract dosimetry.

Several factors influence these doses and the effects, depending on whether they act during inhalation, deposition, or clearance. Breathing rate and tidal volume obviously affect the inhaled dose as well as the deposited dose. In addition, airway geometry and physicochemical characteristics of particles affect deposition and, consequently, the deposited dose. Clearance efficiency in the conducting airways and in the alveolar region of the lung are mainly affected by functions of the mucociliary escalator and by the alveolar macrophages, respectively. Disturbances in these clearance functions significantly alter retention, and thus the retained dose, of inhaled particulate compounds and other materials adsorbed to the particles. Such disturbances can also alter the pathways for clearance, diverting deposited particles into, for example, the interstitium or lymphatic tissue. Figure 3 lists some of the events that could affect or modify effects caused by a dose retained at target sites. These include release of mediators of inflammatory cells, effects of toxicants (or of these mediators) on epithelial integrity and the interaction of different cell types with one another. Furthermore, interaction of metabolites or toxicants with DNA function could become important for neoplastic effects. In addition, normal clearance in the conducting airways may not be as efficient at bifurcations, increasing doses at these sites from both increased deposition and decreased clearance.

The deposited, retained doses in Figure 3 are of different magnitudes for different regions of the respiratory tract. Lung models can be used to predict the deposited dose; however, we have no data that can also predict retained doses of inhaled smoke constituents or asbestos in the human lung. For modeling deposition of mainstream smoke particles in the respiratory tract, we used the typical-path, whole-lung model described by Yeh and Schum (1980) and Schum and Yeh (1980), as modified by Wojciak et al. (1987). With it, we predicted the relative and absolute deposited dose and dose rate in the lung regions and in individual generations of the respiratory tract. We assumed the following respiratory parameters for smokers: tidal volume, 1200 ml; respiratory rate, 10 per minute; respiratory pause, 3 seconds. The size of the mainstream smoke particles was reported by Huber et al. (1981) as having a mass median aerodynamic diameter of 0.5 μm and a geometric standard deviation of 1.4. Because those particles are hygroscopic, they grow after entering the airways; Evans et al. (1987) reported an increase in particle diameter to 1.5 μm. Therefore we considered deposition of both 0.5- and 1.5-μm particles. In addition, it is possible that deposition of mainstream smoke particles entering the airways will be greater than predicted by the model because the high particle concentration modifies the fluid properties of air (Evans et al., 1987). However, this aspect was not considered in our modeling efforts. The concentration of mainstream smoke particles was assumed to average 15 mg/m^3, based on a 1-pack-per-day smoker, assuming 10 mg tar per cigarette.

Figure 4A shows the relative deposition of inhaled mainstream smoke (for both 0.5- and 1.5-μm particles) in different airway generations predicted by the model. Generation 1 represents the trachea, generation 16 the terminal bronchioles, and generation 25 the alveolar ducts. The relative deposition (percent of inhaled dose) is very low for the conducting airways and increases toward the periphery of the lung. However, when expressing the results in terms of deposition rate per cm^2 surface area of the airways (Figure 4B), it can be seen that the upper conducting airways receive a higher dose than the regions of the respiratory zone. The hygroscopically enlarged particles (1.5 μm) increase the dose to the surface area throughout the respiratory tract, but particularly in the upper bronchial generations. One aspect that is not considered here is that the smoke particles will preferentially deposit along the carinal ridges of bifurcations in the conducting airways, as demonstrated by Martonen et al. (this volume), which increases the local tissue dose in those regions significantly. Such deposition along bifurcating ridges has also been observed with fibrous particles in the transitional zone of the rat lung by Brody et al. (1981). In addition, deposition modeling by Asgharian and Yu (in press) showed that fibrous particles preferentially deposited in the alveolar region of the human lung, probably starting at the respiratory bronchioles and extending into the alveolar ducts.

MODIFIERS OF DOSE TO THE LUNG

The results of the deposition modeling described in the previous section reflect the dosimetric situation under normal conditions. The following is a discussion of several factors that can modify doses and effects at target sites. With regard to the tracheobronchial region (Table 2), impaired mucociliary clearance caused by chronic tobacco-smoke exposure (Vastag et al., 1986) leads to increased retention of asbestos fibers as well as of mainstream smoke particles in this region. It is conceivable that PAH adsorbed onto the small particles (and, possibly, onto fibers) are also retained longer than under conditions of normal mucociliary clearance and thus increase the PAH dose to this region. Likewise, prolonged retention of PAH in the lipid-aqueous heterogeneic structure of the bronchial lining layer, as described by Gerde and Scholander (1987), should also be considered. As Mantel (1987) speculated, attachment of radon daughters to smoke particles could introduce another carcinogenic agent in this scenario when cigarette-smoking occurs in rooms in which radon progeny accumulate.

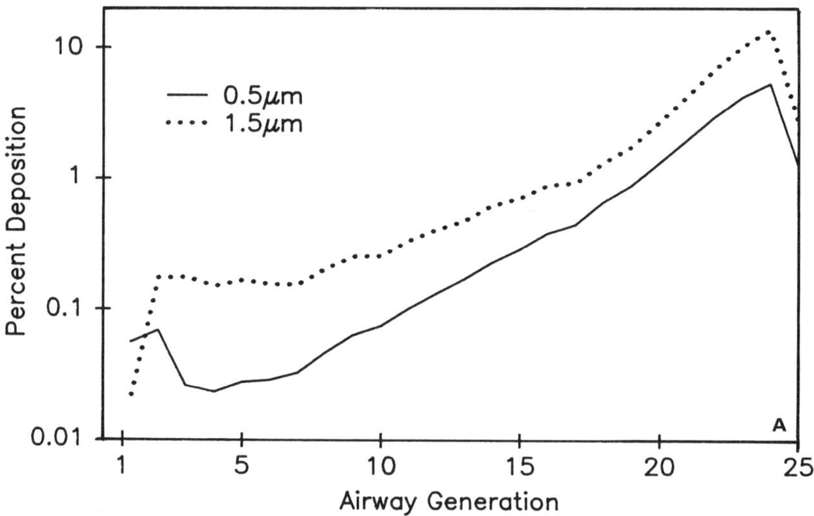

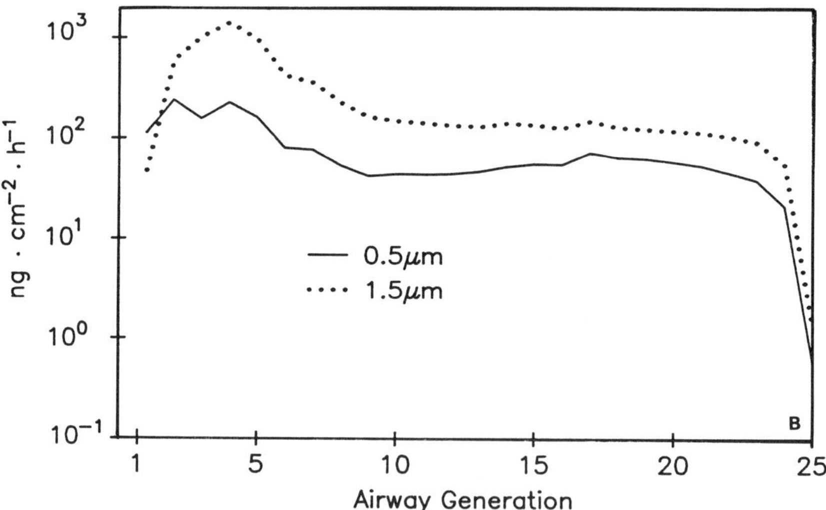

Figure 4. A, Lung model prediction of relative deposition (percent of inhaled amount) of mainstream smoke particles in individual generations of the human respiratory tract. B, Lung model prediction of deposited surface area dose rate in individual generations of the human respiratory tract. (Generation 1 = trachea; Generation 16 = terminal bronchioles; Generation 25 = alveoli. See text for details.

Table 2. Interaction of combined exposure to mainstream cigarette smoke (MS) and asbesetos on target sites in respiratory tract

Region of Interaction	Interaction of Factors That Increase Dose of Carcinogenic and Toxic Agents to Target Sites
Tracheobronchial	Impaired mucociliary clearance
	• Fiber retention, MS retention • Polycyclic aromatic hydrocarbon (PAH) retention (smoke particles, mucus, fibers) • Radon daughters on smoke particles (?)
	Bronchitis
	• Central deposition (decrease in pulmonary dose)
	Release and effect of mediators (e.g., oxidants)
	• Epithelial cells; DNA
Alveolar/ Interstitial	Impaired alveolar macrophage (AM) clearance function
	• Fiber retention, MS retention, PAH (?) • AM chemotactic activity • Access of particles to interstitium • Interaction with interstitial macrophages • Build-up in lymph nodes
	Release of inflammatory cell mediators
	• Epithelial permeability [oxidants (influence of Fe?, proteases)] • Diffusion into interstitium (e.g., platelet-derived growth factor, macrophage-derived growth factor) • Interaction with fibroblasts
Pleural	Access of fibers and MS via interstitial and pleural lymphatics
	• Attraction and activation of intrapleural macrophages • PAH on MS (on fibers, if inhaled together) (?)

Bronchitis, which develops in many smokers, changes the geometry of the conducting airways, i.e., they will become narrower. This results in more central deposition of other inhaled pollutants such as asbestos, thus increasing its dose to that target site. Consequently, this increased deposition in the tracheobronchial region may mean decreased deposition in the alveolar region, i.e., a decrease in pulmonary dose, because fewer particles are available for pulmonary deposition. Furthermore, the release of mediators from inflammatory cells in conducting airways, and the effects, for example, of the resulting oxidants, represent a biochemical mechanism by which epithelial cells, including their DNA, might be affected. This effect occurs to a greater degree when doses of the inhaled toxic particles are increased by mechanisms discussed above.

In the alveolar and interstitial region, the macrophage-mediated clearance of particles may be impaired by inhalation of toxic substances, providing a central mechanism for increasing doses to tissues in this region. Such effects have been reported for exposures to both asbestos and mainstream smoke (Cohen et al., 1979; Bohning et al., 1982; Ferin and Leach, 1976). Combining these exposures might increase retention of asbestos fibers of a size that would otherwise be cleared more efficiently by alveolar macrophages, as shown by Churg et al. (1987). Furthermore, it may increase retention of mainstream smoke particles.

Chemotaxis may be an essential part of the alveolar macrophage clearance function; if alveolar macrophages become less chemotactically active because of the effects of a toxic agent, this will further impair alveolar-macrophage-mediated clearance (Warheit et al., 1988). Consequently, the access of particles to the interstitium will increase, as generally happens when alveolar-macrophage-mediated particle clearance is disturbed (Ferin and Feldstein, 1978). Interaction of the particulate materials with interstitial macrophages increases, and particulate material accumulates in regional lymph nodes.

The release of inflammatory cell mediators within the alveolar space could decrease the barrier function of the alveolar epithelium by the action of, for example, oxidants or proteases (Johnson et al., 1981; Mossman and Landesman, 1983). Thus, access of other released mediators into the interstitium increases (for example, that of platelet-derived or macrophage-derived growth factors), facilitating their interaction with fibroblasts. In this context, iron could be important. It is known from *in vitro* studies (Goodglick and Kane, 1986) that the iron in crocidolite is an important component of its toxicity, possibly through the formation of more-toxic hydroxyl radicals from the less-toxic oxygen radicals released from activated inflammatory cells (modified Haber-Weiss reaction). Whether this can also explain the results of epidemiological studies that show that crocidolite is more effective than other forms of asbestos in causing mesotheliomas (Henderson, 1982) remains to be seen. In any event, formation of the toxic hydroxyl radical, caused by transition metals such as iron and copper, should be taken into account, considering the bioavailability of iron from certain asbestos fibers.

All factors listed in Table 2 for the alveolar/interstitial regions can lead to the increased interaction of asbestos, smoke particles, and released mediators with interstitial fibroblasts. Such events could easily offset any possible decrease in the pulmonary dose of inhaled asbestos that is caused by more central deposition in smokers as a result of bronchitis.

Factors responsible for effects at pleural sites can also modify effects. Depending on their size, fibers can reach the pleura via direct migration through the interstitium or via lymphatic channels (Oberdörster et al., in press). The latter may also be a pathway for mainstream smoke particles, as evidenced by the results of studies with other particulate materials, in which pleural accumulation of dust was attributed to the pleural lymphatic network (Holt, 1983). As in the alveolar region, it is possible that intrapleural macrophages may be activated by fibrous material in the pleural space, which can increase their numbers, as we showed in earlier studies (Oberdörster et al., 1983). Furthermore, the aforementioned increased retention of fibers and other particles in the alveolar space, which is likely to lead to an increase in their dose to the interstitium, could also lead to an increase in their dose to the pleural tissue because of their translocation to the pleura. Perhaps PAH could also reach those sites when smoking and asbestos exposure occur concurrently rather than serially. In that case, the smoke constituents of the gas phase would be adsorbed onto the asbestos fibers during exposure. However, it is not known whether they will have an additional adverse effect.

Although many of the factors discussed are well-known, some are more speculative than others. The former were included intentionally in this presentation to encourage further discussion.

In conclusion, the observed "synergistic" effects of combined exposure to mainstream cigarette smoke and asbestos on lung cancer could be explained by the increased dose to target sites rather than by true synergism. Other adverse effects of combined smoke and asbestos exposure may also be due to increased doses to pulmonary target tissues.

REFERENCES

Asgharian, B, and CP Yu. Deposition of inhaled fibrous particles in the human lung. J Aerosol Med (**in press**).

Bohning, DE, HL Atkins, and SH Cohn. **1982.** Long-term particle clearance in man: Normal and impaired. Ann Occup Hyg 26:259-271.

Bond, JA, JD Sun, CE Mitchell, JS Dutcher, RK Wolff, and RO McClellan. **1985.** Biological fate of inhaled organic compounds associated with particulate matter, pp. 579-592. In: *Aerosols: Research, Risk Assessment and Control Strategies,* SD Lee, T Schneider, LD Grant, and PJ Verberk (eds.). Lewis Publishers, Inc., Chelsea, MI.

Brody, AR, LH Hill, B Adkins, and RW O'Connor. **1981.** Chrysotile asbestos inhalation in rats; deposition pattern and reaction of alveolar epithelium and pulmonary macrophages. Am Rev Respir Dis 123:670-679.

Churg, A, V Tron, and JL Wright. **1987.** Effects of cigarette smoke exposure on retention of asbestos fibers in various morphologic compartments of the guinea pig lung. Am J Pathol 129:385-393.

Cohen, D, SF Arai, and JD Brain. **1979.** Smoking impairs long term clearance from the lung. Science 204:514-517.

Evans, JC, JN Pritchard, A Black, JF Hicks, and JR Morgan. **1987.** Factors influencing accepted deposition patterns, pp. 63-68. In: *Deposition and Clearance of Aerosols in the Human Respiratory Tract,* W Hoffmann (ed.). Facultas Universitätsverlag, Salzburg, Austria.

Ferin, J and M Feldstein. **1978.** Pulmonary clearance and hilar lymph node content in rats after particle exposure. Environ Res 16:342-352.

Ferin, J and LJ Leach. **1976.** The effect of amosite and chrysotile asbestos on the clearance of TiO_2 particles from the lung. Environ Res 12:250-254.

Gerde, P and P Scholander. **1987.** A mathematical model of the penetration of polycyclic aromatic hydrocarbons through the bronchial lining layer. Environ Res 44:321-334.

Goodglick, LA and AB Kane. **1986.** Role of reactive oxygen metabolites in crocidolite asbestos toxicity to mouse macrophages. Cancer Res 46:5558-5566.

Hammond, EC, IJ Selikoff, and H Seidman. **1979.** Asbestos exposure, smoking, and death rates. Ann NY Acad Sci USA 330:473-492.

Harrison, PTC. and JC Heath. **1986.** Apparent synergy in lung carcinogenesis: Interactions between N-nitrosoheptamethyleneimine, particulate cadmium and crocidolite asbestos in rats. Carcinogenesis 7:1903-1908.

Henderson, DW. **1982.** Asbestos related pleuropulmonary diseases: Asbestosis, mesothelioma and lung cancer. Pathology 14:239-243.

Hodgson, E and P Levi. **1987.** *A Textbook of Modern Toxicology.* Elsevier Science Publishing Co., Inc., New York, NY.

Holt, PF. **1983.** Translocation of inhaled dust to the pleura. Environ Res 31:212-220.

Huber, GL, P Davies, GR Zwilling, VE Pochay, WC Hinds, HA Nicholas, VK Mahajan, M Hajashi, and MW First. **1981.** A morphologic and physiologic bioassay for qualifying alterations in the lung following experimental chronic inhalation of tobacco smoke. Bull Eur Physiopathol Respir 17:269-327.

Johnson, K, J Fantone, J Kaplan, and P Ward. **1981.** *In vivo* damage of rat lungs by oxygen metabolites. J Clin Invest 67:983-993.

Jones, JG, P Lawler, JCW Crawley, BD Minty, G Hulands, and N Veall. **1980.** Increased alveolar epithelial permeability in cigarette smokers. Lancet Jan 12:66-68.

Klaassen, CD, MD Amdur, and J Doull (eds.). **1986.** *Casarett and Doull's Toxicology,* 3rd edition. MacMillan Publishing Company, New York, NY.

Mantel, N. **1987.** Re: Passive smoking and lung cancer in Swedish women, Letter to the Editor. Am J Epidemiol 126:1215-1216.

Mossman, BT and JM Landesman. **1983.** Importance of oxygen free radicals in asbestos-induced lung injury to airway epithelial cells. Chest 83S:50S-51S.

Mossman, BT, J Marsh,and M Shatos. **1986.** Alteration of superoxide dismutase activity in tracheal epithelial cells by asbestos and inhibition of cytotoxicity by antioxidants. Lab Invest 54:204-212.

Oberdörster, G and D Hochrainer. **1980.** Lung clearance of Fe_2O_3- and $CdCl_2$ aerosols during chronic CdO inhalation, pp. 198-203. In: *Aerosols in Science, Medicine and Technology - Physical and Chemical Properties of Aerosols,* Vol. 8. Gesellschaft für Aerosolforschung, Mainz, FRG.

Oberdörster, G, J Ferin, NL Marcello, and SH Meinhold. **1983.** Effect of intrabronchially instilled amosite on lavageable lung and pleural cells. Environ Health Perspect 51:41-48.

Oberdörster, G, PE Morrow, and K Spurny. Size dependent lymphatic short-term clearance of amosite fibers in the lung. Ann Occup Hyg (**in press**).

Pylev, LN, FJC Roe, and GP Warwick. **1969.** Elimination of radioactivity after intratracheal instillation of tritiated 3,4-benzopyrene in hamsters. Br J Cancer 23:103-115.

Schum, M and HC Yeh. **1980.** Theoretical evaluation of aerosol deposition in anatomical models of mammalian lung airways. Bull Math Biol 42:1-15.

Tron, V, JL Wright, N Harrison, B Wiggs, and A Churg. **1987.** Cigarette smoke makes airway and early parenchymal asbestos-induced lung disease worse in the guinea pig. Am Rev Respir Dis 136:271-275.

Vastag, E, H Matthys, G Zsamboki, D Kohler, and G Daikeler. **1986.** Mucociliary clearance in smokers. Eur J Respir Dis 68:107-113.

Warheit, DB, LH Overby, G George, and AR Brody. **1988.** Pulmonary macrophages are attracted to inhaled particles through complement activation. Exp Lung Res 14: 51-66.

Weiss, W. **1984.** Cigarette smoke, asbestos and small irregular opacities. Am Rev Respir Dis 130:193-301.

Weiss, W and PA Theodos. **1978.** Pleuropulmonary disease among asbestos workers in relation to smoking and type of exposure. J Occup Med 20:341-345.

Weiss, T, P Dorow, and R Feliz. **1983.** Regional mucociliary removal of inhaled particles in smokers with small airways disease. Respiration 44:338-345.

Wojciak, JF, G Oberdörster, and RH Notter. **1987.** Dosimetric aspects of particle deposition in the respiratory tract of rat and man. Implications for extrapolating from rodent studies, pp. 47-52. In: *Deposition and Clearance of Aerosols in the Human Respiratory Tract,* W Hoffmann (ed.). Facultas Universitätsverlag, Salzburg, Austria.

Yeh, HC and M Schum. **1980.** Models of human lung airways and their application to inhaled particle deposition. Bull Math Biol 42:461-480.

Intrapulmonary Airway Branching and Parenchymal Deposition of Chrysotile Asbestos Fibers*

Kent E. Pinkerton[1] and Chia-Ping Yu[2]

[1]Department of Anatomy and Institute for Environmental Health Research, School of Veterinary Medicine, University of California, Davis, CA 95616

[2]Department of Mechanical and Aerospace Engineering, State University of New York, Buffalo, NY 14260

KEY WORDS: airways, branch points, retention, fiber deposition, chrysotile

---

ABSTRACT

Prolonged exposure to asbestos fibers is associated with marked changes in the lungs. Workers occupationally exposed to asbestos commonly have a diffuse form of fibrosis with alveolar tissue involvement that is highly variable from one region of the lungs to another. In this review, airway characteristics that may influence the deposition of fibers in the lung parenchyma are described in a rodent model for asbestosis. The influence of airway branching on numbers and lengths of asbestos fibers found in anatomically distinct regions of the lung parenchyma is examined and correlated to alveolar tissue changes in rats chronically exposed to asbestos. A theoretical model for fiber deposition is proposed, and calculations for fiber size distribution based on this model are compared to observed values.

INTRODUCTION

The use of asbestos spans several thousand years, but health hazards associated with its inhalation have been recognized only

*This work is supported in part by NIH Grants R29 ES04338, RO1 HL38503 and the American Lung Association.

since the beginning of this century (Murray, 1907; Selikoff and Lee, 1978). Prolonged exposure to asbestos commonly results in a diffuse form of pulmonary fibrosis (Vorwald et al., 1951). The relationship of fibrotic change to fiber concentration in the lung appears to be highly variable from one individual to another as well as from one region to another in the same lung (Ashcroft and Heppleston, 1973; Sebastian et al., 1977; Churg, 1980; Churg and Warnock, 1980; Morgan and Holmes, 1984; Davis et al., 1978). The cause for these differences in parenchymal lung scarring has only recently been addressed (Roggli et al., 1986; Pinkerton et al., 1986). Work in our laboratories suggests that the branching pattern of the airways plays an important role in the deposition of asbestos in the lungs and constitutes an important factor in the pattern of pulmonary fibrosis observed. This paper will review studies in which the parenchymal or alveolar tissue response from different regions of the lung was measured. Each lung region studied was isolated, using airway microdissection techniques. The size distribution of asbestos fibers found within each region of lung parenchyma isolated is described. Also described is a model for predicting the number and size of fibers deposited in parenchymal tissues, based on the characteristics of the airway from which these tissues originate. A correlation between the theoretical and observed values of fiber number and size is discussed.

MATERIALS AND METHODS

The exposure conditions for these experiments are described in detail in publications by Pinkerton et al. (1984, 1986). All studies were performed in specific-pathogen-free, male Fischer-344 rats. Animals were divided into two groups by random selection. One group was exposed to chrysotile asbestos, while the second group was exposed to filtered air only. All animals were housed in pairs in wire cages in stainless-steel exposure chambers of 5-m^3 capacity. Asbestos fibers were aerosolized using a Timbrell generator (Timbrell, 1968). Exposure to asbestos was for 7 hours/day, 5 days/week for 12 months.

Chamber concentrations of asbestos were measured daily. They averaged 11 mg/m^3 for the entire experiment (Pinkerton et al., 1984). Control animals were exposed, during this same period of time, to filtered air only. Animals were maintained in the exposure chambers for approximately 1 week following fiber exposure and then sacrificed. Animals were anesthetized by intraperitoneal injection of pentobarbital, and the lungs were infusion-fixed by intratracheal instillation of 2% glutaraldehyde at a hydrostatic pressure of 20 cm.

Five anatomically distinct regions of the left lung (Figure 1) were isolated using an airway microdissection technique (Plopper et al., 1983). With a pair of fine scissors, forceps, and razor blades, selected airways were followed by longitudinally opening each airway. The pathway selected was the same for all animals. The microdissection procedure was facilitated using a dissecting microscope and fiber-optic lighting system. For simplicity, the five areas isolated are referred to as the dorsal, cranial, lateral, costolateral and caudal regions. Airway characteristics for each of these pathways are given in Table 1. To summarize, the dorsal, cranial and lateral regions represent parenchymal lung tissues that arise from pathways of approximately identical length, while the parenchymal tissues from the costolateral and caudal regions arise from airways of longer path length. All five regions have different airway branching patterns relative to the trachea as well as different numbers of airway branch points (Table 1).

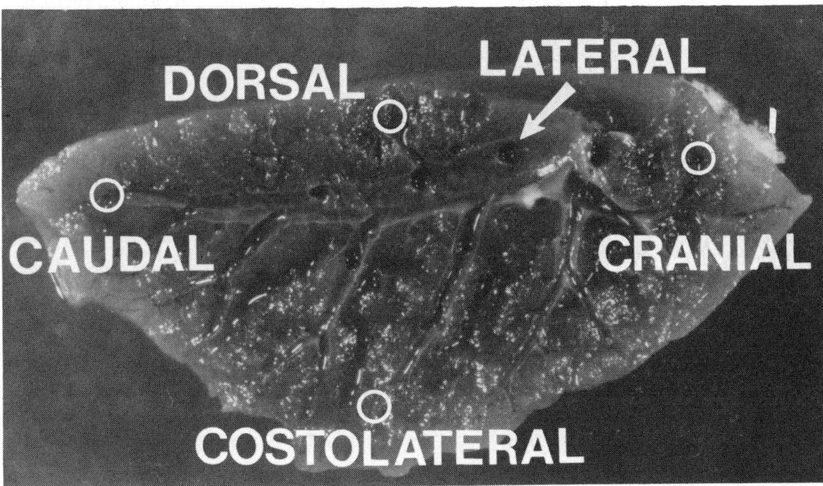

Figure 1. Dissection of the left lung to reveal airways by opening each passage in a longitudinal axis. The five parenchymal regions examined are labeled with four of the five regions studied enclosed by a circle. (From Hayes and Crapo, 1988; reproduced by permission of Academic Press.)

The airways isolated were followed from the trachea to within two to four generations of the terminal bronchiole. Adjacent blocks of tissue were cut just beyond the last dissected airway for tissue digestion and histologic examination. Tissue digestion was used to recover asbestos fibers from the parenchymal tissues. Filtered

5.25% sodium hypochlorite was used to digest the lung tissue in 5-ml sterile plastic syringes. Before digestion, each tissue block was carefully measured to determine its volume. During the process of digestion, the syringe was gently agitated to facilitate the dispersion of fibers. Once all tissue fragments had completely dissolved (usually within 45 to 60 minutes), the solution in the syringe was diluted with double-distilled filtered water and passed through a 0.2-μm Nuclepore® filter. The filter housing unit and syringe were rinsed several times with additional distilled water to enhance the recovery of fibers and to remove any remaining traces of sodium hypochlorite, which might crystallize on the Nuclepore filter following drying (Pinkerton et al., 1986).

Table 1. Characteristics of pulmonary airways isolated from the left lung[a]

Region of Airway Termination	Pathlength from Carina (mm)[b]	Branchpoint Number, Counting from the Trachea	Gravitational Orientation
Dorsal	13.6 ± 1.4	7	Against gravity
Lateral	13.0 ± 0.8	9	None[c]
Cranial	14.0 ± 1.2	10	With gravity
Costolateral	18.3 ± 0.9	16	With gravity
Caudal	22.3 ± 0.3	17	With gravity

[a]Modified from Table 1, Pinkerton et al., 1986.
[b]Values are mean ± SD
[c]This airway path has neither a dorsal nor a ventral orientation in the left lung as do the other microdissected airways. Therefore, the gravitational orientation of this region has not been classified.

Each filter was sputter-coated with a thin layer of gold (approximately 125 Å thick) and examined, using a scanning electron microscope. Fibers were counted by examining random fields on the filter at a magnification of 6,000X. Only those fibers whose midpoints were within the area of each field observed were counted. A total of 200 fibers, or 100 fields, were counted, whichever came first. In a subsequent session, the lengths of 50 fibers were measured for each region of the lung isolated (Roggli and Brody, 1984).

Tissue blocks embedded in Epon® were sectioned to a thickness of 0.5 μm and stained with azure/methylene blue for histologic analysis. To determine the degree of tissue inflation for each isolated region of the lung, the mean alveolar airspace length was determined for each region. Alveolar surface area per unit volume of tissue was also examined.

These studies demonstrated no statistically significant difference between asbestos-exposed and control animals or among the various tissue regions isolated (Pinkerton et al., 1986). This was an important parameter to analyze, because the degree of tissue inflation can significantly affect tissue density.

Parenchymal volume density was measured by dividing the lung parenchyma into three compartments: alveolar air space, alveolar septal tissue, and capillary lumen. The density of each compartment was determined using a simple Weibel test lattice system and applying well-described morphometric counting methods (Weibel, 1979; Pinkerton et al., 1986). The assessment of asbestos-induced tissue responses centered on changes that occurred in the alveolar septal tissue volume density.

The deposition efficiencies resulting from the characteristics of the airways and nose were used to calculate the deposition of fibers in the rat lung. This deposition model, described elsewhere (Asgharian and Yu, 1988a,b), is dependent on the surface area and branchpoint number of airways for predicting fiber deposition. All calculations were based on the whole-lung model of Schum and Yeh (1980). The respiratory conditions used in the calculations were: tidal volume, 1.68 cm^3 and respiratory rate, 98 breaths/minute.

To compare differences in the degree of tissue response and asbestos fiber concentration for each region of the lung, Duncan's multiple range test was used. Intercomparisons with a P value less than 0.05 were considered significantly different.

RESULTS

Changes in alveolar septal tissue volume fraction for each region studied are shown in Figure 2. The greatest degree of change for all regions examined occurred in the cranial region, which had an alveolar tissue volume fraction of 0.154 for asbestos-exposed lung, compared to a control value of 0.054. The lateral region also demonstrated a marked change from control value. The costolateral and dorsal regions had similar values, with an alveolar tissue volume fraction 50% greater than that of controls. With the exception of the caudal region, the histologic appearance of each region is shown in Figure 3.

Asbestos fiber concentration is shown in Figure 4 for each region of the lung. These values are expressed as total numbers of fibers per unit volume of infusion-fixed lung. The highest fiber concentration (450,000 fibers per mm^3 of fixed lung) was found in the dorsal region; 367,000 and 320,000 fibers were present in the lateral and cranial regions, respectively. The costolateral and caudal regions contained significantly less asbestos: 128,000 and 61,000 fibers per mm^3 of fixed lung, respectively.

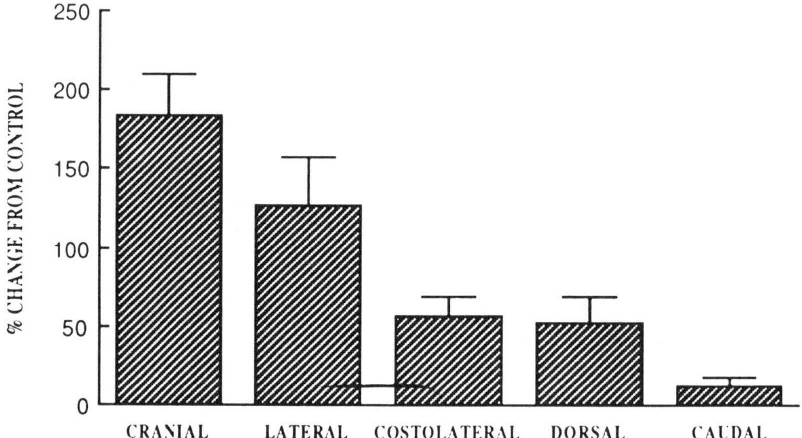

Figure 2. Alveolar septal tissue density changes (% ± SD, compared to controls) for the five regions of the left lung examined. (From Hayes and Crapo, 1988; reproduced by permission of Academic Press.)

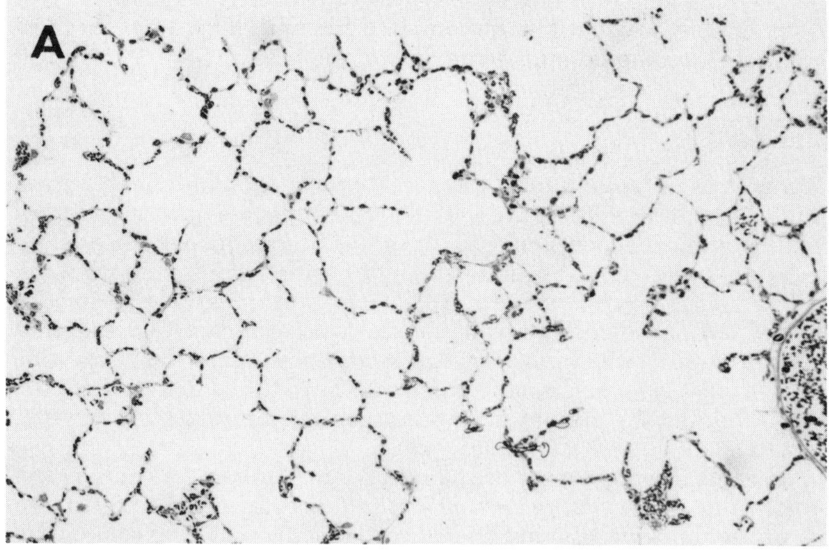

Figure 3. Micrographs of parenchymal lung tissue from five regions of the left lung of asbestos-exposed and control rats: A, control; B, cranial; C, lateral; and D, dorsal regions. Septal tissue thickening (compared to control) is apparent in the cranial and lateral regions. Alveolar septal thickening is more subtle in the dorsal region. Scale bar is 250 μm.

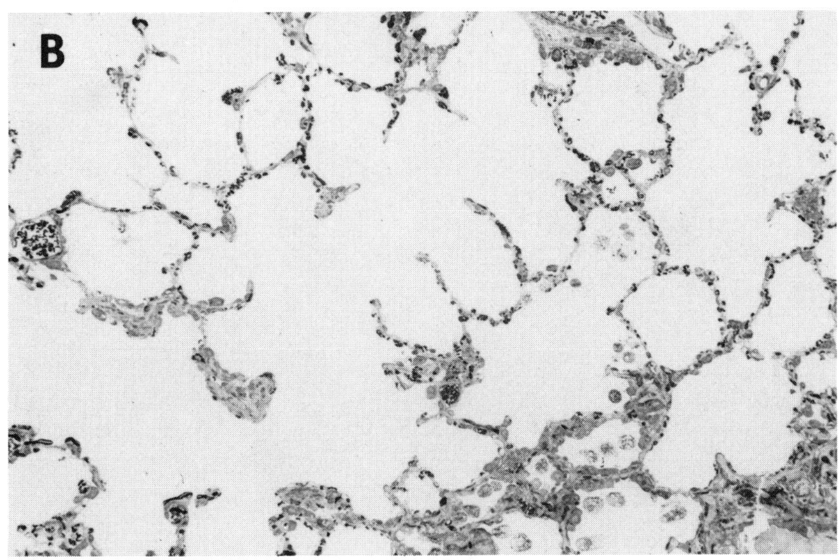

Figure 3B

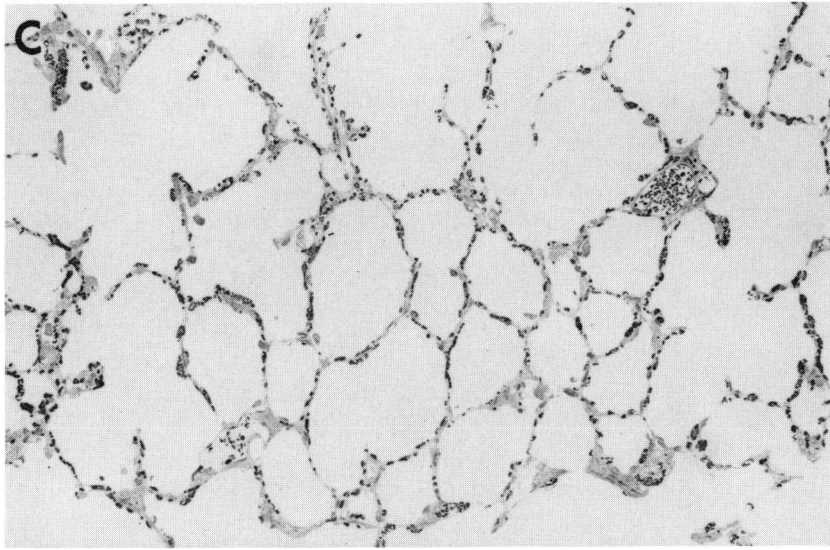

Figure 3C

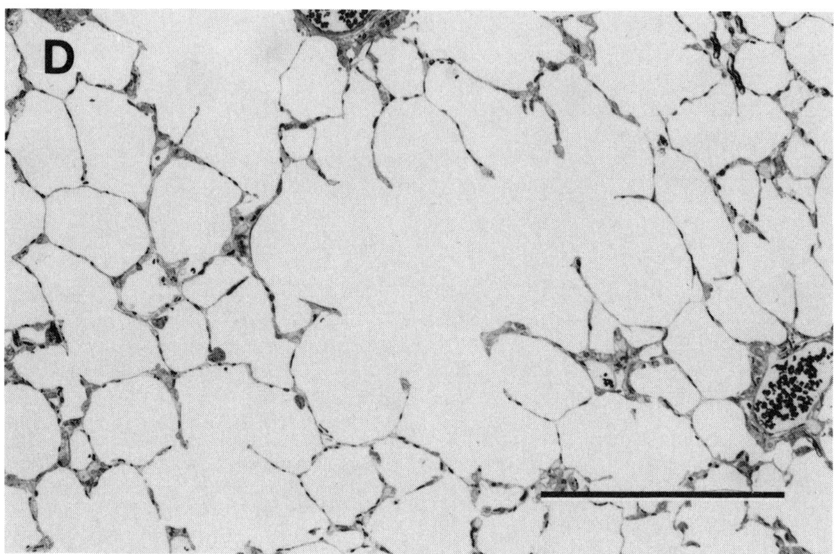

Figure 3D

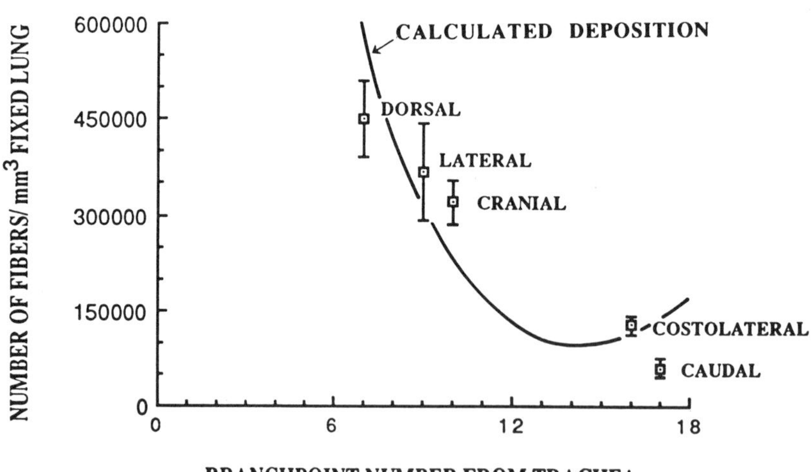

Figure 4. Asbestos fiber concentration (mean ± SD) in five regions of the left lung following chronic inhalation of chrysotile asbestos. (From Hayes and Crapo, 1988; reproduced by permission of Academic Press.)

The observed and calculated length distributions of asbestos fibers in each region of the lung are shown in Figure 5. For all regions examined, the greatest proportion of fibers longer than 20 μm was found in the cranial and lateral regions. The proportion of fibers greater than 20 μm was progressively smaller for the costolateral, dorsal, and caudal regions. For each of these regions, the theoretical model predicted the presence of a greater proportion of fibers longer than 20 μm than was actually observed.

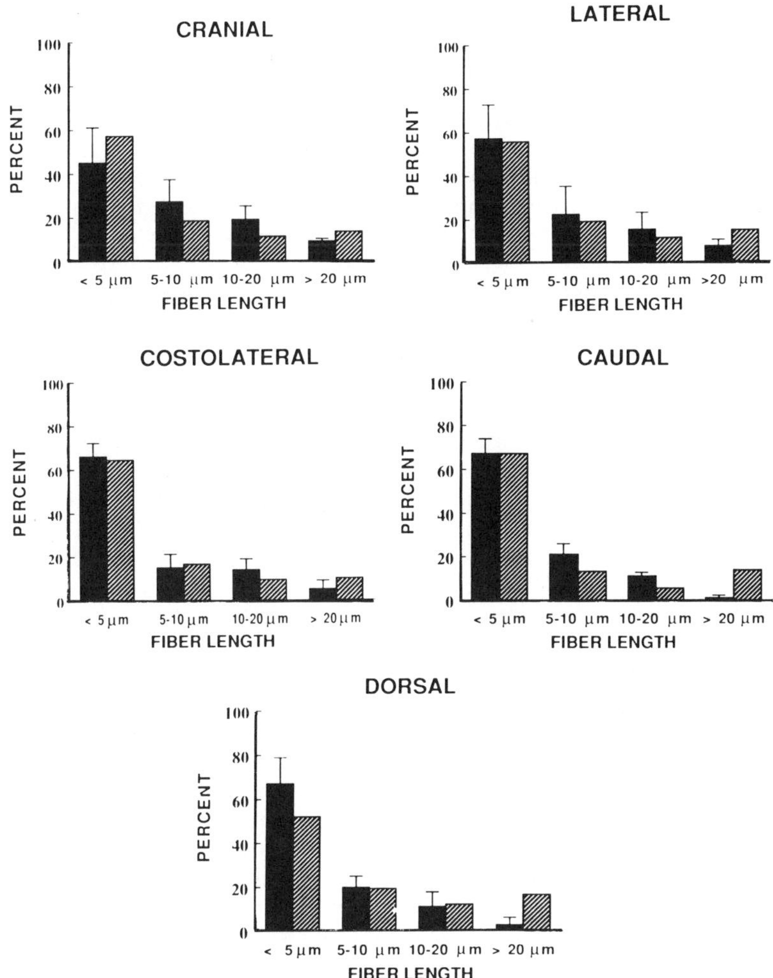

Figure 5. Observed (solid bars) and calculated (crosshatched bars) values (mean ± SD) for distribution of asbestos fiber lengths for five regions of the left lung following prolonged inhalation of chrysotile asbestos in rats.

DISCUSSION

Deposition of asbestos fibers in the gas-exchange region of the lungs is a complex process because of the sequential branching and the changes in orientation of the pathways composing the tracheobronchial tree. Fibers of varying lengths also have a complex behavior when carried through the airways in the airstream. The degree of fiber deposition along the walls of each airway passage depends not only on fiber characteristics, airway dimensions and flow field, but also on the orientation of fibers with respect to the direction of flow (Peterlin, 1938).

Analysis of parenchymal tissues from well-described airway paths has provided a number of interesting observations. First, airway path length plays an important role in the number of asbestos fibers deposited in parenchymal tissues. Second, the number of branchpoints along the airway also affects the number of asbestos fibers deposited within the parenchymal tissue. For pathways containing only a few branch points, the concentration of asbestos fibers that deposit in parenchymal tissues beyond these airways is greater. In contrast, airways of longer path length and more numerous branch points have comparatively fewer numbers of fibers in the alveolar tissues.

Parenchymal lung changes correlate well with asbestos fiber concentrations in each region of the lung, with the exception of the dorsal region. Although this region contained the greatest numbers of asbestos fibers compared to other regions, the septal tissue changes were similar to those in the costolateral region. The dorsal region is unique by virtue of its orientation against gravity. Airflow from the major bronchus must flow upward, or against gravity, along this passage. Compared to other regions, the dorsal region contained the greatest number of fibers shorter than 10 μm. However, the proportion of fibers longer than 20 μm was significantly smaller than that in the cranial and lateral regions but was similar to that in the costolateral and caudal regions. The tissue response of the dorsal region was almost identical to that in the costolateral region but was more marked than that in the caudal region, which contained the least number of asbestos fibers.

These findings in the rat can be placed in perspective when they are compared with studies in workers who were occupationally exposed to asbestos. Sebastien and colleagues (1977) found that asbestos fiber concentrations were generally higher in the apical portions compared to the basilar portions of the lung. In contrast, parenchymal changes were usually more extensive in the basilar regions compared to those in the apical regions. Inhaled particles that move distally in the airway passages that lead to each of these regions clearly go against (apical) or with (basilar) gravity. Fiber size distribution was not analyzed for these regions in the asbestos workers studied. However, extrapolation from our rodent model to humans suggests that differences in asbestos fiber length are likely to be significant in regions where airflow complements gravity, compared to that in regions where airflow opposes gravity. Our rat model may provide a partial explanation for this discrepancy in correlating asbestos fiber burden to the severity of asbestotic lesions in different regions of the human lung.

The theoretical model was remarkably accurate for calculating numbers and proportions of fibers in the lung parenchyma, based on airway surface area and airway branchpoint number. However, some shortcomings of the model are evident with regard to predicting the proportion of fibers of a given length that will be present in certain regions of the lung. Two examples are inaccuracies in predicting numbers of fibers longer than 20 μm for both the dorsal and caudal regions (Figure 5). Other factors, such as influences associated with gravitational effects of particles in the lung or fiber clearance from the lung during periods of prolonged asbestos inhalation, may play important roles and deserve further investigation.

This study presents some of the first tentative evidence of a predilection or selective process for deposition of fibers of discrete sizes in various regions of the lung. The deposition site and numbers of fibers deposited are strongly influenced by the characteristics of the airways from which the parenchymal lung tissues arise. Further investigation of this phenomenon may help in understanding why different regions of the lung show different biological responses to asbestos fibers. These studies strongly support the well-established premise that long fibers are more injurious to the lungs than short fibers (Vorwald et al., 1951).

ACKNOWLEDGMENTS

The authors thank Ms. Melissa Chechowitz and Ms. Patricia Tom for exceptional technical and photographic assistance.

REFERENCES

Asgharian, B, and CP Yu. **1988a.** Deposition of inhaled fibrous particles in the human lung. J Aerosol Med 1:37-50.

Asgharian, B, and CP Yu. **1988b.** Deposition of fibers in the rat lung. Submitted to J Aerosol Sci.

Ashcroft, T and AG Heppleston. **1973.** The optical and electron microscopic determination of pulmonary asbestos fiber concentration and its relation to the human pathological reaction. J Clin Pathol 26:224-234.

Churg, A. **1980.** Asbestos fiber content of the lungs in patients with and without asbestos airway disease. Am Rev Respir Dis 127:470-473.

Churg, A and ML Warnock. **1980.** Asbestos fibers in the general population. Am Rev Respir Dis 122:669-678.

Davis, JMG, ST Beckett, RE Bolton, P Collings, and AP Middleton. **1978.** Mass and number of fibers in the pathogenesis of asbestos-related lung disease in rats. Br J Cancer 37:673-688.

Hayes AW and JD Crapo (eds.). **1988.** *Extrapolation of Dosimetric Relationships for Inhaled Particles and Gases.* Academic Press, New York, NY.

Morgan, A and A Holmes. **1984.** The distribution and characteristics of asbestos fibers in the lungs of Finnish anthophyllite mine-workers. Environ Res 33:62-75.

Murray, M. **1907.** Department committee for compensation for industrial disease. Cmd. 3495-3496. Her Majesty's Stationery Office, London, UK; cited in *Asbestos and Disease,* IJ Selikoff and DH Lee (eds.). Academic Press, New York, NY, 1978.

Peterlin, A. **1938.** Über die Viskosität von verdünnten Lösungen und Suspensionen in Abhängigkeit von der Teilchenform. Z Phys 111:232-263.

Pinkerton, KE, PC Pratt, AR Brody, and JD Crapo. **1984.** Fiber localization and its relationship to lung reaction in rats after chronic inhalation of chrysotile asbestos. Am J Pathol 117:484-498.

Pinkerton, KE, CG Plopper, RR Mercer, VL Roggli, AL Patra, AR Brody, and JD Crapo. **1986.** Airway branching patterns influence asbestos fiber location and the extent of tissue injury in the pulmonary parenchyma. Lab Invest 55:688-695.

Plopper, CG, AT Mariassy, and LO Lollini. **1983.** Structure as revealed by airway dissection: A comparison of mammalian lungs. Am Rev Respir Dis 138:S4-S7.

Roggli, VL and AR Brody. **1984.** Changes in numbers and dimensions of chrysotile asbestos fibers in lungs of rats following short-term exposure. Exp Lung Res 7:133-147.

Roggli, VL, PC Pratt, and AR Brody. **1986.** Asbestos content of lung tissue in asbestos associated diseases: A study of 110 cases. Br J Ind Med 43:18-28.

Schum, M and BC Yeh. **1980.** Theoretical evaluation of aerosol deposition in anatomical models of mammalian lung airways. Bull Math Biol 42:1-15.

Sebastien, P, A Fondimare, J Bignon, G Monchaux, J Desbordes, and G Bonnaud. **1977.** Topographic distribution in relation to occupational and non-occupational exposure, pp. 435-444. In: *Inhaled Particles IV,* WH Walton (ed.). Pergamon Press, Oxford, England.

Selikoff, IJ and DH Lee (eds.). **1978.** *Asbestos and Disease.* Academic Press, New York, NY.

Timbrell, V. **1968.** A simple dispenser for generating dust clouds from standard reference samples of asbestos. Ann Occup Hyg 11:273-281.

Vorwald, AJ, TM Durkan, and PC Pratt. **1951.** Experimental studies of asbestosis. Arch Ind Hyg Occup Med 3:1-43.

Weibel, ER. **1979.** *Stereological Methods,* Vol. 1. Academic Press, New York, NY.

The Effect of Chronic Cigarette Smoke Inhalation on the Long-Term Pulmonary Clearance of Inhaled Particles in the Rat

Joe L. Mauderly,[1] Bean T. Chen,[1] Fletcher F. Hahn,[1] David L. Lundgren,[1] Richard G. Cuddihy,[1] Josef Namenyi,[2] and Alan H. Rebar[3]

[1]Lovelace Inhalation Toxicology Research Institute, Lovelace Biomedical and Environmental Research Institute, P. O. Box 5890, Albuquerque, NM 87185

[2]National Research Institute for Radiobiology and Radiohygiene, Budapest, Hungary

[3]Office of Research Development, College of Veterinary Medicine, Purdue University, West Lafayette, IN 47906

KEY WORDS: cigarette smoke, cerium oxide, inhalation exposure, lung clearance, rat

---

ABSTRACT

The effect of chronic cigarette-smoke inhalation on the long-term retention of relatively insoluble, radiolabeled particles in the lungs of rats was studied. Rats were sham-exposed or exposed nose-only, twice daily, 5 days/week for approximately 12 months to ten 30-second puff cycles of ~1:6 mixture of smoke diluted in air from three type 2R1 research cigarettes puffed simultaneously. After 8 weeks of smoke exposure, all rats were exposed once by inhalation to an aerosol of ^{144}Ce dioxide particles. Group differences in pulmonary retention of ^{144}Ce were examined by comparing retention parameters of radioactivity counts of lungs excised from rats sacrificed serially for up to 315 days after ^{144}Ce dioxide exposure. The variability of retention among individuals was examined by comparing retention parameters of serial whole-body counts of radioactivity. Smoking increased the half-time of short-term clearance of ^{144}Ce by 63% and the half-time of long-term clearance by 106%. The effect of smoking was variable. There was a 3.9-fold range between minimum and maximum values for individual long-term ^{144}Ce clearance half-times in the nine smoke-exposed rats that lived to the end of the study; the coefficient of variation was 47%. In comparison, there was a 1.3-fold range of values for sham-exposed rats and a 10% coefficient of variation. Both the magnitude and variability of the effect of smoking on particle clearance were very similar to those reported from a similar study of humans. These results suggest that rats exposed chronically to cigarette smoke provide a useful model for studying potential interactions between cigarette-smoking and inhaled particles and fibers in man.

INTRODUCTION

Cigarette-smoking is known to alter the mucociliary clearance of innocuous tracer particles and to alter pulmonary macrophage structure and function (reviewed by the U.S. Public Health Service, 1984). Cohen et al. (1979) and Bohning et al. (1982) showed that the long-term clearance of innocuous tracer particles from the lungs of human smokers was slower than that of nonsmokers. It is reasonable to assume that smoking also alters the clearance of potentially toxic particles and fibers from the lungs of smokers, and that this mechanism might be an important factor in the interactions frequently observed between smoking and the effects of inhaled toxicants. Late-occurring health effects, such as carcinogenicity, are likely to be more affected by a smoking-related slowing of the long-term clearance of inhaled toxicants than by alterations of short-term clearance. These observations suggest that the effects of cigarette-smoking on long-term clearance should be considered in toxicological studies of the health risks and mechanisms of effects of inhaled particles and fibers.

Little is known about the effect of chronic cigarette-smoking on the long-term clearance of particles from lungs of animals. Most of the information on the effects of smoke inhalation on the clearance of particles from the respiratory tracts of animals is related to short-term effects on phagocytic cells, bacterial defenses, and mucociliary clearance. Ferin et al. (1965) reported that rats exposed to cigarette smoke before inhalation exposure to SiO_2 had increased amounts of SiO_2 present in their lungs 25 days later compared to the amounts in controls, but only if both exposures occurred on the same day. The rats in that study were not exposed to smoke after inhalation of SiO_2. Bair and Dilley (1965) found little effect of cigarette-smoke exposure on the 3-day clearance of inhaled $^{59}Fe_2O_3$ or $^{51}Cr_2O_3$ from the lungs of rats, regardless of whether smoke exposure occurred before or after exposure to the tracer particles.

The same investigators found no effect of cigarette-smoking on the long-term component of clearance of the same two tracer particles from the lungs of three dogs that had been exposed to cigarette smoke repeatedly, 5 days/week for approximately 1 year (Bair and Dilley, 1965). Albert et al. (1971) reported retarded clearance of radiolabeled iron oxide particles from the lungs of donkeys exposed chronically to cigarette smoke for up to 8 months, but they evaluated clearance of the tracer particles for only 10 hours.

Our study was conducted to examine the effect of chronic cigarette-smoke inhalation on the clearance of relatively insoluble particles from the lungs of rats. The study included a single exposure of rats, by inhalation, to ^{144}Ce dioxide ($^{144}CeO_2$) after the rats were conditioned to repeated smoke exposures. Serial measurements were made of the clearance of the radiolabeled particles during approximately 10 months of continued smoking. This study was a companion to studies conducted in our laboratory to examine the carcinogenicity of inhaled radiocerium (^{144}Ce) in rats (Lundgren et al., 1983, 1987). The amount of $^{144}CeO_2$ inhaled produced negligible radiation-induced lung disease, and the particles were relatively insoluble. Therefore, the results of this study should provide a valuable assessment of the usefulness of the rat as a model for studying interactions between cigarette-smoking and inhaled toxic particles and fibers.

METHODS

Experimental Design

Young-adult rats were assigned to cigarette-smoke-exposed and sham-exposed groups containing equal numbers of males and females (Table 1). The rats were conditioned to smoke or to sham exposures twice daily, 5 days/week for 8 weeks before all rats were exposed once by inhalation to a single concentration of $^{144}CeO_2$ particles (Table 2). Smoke and sham exposures resumed on the sixth day after the $^{144}CeO_2$ exposure. Rats were sacrificed at 2 hours and 7, 14, 29, 90, 180, and 315 days after $^{144}CeO_2$ exposure to determine the ^{144}Ce content in the lung and for histopathologic examination. Whole-body counts of radioactivity were made on the day of $^{144}CeO_2$ exposure, twice weekly for the next 4 weeks, weekly for the next 5 weeks, and bi-weekly thereafter. All remaining rats were sacrificed at 315 days after $^{144}CeO_2$ exposure. Retention curves for ^{144}Ce were constructed from both lung and serial whole-body counting data, and the data were tested for differences in clearance rate as a result of smoke-exposure.

Table 1. Experimental groups and disposition of rats used to study the effects of cigarette-smoke inhalation on clearance of ^{144}Ce inhaled as ^{144}Ce dioxide particles.

Group	Smoke-Exposed Rats			Sham-Exposed Rats		
	Male	Female	Both Sexes	Male	Female	Both Sexes
Total number of animals	21	21	42	18	18	36
Died before $^{144}CeO_2$ exposure[a]	6	3	9	1	0	1
Died during $^{144}CeO_2$ exposure	0	2	2	0	0	0
Exposed to $^{144}CeO_2$	15	16	31	17	18	35
Died after $^{144}CeO_2$ exposure[b]	1	1	2	1	1	2
Sacrificed after $^{144}CeO_2$ exposure	14	15	29	16	17	33

[a]The smoke-exposed males and females died at 21, 28, 36, 43, 44 and 49 and at 28, 38, and 49 days after initiation of smoking, respectively ($^{144}CeO_2$ exposure was on Day 50 after initiation of smoking). The sham-exposed male died at 23 days after initiation of sham-smoke exposure.

[b]The smoke-exposed male and female died at 7 and 24 days, respectively, after $^{144}CeO_2$ exposure. The sham-exposed male and female died at 91 and 2 days, respectively, after $^{144}CeO_2$ exposure.

Table 2. Initial lung burdens of ^{144}Ce achieved by exposing one-half of the rats to ^{144}Ce dioxide during each of two exposures[a]

Group	Exposure A (kBq)		Exposure B (kBq)	
	Male $\bar{X}$ (SD)	Female $\bar{X}$ (SD)	Male $\bar{X}$ (SD)	Female $\bar{X}$ (SD)
Smoke-exposed	422 (89)	348 (93)	270 (44)	222(85)
Sham-exposed	577 (144)	407 (78)	344 (130)	289 (78)

[a]The mean initial lung burdens of the smoke-exposed and sham-exposed groups were not significantly different at the $P < 0.05$ level, as tested by one-way analysis of variance.

Animals and Maintenance

A total of 78 12-week-old male and female F344 rats from the Institute's breeding colony were randomly assigned by weight to the experimental groups listed in Table 1. The rats were housed two/plastic cage, with hardwood-chip bedding and filter tops throughout the study. Feed (Wayne Lab Blox,® Continental Grain Co., Libertyville, IL) and water were provided *ad libitum* except during smoke or sham exposures and whole-body counting. The housing environment was maintained at 18 to 26°C and 35 to 70% relative humidity, on a 12-hour light cycle (on, 0600 to 1800 hours). The rats were weighed bi-weekly.

Cigarette-Smoke Exposures

Rats were smoke- or sham-exposed using Walton Smoke Exposure Machines® (Process Instruments Corp., Brooklyn, NY). Six rats, confined in cylindrical plastic, nose-only, inhalation exposure tubes, were simultaneously attached to the exposure plenum of the machine for each exposure. Each smoke exposure lasted approximately 10 minutes; sham exposures were also conducted for 10 minutes. Three smoke-exposure machines were used; thus, the rats were exposed in groups of 18, twice daily, mornings and afternoons, 5 days/week, for approximately 12 months.

Type 2R1 research cigarettes (high-tar, high-nicotine) were obtained from the Tobacco Health Research Institute, Lexington, KY, in sealed cases of 5000, which were stored at -18°C until used. The cigarettes were removed from the freezer, individual packs were opened, and the cigarettes were conditioned at room temperature and 60% relative humidity for 48 hours prior to use. Up to three cigarettes were placed manually in the puffing mechanism of the Walton machine for each exposure. The machine used positive external pressure to generate a 35-ml puff during 2 seconds, once/minute from each cigarette. The smoke passed into the 675-ml exposure plenum, resulting in dilutions of 5.2, 10.4 and 15.6% smoke, for one, two, and three cigarettes, respectively. The smoke was held in the exposure plenum for 28 seconds, followed by a 30-second purge with clean air. Cigarettes were smoked to a 30-mm butt length, which required approximately 10 puffs. The rats thus received approximately ten 30-second cycles of smoke during each twice-daily exposure.

Rats were conditioned to smoke exposure during a 5-week period, then exposed to smoke, using the final (three cigarettes/exposure) regimen, for 3 weeks before exposure to $^{144}CeO_2$. All rats were placed in the nose-only smoke-exposure tubes twice daily for sham exposures during the first conditioning week. During the second and third weeks, the smoke-exposed rats were placed in the tubes and exposed to smoke from one and two cigarettes (burned simultaneously), respectively. No exposures were conducted during the fourth conditioning week, to match the smoking history of companion groups of rats that were treated at that time to induce pulmonary emphysema (Mauderly et al., 1987). Twice-daily exposures to smoke from two cigarettes burned simultaneously resumed during the fifth week. The final smoke-exposure regimen, twice-daily exposures to smoke from three cigarettes burned simultaneously, started in the sixth week, and continued thereafter except as noted below. Sham-exposed rats were placed in tubes and exposed to clean air on the same schedule.

Cerium Dioxide Exposures

All rats were exposed once by nose-only inhalation to an aerosol of $^{144}CeO_2$ during experimental week 9 (7 weeks after the first smoke exposure). To accommodate the number of rats to be exposed, they were divided into two equal groups, with both sham- and smoke-exposed rats in each group. Both exposure groups were exposed on the same day. The rats were cigarette-smoke- or sham-exposed on Monday, exposed to $^{144}CeO_2$ on Tuesday, and cigarette-smoke and sham exposures were resumed on the following Monday.

Rats were exposed using methods described previously (Lundgren et al., 1982). A suspension of 0.6 M HCl containing 3 mg/ml stable cerium and sufficient ^{144}Ce to achieve an activity of 350 kBq/ml was aerosolized using a Lovelace nebulizer. The aerosol was passed through a two-stage heating column (300 and 1000°C), and the resulting $^{144}CeO_2$ aerosol was diluted with dry, cool air and passed into the nose-only exposure chamber (Raabe et al., 1973). The first and second exposures lasted 40 and 30 minutes, and the chamber activity concentrations were 530 and 660 kBq/L, respectively. The activity median aerodynamic diameter of the particles was determined by a cascade impactor to be 1.16 μm, with a geometric standard deviation of 1.6.

Clearance of ^{144}Ce

Differences between the clearance of ^{144}Ce from the lungs of smoke- and sham-exposed rats were examined by comparing ^{144}Ce retention curves constructed from analyses of radioactivity in lungs excised from rats sacrificed at 2 hours and 7, 14, 28, 90, 180, and 315 days after $^{144}CeO_2$ exposure. Two male and two female rats were selected randomly for sacrifice at each sacrifice time through 180 days after $^{144}CeO_2$ exposure. All remaining rats were sacrificed at 315 days after $^{144}CeO_2$ exposure. The rats were killed by intraperitoneal injection of sodium pentobarbital; a complete necropsy was performed, and the lungs were removed and fixed in 10% netural buffered formalin at a constant perfusion pressure of 20 cm H_2O. The amount of ^{144}Ce in the lungs was determined by scintillation counting. The counting data were fitted to two-component, sum-of-negative exponential functions, using a computerized nonlinear, least-squares fitting routine (SAS Institute, Cary, NC). Clearance curves were constructed by plotting the counting data as percentages of the inital lung burden (ILB) of ^{144}Ce. The ILB (Table 2) was estimated by extrapolating the slope of the whole-body counts between 7 and 56 days after $^{144}CeO_2$ exposure back to the day of exposure. The significance of differences between curves from smoke-exposed and sham-exposed groups was determined using an F test.

The variability of clearance of ^{144}Ce among individual rats was examined by comparing retention curves constructed from the whole-body counting data. All remaining rats were whole-body counted on the schedule described above, using large-volume, deep-well scintillation detectors. Retention of the 7-day whole-body burden of ^{144}Ce was used to construct clearance curves, as described above, from data for five smoke-exposed (two male, three female) and nine sham-exposed (four male and five female) rats that survived to 315 days after $^{144}CeO_2$ exposure. The curves were analyzed as described above for the lung-counting data.

After counting, lungs were embedded in paraffin, sectioned, and stained with hematoxylin-eosin for examination by light microscopy. Detailed examinations were made of the histologic appearance of the lungs of four rats (two males and two females) from the smoke- and sham-exposed groups sacrificed on the day of $^{144}CeO_2$ exposure and at 180 days after $^{144}CeO_2$ exposure, and from five rats (two males and three females) from the final sacrifice at 315 days after $^{144}CeO_2$ exposure. A semi-quantitative scoring system was used to compare the severity of four histologic changes in the lung parenchyma: increased numbers of macrophages; pigmentation of macrophages; inflammation; and alveolar septal thickening. Scores were: 0 = not present; 1 = slight, diffuse change; 1.5 = slight, infrequent focal change; 2 = slight, more frequent change; and 3 = prominent change.

RESULTS

Mortality, Body Weight, and Histopathology

The stress caused by smoke exposures was evident from the mortality that occurred during the smoke-conditioning period before $^{144}CeO_2$ exposure (Table 1). Nine smoke-exposed rats (six males and three females) died at times ranging from 4 to 8 weeks after initiation of smoke exposures (4 weeks to 1 day before $^{144}CeO_2$ exposure). Only one sham-exposed rat (male) died during this period. The smoke-exposed rats were visibly irritated by the smoke, exhibiting erratic breathing and considerable movement during the puff cycle, including attempts to reverse position inside the exposure tubes. Two female smoke-exposed rats died during the 1-hour tube confinement required for the $^{144}CeO_2$ exposure, while none of the sham-exposed rats died. There was no smoke-related difference in survival after $^{144}CeO_2$ exposure; one male and one female in both the smoke- and sham-exposed groups died at times ranging from 2 to 91 days after $^{144}CeO_2$ exposure.

Smoke exposures clearly affected body weight (Figure 1). Group mean body weights were identical before smoke exposures began. At all times after $^{144}CeO_2$ exposure, mean body weights of male and female smoke-exposed rats were significantly lower than those of sham-exposed rats, except for the males weighed at 1, 4, 6, 7, and 9 months.

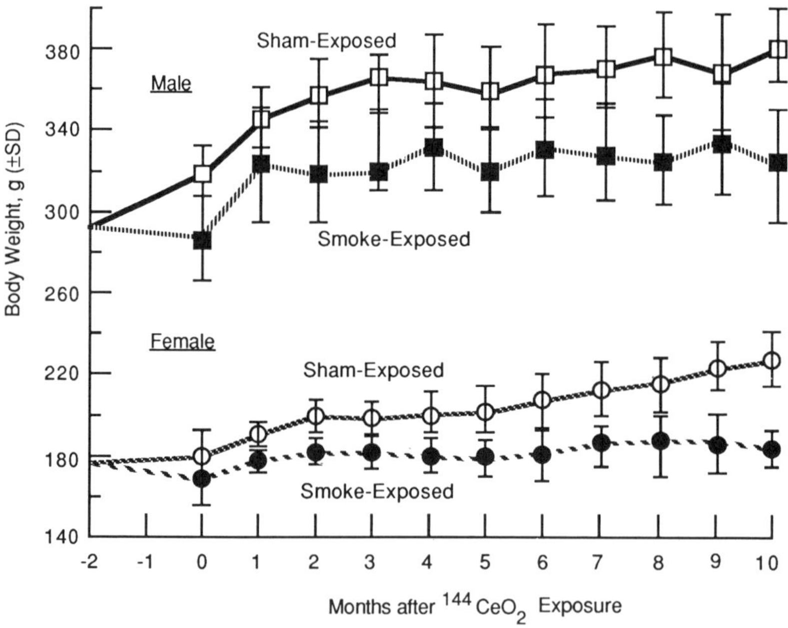

Figure 1. Mean (± SD) body weights of male and female smoke- and sham-exposed rats before smoke exposure, at the time of $^{144}CeO_2$ exposure, and monthly thereafter. Mean weights of smoke-exposed rats were significantly different ($P < 0.05$, analysis of variance) from those of sham-exposed controls at all times after $^{144}CeO_2$ exposure except for males weighed at 1, 4, 6, 7, and 9 months.

There was no histologic evidence of lung injury from the sham smoke exposures and little evidence of lung injury from exposure to $^{144}CeO_2$. No histologic abnormalities were observed in lungs from sham-exposed rats on the day of $^{144}CeO_2$ exposure, which occurred after 8 weeks of sham smoke exposure (Table 3). Three of the four rats sacrificed at 180 days after $^{144}CeO_2$ exposure and three of five rats sacrificed at 315 days after $^{144}CeO_2$ exposure had rare, scattered foci of aggregated alveolar macrophages. These macrophages appeared activated (large and foamy), but were devoid of pigment. A very mild alveolar septal thickening was found adjacent to macrophage aggregates at 315 days after $^{144}CeO_2$ exposure.

Table 3. Summary of scores for histopathologic changes in lung parenchyma of smoke- and sham-exposed rats[a]

Days After $^{144}CeO_2$ Exposure	Increased Macrophages, $\bar{X}$ (Minimum-Maximum)	Macrophage Pigmentation, $\bar{X}$ (Minimum-Maximum)	Inflammation, $\bar{X}$ (Minimum-Maximum)	Septal Thickening, $\bar{X}$ (Minimum-Maximum)
Sham-Exposed				
0	0	0	0	0
180	1.00 (0-1.5)	0.25 (0-1)	0.50 (0-1)	0.50 (0-1)
315	0.90 (0-1.5)	0.40 (0-1)	0.90 (0-1.5)	0
Smoke-Exposed				
0	0.25 (0-1)	0.25 (0-1)	0	0
180	2.25 (2-3)	2.25 (2-3)	1.00 (0-2)	1.50 (0-2)
315	2.20 (2-3)	2.00 (2-2)	1.80 (0-3)	0.60 (0-2)

[a]Semi-quantitative scoring system: 0 = No change; 1 = Slight, diffuse change; 1.5 = Slight, infrequent focal change; 2 = Slight but more frequent focal change; 3 = Prominent change.

One of the smoke-exposed rats had a slight diffuse increase in alveolar macrophage numbers on the day of $^{144}CeO_2$ exposure; the other three rats had no lesions. At 180 days after $^{144}CeO_2$ exposure, all smoke-exposed rats had prominent aggregates of large, foamy macrophages containing brown pigment in alveoli adjacent to the pleura or terminal bronchioles. Neutrophils and lymphocytes were occasionally admixed with the macrophages (inflammation).

Alveolar septal walls adjacent to these aggregates were occasionally thickened, and occasional Type II cell hyperplasia was observed. At 315 days after $^{144}CeO_2$ exposure, all smoke-exposed rats had these lesions.

The histopathological scores listed in Table 3 reflect the differences between the frequency and severity of changes observed in smoke-and sham-exposed rats. The scores also indicate that the macrophage and inflammatory responses were similar at 180 and 315 days after $^{144}CeO_2$ exposure, but that there was some progression of alveolar septal thickening during that period.

Clearance of ^{144}Ce

The ILB achieved by the second of the two $^{144}CeO_2$ exposures was approximately 35% less than that achieved by the first (Table 2); however, rats of both sexes and from both sham- and smoke-exposed groups were included in both exposures. The mean ± SD body-weight-adjusted ILB of all sham- and smoke-exposed rats were 1710 ± 620 and 1470 ± 570 kBq/kg, respectively, values which were not significantly different.

The ^{144}Ce retention curves fitted to the counting data for the ^{144}Ce content of excised lungs are shown in Figure 2, and the values for retention parameters are summarized in Table 4. Chronic inhalation of cigarette smoke retarded clearance of ^{144}Ce from the lung, with the primary effect on the long-term clearance component. The fractions of ILB cleared in the short- and long-term components were not affected by smoke exposure; approximately 40% of the ILB was in the long-term component of both groups. The half-time of the short-term component was increased 63% from 8 to 13 days by smoking, while that of the long-term component was doubled from 86 to 177 days. The difference between the curves of sham- and smoke-exposed groups was significant at $P < 0.01$.

The variability in clearing the 7-day ^{144}Ce whole-body burden among rats sacrificed at 315 days after $^{144}CeO_2$ exposure is illustrated by the individual retention curves in Figure 3. The variability and the difference in clearance half-time between the groups are also demonstrated by Table 5, which lists the half-times of the long-term components (those measured between 56 and 315 days after $^{144}CeO_2$ exposure) of individual rats. The mean half-times of the sham- and smoke-exposed groups were 52 and 164 days, respectively. This difference was threefold, even greater than the twofold difference between the group mean long-term half-times of the lung ^{144}Ce content data. The difference between the mean long-term half-times of the whole-body counts of the two groups was significant at $P < 0.02$ by a one-tailed *t*-test.

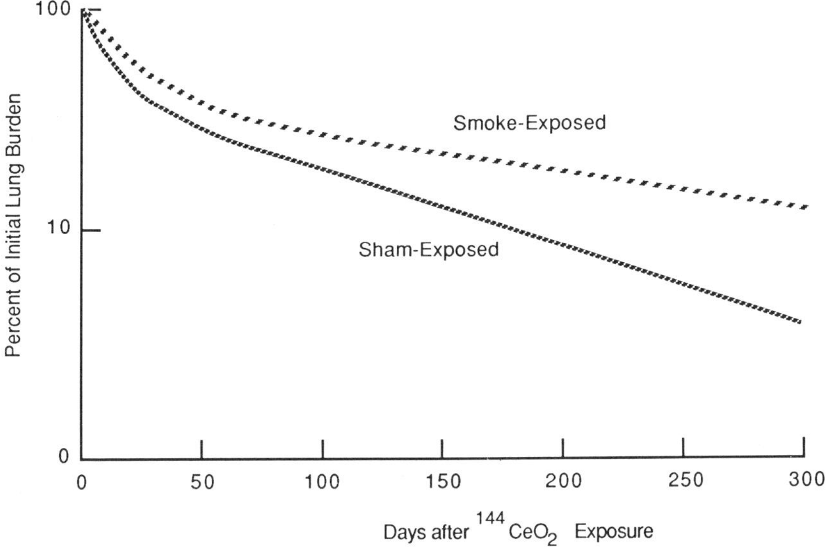

Figure 2. Retention curves of ^{144}Ce of smoke- and sham-exposed rats, based on counts of radioactivity in lungs excised from four rats/group sacrificed at 0.02, 7, 14, 28, 90, 180 and 315 days after $^{144}CeO_2$ exposure. Curves were fitted to data expressed as percentages of initial lung burden, which was estimated by extrapolating the slope of the whole-body counting data between 7 and 56 days after $^{144}CeO_2$ exposure back to the day of exposure. It was assumed that rapid airway clearance was complete by 7 days.

Table 4. Values for retention function of cigarette-smoke-exposed and sham-exposed rats, based on counts of radioactivity in excised lungs of sacrificed rats[a]

Group	Number of Rats	A_1 (%)	T_1 (Days)	A_2 (%)	T_2 (days)
Smoke-exposed	28	61[b]	13(2)[c]	39(7)	177(35)
Sham-exposed	31	59	8(2)	41(4)	86 (4)

[a]Retention was described by the equation: $Y(t) = A_1e^{-0.693t/T_1} + A_2e^{-0.693t/T_2}$, where Y(t) was the lung retention of ^{144}Ce, expressed as a percentage of the initial lung burden. A_1 and A_2 are the percentages of the clearance falling in the short- and long-term components, respectively. T_1 and T_2 are the half-times of the short-and long-term clearance components, respectively. Data were not corrected for radioactive decay.

[b]The standard deviation for A_1 was not determined, because the sum of A_1 and A_2 was forced to equal 100%.

[c]SD

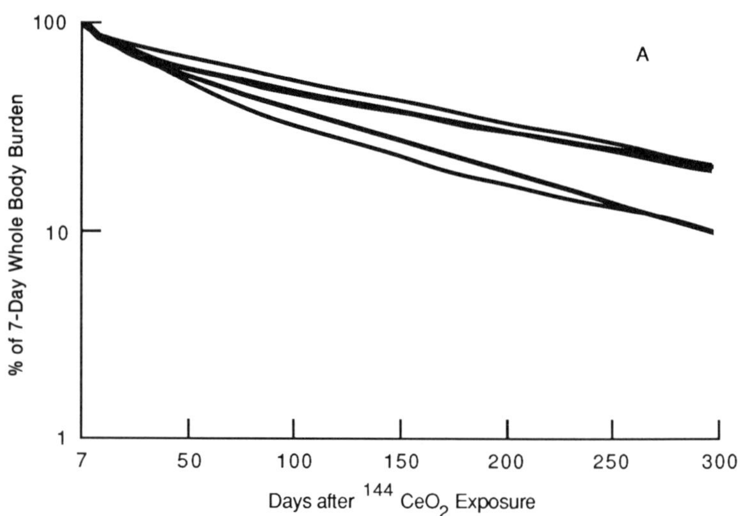

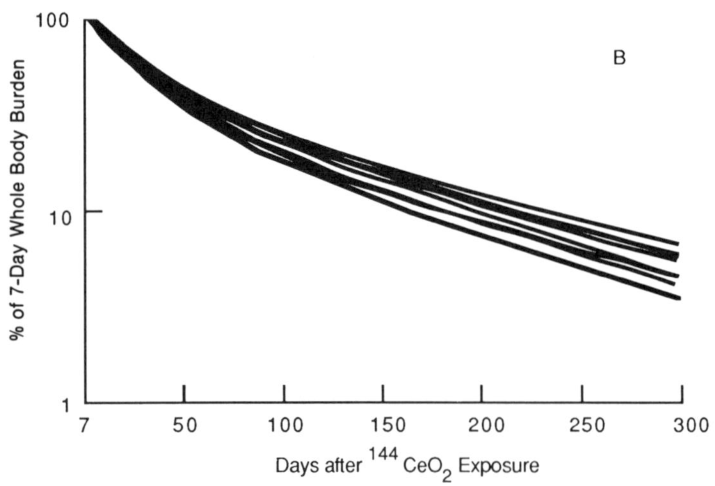

Figure 3. Retention curves for ^{144}Ce, inhaled by smoke- and sham-exposed rats, based on whole-body radioactivity. Individual curves are shown for five smoke-exposed rats (A) and nine sham-exposed rats (B). The curves were fitted to data expressed as percentages of the whole-body burden of ^{144}Ce at 7 days after $^{144}CeO_2$ exposure.

Table 5. Half-times (days) of the long-term clearance components of individual ^{144}Ce retention curves based on whole-body counting data.[a]

	Smoke-Exposed	Sham-Exposed
	67	47
	115	49
	166	49
	209	49
	261	50
		51
		54
		56
		60
Mean	164	52
SD	76	5

[a]Half-times of the long-term component of the whole-body retention curves (the portion betwen 56 and 315 days after $^{144}CeO_2$ exposure).

There was considerably more variability in the half-time of the long-term clearance component of the smoke-exposed rats than in that of the sham-exposed group. The half-times of the smoke-exposed group ranged from 67 to 261 days and had a percentage coefficient of variation (SD x 100/mean) of 46%, while the half-times of the sham-exposed group ranged from 47 to 61 days and had a coefficient of variation of only 10%.

DISCUSSION

Chronic inhalation of cigarette smoke retarded the clearance of ^{144}Ce from the lungs of rats. Both short-term and long-term clearance were slowed, but the effect on long-term clearance was greater. The magnitude of the clearance impairment varied considerably among individuals. The small, nonprogressive macrophage and inflammatory response and lack of progressive septal thickening observed in the sham-smoke-exposed group suggested that the $^{144}CeO_2$ particles were of low toxicity and caused little radiation-induced lung damage.

These results present a good opportunity to compare smoking-related clearance impairments in rats and humans. The methods employed in the present study were similar to those used by

Bohning et al. (1982) in perhaps the most thorough study to date of smoking effects on long-term pulmonary clearance in man. In the Bohning et al. study, five nonsmoking and eight smoking human volunteers were exposed once for 10 minutes to an aerosol of 3.6-μm diameter (4.0-μm aerodynamic diameter) polystyrene microspheres labeled with ^{85}Sr. Retention of ^{85}Sr was examined by serial whole-body counts, extending over an approximately 8-month period. Two-component retention curves were fitted to the data, and values for half-times of the long-term components of individual curves were derived using methods similar to those used in our study.

The mean half-time of the long-term retention component of the smokers in the Bohning et al. study was increased 1.8-fold from 292 to 534 days. That increase was similar to the twofold increase observed in the lung ^{144}Ce content curves in our study but less than the threefold increase observed in the whole-body counting curves. The coefficient of variation of the long-term retention half-times of the Bohning et al. subjects was 15% for nonsmokers and 56% for smokers, values similar to the 10 and 46% we observed for nonsmoking and smoking rats, respectively. The minimum-maximum values for long-term half-times of smokers in the Bohning et al. study were 270 and 1169 days, a 4.3-fold range. The minimum-maximum values for smoke-exposed rats in our study were 67 and 261 days, a 3.9-fold range.

These similarities between the effects of smoking on the clearance of relatively insoluble, spherical particles from the lungs of rats and the humans in the Bohning et al. study are striking, while the differences are minor. The observation of shorter clearance half-times in the rats than in the humans is consistent with species differences reported previously (Snipes et al., 1984). The significance of the finding that smoking induced a delay in long-term clearance of a greater magnitude in the rats than in the humans is difficult to judge. There were several differences in methodology, such as the size of the tracer particles (aerodynamic diameters were 1.16 μm for particles inhaled by rats, 4.0 μm for those inhaled by humans). Moreover, in contrast to the rats, the smoking humans were not a homogenous population with respect to age or smoking history.

The effects of smoking on pulmonary clearance of rats in our study were also qualitatively similar to those observed in man by Cohen et al. (1979). Those investigators used serial magnetometry to measure the clearance of Fe_3O_4 particles from lungs of smokers and nonsmokers. Clearance curves for three smokers and nine nonsmokers were presented, but clearance half-times were not reported. Extrapolating from the published curves, it can be estimated that the percentage of the 2-day lung burden of Fe_3O_4 remaining in the lungs at 10 months after exposure was approximately 4.7-fold greater for smokers than for nonsmokers. In our study, the percentage of the 7-day whole-body burden of ^{144}Ce remaining at 10 months after exposure was approximately threefold greater in smoke-exposed rats than in sham-exposed rats. Although differences in methodology preclude a more precise comparison, it is clear that cigarette-smoke exposure slowed long-term clearance in rats and man by the same order of magnitude.

It is interesting that such a mild smoking regimen produced a substantial effect on particle clearance in our study. The rats were exposed to smoke for approximately 10 minutes/day, 5 days/week (twice-daily exposures to ten 30-second puff cycles) for approximately 12 months. Other investigators, using similar nose-only smoke-exposure machines and identical puffing profiles, have exposed rats chronically for 10 minutes, seven times daily, 5 days/week for 30 months (Dalbey et al., 1980), or eight times daily, 7 days/week for 24 months (Wehner et al., 1981), in attempts to simulate the exposures of human heavy smokers. The histopathological lesions described by those authors were similar to those observed in our study, but they were more severe, including greater increases in pigmented macrophages and greater tissue proliferative and fibrotic responses. Those reports did not describe lesions after 1 year of smoke exposure, the approximate length of exposure in our study. It is likely that exposure length was a major factor in the differences in lesion severity. However, although septal thickening appeared to progress in our study between 180 and 315 days after $^{144}CeO_2$ exposure (Table 3), macrophage accumulation and inflammation did not. It would therefore appear that the differences in severity of lesions between the studies were also related to the number of exposures/week.

It is interesting that the smoke-related reduction of body weight observed in our study was similar to those observed in the studies employing more frequent exposures. At the end of our study, body weights of smoke-exposed rats were approximately 14% lower than those of sham-exposed rats. After approximately the same length of exposure (370 days after initiation), body weight reductions in the Dalbey et al. and Wehner et al. studies were approximately 10 and 14%, respectively. This comparison suggests that the overall stress induced by the exposures in our study was similar to that induced in the studies using more frequent exposures. Perhaps the 15.6% smoke used in our study caused greater stress per exposure than the "10%" smoke (one cigarette at a time) used in the previous studies.

In summary, the results of our study indicate that chronic cigarette-smoke inhalation retarded particle clearance from the lungs of rats, closely mimicking the effect observed in man. This finding suggests that the smoke-exposed rat is a useful model for studying the potential effects of smoking on particle and fiber clearance and the resulting exacerbation of toxicity in humans. Furthermore, the results of our study suggest that a relatively low-intensity smoke-exposure regimen is sufficient for inducing a clearance delay similar to that observed in man.

ACKNOWLEDGMENTS

The authors thank the numerous members of the Institute's staff who contributed to this research. They particularly thank Ms. Dolores Esparza for coordinating numerous experimental events during the study and for the majority of the data summaries and analyses. Ms. Katheryn Callahan, Mr. David Schwarting, and Mr. Terry Zimmerman conducted the cigarette-smoke exposures, with the assistance of Mr. Andrew Baca. Mr. Eloy Salas performed the whole-body and tissue counting. This research was supported by the Office of Defense Programs, U.S. Department of Energy, under Contract No. DE-AC04-76EV01013, and conducted in facilities fully accredited by the American Association for Accreditation of Laboratory Animal Care.

REFERENCES

Albert, RE, D Alessandro, M Lippman, and J Berger. **1971.** Long-term smoking in the donkey. Arch Environ Health 22:12-19.

Bair, WJ and JV Dilley. **1965.** Pulmonary clearance of $^{59}Fe_2O_3$ and $^{51}Fe_2O_3$ in rats and dogs exposed to cigarette smoke, pp. 251-268. In: *Inhaled Particles and Vapours. II,* CN Davis (ed.). Pergamon Press, London, England.

Bohning, DE, HL Atkins, and SH Cohn. **1982.** Long-term clearance in man: Normal and impaired. Ann Occup Hyg 26:259-271.

Cohen, D, SF Arai, and JD Brain. **1979.** Smoking impairs long-term dust clearance from the lung. Science 204:514-517.

Dalbey, WE, P Nettesheim, R Griesemer, JE Caton, and MR Guerin. **1980.** Chronic inhalation of cigarette smoke by F344 rats. J Natl Cancer Inst 64:383-390.

Ferin, J, G Urbankova, and A Vlckova. **1965.** Influence of tobacco smoke on the elimination of particles from the lungs. Nature 206:515-516.

Lundgren, DL, FF Hahn, and RO McClellan. **1982.** Effects of single and repeated inhalation exposure of Syrian hamsters to aerosols of $^{144}CeO_2$. Radiat Res 90:374-394.

Lundgren, DL, FF Hahn, and RO McClellan. **1983.** Effects of repeated inhalation exposure of rats to aerosols of $^{144}CeO_2$: A preliminary report, pp. 83-89. In: *Current Concepts in Lung Dosimetry,* DR Fisher (ed.), Pt. 1. CONF-820492, NTIS, Springfield, VA.

Lundgren, DL, FF Hahn, WC Griffith, RG Cuddihy, PJ Haley, and BB Boecker. **1987.** Effects of relatively low-level exposure of rats to inhaled $^{144}CeO_2$, pp. 308-312. In: *Inhalation Toxicology Research Institute Annual Report,* JA Mewhinney and JD Sun (eds.). Lovelace Inhalation Toxicology Research Institute, Albuquerque, NM. NTIS, Springfield, VA.

Mauderly, JL, DL Lundgren, J Namenyi, and TB Chen. **1987.** The effects of cigarette smoke and pulmonary emphysema on long-term pulmonary retention of ^{144}Cerium oxide, pp. 430-435. In: *Inhalation Toxicology Research Institute Annual Report,* JA Mewhinney and JD Sun (eds.). Lovelace Inhalation Toxicology Research Institute, Albuquerque, NM. NTIS, Springfield, VA.

Raabe, OG, JE Bennick, ME Light, CH Hobbs, RL Thomas, and MI Tillery. **1973.** An improved apparatus for acute inhalation exposure of rodents to radioactive aerosols. Toxicol Appl Pharmacol 26:264-273.

Snipes, MB, BB Boecker, and RO McClellan. **1984.** Respiratory tract clearance of inhaled particles in laboratory animals, pp. 63-71. In: *Lung Modeling for Inhalation of Radioactive Materials,* H Smith H and G Gerber (eds.), EUR 9384 EN. Commission of the European Communities, Luxembourg.

U.S. Public Health Service. 1984. *The Health Consequences of Smoking: Chronic Obstructive Lung Disease,* A Report of the Surgeon General, Public Health Service, Office on Smoking and Health, U.S. Department of Health and Human Services, Washington, DC. U.S. Government Printing Office, Washington, DC.

Wehner, AP, GE Dagle, EM Milliman, DW Phelps, DB Carr, JR Decker, and RE Filipy. **1981.** Inhalation bioassay of cigarette smoke in rats. Toxicol Appl Pharmacol 61:1-17.

Comparison of Particle Deposition Patterns and Functional Responses of Pulmonary Macrophages in Small Rodent Species

David B. Warheit and Mark A. Hartsky

E.I. du Pont de Nemours and Co., Inc., Haskell Laboratory for Toxicology and Industrial Medicine, Newark, DE 19714

KEY WORDS: alveolar macrophages, phagocytosis, chemotaxis, interspecies comparisons, rat, hamster, mouse, guinea pig, particle deposition pattern

---

ABSTRACT

A major challenge for inhalation toxicologists is to define the mechanisms of particle-associated lung toxicity and extrapolate the results of animal data to humans. In carrying out toxicology studies on inhaled materials, a variety of species has been used, although species differences in pulmonary defense mechanisms are known to exist. Since pulmonary macrophages (PM) form the first line of defense against inhaled particulates, we carried out a comparative study to evaluate PM functional responses and inhaled particle deposition patterns in four rodent species.

One strain each of rat, mouse, hamster and guinea pig was lavaged for *in vitro* PM studies or perfused to assess deposition patterns. Cellular differential data demonstrated that PM in all species except the guinea pig accounted for >97% recoverable free lung cells, which contained a resident population of eosinophils. Cell morphology studies indicated that hamster PM were the most active and demonstrated the highest phagocytic activity, while mouse PM phagocytosis was significantly depressed ($P < 0.05$). Chemotaxis studies showed that rat PM migrated most readily to particle-generated chemoattractants, while the chemotactic response to n-formyl peptides was enhanced in hamsters.

To test the predictive value of our *in vitro* findings, all species were exposed to aerosols of carbonyl iron (CI) particles for 1 hour at identical exposure concentrations (i.e., 100 mg/m^3). Analysis of dissected lung tissue by scanning electron microscopy revealed that increased numbers of CI particles were deposited in rats, mice and hamsters, compared to guinea pigs. In addition, increased percentages of rat PM phagocytized CI particles *in vivo,* compared to the other three species. The *in vivo* phagocytosis results correlate with our *in vitro* chemotaxis data and suggest that the rat may be the most efficient species for clearing inhaled CI particles. Whether the rat model best simulates humans remains to be determined.

INTRODUCTION

Inhalation toxicology studies are carried out to evaluate the toxic hazards of inhaled chemicals on the lung and other organs. Although numerous animal models are employed in these investigations, strain and species differences in lung responses to inhaled materials are known to exist. Because risk estimates for humans are formulated as a consequence of the experimental studies, it is clear that a fundamental knowledge of species similarities and differences of pulmonary defense mechanisms is essential. In this regard, several recent studies have examined comparative differences in lung deposition (Brody and Roe, 1983; Lippmann and Schlesinger, 1984) and clearance patterns (Lee et al., 1983; Lippmann and Schlesinger, 1984).

Pulmonary macrophages (PM) form the first line of defense in clearing inhaled particles and bacteria from the distal lung (Brain, 1985). Macrophage movements and phagocytic capacities are essential components of the lung clearance process (Warheit et al., 1988). The comparative studies of PM physiological responses presented here were undertaken to evaluate phagocyte functions *in vitro* to better predict the efficiency of macrophage clearance responses *in vivo* following particle deposition.

MATERIALS AND METHODS

Animals

One strain each of rat, mouse, hamster and guinea pig, all males and 7 to 9 weeks of age, was used in this study. The CD rats (strain, Crl:CD BR), CD-1 mice (strain, Crl:CD-1 BR), and Hartley guinea pigs (strain, Crl:[HA] BR VAF/PLUS) were obtained from Charles River Breeding Laboratory, Kingston, NY. Syrian Golden hamsters (strain, Lak:LVG [SYR]) were purchased from Charles River Breeding Laboratory, Wilmington, MA. All animals were virus-antibody free, and no evidence of viral or other infectious disease was discovered during regular screening of the animals by members of the American Association for Accreditation of Laboratory Animal Care (AAALAC)-approved animal care facility at our institution. Lungs from randomly selected animals were monitored routinely by conventional histopathologic evaluation.

Pulmonary Lavage

All species were anesthetized by intraperitoneal injection of sodium pentobarbital, and the tracheas were isolated and clamped. An incision was made two rings below the larynx, and a butterfly catheter was secured in place. The catheter was connected to a reservoir located 10 cm above the thorax of the animal. The lungs were lavaged with 10 ml of a warmed phosphate-buffered saline solution (Ca^{++}- and Mg^{++}-free), which flowed into the lungs by gravity. This procedure was repeated at least five times per animal.

Preparation of Macrophage Monolayers

The lavaged samples were centrifuged at 250 x g, and the cell pellets were resuspended in Eagle's minimal essential media (Eagle's MEM; F-11, GIBCO, Grand Island, NY) supplemented with penicillin and streptomycin. Cell numbers and viabilities were assessed on a hemocytometer, using a 0.4% trypan blue solution as the vital dye. Cellular differential counts were quantified on cytocentrifuge preparations of lavaged cells stained by a Wright-Giemsa solution. After an additional wash in Eagle's MEM, a suspension of approximately 2.5×10^5 cells was plated onto Thermanox® coverslips (Lux-Miles Scientific, Naperville, IL) placed inside Falcon culture dishes (35 x 10 mm) and incubated for 45 minutes in a CO_2 incubator (5% CO_2-95% humidified room air) at 37°C. After the initial incubation, the monolayers were rinsed vigorously in Eagle's MEM and either immersed in Karnovsky's fixative or processed for phagocytosis experiments (see below). Results of a pilot study showed that the plating efficiency for all species exceeded 90%, as previously reported (Warheit et al., 1984a).

Phagocytosis of Carbonyl Iron (CI) Particles

A suspension of CI powder (GAF Corp., New York, NY) ranging from 0.3 to 2.0 μm in particle size was incubated for 1 hour in Eagle's MEM at 40°C and sonicated to reduce clumping. Final concentrations of 1.75 mg/ml (204 $\mu g/cm^2$) were used in these studies.

After the macrophages were plated for 45 minutes, the monolayers were rinsed in Eagle's MEM to remove nonadherent cells, then immersed in the CI-MEM suspension. Phagocytosis was carried out for 1 hour at 37°C in an incubator. The 1-hour incubation period was selected as a result of a time-course experiment which demonstrated that maximal uptake occurred within 1 hour (Warheit et al., 1984a). Subsequently, the coverslips were vigorously washed in Eagle's MEM to remove extraneous iron and immersed in Karnovsky's fixative prior to processing for electron microscopy.

Scanning Electron Microscopy (SEM)

Following completion of fixation, coverslips were cleared in a cacodylate-buffered sucrose solution, then placed through a series of graded dehydration steps in ethanol. Samples were critical-point-dried, using carbon dioxide as the transitional fluid. The coverslips were mounted on carbon stubs, gold-sputtered, and placed in a JEOL 840 scanning electron microscope for study and photography.

SEM Analysis of Macrophage Morphology and Phagocytosis

The morphology and phagocytosis patterns of representative macrophages were studied in a random fashion. A minimum of 250 cells per monolayer was analyzed and recorded according to its shape, surface morphology (i.e., ruffled membranes or smooth-surfaced, unruffled membranes) and phagocytic profile. The numbers of interiorized CI particles in individual macrophages were recorded, using secondary and backscattered electron-imaging modes (Warheit et al., 1983). Population distributions were tabulated according to the number of ingested CI particles following completion of the SEM analysis.

Activation of Autologous Sera by Zymosan Particles

For each experiment, 1 ml of autologous serum was incubated with zymosan particles (10 mg/ml serum), a well-known activator of complement (Snyderman et al., 1969), for 45 minutes at 37°C in a shaking water bath. Subsequently, the "activated" serum samples were decomplemented by incubating them in a water bath at 56°C for 30 minutes. Negative controls included sera incubated without particles (37°C for 45 minutes) and heat-decomplemented serum samples (56°C for 30 minutes), which were then incubated with zymosan particles. The decomplementation procedure was carried out to ensure that no additional complement-dependent chemoattractant generation would occur following removal of zymosan particles from the incubation mixture or during the assay procedure. Following incubation, the serum-particle solutions were centrifuged at 1000 x g for 15 minutes, and the supernatant was removed and stored in a freezer.

In one set of experiments, the synthetic chemotactic tripeptide N-formyl-leucyl-phenylalanine (FMLP; Sigma Chemical Co., St. Louis, MO) was used as the chemotactic agent. Sequential dilutions at molar concentrations of 10^{-5} through 10^{-9} M were used in these experiments.

PM Chemotaxis

The chemotactic response of PM was assessed using polycarbonate filters inserted into blind-well chambers (Warheit et al., 1984b). The cells were plated in the upper portion of the chamber and incubated for 3.5 hours. Following termination of the assay, the filters (pore size, 5 μm) were fixed with ethanol and stained for light microscopy. To quantify macrophage migration, macrophages that had migrated from the top to the opposite side of the polycarbonate filters were counted in 20 predetermined high-power fields.

Inhalation Studies

Animals were exposed nose-only to aerosolized CI particles for 1 hour at a concentration of 100 mg/m^3. Control animals were sham-exposed to room air. Immediately after cessation of exposure, the lungs of animals were perfusion-fixed through the pulmonary vasculature to assess qualitative and quantitative aspects of particle deposition in the alveolar regions of the lung. The fixed lung tissue was then dissected for SEM as previously described. To quantify macrophage phagocytosis of inhaled CI particles, the lungs of CI-exposed animals were lavaged at 0, 24, 48 and 172 hours after exposure, and the percentages of iron-containing macrophages were assessed by SEM, as described above for the *in vitro* phagocytosis assay.

RESULTS AND DISCUSSION

Cellular differentials from lavaged specimens are given in Table 1. The PM comprised >97% of recoverable cells in rats, mice and hamsters. In contrast, eosinophils accounted for 12.5% of free lung cells recovered by lavage in guinea pigs (Figure 1). These data confirm the earlier findings of Gorenberg and Daniele (1976), who reported that eosinophils accounted for 19% of the recoverable guinea pig lung cells. Because it is well known that increased numbers of mast cells, basophils and eosinophils reside in the guinea pig airways (Karol et al., 1985), it is not surprising that this experimental model is frequently used to simulate human airway responses in cellular hypersensitivity reactions.

Table 1. Summary of cellular interspecies differentials in lavage fluid[a]

Species	Number of Animals	Pulmonary Macrophages	Polymorphonuclear Leukocytes	Lymphocytes	Eosinophils
CD-1 mouse	7	99.2 ± 0.4	0.3 ± 0.2	0.4 ± 0.5	0.1 ± 0.4
CD rat	15	97.3 ± 0.9	1.8 ± 0.8	0.6 ± 0.7	0.3 ± 0.5
Guinea pig	7	86.4 ± 4.0	0.3 ± 0.2	0.8 ± 0.3	12.5 ± 4.3[b]
Hamster	6	98.3 ± 2.2	1.1 ± 2.0	0.2 ± 0.3	0.4 ± 0.3

[a]Values given are mean percentage ± standard deviation
[b]$P < 0.001$ compared to all other groups (Student's *t* test)

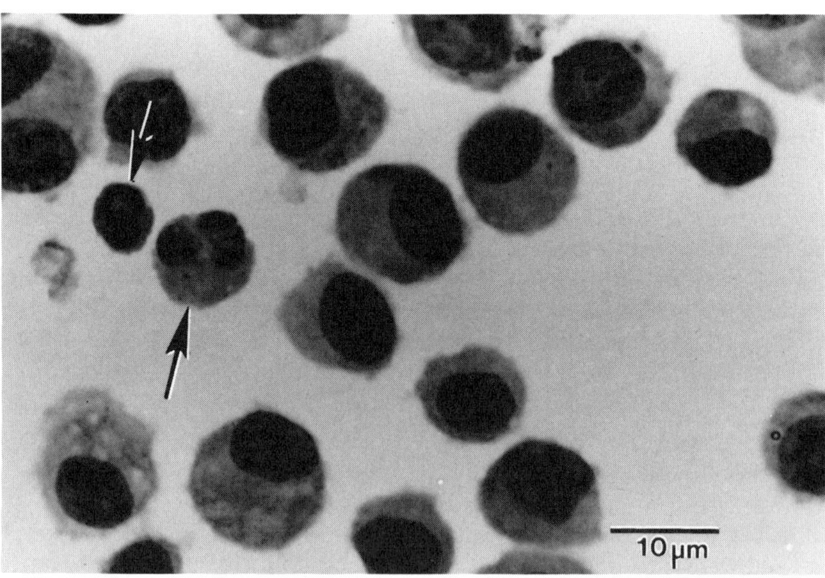

Figure 1. Cytocentrifuge preparation from a lavaged guinea pig. The majority of cells are macrophages, but eosinophils (arrows) comprise 12.5% of the cellular population.

Scanning electron micrographs of PM morphology and phagocytosis of CI particles are illustrated in Figures 2 and 3, respectively. Species comparisons of macrophage morphology and phagocytosis are enumerated in Table 2. Hamster PM demonstrated the highest phagocytic activity, and this correlated with enhanced percentages of ruffled macrophages. In contrast, the phagocytic capacity of mouse PM was depressed compared to that of the rat, hamster, and guinea pig. Previously, we demonstrated a correlation between macrophage morphology and functional capacity; i.e., macrophages with ruffled membranes phagocytized particles at a greater rate than corresponding smooth-surfaced, unruffled PM (Warheit et al., 1984a). Surface morphology, phagocytosis and motility of PM are functions of intracellular cytoskeletal components (Lazarides, 1976; Stossel and Hartwig, 1976). Actin-containing microfilaments form the cytoskeletal constituents of ruffled membranes, providing the motive power for cell migration. These microfilaments are responsible for the infolding of plasma membranes (i.e., ruffles) that facilitate phagocytosis (Painter and McIntosh, 1979; Trotter, 1981). Therefore, the finding of increased percentages of ruffled PM and corresponding phagocytic capacities in the hamster confirms the interrelationship between cell morphology and functional activity.

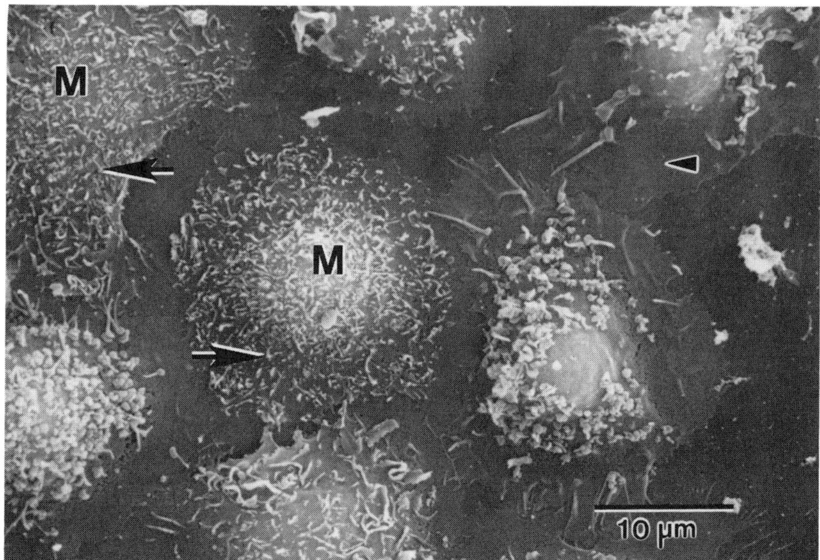

Figure 2. Scanning electron micrograph of lavage-recovered pulmonary macrophages (M) cultured on Thermanox® coverslips for 45 minutes. Ruffled macrophages can be observed.

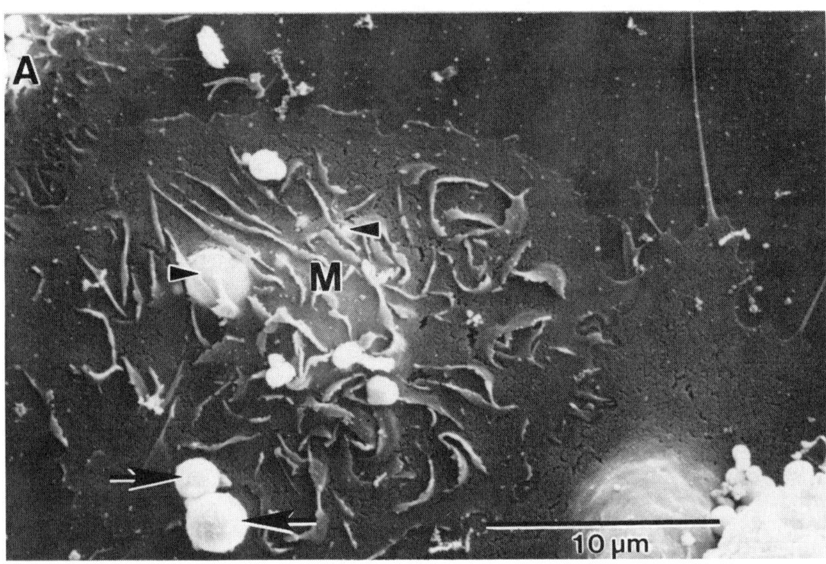

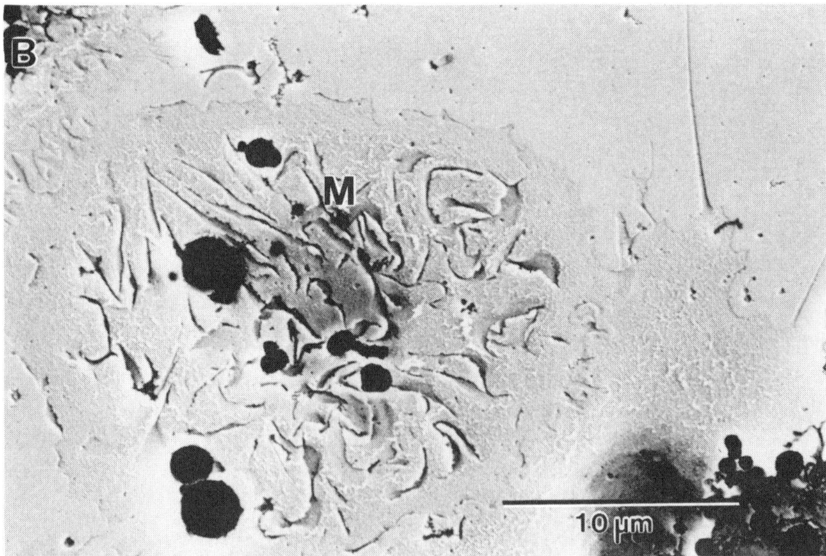

Figure 3. Scanning electron micrograph of carbonyl iron phagocytosis by a ruffled macrophage (M) in secondary (A) and backscatter (B) electron images. The phagocytized beads (arrowheads) can be distinguished from the bead attached to the surface of the cell (arrows).

Table 2. Species comparisons of pulmonary macrophage (PM) morphology and phagocytic capacities[a]

Species	Percentage of Cells Phagocytizing Beads			Cell Morphology (%)	
	0	1-4	>5	Ruffled	Smooth PM
CD-1 mouse	38.2 ± 1.7	23.7 ± 7.3	38.1 ± 9.0	81.7 ± 6.6	18.3 ± 6.6
CD rat	20.6 ± 1.1	47.3 ± 0.8	32.1 ± 1.4	85.2 ± 4.5	14.8 ± 4.5
Guinea pig	31.7 ± 1.9	16.3 ± 5.4	51.9 ± 7.2	83.8 ± 0.8	16.2 ± 0.8
Hamster	13.1 ± 1.8	54.0 ± 2.8	32.9 ± 4.7	90.8 ± 2.4	9.2 ± 2.4

[a]Values given are mean percentages of phagocytic, ruffled or smooth macrophages ± SD for two experiments (two animals/experiment)

The results of chemotaxis studies indicated that PM from the CD rat were the most responsive to zymosan-activated sera, while hamster PM migrated most readily to n-formyl peptides (Table 3). Previously, we demonstrated that a variety of particles activate complement both *in vitro* and *in vivo* following particle deposition, thus generating complement-derived chemotactic factors as a by-product of the activation (Warheit et al., 1988). Because rat PM migrated most readily to zymosan-activated sera, a well-known activator of complement-dependent chemoattractants, it appears reasonable to predict that rat PM are rapidly recruited to sites of particle deposition. Conversely, hamster PM responded vigorously to n-formyl peptides, which simulate bacterial chemotactic factors. Therefore, it is conceivable that hamster PM may rapidly accumulate at deposition sites of inhaled bacteria.

Qualitative data on particle deposition demonstrated that for all species examined, inhaled particles deposited preferentially on alveolar duct bifurcations. In addition, numbers of CI particles deposited on alveolar duct bifurcations of rats, mice and hamsters were greater than those in guinea pigs (Table 4). These data are in agreement with those of Raabe et al. (in press), who evaluated the regional deposition patterns of inhaled aerosols and reported that the depositional fraction of respirable particles in the pulmonary regions of rats was significantly increased in comparison to that for guinea pigs. It is conceivable that the reduced particle deposition in guinea pigs could be attributed to a decreased respiratory rate and/or increased muscle tone (i.e., bronchoconstriction; Jones et al., 1980) in guinea pig airways.

Table 3. Interspecies comparisons of pulmonary macrophage responses to complement-dependent chemoattractants or n-formyl peptides.

Responses to Complement-Derived Chemotactic Factors (Zymosan-Activated Sera)

Species	Number of Animals	Numbers of Migrating Macrophages/ 20 High-Power Fields			
		0.5%	1%	5%	10%[a]
CD-1 mouse	9	ND[b]	85 ± 27	150 ± 44	97 ± 24
CD rat	6	152 ± 34	468 ± 97	693 ± 80	487 ± 76
Guinea pig	9	2 ± 1	51 ± 13	37 ± 9	28 ± 3
Hamster	9	ND	55 ± 10	50 ± 17	35 ± 6

Responses to N-Formyl Peptides

Species	Number of Animals	Numbers of Migrating Macrophages/ 20 High-Power Fields (%)			
		10^{-5} M	10^{-7} M	10^{-8} FMLP[b]	10^{-9} FMLP[c]
CD-1 mouse	9	2 ± 1	60 ± 12	54 ± 7	7 ± 2
CD rat	6	ND	1 ± 1	2 ± 1	2 ± 1
Guinea pig	9	14 ± 2	40 ± 8	32 ± 9	14 ± 3
Hamster	9	78 ± 22	495 ± 87	163 ± 28	36 ± 7

[a]Percentage of zymosan-activated serum
[b]ND = Not determined
[c]N-Formyl methionine leucine phenylalanine

Table 4. Species comparisons of particle deposition patterns in the distal lungs of rodents.

Species[a]	Number of Bifurcations Examined	Mean Number of Particles Deposited ± SD
CD-1 mouse	14	20.1 ± 11.6[b]
CD rat	18	19.8 ± 9.4[b]
Guinea pig	24	8.0 ± 5.3
Hamster	27	15.2 ± 7.3[b]

[a]Three animals per species
[b]$P < 0.01$, when compared with guinea pig

Time-course studies showed that increased percentages of rat PM phagocytized CI particles *in vivo* at 24 and 48 hours after exposure. In contrast, endocytic responses of mouse PM were significantly reduced (Table 5). These results correlated with our *in vitro* findings, where rat PM migrated most readily to complement-dependent chemotactic factors and the phagocytic response of mouse PM was depressed. These data confirm the predictive value of PM functional assessments *in vitro* and suggest that the rat may be the most efficient species of those studied in clearing inhaled CI particles. Whether the rat model best simulates humans remains to be determined.

Table 5. Summary of interspecies comparison of *in vivo* phagocytosis following 6-hour carbonyl iron exposure (concentration, 100 mg/m³).[a]

	Percentage of Phagocytic Pulmonary Macrophages (Hours after Exposure)			
Species	0	24	48	172
CD rat	37.9 ± 3.2	59.0 ± 7.6	58.3 ± 3.2	37.6 ± 10.5
CD-1 mouse	14.9 ± 5.1	24.4 ± 8.0	22.9 ± 4.1	11.5 ± 1.3
Guinea pig	35.1 ± 3.3	36.1 ± 0.4	45.8 ± 4.0	ND[b]
Hamster	35.7 ± 11.5	40.7 ± 16.1	40.5 ± 9.5	44.1 ± 1.9

[a]Values are based on a minimum of two animals per time point
[b]ND = Not determined

ACKNOWLEDGMENTS

The authors wish to acknowledge Mary Stefaniak, Mike L. Van Kavelaar, and John Bamberger for their expert technical assistance.

REFERENCES

Brain, JD. **1985.** Physiology and pathophysiology of pulmonary macrophages, pp. 315-337. In: *The Reticuloendothelial System,* Vol. 7B, SM Reichard and J Filkins (eds.). Plenum Press, New York, NY.

Brody, AR and MW Roe. **1983.** Deposition patterns of inorganic particles at the alveolar level in the lungs of rats and mice. Am Rev Respir Dis 128:724-729.

Gorenberg, DJ and RP Daniele. **1976.** Characterization of immunocompetent cells recovered from the respiratory tract and tracheobronchial lymph node of normal guinea pigs. Am Rev Respir Dis 114:1099-1105.

Jones, RT, MS Kannan, and EE Daniel. **1980.** Ultrastructural study of guinea pig tracheal smooth muscle and its innervation. Can J Physiol Pharmacol 58:974-975.

Karol, MH, J Stadler, and C Magreni. **1985.** Immunotoxicologic evaluation of the respiratory system: Animal models for immediate and delayed-onset pulmonary hypersensitivity. Fundam Appl Toxicol 5:459-47.

Lazarides, E. **1976.** Two general classes of cytoplasmic actin filaments in tissue culture cells. The role of tropomyosin. J Supramol Struct 5:531-563.

Lee, PS, TL Chan, and WE Hering. **1983.** Long-term clearance of inhaled diesel exhaust particles in rodents. J Toxicol Environ Health 12:801-813.

Lippmann, M and RB Schlesinger. **1984.** Interspecies comparisons of particle deposition and mucociliary clearance in tracheobronchial airways. J Toxicol Environ Health 13:441-469.

Painter, RG and AY McIntosh. **1979.** The regional association of actin and myosin with sites of particle phagocytosis. J Supramol Struct 12:369-384.

Raabe, OG, MA Al-Bayati, SV Teague, and A Rasolt. Regional deposition of inhaled monodisperse coarse and fine aerosol particles in small laboratory animals. Ann Occup Hyg (**in press**).

Snyderman, R, HS Shin, JK Phillips, H Gewurz, and SE Mergenhagen. **1969.** A neutrophil chemotactic factor derived from C′5 upon interaction of guinea pig serum with endotoxin. J Immunol 103:413-422.

Stossel, TP and JH Hartwig. **1976.** Interactions of actin, myosin, and a new actin binding protein of rabbit pulmonary macrophages. II. Role in cytoplasmic movement and phagocytosis. J Cell Biol 68:602-618.

Trotter, JA. **1981.** The organization of actin in spreading macrophages. Exp Cell Res 132:235-248.

Warheit, DB, LH Hill, and AR Brody. **1983.** Pulmonary macrophage phagocytosis: Quantification by secondary and backscattered electron imaging. Scanning Electron Microsc 1:431-437.

Warheit, DB, LH Hill, and AR Brody. **1984a.** Surface morphology and correlated phagocytic capacity of pulmonary macrophages lavaged from the lungs of rats. Exp Lung Res 6:71-82.

Warheit, DB, LY Chang, LH Hill, GER Hook, JD Crapo, and AR Brody. **1984b.** Pulmonary macrophage accumulation and asbestos-induced lesions at sites of fiber deposition. Am Rev Respir Dis 129:301-310.

Warheit, DB, LH Overby, G George, and AR Brody. **1988.** Pulmonary macrophages are attracted to inhaled particles through complement activation. Exp Lung Res 14:51-66.

Lung Clearance of Inhaled Particulates: Mechanism of Macrophage Recruitment and Phagocytosis at Sites of Particle/Fiber Deposition

David B. Warheit,[1] Mark A. Hartsky,[1] and Arnold R. Brody[2]

[1]E.I. du Pont de Nemours and Co., Inc., Haskell Laboratory for Toxicology and Industrial Medicine, Newark, DE 19714

[2]Laboratory of Pulmonary Pathobiology, National Institute of Environmental Health Sciences , Research Triangle Park, NC 27709

KEY WORDS: lung clearance, alveolar macrophages, phagocytosis, complement activation, chemotaxis

---

ABSTRACT

Pulmonary macrophages (PM) play a critical role in maintaining normal lung physiology by phagocytizing and removing inhaled particles and bacteria. Phagocyte motility and endocytic capacities in the lung are prerequisites for efficient clearance of inhaled mineral fibers. The mechanism(s) through which PM are recruited to sites of fiber deposition have not been well understood. Recently, we demonstrated that inhaled asbestos fibers generate complement-derived chemotactic factors in the lungs of exposed rats. To determine whether this mechanism was common to inorganic particulates, we tested the hypothesis that a variety of inhaled particulates "signal" their presence to PM in the distal lung by generating chemoattractants, thus facilitating their own clearance at sites of particle deposition.

A number of inorganic particles and fibers were tested for chemotactic factor activity *in vitro,* and these data were correlated with measurements of fiber-induced PM chemotaxis *in vivo.* Our results demonstrated that significant complement-dependent chemotactic activity was generated both in rat serum and in concentrated lavaged proteins by iron-treated chrysotile and crocidolite asbestos, fiberglass, and wollastonite fibers, as well as by carbonyl iron particles. Ash from the Mount St. Helens volcano and decomplemented sera, which did not induce chemotactic activity *in vitro,* provided negative controls. To correlate our *in vitro* results with inhalation studies, rats were exposed to aerosols of each of the particulates listed above. Time-course studies showed that all of the particles except Mount St. Helens ash induced significant accumulations of PM at sites of deposition. We conclude that complement activation is a mechanism through which PM detect inhaled mineral fibers on alveolar surfaces, thus facilitating particle clearance from the lung.

INTRODUCTION

Pulmonary macrophages (PM) play a pivotal role in maintaining the sterility of the lung by phagocytizing and clearing inhaled particles and bacteria (Brain, 1985). Along with phagocyte motility and endocytic functions, particle identification by macrophages in the distal lung is an important prerequisite for efficient particle clearance. However, little information exists regarding the mechanisms through which lung macrophages detect the presence of inhaled particles on alveolar surfaces.

In previous studies we demonstrated that rat PM migrate to sites of asbestos fiber deposition within 24 hours after exposure and phagocytize the inhaled fibers (Warheit et al., 1984a). In attempting to discern the mechanisms through which these phagocytes are recruited to alveolar duct bifurcations, we showed that chrysotile asbestos fibers interact with complement proteins on lung surfaces to chemotactically attract PM (Warheit et al., 1985). In addition to asbestos, a variety of inorganic dusts have been shown to activate complement *in vitro* (Olenchock et al., 1978; Hill et al., 1982; Warheit et al., 1984b). Therefore, the current study was undertaken to test the hypothesis that inorganic particulates, which activate complement *in vitro,* generate chemotactic factors for macrophages *in vivo,* thus providing a mechanism by which inhaled particulates are detected by PM in the alveolar regions of the lung.

MATERIALS AND METHODS

Pulmonary Lavage and Preparation of Macrophage Monolayers

Rats (strain Crl:CD BR; Charles River Breeding Laboratories, Wilmington, MA) were anesthetized by intraperitoneal injections of Nembutal.® The methods used for bronchoalveolar lavage have been previously reported (Warheit et al., 1984c). Fluid recovered by lavage was centrifuged (250 x g for 10 minutes), and the supernatant (i.e., lavage fluid) was removed and concentrated for chemotaxis studies. The cell pellet was resuspended in Eagle's minimal essential medium (Eagle's MEM; F-11 GIBCO, Grand Island, NY) supplemented with penicillin and streptomycin. Cell numbers and viabilities were quantified using a hemoctyometer and trypan blue solution. Cell differential counts were carried out on Wright-Giemsa-stained cytocentrifuge preparations.

After an additional wash, a suspension of macrophages containing 2 x 10^5 cells was plated on Thermanox® coverslips (Lux-Miles Scientific, Naperville, IL) placed inside Falcon® culture dishes. The cells were incubated for 45 minutes in a CO_2 incubator (5% CO_2/95% humidified room air) at 37°C. Subsequently, the monolayers were rinsed vigorously in Eagle's MEM to remove nonadherent cells and either placed in fixative or further processed for phagocytosis studies.

To carry out *in vitro* phagocytosis studies, a suspension of carbonyl iron particles was incubated with either zymosan-activated, normal heated, or decomplemented rat serum for 1 hour at 40°C and sonicated to reduce aggregations of particles. The iron particles ranged in diameter from 0.3 to 2.0 μm. A final concentration of 1.75 mg/ml (204 $\mu g/cm^2$) was added to the monolayers. Phagocytosis of iron particles was carried out at 37°C in the CO_2 incubator for 1 hour. The coverslips were then rinsed in Eagle's MEM to remove residual carbonyl iron and fixed in Karnovsky's solution before proccessing for scanning electron microscopy (SEM), as described below.

After fixation, coverslips were rinsed in a cacodylate-sucrose-buffered solution and dehydrated through a series of ethanol steps. Samples were critical-point-dried using carbon dioxide as the transitional fluid. Coverslips were mounted on carbon stubs, gold-coated, and studied in a JEOL 35 or 840 scanning electron microscope.

Studies of the morphology and phagocytic capacities of PM were carried out using SEM of randomly selected cultured cells, as previously described (Warheit et al., 1984c). Initially, a field of view was selected at low magnification to avoid observer bias. Then each cell in the field of view was analyzed at higher magnification. The characteristic shape and surface morphology of each cell was recorded. Cells were categorized according to their ruffled membranes or unruffled, smooth surface characteristics. The surfaces of smooth macrophages were devoid of ruffled membranes but frequently contained blebs or other irregularities. Endocytosed carbonyl iron beads were quantified in individual macrophages using secondary and backscattered electron imaging modes of the SEM.

Particulates

Chrysotile asbestos fibers, obtained from the Jeffrey Mine in Quebec, Canada, have been previously characterized (Pinkerton et al., 1983). An aliquot of these fibers was treated with ammonium ferrous sulfate according to the method of Flowers (1982) to obtain iron-treated chrysotile asbestos. The crocidolite asbestos fibers were obtained from a UICC sample previously characterized (Warheit et al., 1984b). The glass fibers (Code 100) were provided by Dr. James Leineweber (Johns Manville Co., Denver, CO). The frequency distribution of lengths and diameters of Code 100 glass fibers were reported by Hesterberg and Barrett (1984). Carbonyl iron particles were purchased from GAF Corp. (New York, NY). Ash from the Mount St. Helens volcano eruption (in May 1980), obtained from the U.S. Environmental Protection Agency, is a heterogeneous mix of mineral particles. The major minerals in the ash are feldspar and orthopyroxene (Fruchter et al., 1980).

In Vitro Chemotaxis Studies

Pulmonary macrophage chemotaxis was the indicator for complement activation in response to both activated serum and lavaged proteins (Warheit et al., 1985). Briefly, fresh serum or lavaged proteins (concentration, 1.2 mg/ml) were incubated with either crocidolite asbestos, iron-treated chrysotile asbestos fibers, fiberglass, wollastonite fibers, carbonyl iron particles, or Mount St. Helens ash particles at concentrations of 25 mg/ml sera. The serum-particle or particle-lavaged protein suspensions were incubated in conical tubes for 45 minutes in a shaking water bath at 37°C. The "activated" sera or lavaged proteins were subsequently incubated for an additional 30 minutes at 56°C to prevent any further activation, then centrifuged to remove the particles (250 x g for 10 minutes). Normal heated serum (37°C for 40 minutes) and decomplemented sera (56°C for 30 minutes, then incubated with either chrysotile asbestos or fiberglass after decomplementation) were used as negative controls. The activated preparations of sera and lavaged proteins were diluted to concentrations of 1, 5, and 10% (v/v) in an RPMI 1640 buffer solution containing 10 mM Hepes and 1% bovine serum albumin. Chemotaxis was assessed using polycarbonate filters inserted into blind-well chambers (Warheit et al., 1984a). The macrophages (concentrations, 1.5×10^6 cells/ml) were plated in the upper portion of the chambers and incubated for 3.5 hours in a CO_2 incubator. Following completion of the assay, the filters (pore size, 5 μm) were removed from the blind-well chambers, fixed with ethanol, and stained for light microscopic analysis. To quantify cell migration, the numbers of PM that had migrated from the top to the opposite side of the polycarbonate filters were counted in 20 predetermined high-power fields (HPF; only 10 HPF for assessment of dust-activated lavaged proteins).

Inhalation Studies

Rats were exposed to aerosolized concentrations of either crocidolite, chrysotile (data not shown), iron-treated chrysotile asbestos fibers, wollastonite fibers, fiberglass, carbonyl iron particles, or Mount St. Helens volcanic ash particles ranging from 10 to 15 mg/m^3 for 1, 3, or 5 hours in wire-mesh cages contained within inhalation chambers. Control rats were similarly sham-exposed to room air. Twenty-four or 48 hours after exposure to the particulate aerosol, the rats were anesthetized with a lethal dose of pentobarbital. The lungs were infused with fixative (1% paraformaldehyde, 1% glutaraldehyde) through the airway at a pressure of 15 cm of water. The fixed lung tissue was prepared for SEM to facilitate quantification of PM recruitment to sites of particulate deposition. All bifurcation surfaces revealed by random dissection of critical-point-dried lung tissue were evaluated as previously described (Warheit et al., 1984a). The numbers of macrophages which had migrated to alveolar duct bifurcations were recorded in rats exposed to crocidolite asbestos, iron-treated chrysotile asbestos, fiberglass, wollastonite, carbonyl iron, or Mount St. Helens ash.

RESULTS AND DISCUSSION

In Vitro Chemotaxis and Phagocytosis

PM chemotaxis was used as a bioassay for complement activation. Addition of either crocidolite asbestos, iron-treated chrysotile asbestos fibers, fiberglass, wollastonite fibers, or carbonyl iron particles to rat sera enhanced chemotactic responses in comparison to serum incubated with Mount St. Helens ash particles (Figures 1 and 2). Normal heated sera and sera decomplemented prior to incubation with fiberglass provided additional controls. Similarly, increased chemotactic activity was detected in cell-free lavaged proteins following activation with either crocidolite or iron-treated chrysotile asbestos, wollastonite or carbonyl iron particles (Table 1). As demonstrated in the chemotaxis studies with dust-activated sera, Mount St. Helens ash particles did not activate complement in lavaged lung proteins, thus providing an additional negative control.

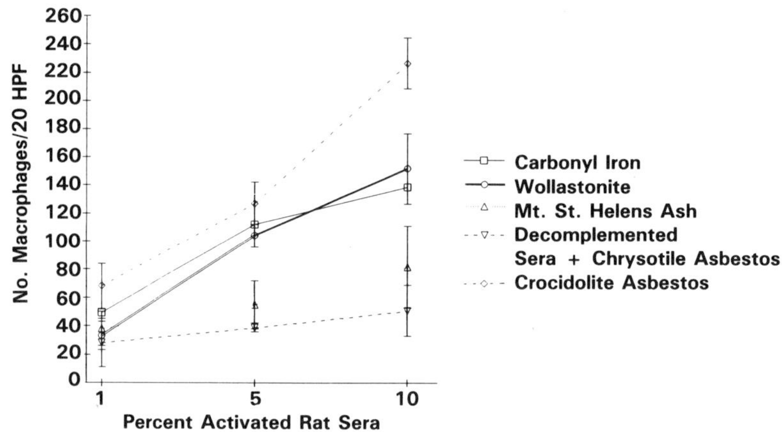

Figure 1. Pulmonary macrophage chemotaxis in response to varying concentrations of sera activated by crocidolite asbestos, wollastonite fibers, carbonyl iron particles, Mount St. Helens ash, or decomplemented sera. Values given are mean ± SD/20 high-power fields for two experiments each. Macrophages clearly were more responsive to serum activated by crocidolite, wollastonite, and carbonyl iron, in comparison to Mount St. Helens ash particles or controls.

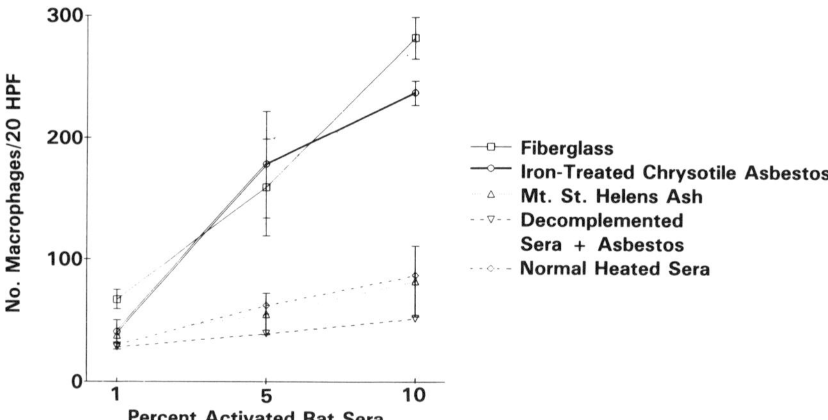

Figure 2. Pulmonary macrophage chemotaxis in response to varying concentrations of sera activated by fiberglass, iron-treated chrysotile asbestos, Mount St. Helens ash, normal heating, or decomplementation. Values given are mean ± SD/20 high-power fields for two experiments each. Macrophages clearly were more responsive to serum activated by fiberglass and iron-treated chrysotile asbestos, compared to Mount St. Helens ash particles or controls. These results (Figures 1 and 2) demonstrate that the incubation of a variety of particulates with serum produces complement activation.

Table 1. Chemotactic response of pulmonary macrophages to dust-activated lavaged proteins[a]

	Numbers of Migrating Macrophages/10 High-Power Fields ($\bar{x} \pm SD$)
Iron-treated chrysotile asbestos	29.5 ± 6.4[b]
Crocidolite asbestos	22.7 ± 3.5[b]
Carbonyl iron	20.7 ± 6.0
Wollastonite	20.5 ± 2.1[b]
Mount St. Helens ash	15.5 ± 0.7
Normal heat-activated lavage	15.3 ± 1.5
Decomplemented sera plus fiberglass	8.5 ± 2.1

[a]Values given are mean numbers of migrating macrophages from six filters (two experiments)
[b]$P < 0.05$ (Student's *t*-test) compared to ash-activated lavaged proteins

To assess the effects of complement activation on PM phagocytosis, carbonyl iron particles were opsonized with either normal heated sera, heat-decomplemented sera, or zymosan-activated sera, a well-known activator of complement (Snyderman et al., 1969). Macrophage monolayers were incubated with suspensions of opsonized carbonyl iron particles for 1 hour. The results showed that PM phagocytized zymosan-activated, opsonized carbonyl iron particles at a greater rate than normal or decomplemented serum-opsonized particles (Figures 3A and B; Table 2). These results support the hypothesis that complement activation enhances particle phagocytosis by PM.

Macrophage Accumulation *In Vivo*

Scanning electron microscopic techniques were used to evaluate particle deposition patterns and to quantify corresponding PM recruitment responses following brief exposure to aerosolized dusts. As previously described (Brody and Roe, 1983), inhaled particulates, regardless of shape or composition, deposit preferentially on alveolar duct bifurcations (Figures 4 and 5). Within 24 hours after exposure, PM migrated to alveolar duct bifurcations in the lungs of rats exposed to crocidolite and iron-treated chrysotile asbestos, wollastonite, fiberglass, and carbonyl iron (Figures 6A and B). In contrast, macrophages did not accumulate at sites of particle deposition in animals exposed to aerosolized Mount St. Helens ash. This correlated with the inability of the volcanic ash to activate complement in serum or lavaged proteins (Table 3).

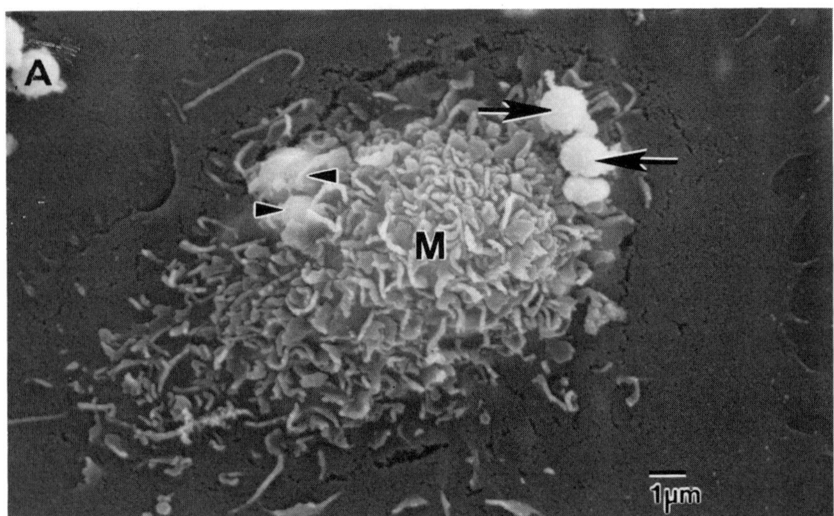

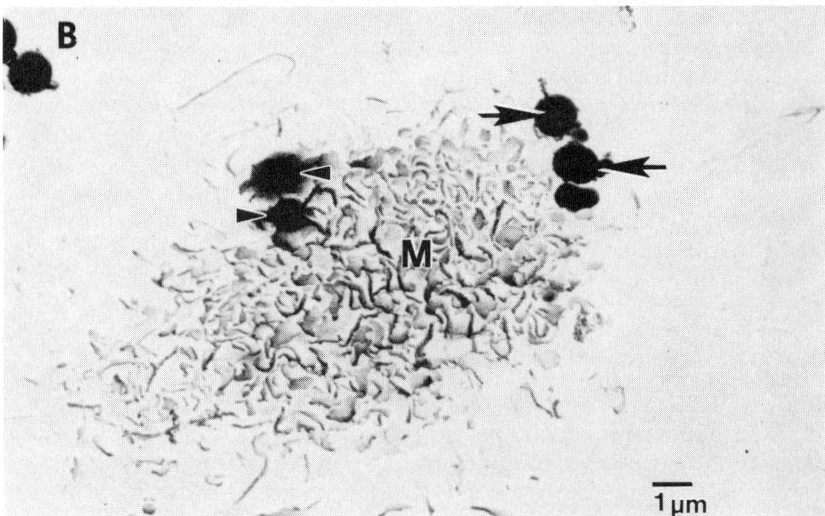

Figure 3. Scanning electron micrograph of a flat-ruffled pulmonary macrophage (M) containing iron beads in secondary (A) and backscatter (B) images. Note that the backscatter image is particularly useful in differentiating between internalized beads (arrowheads) and beads adsorbed to the surface of the cell (arrows).

Table 2. Effects of serum complement activation on macrophage morphology and phagocytic capacities[a]

Carbonyl Iron Particles Opsonized with	Percentage of Cells Phagocytizing Iron Beads			Cell Morphology	
	0	1-4	≥5	Percent Ruffled	Percent Smooth
Zymosan-activated sera	20.4 ± 3.3	22.6 ± 11.2	57.1 ± 8.0	81.8 ± 4.5	18.2 ± 4.9
Normal heated sera	30.7 ± 3.2	31.4 ± 5.7	38.0 ± 8.9	75.5 ± 1.4	24.5 ± 1.6
Decomplemented sera	53.0 ± 6.4	25.0 ± 0.4	22.1 ± 6.1	73.3 ± 3.3	26.7 ± 3.6

[a]All values represent mean ± SD of two experiments. Number of cells analyzed per monolayer, 250; dose of serum-coated carbonyl iron, 204 μg/cm²; two animals per experiment.

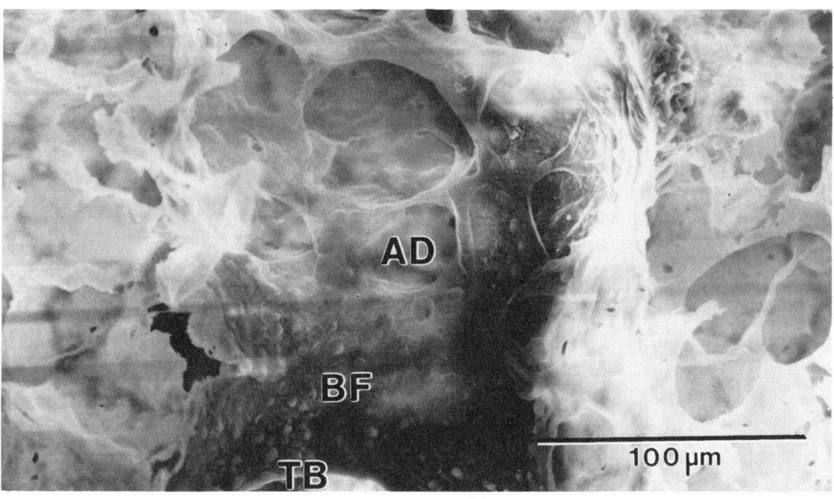

Figure 4. Scanning electron micrograph of critical-point-dried lung tissue from a CD rat that inhaled chrysotile asbestos. This low magnification illustrates a terminal bronchiole (TB) that leads to an alveolar duct (AD). A first alveolar duct bifurcation is labeled BF; a similar region is enlarged in Figure 5.

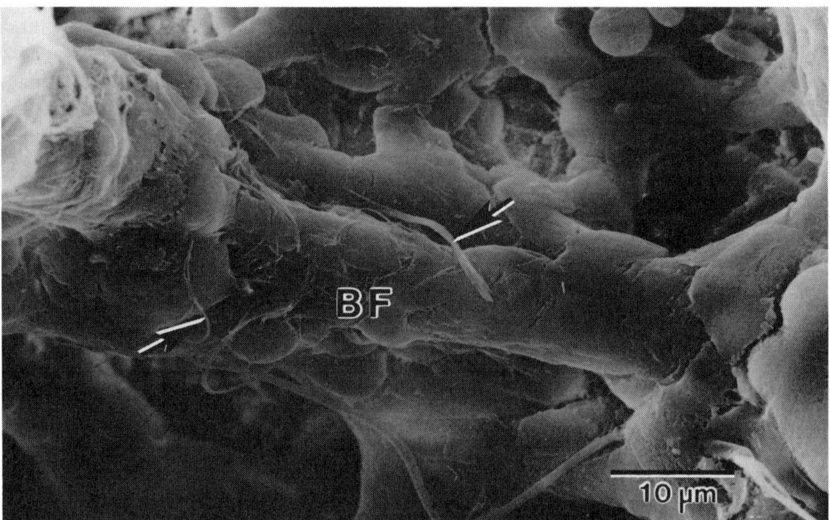

Figure 5. Scanning electron micrograph of a first alveolar duct bifurcation (BF), taken immediately following a 1-hour inhalation exposure to chrysotile asbestos. Asbestos fibers have deposited on the bifurcation surface, while adjacent alveolar duct surfaces are devoid of fibers.

We have previously demonstrated in rats and mice that PM migrate electively to sites of chrysotile asbestos deposition and phagocytize inhaled fibers (Warheit et al., 1985, 1986). In attempting to elucidate the mechanisms through which macrophages respond following a brief asbestos exposure, we showed that the inhaled fibers activate a complement-dependent chemoattractant at sites of fiber deposition. The studies reported here were carried out to determine whether chemotactic factor generation *in vivo* is unique to chrysotile-asbestos-exposed animals or, alternatively, whether activation of complement by inhaled particulates represents a common mechanism through which PM migrate to sites of particle deposition. Our results indicate that a variety of inhaled particulates activate complement in both serum and lung fluids *in vitro*. Furthermore, when inhaled, these particles deposit at alveolar duct bifurcations and activate complement, generating complement-derived chemoattractants as by-products of this reaction, thus facilitating macrophage accumulation at sites of particle deposition (Table 4). It is interesting that, as previously reported (Olenchock and Mull, 1981; Yano et al., 1985), Mount St. Helens ash particles did not activate complement *in vitro*. In the studies presented here, we have extended these results to show that volcanic ash did not stimulate macrophage chemotaxis *in vivo* following particle exposure.

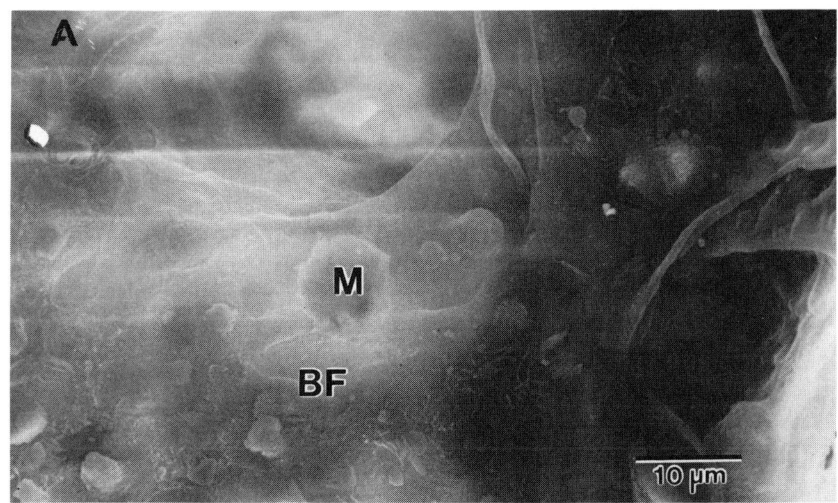

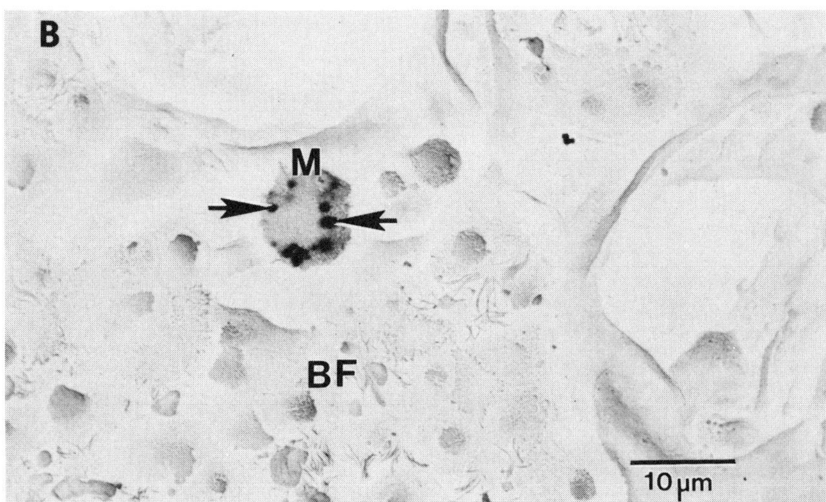

Figure 6. Secondary (A) and backscatter (B) images of an alveolar duct bifurcation (BF) 48 hours after a 3-hour exposure to carbonyl iron particles. A pulmonary macrophage (M) has migrated to the bifurcation and has phagocytized several carbonyl iron particles (arrows).

Table 3. Number and distribution of pulmonary macrophages (PM) at alveolar duct bifurcations in rats exposed to various inhaled particulates[a]

Exposure	Number of Animals	Number of Bifurcations Examined	Number of PM ($\bar{x} \pm$ SD)	Percentage of Bifurcations Containing		
				0 PM	1 PM	2 to 10 PM
Sham						
3-hour exposure to room air, no recovery	3	28	0.3 ± 0.5	75.0	21.4	3.6
3-hour exposure to room air, 24-hour recovery	4	18	0.2 ± 0.3	78.6	14.3	7.1
3-hour exposure to room air, 48-hour recovery	6	43	0.3 ± 0.6	67.0	27.0	6.0
Mount St. Helens Ash						
3-hour exposure to dust, no recovery	4	29	0.2 ± 0.4	82.8	17.2	—
3-hour exposure to dust, 24-hour recovery	3	36	0.3 ± 0.4	71.4	28.6	—
3-hour exposure to dust, 48-hour recovery	5	34	0.2 ± 0.5	73.6	21.1	5.3
Carbonyl Iron Particles						
3-hour exposure to dust, no recovery	3	18	0.5 ± 0.7	61.1	27.8	11.1
3-hour exposure to dust, 24-hour recovery	3	30	0.9 ± 0.6[b]	23.3	60.0	16.7
3-hour exposure to dust, 48-hour recovery	4	25	1.5 ± 0.9[c]	8.0	48.0	44.0
Crocidolite Asbestos Fibers						
1-hour exposure to dust, 48-hour recovery	3	15	1.3 ± 1.0[b]	23.4	41.3	35.2
5-hour exposure to dust, 48-hour recovery	2	7	1.7 ± 1.2[c]	10.1	48.3	48.2
Wollastonite Fibers						
3-hour exposure to dust, no recovery	3	25	0.6 ± 0.7	52.0	36.0	12.0
3-hour exposure to dust, 24-hour recovery	4	15	1.1 ± 0.7[b]	20.0	53.3	26.7
3-hour exposure to dust, 48-hour recovery	4	21	1.6 ± 1.0[c]	14.3	38.1	47.6
Fiberglass						
3-hour exposure to dust, 24-hour recovery	3	11	1.4 ± 0.8[b]	31.3	32.3	36.4
3-hour exposure to dust, 48-hour recovery	2	6	2.2 ± 1.6[c]	9.2	30.4	60.5
Iron-Treated Chrysotile Asbestos Fibers						
1-hour exposure to dust, 48-hour recovery	3	10	2.8 ± 1.8[c]	12.2	40.5	47.3

[a]Values are mean number of accumulated PM ± SD
[b]$P < 0.05$ when compared to sham- or Mount St. Helens ash values (Student's *t*-test)
[c]$P < 0.01$ when compared to sham- or Mount St. Helens ash values

Table 4. Correlation between complement activation by inorganic particles *in vitro* and pulmonary macrophage (PM) chemotactic responses *in vivo.*

Species	Particle	Complement Activation[a] Serum	Lavage	PM Accumulation *In Vivo*
Mouse, Rat	Zymosan-activated serum	+ + +	+ +	Not determined
Mouse	Chrysotile asbestos	+ +	+	+ +
Rat	Chrysotile asbestos	+ + +	+	+ + +
Rat	Crocidolite asbestos	+ +	+	+
Rat	Fiberglass	+ +	Not determined	+ +
Rat	Iron-treated chrysotile asbestos	+ +	+	+ +
Rat	Carbonyl iron	+ +	+	+ +
Rat	Wollastonite	+ +	+	+ +
Rat	Mount St. Helens ash	Not significant	Not significant	Not significant

[a] + = $P < 0.05$ compared to sham-control by Student's *t*-test
+ + = $P < 0.01$
+ + + = $P < 0.001$

Complement proteins play an important role in facilitating bacterial clearance from the lung by modulating pulmonary inflammatory responses and phagocytosis through anaphylotoxin activity as well as by mediating opsonic and chemotactic effects (Heidbrink et al., 1982; Joiner et al., 1984). In support of this idea, several investigators have shown that pulmonary clearance of *Streptococcus pneumoniae* or *Pseudomonas aeruginosa* was impaired in complement-deficient mice (Larsen et al., 1982; Toews and Vial, 1984). Because a variety of particles and bacteria are known to activate complement *in vitro,* it seems likely that chemotactic factor generation *in vivo* may attract macrophages to sites of deposition.

In summary, PM play a central role in maintaining normal lung physiology by phagocytizing and removing inhaled particulates and bacteria. Macrophage motility and phagocytosis are prerequisites for efficient clearance of inhaled dusts (Warheit et al., 1988). The mechanisms through which macrophages identify inhaled particulates in the distal lung are not well understood. We have proposed a possible mechanism by which the inhaled particles and fibers may stimulate their own clearance from the lung through activation of complement and consequent generation of chemotactic factors.

ACKNOWLEDGMENTS

The authors wish to acknowledge Dr. Bernard Adkins, Jr., Robert O'Connor, and Cindy Crawford of Northrop Services, Inc. for their expert handling of dust inhalation procedures. We especially acknowledge Lila H. Overby for contributing important insights and technical expertise during the course of this work. D. B. Warheit was supported by a Parker B. Francis Fellowship from the Puritan Bennett Foundation.

REFERENCES

Brain, JD. **1985.** Physiology and pathophysiology of pulmonary macrophages, pp. 315-337. In: *The Reticuloendothelial System,* Vol. 7B, SM Reichard and J Filkins (eds.). Plenum Press, New York, NY.

Brody, AR and MW Roe. **1983.** Deposition patterns of inorganic particles at the alveolar level in the lungs of rats and mice. Am Rev Respir Dis 128:724-729.

Flowers, ES. **1982.** New chemical process for asbestos treatment. Asbestos 64:5-10.

Fruchter, JS, DE Robertson, JC Evans, et al. **1980.** Mount St. Helens ash from the May 18, 1980 eruption: Chemical, physical, mineralogical and biological properties. Science 209:1116-1125.

Heidbrink, PJ, GB Toews, GN Gross, and AK Pierce. **1982.** Mechanisms of complement-mediated clearance of bacteria from the murine lung. Am Rev Respir Dis 125:517-520.

Hesterberg, TW and JC Barrett. **1984.** Dependence of asbestos and mineral dust-induced transformation of mammalian cells in culture on fiber dimension. Cancer Res 44:2170-2180.

Hill, JO, SJ Rothenberg, GM Kanapilly, RL Hanson, and BR Scott. **1982.** Activation of immune complement by fly ash particles from coal combustion. Environ Res 28:113-122.

Joiner, KA, EJ Brown, and MM Frank. **1984.** Complement and bacteria: Chemistry and biology in host defense. Ann Rev Immunol 2:461-491

Larsen, GL, BC Mitchell, TB Harper, and PM Henson. **1982.** The pulmonary response of C5 sufficient and deficient mice to *Pseudomonas aeruginosa.* Am Rev Respir Dis 126:306-311.

Olenchock, SA and JC Mull. **1981.** Volcanic ash and human complement. Life Sci 28:791-794.

Olenchock, SA, JC Mull, PC Major, MJ Peach, III, MD Gladish, and G Taylor. **1978.** *In vitro* activation of the alternative pathway of complement by settled grain dust. J Allergy Clin Immunol 62:295-302.

Pinkerton, KE, AR Brody, DA McLaurin, B Atkins, Jr, RW O'Connor, PC Pratt, and JD Crapo. **1983.** Characterization of three types of chrysotile asbestos after aerosolization. Environ Res 31:32-53.

Snyderman, R, HS Shin, JK Phillips, H Gewurz, and SE Mergenhagen. **1969.** A neutrophil chemotactic factor derived from C′5 upon interaction of guinea pig serum with endotoxin. J Immunol 103:413-422.

Toews, GB and WC Vial. **1984.** The role of C5 in polymorphonuclear recruitment in response to *Streptococcus pneumoniae.* Am Rev Respir Dis 129:82-86.

Warheit, DB, LY Chang, LH Hill, GER Hook, JD Crapo, and AR Brody. **1984a.** Pulmonary macrophage accumulation and asbestos-induced lesions at sites of fiber deposition. Am Rev Respir Dis 129:301-310.

Warheit, DB, LH Hill, and AR Brody. **1984b.** *In vitro* effects of crocidolite asbestos and wollastonite on pulmonary macrophages and serum complement. Scanning Electron Microsc II:919-926.

Warheit, DB, LH Hill, and AR Brody. **1984c.** Surface morphology and correlated phagocytic capacity of pulmonary macrophages lavaged from the lungs of rats. Exp Lung Res 6:71-82.

Warheit, DB, G George, LH Hill, R Snyderman, and AR Brody. **1985.** Inhaled asbestos activates a complement-dependent chemoattractant for macrophages. Lab Invest 52:505-514.

Warheit, DB, LH Hill, G George, and AR Brody. **1986.** Time course of chemotactic factor generation and the corresponding macrophage response to asbestos inhalation. Am Rev Respir Dis 134:128-133.

Warheit, DB, LH Overby, G George, and AR Brody. **1988.** Pulmonary macrophages are attracted to inhaled particles through complement activation. Exp Lung Res 14:51-66.

Yano, E, A Takeuchi, S Nishii, et al. **1985.** *In vitro* biological effects of volcanic ash from Mount Sakurajima. J Toxicol Environ Health 16:127-135.

Incorporation of Tritiated Thymidine by Vascular, Epithelial, and Interstitial Cells in Asbestos-Exposed Animals

Arnold R. Brody and Patricia D. McGavran

Laboratory of Pulmonary Pathobiology, National Institute of Environmental Health Sciences, P. O. Box 12233, Research Triangle Park, NC 27709

KEY WORDS: growth factors, macrophages

ABSTRACT

Inhaled asbestos causes progressive interstitial lung disease. We have carried out studies to elucidate the initial pathogenetic events at sites of fiber deposition, i.e., alveolar duct bifurcations in asbestos-exposed rats.

Here we report that a single 5-hour exposure to chrysotile asbestos induced significant increases in incorporation of tritiated thymidine (^{3}HTdR) in nuclei of vascular endothelial and smooth muscle cells, as well as epithelial and interstitial cells of bronchioloalveolar regions. No cell population in air-exposed or carbonyl-iron-exposed control animals exhibited more than 1% labeling at any time. Immediately after the 5-hour asbestos exposure, incorporation was normal. By 12 hours after exposure there was a significant increase in incorporated ^{3}HTdR, particularly by Type II epithelial cells of the first alveolar duct bifurcations. The greatest increase was observed between 12 and 20 hours after exposure, and increased percentages of ^{3}HTdR-labeled cells were maintained through the 48-hour postexposure period. Labeling was normal by 8 days after exposure, and remained normal through the 1-month period studied. This apparent mitogenic response correlated with increased numbers of bronchioloalveolar cells, demonstrated by ultrastructural morphometry in related studies.

We speculate that the incorporation of 3HTdR could be induced by the direct effects of inhaled fibers or by mitogenic factors released from macrophages attracted to the inhaled asbestos. No data are available on the interactive effects of fibers and gases on pulmonary cell proliferation.

INTRODUCTION

It is clear that inhalation of toxic particles, such as asbestos and silica, causes a variety of cellular alterations in the lung. To determine the mechanisms through which the inhaled materials induce fibrogenic or neoplastic sequelae, it is essential to firmly establish the pathogenetic sequence of events that follow exposure. This is particularly relevant for analyzing the effects of exposures to mixtures of particles and gases, where each component can induce its own pattern of injury. We have attempted to define the earliest cellular and biochemical responses to asbestos inhalation in a rat model (Brody, 1986; Chang et al., 1988). Here, we report that brief inhalation of asbestos causes rapid incorporation of tritiated thymidine (^{3}HTdR) by a variety of cell types at the bronchioloalveolar junctions. We speculate that this reaction is mediated by macrophage-derived growth factors.

MATERIALS AND METHODS

Male (CD white) rats, 8 weeks old, were exposed (five animals per group) to room air (sham) or to an aerosol of chrysotile asbestos (10 mg/m^3 respirable mass) for 5 hours in open cages, as previously described (Warheit et al., 1985, 1986). Following recovery periods of 0, 19, 24, 33, 48 hours and 1, 2 and 4 weeks after inhalation, ^{3}HTdR (2 μCi/g) was administered intraperitoneally (IP) to the asbestos- and sham-exposed animals. They were sacrificed 4 hours after administration of the ^{3}HTdR by IP injection of 1 ml sodium pentobarbital (50 mg/ml). Animals were then perfused through the pulmonary artery with fixative (1% glutaraldehyde, 1% paraformaldehyde) at 23 cm H_2O pressure for 5 minutes. The whole lungs were removed from the chest and immersed in fixative overnight.

After the tissues were fixed, slices (2 x 5 x 10 mm) were taken at right angles to each mainstem bronchus from both right and left lungs and postfixed with 0.5% osmium tetroxide in veronal acetate buffer. The slices were embedded in soft Epox 812 and polymerized at 60°C for 15 hours. These plastic blocks were softened on a warming tray at 40°C, and 0.5-mm-thick slices were cut parallel to the large tissue face with a double-edged razor blade. A terminal bronchiole with its attached alveolar ducts, including the bifurcation between the ducts, was selected under a dissecting microscope and excised from the warmed plastic block. Two terminal bronchiolo-alveolar duct regions per animal were selected, for a total of 10 anatomical units per treatment group. The selected tissue was mounted on a BEEM blank with epoxy glue. For light microscope autoradiography, 0.6-μm sections were cut with a diamond knife on a MT5000 microtome and, from the first two blocks sectioned at each time point, a thin section for electron microscopy was cut adjacent to the thick section taken for autoradiography. The thin sections were mounted on slotted grids (0.2 x 1 mm), stained with uranyl acetate and lead citrate, and photographed with a JEOL 100CX electron microscope. The thick sections for autoradiography were placed on glass slides, coated with Ilford L4 emulsion, exposed for 3 weeks, developed with D-19 (Kodak, Rochester, NY), and stained with toluidine blue. For each treatment group, labeled nuclei (six or more grains over a nucleus) were counted by light microscopy at 100X magnification in the epithelium and interstitium of the following four anatomical units of the terminal bronchioloalveolar duct regions: (1) terminal bronchiole, (2) alveolar duct walls between the terminal bronchiole and first alveolar duct bifurcation, (3) first alveolar duct bifurcation, and (4) ducts distal to the bifurcation (Figure 1).

Data were analyzed by Wilcoxon's rank sum test for nonparametric values, and statistical significance was reached at a level of $P < 0.05$.

RESULTS AND DISCUSSION

As previously described for normal animals (Shami et al., 1986; Tryka et al., 1986), sham-exposed rats and mice showed no increases in ^{3}HTdR incorporation at any time after exposure. All anatomical regions had a labeling level of about 1% (Figure 2).

A 5-hour exposure to chrysotile induced clear incorporation of ^{3}HTdR by about 20 hours after exposure (Figures 1 through 3). Immediately after exposure, percentages of labeled cells remained at normal levels (Figure 2). These percentages rose significantly through a 12- to 20-hour period and reached a peak by 24 to 33 hours after exposure (Figure 2). Percentages of labeled cells declined to normal levels by 1 week after exposure and remained normal throughout the 1-month period studied (Figure 2).

The cell types labeled included smooth muscle cells and endothelial cells of small parenchymal vessels (Figure 3), and cuboidal epithelial cells and interstitial cells of the terminal bronchioles (Figure 3), as well as Type II epithelial and undefined interstitial cells at the alveolar level (Figure 1). Here, cells of the proximal alveolar ducts and first alveolar duct bifurcations exhibited significantly increased levels of ^{3}HTdR incorporation. No increases were observed in any cells distal to the first duct bifurcations. These findings are consistent with ultrastructural morphometric studies on rats that showed that epithelial and interstitial cells of the first alveolar duct bifurcations increased in number and volume only 48 hours after a 1-hour exposure to chrysotile asbestos (Chang et al., 1988). Interestingly, these morphometric studies show that an interstitial lesion at the bifurcations progresses through the 1-month period studied, but tissues distal to the first alveolar duct bifurcations apparently remain unaffected (Chang et al., 1988).

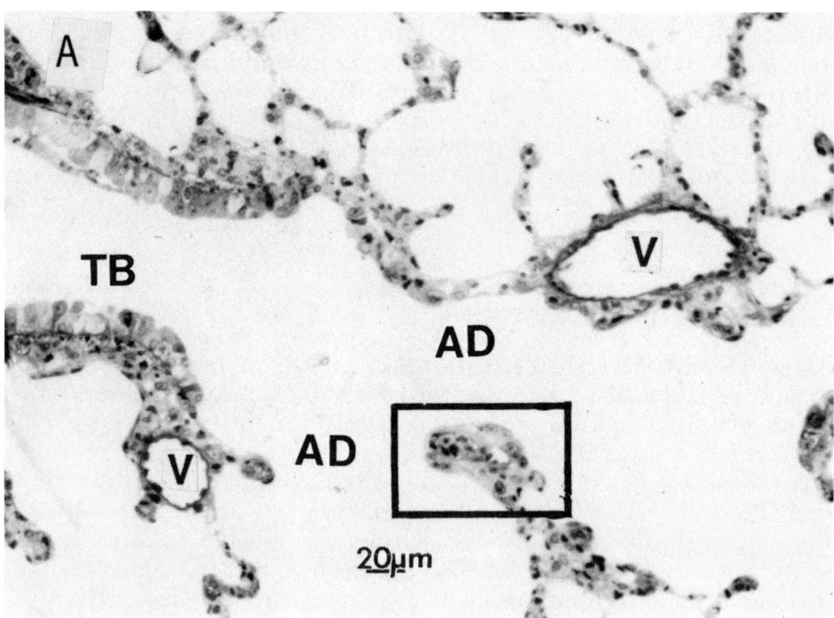

Figure 1. (A) Section of plastic-embedded rat lung tisue showing the anatomic regions in which cells were assessed for tritiated thymidine (^{3}HTdR) incorporation. Tissue from an animal sacrificed 48 hours after a 5-hour exposure to chrysotile asbestos exhibits a terminal bronchiole (TB) that opens into alveolar ducts (AD). The first alveolar duct bifurcation (rectangle) is enlarged in Figure 1B. The small vessels (V) adjacent to bronchioloalveolar regions commonly exhibited ^{3}HTdR-labeled cells (see Figure 3).

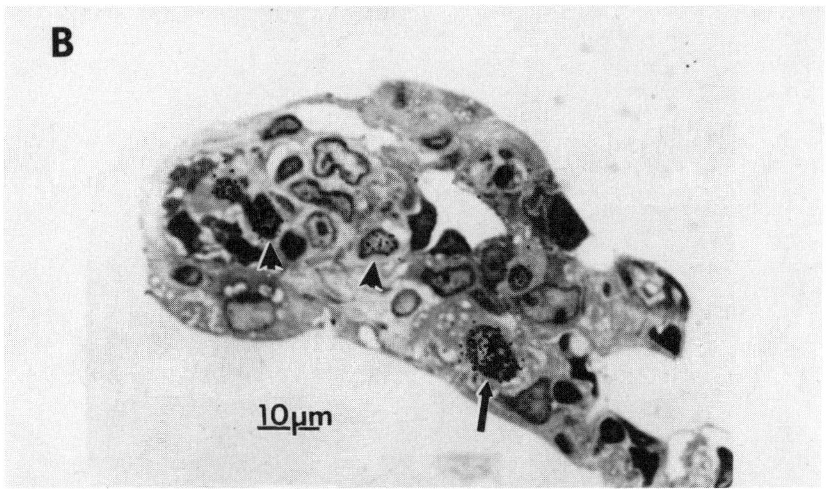

Figure 1. (B) The first alveolar duct bifurcation, enlarged from Figure 1A. Several cells are clearly labeled with ^{3}HTdR. One is a Type II epithelial cell (arrow), characterized by its large size and position on the alveolar wall. The other two cells (arrowheads) are interstitial, and their precise identity remains undefined. This entire bifurcation region is hypercellular and enlarged as determined by ultrastructural morphometry (see Chang et al., 1988).

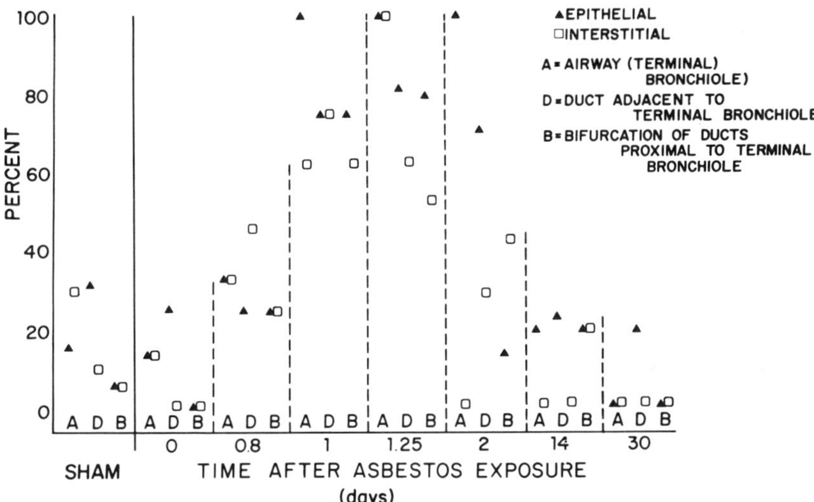

Figure 2. Percentages of the various anatomic region that contained at least one labeled cell at each of the time points studied. The sham-exposed animals showed no significant variations over time.

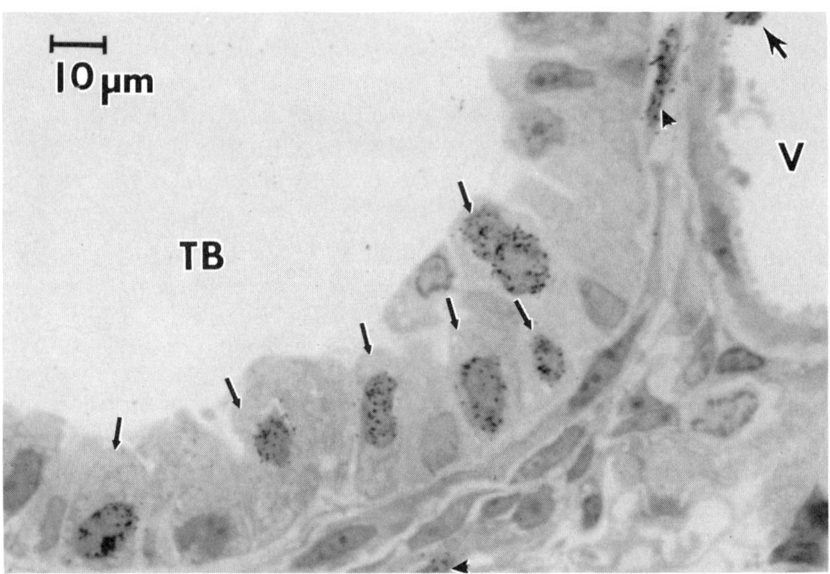

Figure 3. Light microscopic autoradiograph, showing a high percentage of terminal bronchiolar (TB) epithelial cells (arrows) that have incorporated tritiated thymidine (^{3}HTdR) in an asbestos-exposed mouse. Quantitative data showed up to 18-fold increases in labeling over that in sham-exposed controls. Attenuated fibroblast-like submucosal cells (arrowheads) were also labeled. In addition, smooth muscle cells and endothelial cells (short arrows) of small parenchymal vessels (V) incorporated ^{3}HTdR at a significantly higher rate in asbestos-exposed animals than in those sham-exposed.

The autoradiographic findings presented here and the morphometric studies support our hypothesis that asbestos fibers originally deposited on the surfaces of alveolar duct bifurcations (Brody and Roe, 1983) induce rapid cellular responses and consequent development of an interstitial lesion (Chang et al., 1988). The basic biological mechanisms that mediate the progression of the lesion are uncertain. It is clear that increased numbers of macrophages are attracted to the sites of fiber deposition (Chang et al., 1988; Warheit et al., 1985, 1986), and some of the cells that have incorporated ^{3}HTdR are apparently interstitial macrophages, several of which contain asbestos (Brody and Overby, in press). Furthermore, because complement-deficient mice exhibit a reduced macrophage response to asbestos inhalation (Warheit et al., 1985), we hoped that autoradiographic studies would shed some light on the role macrophages might play in the early cell responses. At this point in our studies, no apparent differences in macrophage function have been discerned between normal and complement-deficient mice at the early time points. However, it was interesting that, by 1 month after exposure, the complement-deficient mice had significantly fewer interstitial lesions compared with those of the normal controls (Morgan, unpublished observations). Further autoradiographic and ultrastructural comparisons are being carried out in this model system.

Thus, at least two alternative, although not mutually exclusive, hypotheses can explain mechanisms controlling the pathogenesis of the asbestos-induced cellular alterations. First, it is clear that inhaled asbestos fibers are deposited at all levels of the respiratory tract (Morgan et al., 1975). It is conceivable that the fibers on epithelial membranes that are taken into the cytoplasm of Type I alveolar epithelial cells (Brody et al., 1981) could directly provoke a mitogenic response by the Type II epithelium. Even though Type II cells very rarely take up fibers (Pinkerton et al., 1984), the reaction of Type I cells can dictate a proliferative response in Type II cells. This has been shown clearly in studies where injury to Type I cells by oxygen or NO_2 (Crapo et al., 1984) results in a mitogenic response by Type II cells. The fact that the Type I cells rapidly become thicker (Chang et al., 1988), together with the development of a small but significant leak of serum proteins into the lung (Warheit et al., 1986), support the notion that the inhaled asbestos could induce a mitogenic effect through direct membrane interactions with epithelial cells. On the other hand, direct effects on the bronchiolar epithelium are more difficult to envision. These cells, which are covered by a layer of secreted proteins, lipids and carbohydrates, have not been shown to phagocytize asbestos fibers *in vivo*.

A second possibility to be considered as a source of the mitogenic stimulus is the population of pulmonary macrophages, which responds to the inhaled asbestos (Warheit et al., 1985, 1986). An alveolar macrophage-derived factor has been shown to induce ^{3}HTdR incorporation by Type II cells *in vitro* (Leslie et al., 1986). Recently, it has been found that lung macrophages produce TGFα, a potent epithelial mitogen (Madtes et al., 1988), and macrophage-derived growth factors for fibroblasts have been clearly demonstrated (Ross et al., 1986). Recent work in our laboratory has shown that pulmonary macrophages secrete a platelet-derived growth factor homologue that binds specifically to receptors on rat lung fibroblasts (Kumar et al., 1988). Because increased numbers of pulmonary macrophages accumulate in the bronchioloalveolar regions during the 48-hour postexposure period (Warheit et al., 1985, 1986), it is conceivable that these cells synthesize and secrete mitogenic factors that induce the epithelial and interstitial cells to incorporate ^{3}HTdR during proliferation. This hypothesis remains to be proven; however, the anatomical distribution of alveolar and interstitial macrophages appears to be appropriate. It is clear that asbestos fibers cause early significant incorporation of ^{3}HTdR by a variety of pulmonary cells.

In conclusion, we have shown that a brief exposure to chrysotile asbestos fibers induces a proliferative response by epithelial and interstitial cells associated with sites of initial dust deposition in rats and mice. These findings correlate with earlier morphometric studies showing progression of an interstitial lesion (Chang et al., 1988). This shows that even brief exposures, such as those that might occur while workers demolish or remove buildings that contain asbestos, induce cellular responses and subsequent bronchioloalveolar lesions. Whether or not similar lesions occur in humans who have been exposed to other toxic agents such as cigarette smoke, and whether such lesions progress and have pathological sequelae, has not yet been determined.

ACKNOWLEDGMENTS

We are indebted to the highly cooperative individuals from Northrop Services, Inc. who operate the NIEHS Inhalation Exposure Facility under contract to the National Toxicology Program.

REFERENCES

Brody, AR. **1986.** Pulmonary cell interactions with asbestos fibers *in vivo* and *in vitro*. Chest 89:155-159.

Brody, AR, LH Hill, B Adkins, and R O'Connor. **1981.** Chrysotile asbestos inhalation in rats: Deposition pattern and reaction of alveolar epithelium and pulmonary macrophages. Am Rev Respir Dis 123:670-679.

Brody, AR and LH Overby. Incorporation of tritiated thymidine by epithelial and interstitial cells in bronchiolar-alveolar regions of asbestos-exposed rats. Am J Pathol (**in press**).

Brody, AR and MW Roe. **1983.** Deposition pattern of inorganic particles at the alveolar level in the lungs of rats and mice. Am Rev Respir Dis 128:724-729.

Chang, LY, LH Hill, AR Brody, and JD Crapo. **1988.** Progressive lung cell reactions and extracellular matrix production after a brief exposure to asbestos. Am J Pathol 131:156-170.

Crapo, JD, BE Barry, L Chang, and RR Mercer. **1984.** Alterations in lung structure caused by inhalation of oxidants. J Toxicol Environ Health 13:301-321.

Kumar, RK, RA Bennett, and AR Brody. **1988.** A homologue of platelet-derived growth factor produced by rat alveolar macrophages. Fed Am Soc Exp Biol J 2:2272-2277.
Leslie, CL, K McCormick-Shannon, JL Cook, and RJ Mason. **1986.** Macrophages stimulate DNA synthesis in rat alveolar Type II cells. Am Rev Respir Dis 132:1246-1252.
Madtes, DK, EW Raines, KS Sakariassen, RK Assoian, MB Sporn, GI Bell, and R Ross. **1988.** Induction of transforming growth factor α in activated human alveolar macrophages. Cell 53:285-293.
Morgan, A, JC Evans, RJ Evans, RF Hounam, A Holmes, and S Doyle. **1975.** Studies on the deposition of inhaled fibrous material in the respiratory tract of the rat and its subsequent clearance using radioactive tracer techniques. II. Deposition of UICC standard reference samples of asbestos. Environ Res 10:196-207.
Pinkerton, KE, PC Pratt, AR Brody, and JD Crapo. **1984.** Fiber localization and its relationship to lung reactions in rats after chronic exposure to chrysotile asbestos. Am J Pathol 117:484-493.
Ross, R, EW Raines, and DF Bowen-Pope. **1986.** The biology of platelet-derived growth factor. Cell 46:155-169.
Shami, SG, MJ Evans, and LA Martinez. **1986.** Type II cell proliferation related to migration of inflammatory cells into the lungs. Exp Mol Pathol 44:344-352.
Tryka, AF, H Witschi, DG Gosslee, AH McArthur, and NK Clapp. **1986.** Patterns of cell proliferation during recovery from oxygen injury. Am Rev Respir Dis 133:1055-1059.
Warheit, DB, G George, LH Hill, R Snyderman, and AR Brody. **1985.** Inhaled asbestos activates a complement-dependent chemoattractant for macrophages. Lab Invest 52:505-514.
Warheit, DB, LH Hill, G George, and AR Brody. **1986.** Time course of chemotactic factor generation and the corresponding macrophage response to asbestos inhalation. Am Rev Respir Dis 134:128-133.

The Effects of Amphibole and Serpentine Asbestos Inhalation on the Distribution and Functional State of Alveolar Macrophage Subpopulations*

Elliott Kagan, Tamio Inamoto, and M. Mala Georgian

Department of Pathology, Georgetown University School of Medicine, 3900 Reservoir Road, NW, Washington, DC 20007

KEY WORDS: amphiboles, serpentine asbestos, macrophage function

---

ABSTRACT

There is considerable evidence that implicates the alveolar macrophage in the pathogenesis of asbestosis. Thus, both clinical and experimental studies have shown that inhalation of asbestos fibers leads to the accumulation of alveolar macrophages at intrapulmonary sites of asbestos deposition. Furthermore, we have shown previously that asbestos exposure is associated with enhanced release of alveolar macrophage-derived inflammatory mediators such as chemoattractants and immunostimulatory molecules. It is conceivable that the presence of alveolar macrophages at sites of asbestos-mediated pulmonary injury may reflect increased proportions of newly recruited immature and/or "activated" macrophages. To test this hypothesis, we have studied the effects of *in vivo* asbestos exposure on the distribution of alveolar macrophage subpopulations defined by continuous iso-osmotic Percoll gradients (density range: 1.006 to 1.123 g/ml). Two groups of rats were exposed by intermittent inhalation (6 hours/day for 5 days/week over 4 weeks) to either amphibole (crocidolite) or serpentine (chrysotile) asbestos. A group of control rats was sham-exposed to clean air only. Equal numbers of rats from each group were sacrificed on days 7 and 16 during exposure and at

*Supported by U.S. Environmental Protection Agency Grant #R812036-01-0.

2 to 3 weeks and 2 to 5 months, respectively, after the cessation of exposure. The lungs of animals sacrificed at these times were examined histologically for evidence of asbestosis. Alveolar macrophages obtained from three exposure groups by bronchoalveolar lavage were collected in 10 Percoll fractions, then examined morphologically and for evidence of functional "activation." The functional characteristics of alveolar macrophages in various density-defined fractions were evaluated by analysis of surface immune-associated (Ia) antigen expression (a marker of macrophage activation) and by measuring secretion of the immunostimulatory molecule interleukin-1 in a murine bioassay.

During exposure, distinct differences were noted between the sham-exposed group and both groups of asbestos-exposed rats with respect to the recovery of alveolar macrophages from corresponding density-defined fractions. These differences appeared within 7 days of asbestos exposure, and some of these findings persisted in the crocidolite-exposed group for as long as 2 to 5 months after the cessation of exposure. Furthermore, both amphibole and serpentine asbestos inhalation were associated with enhanced activation of alveolar macrophages in the majority of Percoll density fractions. Thus, relatively greater proportions of Ia-positive cells were detected in several density fractions obtained from both asbestos-exposed groups (especially the crocidolite-exposed group). Augmented secretion of interleukin-1 was detected in culture supernatants of all Percoll fractions from both groups of asbestos-exposed rats. Multinucleated alveolar macrophages were an uncommon finding in sham-exposed rats but were seen frequently in all Percoll fractions after both types of asbestos inhalation. Interestingly, after asbestos exposure, a significant proportion of multinucleated alveolar macrophages in these fractions expressed surface Ia-positivity. The morphologic and functional abnormalities observed in this study preceded histologic development of asbestosis (which was first evident approximately 2 to 3 months after the cessation of asbestos exposure) and also persisted after the establishment of interstitial pulmonary fibrosis. These changes in the distribution and functional properties of alveolar macrophage subpopulations may have important pathogenetic implications for the initiation and perpetuation of asbestos-mediated pulmonary injury.

INTRODUCTION

Asbestosis is a form of diffuse interstitial pulmonary fibrosis caused by inhalation of asbestos fibers. There is considerable evidence that alveolar macrophages play a pivotal role in the pathogenesis of asbestosis (Kagan, 1985, 1988), because these phagocytic cells are a notable feature of histologic lesions at sites of asbestos deposition in the lungs (Davis, 1963; Brody et al., 1981; Oghiso et al., 1984). Multinucleated giant cells are also a prominent component of the macrophage response to inhaled asbestos (Kagan et al., 1983a; Kagan, in press). It is conceivable that the accumulation of alveolar macrophages in evolving asbestotic lesions may reflect a localized tissue response to the release of asbestos-induced chemotactic stimuli within the lungs. Support for this concept is provided by experimental studies that have demonstrated that asbestos inhalation can evoke the release of chemoattractants for alveolar macrophages (Kagan et al., 1983b; Warheit et al., 1985).

Asbestos exposure is also associated with enhanced expression of immune-associated (Ia) surface antigens on alveolar macrophages and with augmented production of the immunostimulatory monokine interleukin-1 (Hartmann et al., 1984a,b). Since the surface expression of Ia antigens on macrophages is a useful morphologic correlate of macrophage activation (Garrett et al., 1984; Kunkel et al., 1984), these findings collectively suggest that contact with asbestos may induce alveolar macrophages to become functionally activated.

Studies in several species, using continuous or discontinuous density gradients, have shown that pulmonary alveolar macrophage populations are heterogeneous in nature, comprising subsets of both young and functionally more mature macrophages (Murphy and Herscowitz, 1984; Shellito and Kaltreider, 1984; Chandler et al., 1986; Ferro et al., 1987). It is possible that alveolar macrophages that aggregate at sites of intrapulmonary asbestos deposition may reflect increased proportions of newly recruited, immature cells, as well as increased percentages of activated phagocytic cells. Our study was designed to test this hypothesis by examining the effects of chrysotile (i.e., serpentine) and crocidolite (i.e., amphibole) asbestos inhalation on the distribution of alveolar macrophage subpopulations in the rat, defined by continuous, iso-osmotic Percoll gradients.

MATERIALS AND METHODS

Experimental Animals and Exposure Protocol

The study entailed a comparison of three matched groups of adult male, inbred Fischer-344 rats. One group of rats was exposed to a time-weighted average concentration of 10.52 mg/m^3 of crocidolite asbestos. A second group of rats received a time-weighted concentration of 10.23 mg/m^3 of crocidolite asbestos. A control group of rats was sham-exposed only to filtered clean air. The exposures were performed under contract at the University of Vermont. The rats were exposed by intermittent inhalation for 6 hours/day, 5 days/week, over 4 weeks. Some animals were sacrificed on days 7 or 17, respectively, of the exposure regimen, whereas others were sacrificed at 2 to 3 weeks or 2 to 5 months, respectively, after the cessation of exposure.

Bronchoalveolar Lavage Studies

Bronchoalveolar cells were obtained by bronchoalveolar lavage, as described previously (Kagan et al., 1983a).

Fractionation of Alveolar Macrophages on Percoll Gradients

A continuous, iso-osmotic Percoll density gradient (Pharmacia, Piscataway, NJ) was generated, using a two-chamber gradient mixer (Chandler et al., 1986). The density of the gradient varied from 1.006 to 1.123 g/ml (Table 1). Unfractionated alveolar macrophage populations (containing at least 1 x 10^7 cells) were then layered on the linear density gradient and centrifuged at 800 x g for 30 minutes at 4°C. Using a sterile, dense sucrose solution (1.45 g/ml) to displace the gradient, 10 Percoll density-defined alveolar macrophage fractions were collected in 6-ml volumes in plastic tubes, then washed twice in Ca^{++}- and Mg^{++}-free phosphate-buffered saline.

Table 1. Continuous iso-osmotic Percoll gradients

Fraction Number	Density Range (g/ml)
1	$<$ 1.018
2	1.018 to 1.028
3	1.028 to 1.037
4	1.037 to 1.046
5	1.046 to 1.055
6	1.055 to 1.064
7	1.064 to 1.072
8	1.072 to 1.081
9	1.081 to 1.090
10	$>$ 1.090

Macrophage Morphologic Assessment

The composition of unfractionated and density-defined cell fractions (including the proportion of multinucleated macrophages) was enumerated by proportional analysis on Giemsa-stained cytospin preparations. The various fractions comprised approximately 90 to 99% macrophages in virtually all instances, as defined by nonspecific esterase positivity and by morphologic criteria. Determinations were also made of the macrophage yield (i.e., the proportion of unfractionated macrophages recoverable) in each density-defined fraction.

Assessment of Ia Surface Antigen Expression on Macrophages

The surface expression of Ia antigen on rat alveolar macrophages was determined by an immunoperoxidase technique on cytospin preparations, as described previously (Hartmann et al., 1984a). For this purpose, a monoclonal mouse IgG anti-rat Ia antiserum (Accurate Chemicals, Westbury, CT) was used as the primary antibody, and a biotin-labeled horse anti-mouse IgG antiserum (Vector Laboratories, Burlingame, CA) as the secondary antibody.

Functional Interleukin-1 Assays

For the assessment of interleukin-1 production, various density-defined alveolar macrophage fractions (2.5×10^6 macrophages/ml) were allowed to attach to 24-well microtiter plates (Costar Plastics, Vineland, NJ) for 2 hours at 37°C. After washing twice, the macrophages were then cultured in serumless Neuman and Tytell medium (GIBCO, Grand Island, NY) for 24 hours at 37°C. Thereafter, the macrophage culture supernatants were assayed for interleukin-1 activity by a standard functional assay, using C_3H/HeJ mouse thymocytes (Mizel, 1981). The presence of interleukin-1 was assayed in parallel cultures containing either unstimulated macrophages or macrophages stimulated with 100 μg/ml of bacterial lipopolysaccharide (LPS; Difco Laboratories, Detroit, MI).

Interpretation of Data

Results were expressed as the mean ± standard error of the mean of three to five experiments. Statistical comparisons were made using Student's *t*-test.

RESULTS

Density-Defined Distribution of Alveolar Macrophages

When unfractionated alveolar macrophages from the three groups of exposed rats were layered on continuous, iso-osmotic Percoll gradients, the majority (i.e., more than 70%) of the cells were recoverable from density fractions 6 and 7. There were, nevertheless, distinct differences between sham-exposed and asbestos-exposed groups of rats with respect to the density-defined distribution of alveolar macrophage subpopulations. Thus, when rats were sacrificed on days 7 and 17 during exposure, significantly greater proportions of alveolar macrophages were recoverable in the highest density fractions (i.e., fractions 8 to 10) after crocidolite exposure than after sham exposure ($P < 0.01$). Similar, albeit less striking, changes were detectable after chrysotile inhalation ($P < 0.05$). The crocidolite-related effect persisted and was detectable in rats sacrificed at 2 to 3 weeks and 2 to 5 months, respectively, after the cessation of exposure ($P < 0.05$).

Proportions of Multinucleated Alveolar Macrophages

Both crocidolite and chrysotile exposures were associated with significantly increased numbers of multinucleated alveolar macrophages recoverable by bronchoalveolar lavage, when compared with those in sham-exposed controls. It is noteworthy that the proportion of multinucleated macrophages was significantly increased in virtually all density-defined fractions after both types of asbestos exposure (Table 2). This effect occurred within 7 days of the onset of asbestos exposure and persisted throughout the entire period of the study.

Ia Surface Antigen Expression on Alveolar Macrophages

The proportion of Ia antigen-bearing alveolar macrophages was also significantly increased after asbestos exposure in several density-defined fractions (Table 3). Although this finding was noted in the context of both types of asbestos exposure, it was more prominent after crocidolite than after chrysotile exposure. Once again, the effect could be detected within 7 days of beginning asbestos inhalation and, in the case of crocidolite, persisted throughout the entire course of the study. Furthermore, when consideration was given to the presence of Ia-positive multinucleated alveolar macrophages in the various density-defined fractions, both types of asbestos inhalation were associated with relatively large proportions of such cells. Thus, approximately 2 to 32% of multinucleated macrophages expressed the Ia surface marker in different density-defined fractions. By contrast, Ia-positive multinucleated cells were almost never detected in any Percoll fraction after sham exposure.

Table 2. Proportions (%) of multinucleated alveolar macrophages[a]

	Fraction Number	Rat Exposure Group		
		Sham-Exposed	Chrysotile-Exposed	Crocidolite-Exposed
During Exposure (Days 7-17)	Unfractionated	1.31 ± 0.47	6.04 ± 1.10[b]	8.03 ± 0.85[b]
	1	—	1.67 ± 1.67	8.89 ± 6.48
	2	0.74 ± 0.53	3.55 ± 1.58	3.08 ± 0.98[c]
	3	1.04 ± 0.50	6.87 ± 1.52[b]	5.10 ± 1.42[b]
	4	1.09 ± 0.37	5.99 ± 1.06[b]	6.29 ± 1.33[b]
	5	1.02 ± 0.41	5.34 ± 0.95[b]	5.77 ± 1.40[b]
	6	0.86 ± 0.33	4.90 ± 0.93[b]	5.84 ± 0.61[b]
	7	0.91 ± 0.40	5.90 ± 0.98[b]	5.97 ± 1.37[b]
	8	0.77 ± 0.26	7.88 ± 1.30[b]	8.51 ± 1.11[b]
	9	0.95 ± 0.57	6.95 ± 1.11[b]	10.64 ± 1.35[b]
	10	0.23 ± 0.23	7.45 ± 1.61[b]	12.84 ± 1.41[b]
2 Weeks to 5 Months after Exposure	Unfractionated	1.71 ± 0.41	5.31 ± 1.60[c]	5.27 ± 1.28[c]
	1	1.00 ± 1.00	3.94 ± 3.70	1.89 ± 1.89
	2	1.83 ± 1.32	3.23 ± 1.06	1.19 ± 0.70
	3	0.74 ± 0.40	7.21 ± 0.97[b]	3.93 ± 1.02[b]
	4	0.95 ± 0.31	5.20 ± 1.08[b]	4.65 ± 0.80[b]
	5	1.56 ± 0.43	6.14 ± 0.80[b]	4.70 ± 1.09[b]
	6	1.02 ± 0.31	4.92 ± 0.70[b]	4.01 ± 0.53[b]
	7	0.73 ± 0.39	5.26 ± 1.03[b]	5.02 ± 0.93[b]
	8	1.73 ± 0.71	7.65 ± 2.19[b]	6.58 ± 1.32[b]
	9	1.13 ± 0.44	8.39 ± 2.45[c]	11.77 ± 2.06[b]
	10	0.51 ± 0.45	6.78 ± 0.90[b]	13.28 ± 1.20[b]

[a]Results are expressed as mean ± SEM of 10 experiments
[b]$P < 0.01$ (sham-exposed versus asbestos-exposed)
[c]$P < 0.05$ (sham-exposed versus asbestos-exposed)

Table 3. Proportions (%) of immune-associated (Ia)-positive alveolar macrophages[a]

	Fraction Number	Rat Exposure Group: Sham-Exposed	Chrysotile-Exposed	Crocidolite-Exposed
During Exposure (Days 7-17)	Unfractionated	3.12 ± 1.58	7.28 ± 1.25[b]	9.90 ± 2.01[b]
	1	—	—	—
	2	0.58 ± 0.58	0.80 ± 0.51	0.21 ± 0.21
	3	0.98 ± 0.65	3.44 ± 1.19[c]	2.15 ± 0.64[c]
	4	1.39 ± 0.75	4.19 ± 1.25[c]	3.04 ± 1.32
	5	2.19 ± 1.19	6.47 ± 2.31[c]	6.06 ± 2.01[c]
	6	1.51 ± 0.78	4.98 ± 2.12	7.04 ± 1.74[b]
	7	1.55 ± 0.89	4.82 ± 1.34[c]	6.02 ± 2.03[c]
	8	1.66 ± 0.51	2.47 ± 0.71[c]	4.26 ± 1.51[c]
	9	1.31 ± 1.31	2.14 ± 0.88	6.51 ± 3.16[c]
	10	1.42 ± 1.27	2.96 ± 1.69	4.01 ± 1.17[b]
2 Weeks to 5 Months after Exposure	Unfractionated	2.83 ± 1.21	9.88 ± 2.81[c]	16.68 ± 3.62[b]
	1	0.68 ± 0.68	1.16 ± 1.16	2.50 ± 2.50
	2	0.96 ± 0.96	1.51 ± 1.14	4.21 ± 3.44
	3	2.43 ± 1.03	2.87 ± 2.02	4.67 ± 2.00
	4	2.67 ± 1.10	6.60 ± 2.89	8.38 ± 2.25[c]
	5	2.64 ± 1.12	6.24 ± 3.27	10.80 ± 2.07[b]
	6	1.31 ± 0.50	6.39 ± 4.02	9.70 ± 3.81[c]
	7	1.60 ± 0.43	7.34 ± 4.22	8.97 ± 2.30[b]
	8	3.67 ± 0.68	5.14 ± 2.43	7.46 ± 1.62[b]
	9	3.72 ± 1.83	6.21 ± 3.41	9.81 ± 3.53
	10	5.38 ± 1.93	10.44 ± 4.68	14.09 ± 4.74[c]

[a]Results are expressed as mean ± SEM of 10 experiments
[b]$P < 0.01$ (sham-exposed versus asbestos-exposed)
[c]$P < 0.05$ (sham-exposed versus asbestos-exposed)

Interleukin-1 Production by Alveolar Macrophages

Both types of asbestos exposure were associated with greatly enhanced production of interleukin-1 by alveolar macrophages when compared with sham exposure. These differences were already evident within 7 days of the beginning of exposure and were most striking in LPS-stimulated cultures. However, differences between asbestos- and sham-exposed rats were also evident in unstimulated cultures. Thus, LPS-directed functional interleukin-1 activity was usually less than 100 units/ml, and never exceeded 400 units/ml, in culture supernatants from any density-defined fraction obtained from sham-exposed rats. By contrast, similar culture supernatants from crocidolite- and chrysotile-exposed animals frequently contained functional interleukin-1 levels ranging from 500 to 1,600 units/ml. In general, these asbestos-related effects were most pronounced in the higher density-defined macrophage fractions (i.e., fractions 6 to 10).

DISCUSSION

The study has demonstrated that the deposition of asbestos fibers in the lungs produces striking changes in the composition and distribution of alveolar macrophage subpopulations defined by continuous, iso-osmotic Percoll gradients. These alterations are characterized by increased proportions of multinucleated and higher-density macrophages after asbestos exposure. Alveolar macrophages in the higher-density fractions have been shown to be developmentally immature (Shellito and Kaltreider, 1984; Elias et al., 1985). Thus, the finding of enriched numbers of higher-density phagocytes in bronchoalveolar lavage cell subpopulations from asbestos-exposed rats may reflect the presence of newly recruited, immature monocytes and/or macrophages at sites of intrapulmonary asbestos deposition. Studies demonstrating the presence of asbestos-related chemoattractants for alveolar macrophages give credence to this notion (Kagan et al., 1983b; Warheit et al., 1985).

Because alveolar macrophage populations are heterogeneous in nature, their overall function is dependent on mixtures of cells with variable functional capabilities. A disproportionate increase in the number of functionally activated phagocytic cells can result in macrophage-mediated lung injury, as has been shown for sarcoidosis and other granulomatous pulmonary diseases (Garrett et al., 1984; Kunkel et al., 1984). A similar mechanism may pertain to asbestosis, because this study has demonstrated interleukin-1 production in several density-defined fractions after asbestos exposure. This is especially noteworthy because this effect was noted both spontaneously and in LPS-stimulated cultures. The enhancement of Ia antigen expression in most density-defined alveolar macrophage fractions provides an additional morphologic correlate of functional macrophage activation induced by asbestos. This phenomenon was particularly prominent among multinucleated alveolar macrophage subpopulations. Although the significance of these multinucleated cells in asbestosis has not been established, they may represent a distinct subset of functionally activated phagocytes. Their appearance may result from the fusion of macrophage membranes induced by γ-interferon (Nagasawa et al., 1987).

Both amphibole and serpentine exposure are capable of inducing the changes seen in this study, and these effects develop shortly (i.e., by day 7) after the start of asbestos exposure. However, the effects of crocidolite exposure tend to be more prominent and to persist for a longer period after the cessation of asbestos inhalation. These variations in the biological effects of the two asbestos fiber types may relate to the relatively more efficient clearance and greater solubility of chrysotile, compared with that of crocidolite (Becklake, 1982; Kagan, in press).

In summary, this study has demonstrated that asbestos inhalation can induce dramatic alterations in the composition and distribution of alveolar macrophage subpopulations. Given the pivotal role played by the alveolar macrophage in asbestos-related lung injury, these findings may have biological relevance to the pathogenesis of asbestosis.

REFERENCES

Becklake, MR. **1982.** Asbestos-related diseases of the lungs and pleura. Am Rev Respir Dis 127:187-194.

Brody, AR, LH Hill, B Adkins, Jr, and RW O'Connor. **1981.** Chrysotile asbestos inhalation in rats: Deposition pattern and reaction of alveolar epithelium and pulmonary macrophages. Am Rev Respir Dis 123:670-679.

Chandler, DB, WC Fuller, RM Jackson, and JD Fulmer. **1986.** Studies of membrane receptors and phagocytosis in subpopulations of rat alveolar macrophages. Am Rev Respir Dis 133:461-467.

Davis, JMG. **1963.** An electron microscopy study of the effect of asbestos dust on the lung. Br J Exp Pathol 44:454-464.

Elias, JA, AD Schreiber, K Gustilo, P Chien, MD Rossman, PJ Lammie, and RP Daniele. **1985.** Differential interleukin 1 elaboration by unfractionated and density fractionated human alveolar macrophages and blood monocytes: Relationship to cell maturity. J Immunol 135: 3198-3204.

Ferro, TJ, JA Kern, JA Elias, M Kamoun, RP Daniele, and MD Rossman. **1987.** Alveolar macrophages, blood monocytes, and density fractionated alveolar macrophages differ in their ability to promote lymphocyte proliferation to mitogen and antigen. Am Rev Respir Dis 135:682-687.

Garrett, KC, HB Richerson, and GW Hunninghake. **1984.** Pathogenesis of the granulomatous lung diseases. II. Mechanism of granuloma formation. Am Rev Respir Dis 130:477-483.

Hartmann, DP, MM Georgian, and E Kagan. **1984a.** Enhanced alveolar macrophage Ia antigen expression after asbestos inhalation. J Immunol 132:2693-2695.

Hartmann, DP, MM Georgian, Y Oghiso, and E Kagan. **1984b.** Enhanced interleukin activity after asbestos inhalation. Clin Exp Immunol 55:643-650.

Kagan, E. **1985.** Current perspectives in asbestosis. Ann Allergy 54:464-473.

Kagan, E. **1988.** Current issues regarding the pathobiology of asbestosis: A chronologic perspective. J Thorac Imag 3: 4.

Kagan, E, Y Oghiso, and DP Hartmann. **1983a.** The effects of chrysotile and crocidolite asbestos on the lower respiratory tract: Analysis of bronchoalveolar lavage constituents. Environ Res 32:382-397.

Kagan, E, Y Oghiso, and DP Hartmann. **1983b.** Enhanced release of a chemoattractant for alveolar macrophages after asbestos inhalation. Am Rev Respir Dis 128:680-687.

Kunkel, SL, SW Chensue, M Plewa, and GI Higashi. **1984.** Macrophage function in the *Schistosoma mansoni* egg-induced pulmonary granuloma: Role of arachidonic acid metabolities in Ia antigen expression. Am J Pathol 114:240-249.

Mizel, SB. **1981.** Production and quantitation of lymphocyte-activating factor (interleukin 1), pp. 407-416. In: *Manual of Macrophage Methodology: Collection, Characterization and Function,* HB Herscowitz, HT Holden, JA Bellanti, and A Ghaffar (eds.). Marcel Dekker, New York, NY.

Murphy, MA and HB Herscowitz. **1984.** Heterogeneity among alveolar macrophages in humoral and cell mediated immune responses: Separation of functional subpopulations by density gradient centrifugation on Percoll. J Leukocyte Biol 35:39-54.

Nagasawa, H, C Miyaura, E Abe, T Suda, M Horiguchi, and T Suda. **1987.** Fusion and activation of human alveolar macrophages induced by recombinant interferon-γ and their suppression by dexamethasone. Am Rev Respir Dis 136:916-921.

Oghiso, Y, E Kagan, and AR Brody. **1984.** Intrapulmonary distribution of inhaled chrysotile and crocidolite asbestos: Ultrastructural features. Br J Exp Pathol 65:467-484.

Shellito, J and HB Kaltreider. **1984.** Heterogeneity of immunologic function among subfractions of normal rat alveolar macrophages. Am Rev Respir Dis 129:747-753.

Warheit, DB, G Georg, LH Hill, R Snyderman, and AR Brody. **1985.** Inhaled asbestos activates a complement-dependent chemoattractant for macrophages. Lab Invest 52:505-514.

FIBER-INDUCED CHANGES

Characterization of Dusts from Machining of Fiber-Epoxy Composites and Biological Responses to Respirable Fractions*

Daniel L. Luchtel,[1] Thomas R. Martin,[2] and Edwin S. Boatman[1]

[1]Department of Environmental Health, School of Public Health and Community Medicine, University of Washington, Seattle, WA 98195

[2]Medical Research Service of the Seattle Veterans Administration Medical Center and the Division of Pulmonary and Critical Care Medicine, Department of Medicine, School of Medicine, University of Washington, Seattle, WA 98195

KEY WORDS: fiber-epoxy composites, quartz, aluminum oxide, intratracheal injection, lung lesions, machining

ABSTRACT

It is of current concern whether respirable dusts derived from machining composite materials pose a health risk to workers. Dust samples representative of a number of composites were collected at tool faces, and aerodynamically sized and fractionated. Bulk and fractionated (i.e., respirable) samples were examined by light and electron microscopy and analyzed chemically by thermogravimetric analysis (TGA), gas chromatography (GC) and mass spectrometry (MS). Using scanning electron microscopy, bulk particles were observed to range from 7 to 10 μm in diameter, with mean aspect ratios of 6:1 to 26:1. Aerodynamic diameters of respirable particles ranged from 0.8 to 2.1 μm. The respirable fraction of the total mass of the bulk samples ranged from less than 1 to about 3%. By TGA, the weight loss of fractionated material was negligible below 250° C; it was variable but increased at higher temperatures, up to 860° C. In assays of vapors released from bulk material at 250° C, GC/MS indicated a variety of compounds, in differing amounts for each sample.

*Supported in part by a contract from the Boeing Co., Seattle, WA.

We studied the potential pulmonary toxicity of these materials, using the respirable fractions. A single intratracheal 5-mg bolus of each sample was injected in rats. Quartz and aluminum oxide were injected as positive and negative controls, respectively. After a 1-month exposure, lungs were evaluated for histopathology. The fiber-epoxy composite materials showed a continuum of lung injury that was intermediate between that of the positive and negative controls. None of the composite dusts had effects as severe as those of quartz; however, four produced small fibrotic nodules, an effect that was not seen after exposure to aluminum oxide. Lavage and *in vitro* cytotoxicity studies also indicated that the composite dusts had intermediate effects. Their place on the spectrum from highly toxic (quartz) to inert (Al_2O_3) appeared to be much closer to the latter.

We do not know which component or mixture of components in the various fiber-epoxy composite materials caused the tissue responses. Variables include the graphite type, the epoxy composition, and the type of machining operation that produced the dust. As far as we are aware, ours is the first study to evaluate possible pulmonary effects of composite dusts. A synergistic or other interaction of cigarette smoke with these fibers has not been studied. One can only speculate that interactions might occur between these two materials, given the adsorptive properties of different kinds of amorphous carbon, such as activated charcoal or lampblack.

INTRODUCTION

The use of carbon, graphite, or glass fibers combined with a binder derived from an assortment of plastics or epoxy resins is rapidly increasing in the manufacture of components for the aerospace, military, automobile, and sporting goods industries. The term "carbon fiber" applies to carbonaceous fibrous material pyrolyzed at 1200°C that consists essentially of amorphous carbon. Graphite fibers are carbon fibers heated to between 2200 and 2700°C, resulting in a crystalline fiber structure often referred to as graphite yarn (Zumwalde and Harmison, 1980). The derived fibers are chemically inert and resistant to high temperatures, have high mechanical strength, are lightweight, and are good electrical conductors. When combined with a binder, the composite material can be molded and machined in a variety of ways (Saracco et al., 1981; Jones et al., 1982). At various stages during manufacture, fibers may be inadvertently released into the ambient air. During the machining stage, released particles will be coated with residues of binder chemicals that, if heated to more than 400°C, will vaporize and generate condensation aerosols (Mazumder et al., 1982), often in the form of spheroids (Boeing Co., unpublished observations).

Although much is known about the constituents and the production of carbon/graphite composite materials (Saracco et al., 1981; Jones et al., 1982; Chou et al., 1986), only scanty data exist on the characteristics of the airborne fibers that are released during manufacturing processes (Conner, 1981; Peters et al., 1981; Mazumder et al., 1982) and their possible effects on human health (Kowalska, 1982) or in experimental animals (Fedyakina, 1984; Owen et al., 1986; Troickaja et al., 1984).

In view of the immense potential for the use of carbon/graphite fiber-epoxy composite materials, a comprehensive study of such materials is timely and appropriate. In the workplace we investigated, composite dusts (primarily particulates) are generated in lay-up work and in curing, sanding, sawing, cutting, grinding, casting, and machining operations. The study we undertook is in three parts, involving (1) the physical, chemical and morphological characterization of dusts derived from the machining of composite materials (Boatman et al., 1988), (2) exposure of animals to respirable fractions of the dusts (Luchtel et al., in press), and (3) evaluation of dusts for cytotoxicity by using cell-culture and lung-lavage procedures (Martin et al., manuscript in preparation). This paper summarizes our findings.

MATERIALS AND METHODS

Collection and Characterization of Samples

Samples of prefabricated graphite fiber-epoxy and fiberglass/epoxy composite components of differing composition were subjected to routine machining operations. The resultant dusts were collected at the tool face using a Nilfisk GS 80 industrial vacuum cleaner (Malvern, PA) equipped with a bag filter and a Gore-Tex® (Elkton, MD) 0.3-μm microfilter (99.95% collecting efficiency) positioned at its exhaust end. Samples selected were representative of a variety of key structural forms, and of materials most commonly used by this manufacturer. All bulk samples were redispersed to the aerosol phase by use of a fluidized-bed aerosol generator (TSI, Model 9310; St. Paul, MN) connected to a 10-cm-diameter cyclone. The generator output flow and total cyclone flow were adjusted to achieve a size segregation such that at least 90% by mass and more than 90% by number of the particles were less than 10 μm in aerodynamic diameter (D_{ae}).

Samples of aerodynamically defined material were collected on 25-mm-diameter, 2.0-μm-pore-size Nuclepore® filters in open-faced cassettes at a flow of 4 L/min for morphological analysis (using a JEOL JSM 35U scanning electron microscope). Other samples were collected for chemical and biological analysis on 37-mm-diameter, 3.0-μm-pore-size Teflon filters (Membrana, Inc.; presently available from Gelman Sciences, Ann Arbor, MI) with fiber backup disks, at a flow of 20 L/min.

Chemical Analysis

The methods used for analysis of chemical vapors released from plastics have been reported previously (Kalman, 1986). Weight-loss-versus-temperature profiles of each composite material, obtained by thermogravimetric analysis (TGA), were used to establish the quantity of vaporous products produced under controlled heating. The volatilizable organic fraction was then collected under isothermal conditions by dynamic headspace sampling with cryogenic focusing on fused silica capillary gas chromatographic columns for quantitative and qualitative gas chromatography/mass spectrometry (GC/MS) analysis.

Animal Experiments

Male pathogen-free Charles River rats (200 g in weight) were obtained from Charles River Laboratories, Inc. (Wilmington, MA) and randomly placed in groups of five. Each animal received a single, 5-mg intratracheal injection of a respirable fraction of composite or control material in 0.25 ml of pyrogen-free phosphate-buffered saline (PBS).

The following vehicle, controls, and composite materials were tested: (1) PBS, (2) quartz (fibrogenic control), (3) aluminum oxide (inert mineral control), and (4) composite respirable fractions #1, 2, 3, 4, 5, and 6. One month later, all animals were sacrificed by peritoneal injection of pentobarbital, and the lungs were collected. The right lungs were lavaged to recover airway cells and extracellular proteins, then vacuum-dried and weighed. The left lungs were fixed for microscopic analyses by intratracheal instillation of 2% glutaraldehyde and 1% formaldehyde in 0.1M cacodylate buffer, pH 7.4, at 20 cm water pressure for 2 hours at room temperature. After overnight storage at 4°C, the entire left lung was sectioned longitudinally, rinsed in cacodylate buffer, dehydrated in ethanol, and embedded in paraffin. Six-micrometer sections were cut and stained with hematoxylin and eosin. In addition, small cubes of tissue from these fixed lungs were postfixed in osmium and embedded in epon. One-micrometer sections were cut and stained with toluidine blue. Six slides (one from the paraffin block and one from each of five epon blocks) were evaluated for each animal. Selected blocks were thin-sectioned for electron microscopy and examined in a JEOL 100S transmission electron microscope.

Microscopy and Pathology

The sections were analyzed by the first author (DL) without knowledge of the group to which the animal belonged. The following semiquantitative scale of 0 to 4 was used to indicate the range of pathological changes seen on the sections:

Grade	Changes
0	No pathological changes evident: no trace of inflammation or fibrosis
1	Few or seemingly incidental pathological changes: an apparent increase in number of alveolar macrophages (AM) due to particle load; a few small localized areas of mild interstitial fibrosis
2	Definite pathological changes present: alveolar cellular infiltration, including macrophages, neutrophils and lymphocytes, a few small but discrete fibrotic nodules
3	Moderate degree of pathological changes: more extensive areas of alveolar infiltration; epithelial necrosis in alveoli and bronchioles; larger and more numerous fibrotic nodules in alveoli and along alveolar ducts
4	Marked pathological changes: extensive rather than focal areas of alveolar infiltration with striking accumulation of AM, neutrophils and lymphocytes; extensive interstitial fibrosis and numerous fibrotic nodules; alveolar proteinosis

Thus, the final score for each group is a numerical representation of the histopathologic observations that combines the types of lesions seen and the approximate number of such lesions.

Lavage Cell Counts

The right lungs were lavaged 10 times with PBS to recover airway cells and proteins, then vacuum-dried and weighed. The lavage fluids were centrifuged at 200 x g and the supernatant was decanted and frozen at -70°C. The cell pellets were resuspended in PBS, and total cell counts were performed with a hemocytometer. Differential counts were performed on cytocentrifuged preparations stained with Diff-Quik® (Scientific Products, McGaw Park, IN). Differences in results between groups were tested for statistical significance using one-way analysis of variance.

Cytotoxicity Studies

Composite and control dusts were incubated with normal rabbit (male New Zealand White) alveolar macrophages (AM) *in vitro,* and cytotoxicity was measured by ^{51}Cr release. Each rabbit was killed with an intravenous injection of pentobarbital and exsanguinated by cardiac puncture. The thorax was opened, and the lungs were removed *en bloc* and lavaged 10 times with 50 ml of phosphate-buffered 0.9% NaCl containing 0.6 mM EDTA to recover lung macrophages. Lavage fluids were centrifuged for 10 minutes at 300 x g, and the cell pellets were incubated with ^{51}Cr for 1 hour to label intracellular proteins. Cell pellets were washed three times in Tyrode's buffer and resuspended to give 1 x 10^6 viable AM/ml in RPMI medium containing 5% heat-inactivated fetal calf serum, L-glutamine, penicillin (100 IU/ml), and streptomycin (100 IU/ml). The labeled AM were then dispensed into 24-well tissue culture plates at 2.5 x 10^5 cells/well, and aliquots of each fractionated composite sample and control mineral were added so that the final composite and mineral concentration was 500 μg/well.

Cells and test materials were incubated at 37°C in air containing 5% CO_2. At 2 and 48 hours, cells and supernatants in some wells were harvested by scraping the bottoms of the wells gently to resuspend adherent cells and aspirating the supernatants. The supernatants were then centrifuged to remove cells, and the radioactivity in the supernatants was measured in a gamma scintillation counter. To determine the total counts in the wells, both cell pellets and supernatants of the control wells that contained only medium were counted. The results were added to yield 100% activity. The counts in each supernatant were then divided by this value at each time to yield the percentage ^{51}Cr release in each supernatant. Triplicate samples were collected from wells for each experimental condition in each experiment, and these results were averaged within each experiment. Each complete experiment was repeated three or four times, and the differences among the various test conditions at each time were analyzed by a one-way analysis of variance.

RESULTS

Dust Characterization

Sample identification numbers, material compositions, and machining operations are listed in Table 1. For the dusts released at the tool faces, fiber lengths ranged from a few to several hundred micrometers; fiber widths, from 7 to 10 μm (Table 2 and Figure 1). Aspect ratios also varied widely. All dust samples contained respirable fractions, defined as a measurable particle-number concentration of less than 10 μm in D_{ae}. The respirable fraction of the total mass of the bulk sample ranged from less than 1%, in the case of sample #2, to a few percent for samples #4, 5, and 6. Precise quantitative determinations were considered inappropriate because of the large number of nonrespirable particles present. The size statistics are presented in Table 3; an example of a respirable fraction is shown in Figure 2. Because of the nongaussian form of the distributions, it is not valid to express them in terms of simple mean and standard deviation parameters.

Table 1. Composition of composite materials examined[a] (modified from Boatman et al., 1988).

Sample #	Fiber Type	Binder Composition	Equipment	Speed (rpm)
1	Graphite-P[b]	PEEK[c]	Spindle shaper	10,000
2	Fiber glass	Epoxy + amine curing agent	Spindle shaper	3,450
3	Graphite-PAN[d]/Kevlar®	Epoxy + amine curing agent	Hand router Saber saw Spindle shaper	23,000 3,450
4	Graphite-PAN	Epoxy + aromatic amine curing agent	Hand router	23,000
5	Graphite-pitch[e]	Epoxy + aromatic amine curing agent	Spindle shaper	3,450
6	Graphite-PAN	Epoxy + amine curing agent	Hand router	23,000

[a]All materials were preimpregnated, i.e., resin impregnation of bundled continuous filaments to form a continuous tape of fabric, which is later plied in layers of the same or different alignments.
[b]Proprietary material
[c]Nonepoxy polyetheretherketone thermoplastic
[d]Polyacrylonitrile precursor
[e]Pitch graphite-precursor

Table 2. Average fiber lengths (range) and diameters of bulk composite dusts examined by scanning electron microscopy (modified from Boatman et al., 1988).

Sample #	Dimensions: Length (μm)	Dimensions: Diameter (μm)	Aspect Ratio
1	71 (23 - 342)	7	10:1
2	262 (32 - 2500)	10	26:1
3	109 (28 - 340)	9	12:1
4	87 (28 - 264)	8	11:1
5	63 (34 - 120)	10	6:1
6	210 (26 - 1307)	8	26:1

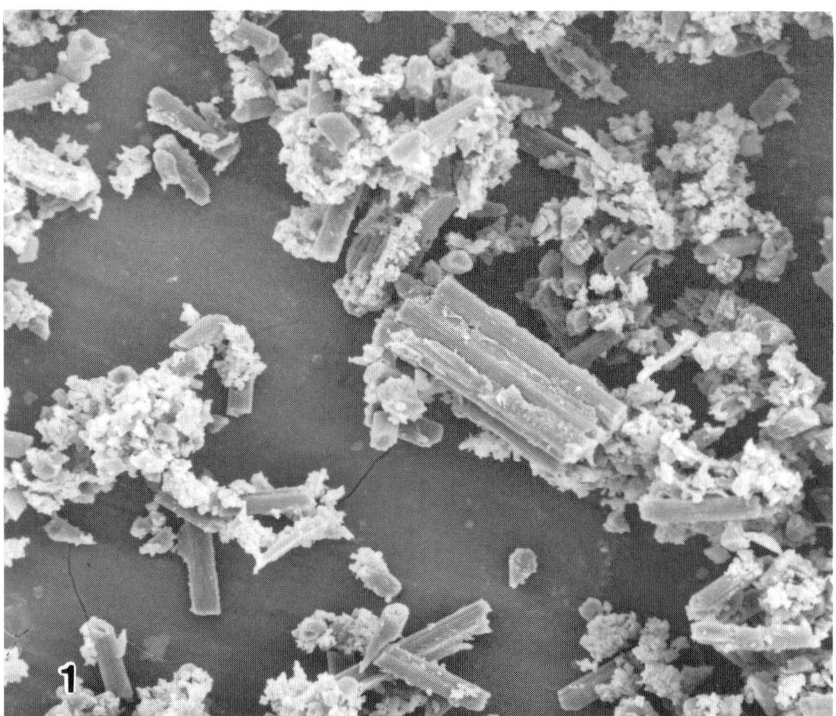

Figure 1. Scanning electron micrograph of bulk dust of composite #4, collected from a manual routing-machine operation. The dust contains a heterogenous population of fractured graphite fibers (20 to 200 μm in length by 8 to 10 μm in diameter) and epoxy debris. Magnification, 530X.

Table 3. Number/size distributions of respirable composite dusts examined (modified from Boatman et al., 1988).

Sample #	Aerodynamic Diameter (μm) Modal Size	Aerodynamic Diameter (μm) Mean Size	Geometric Diameter[a] (μm) Mean Size
1	1.0	1.3	1.6
2	1.1, 3.5[b]	2.1	2.6
3	1.2	1.5	1.9
4	1.2	1.4	1.8
5	0.9	1.3	1.6
6	0.8	0.9	1.1

[a]Corrected for density and shape factors
[b]Bimodal distribution

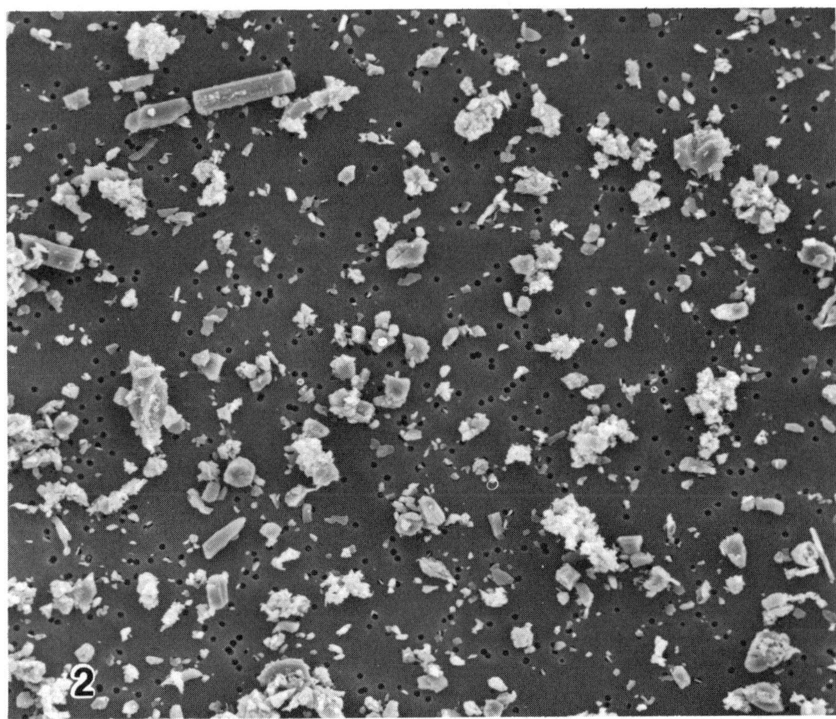

Figure 2. Scanning electron micrograph of the respirable fraction of composite #4. The mean aerodynamic diameter of the particles is 1.4 μm, and the mean geometric diameter is 1.8 μm. Magnification, 530X.

Vapor samples were obtained from a known weight of unfractionated bulk material subjected to isothermal desorption in an inert atmosphere at 250°C and analyzed by GC/MS. The various compounds found, in differing amounts, for each type of sample, are summarized according to chemical class in Table 4. Also shown is a quantitative comparison of the yields of selected compounds in all six samples that are of possible concern to human health.

Animal Studies

Figure 3 shows a longitudinal section of an entire left rat lung. By studying such sections in detail, we were able to identify and enumerate any lesions that occurred along the entire apical-basal length of the lung. Figures 4 through 9 illustrate typical lesions that were observed. Lungs exposed to Al_2O_3 (Figure 4) showed an increased number of macrophages in the air spaces but had no fibrotic lesions. Lungs exposed to quartz showed a striking accumulation of proteinaceous material and macrophages in the alveoli; numerous fibrotic lesions were also seen (Figure 5). The microscopic appearance of lungs exposed to composite materials #1 and 3 (not shown) was very similar to that of the Al_2O_3 controls; both materials stimulated a low histopathological response. Composite samples #5 and 6, as well as #2 and 4, induced small fibrotic nodules in the lung. Examples are shown in Figures 6 and 7. Hypercellularity and fibrotic nodules typically occurred in the area of terminal bronchioles and first- and second-generation alveolar ducts (Figure 8). An example of the phagocytic response of AM to the particulate material is shown in Figure 9.

Table 4. Chemical analysis of composite dusts (modified from Boatman et al., 1988).

Sample #:	1	2	3	4	5	6
	Percentage of Identified Constituents					
Oxygenates	40.1	36.6	29.7	95.4	46.5	89.3
Chlorinates	13.7	59.8	48.5	3.4	7.3	BD[a]
Aromatics	8.7	2.3	2.6	BD	1.7	BD
N-containing compounds	0.1	0.7	BD	BD	BD	BD
Alkenes/alkanes	37.4	0.6	19.2	1.2	55.5	10.7

[a]BD = Below level of detection

Number of Components Identified:	117	29	39	14	44	17
	Yield (μg/g) of Compounds of Principal Human Health Concern					
Chloroaniline	—	—	142	—	—	—
Dichloroaniline	—	8250	5340	—	—	—
Dichloronitrobenzene	—	—	22	—	—	—
Tributyl phosphate	—	—	147	150	—	9
Diphenylphosphine oxide	379	—	58	—	—	—
Dibenzofuranamine	—	—	—	—	—	78
Benzofuran	80	—	—	—	—	—
Biphenyl	95	—	—	—	—	—
Diphenyl hydrazine	162	—	—	—	—	—
Benzothiazone	542	—	—	—	—	—
Triphenylphosphine oxide	—	155	—	355	—	—

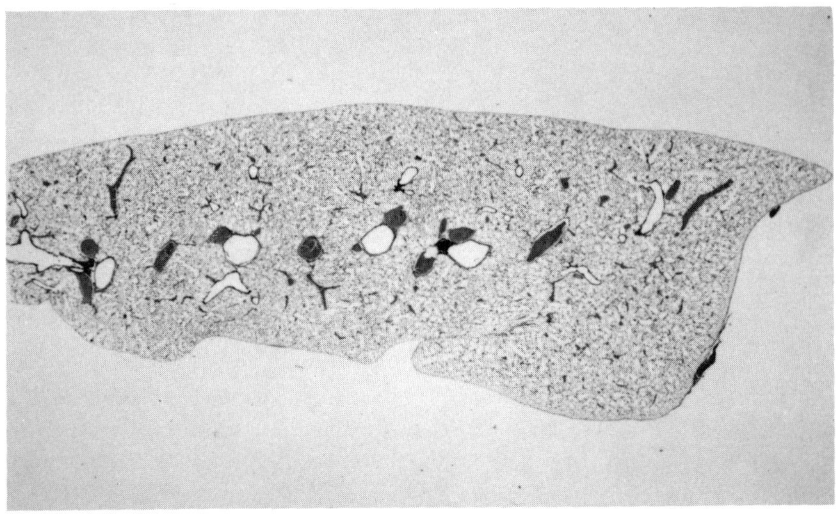

Figure 3. Low magnification of a light micrograph of a longitudinal paraffin section through the entire left lung of a rat exposed to composite #6 for 1 month. While the overall lung architecture appears normal at this low magnification, phagocytic cell hypercellularity and small fibrotic nodules were seen at higher magnification. Magnification, 3.5X.

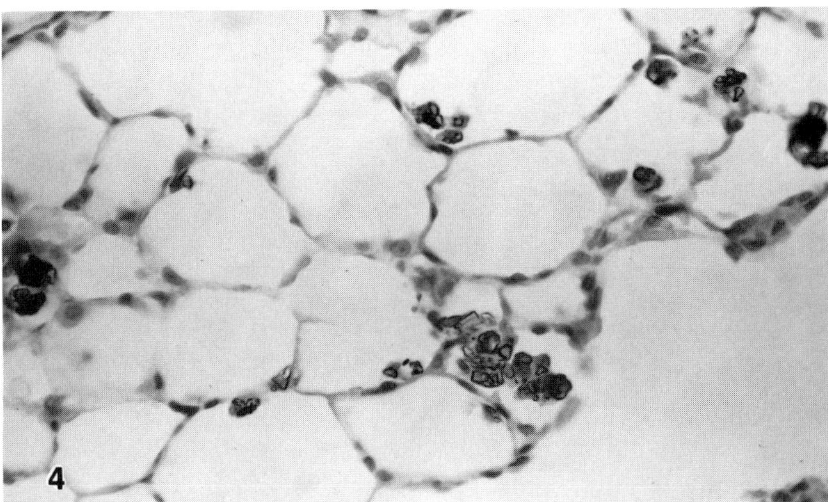

Figure 4. Light micrograph of rat lung after a 1-month exposure to Al_2O_3. Most of the material, in the form of both free particles and particles phagocytized by macrophages, has remained on surfaces of alveoli and alveolar ducts. Some particles appear to have aggregated in the alveolar interstitium, but a fibrotic response has not been induced. Magnification, 620X.

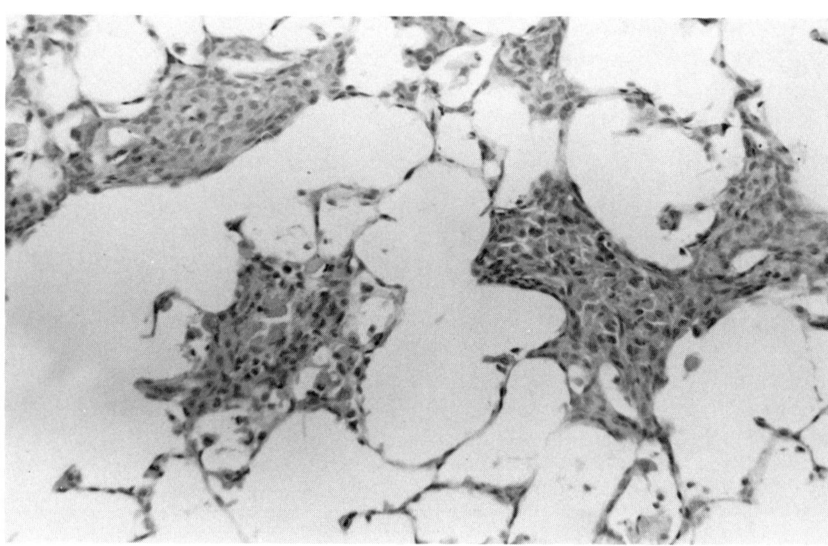

Figure 5. Light micrograph of rat lung after a 1-month exposure to free crystalline silica. Several fibrotic nodules appear in alveolar areas or along walls of alveolar ducts. Individual silica particles are difficult to visualize with bright-field optics, but a few can be seen in nodules as small, clear, reticular shapes. Magnification, 290X.

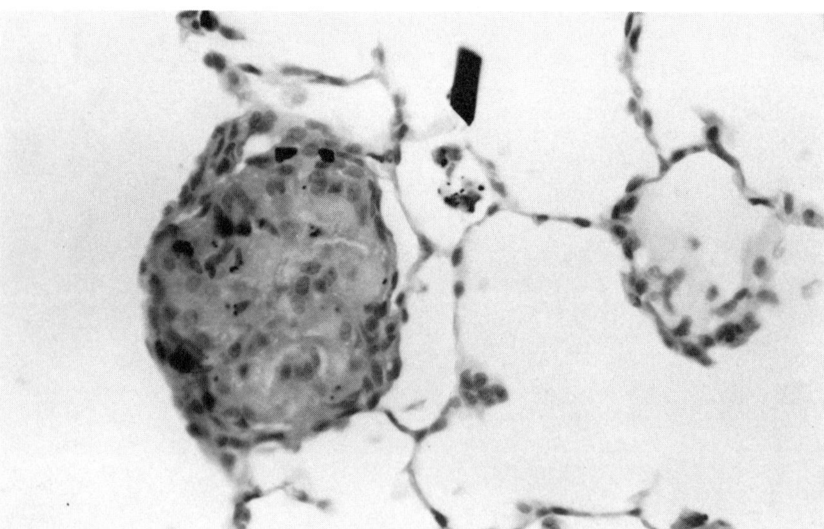

Figure 6. Light micrograph of rat lung after a 1-month exposure to composite #6. A fibrotic nodules is shown in the wall of an alveolar duct (left center of micrograph); a number of small dark particles are embedded in the nodule. Most of the intra-alveolar particles have been phagocytized, although some remain free on the alveolar surface. Magnification, 620X.

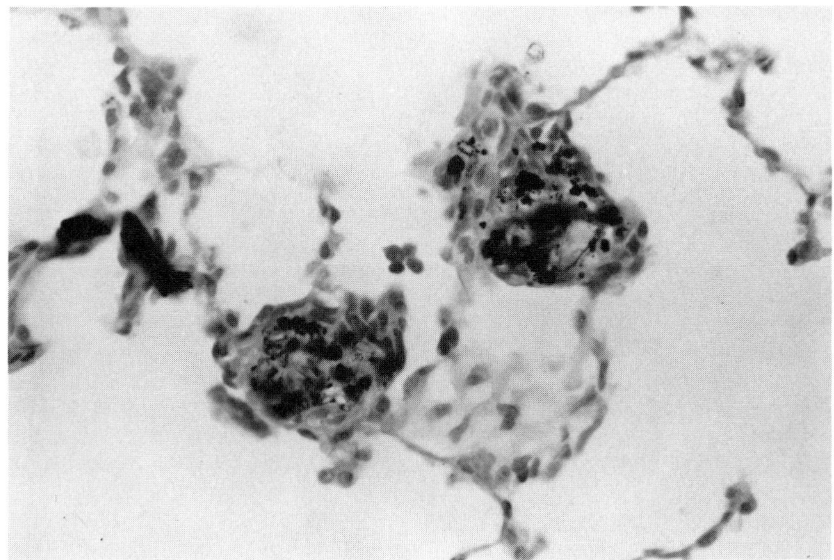

Figure 7. Light micrograph of lung after a 1-month exposure to composite #4. The two fibrotic nodules shown contain fibrous particulates as well as clear, black, refractile, nonfibrous particulates. Magnification, 620X.

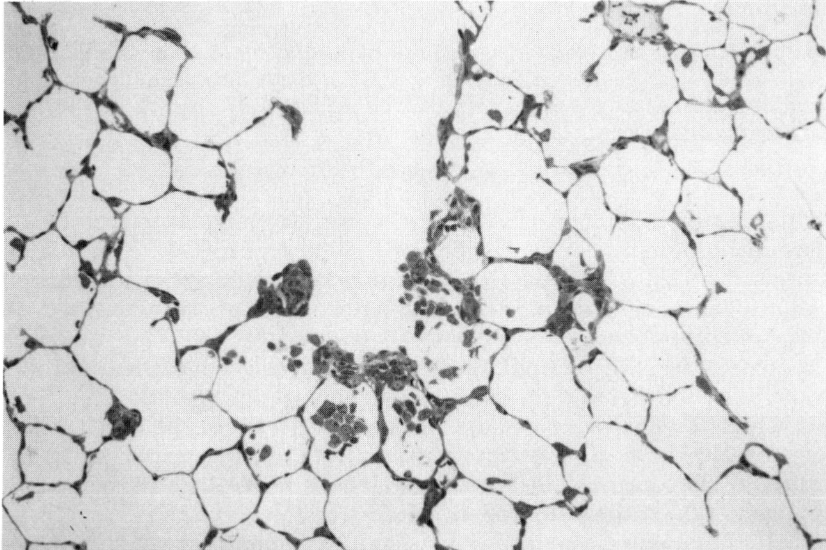

Figure 8. Light micrograph of a 1-μm-thick Epon section showing alveolar duct and adjacent alveoli from a rat exposed to composite #5 for 1 month. Such an area is a preferred site for phagocytic cell hypercellularity and for development of small fibrotic lesions. Magnification, 240X.

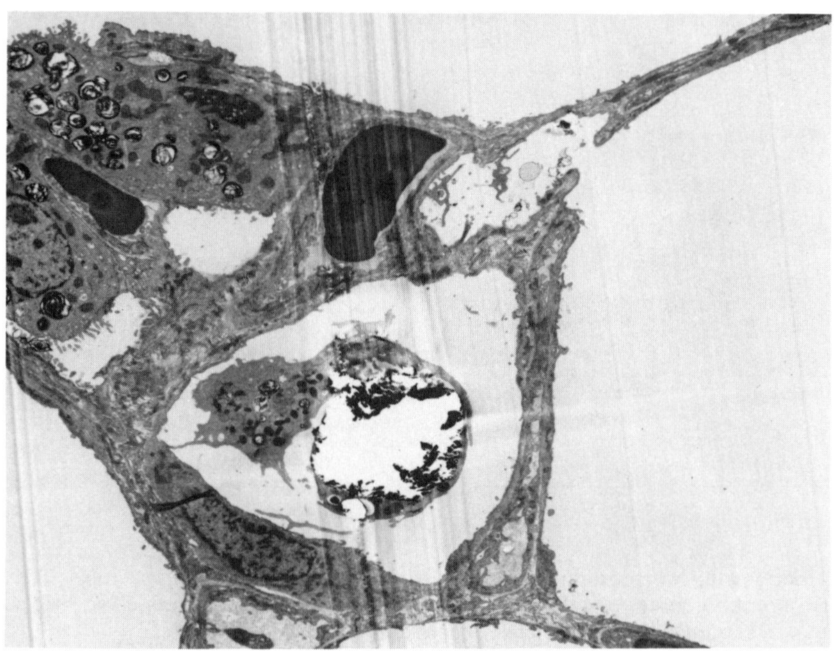

Figure 9. Transmission electron micrograph of rat lung after a 1-month exposure to composite #5. An apparent graphite fiber is surrounded by pseudopodia of a macrophage. Fiber tended to shatter out of the section, and its hard, brittle nature has scratched the Epon. Magnification, 3500X.

The negative and positive controls had the lowest and highest histopathological scores, respectively, whereas the six composite samples had intermediate scores (Figure 10). Although the grading system was only semiquantitative, the control groups spanned a range of injury from 0 for PBS and 1.1 for Al_2O_3, to 3.7 for quartz. The scores for the composite materials covered a continuum of injury that fell between these two extremes.

Overall, it was difficult to distinguish the tissue response to composite samples #1 and 3 from that of the Al_2O_3 negative control group. A distinguishing feature for these three groups was the apparent "inertness" of the injected particles. That is, after 1 month of exposure, the majority of the particles that remained in the alveoli were phagocytized by macrophages, and a minimal fibrotic response was elicited by samples #1 and 3. The definitive presence of fibrotic nodules distinguished groups #2, 4, 5, and 6 from #1 and 3; the number of such nodules was somewhat higher in groups #2 and 4. A large number of fibrotic lesions, prominent alveolar infiltration by macrophages, neutrophils and lymphocytes, and alveolar proteinosis distinguished the quartz positive control group from all other groups.

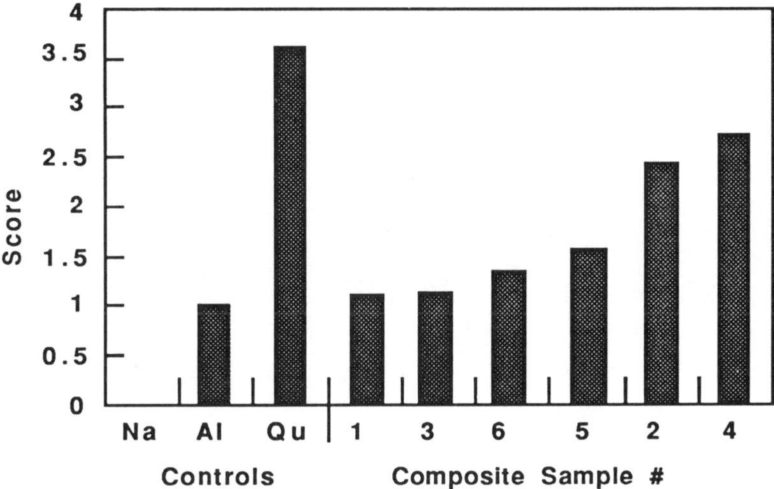

Figure 10. Scale of pathological changes in rats exposed to composite dusts, and controls: 0 = none, 4 = marked. (See Materials and Methods.) NA = saline injection; Al = Al_2O_3; Qu = quartz.

Other measurements are compared with the results of the microscopic examinations in Figures 11 through 15. These figures are constructed similarly to Figure 10 to allow convenient comparisons. That is, on all these figures, a measurement or value is shown on the y-axis, and the three control groups and six composite groups are always shown in the same order (from left to right) on the x-axis.

Figure 11 shows the average dry weight for the right lung in each of the groups at the end of the 1-month exposure. The PBS control had the highest lung weight, while the lung weights of animals exposed to the composite dusts were lower than those of Al_2O_3- and quartz-exposed animals. Figure 12 shows average body weights after the 1-month exposure. The quartz and composite groups are strikingly lower than either the PBS or Al_2O_3 control groups.

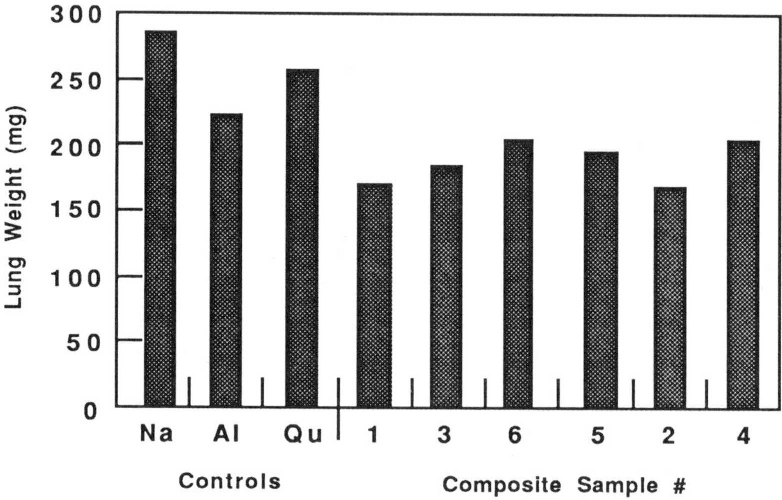

Figure 11. Mean lung weights of rats in control and composite groups after a 1-month exposure. NA = saline injection; Al = Al_2O_3; Qu = quartz.

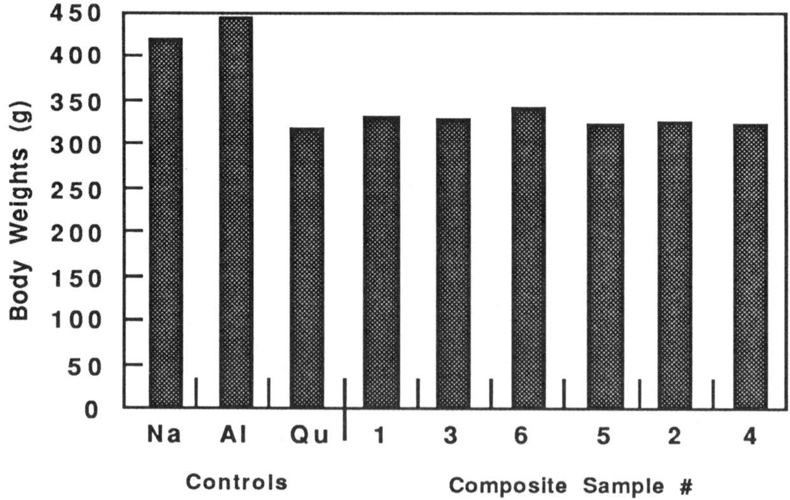

Figure 12. Mean body weights of rats in control and composite groups after a 1-month exposure.

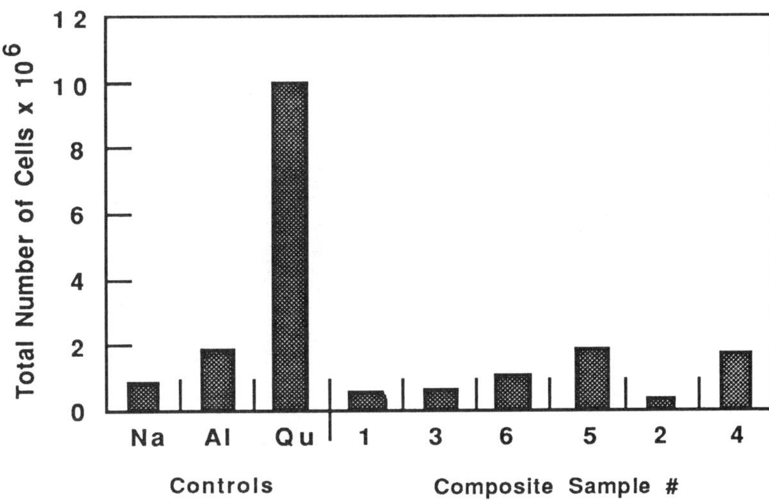

Figure 13. Total number of cells lavaged from right lung of rats in control and composite groups after a 1-month exposure.

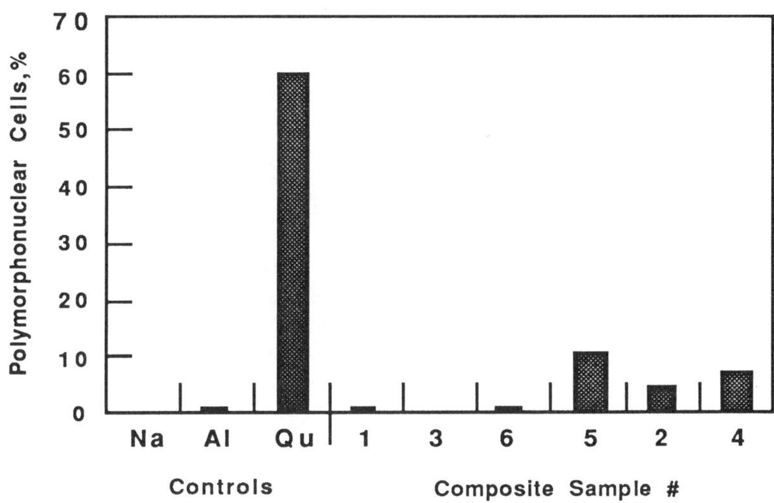

Figure 14. Percentage of polymorphonuclear cells (neutrophils) in lavages from control and composite groups after a 1-month exposure.

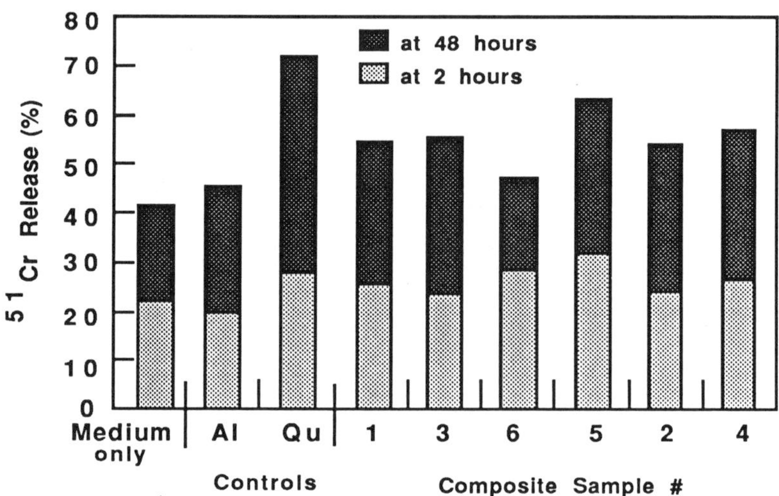

Figure 15. Percentage of ^{51}Cr release from preloaded rabbit alveolar macrophages at 2 and 48 hours of exposure to control or composite dusts in culture medium.

Lavage and Cytotoxicity Studies

Results of the lavage studies are shown in Figures 13 and 14. Animals injected with NaCl had approximately 1 x 10^6 recoverable airway cells, consisting of 98.3 ± 2.9% AM and no identifiable neutrophils. In contrast, quartz, a known fibrogenic agent, caused a highly significant ($P < 0.0001$) 10-fold increase in recoverable cells, the majority of which were neutrophils (66.0 ± 8.8%). The Al_2O_3, used as an inert mineral control, caused doubling of recoverable cells but no increase in lavaged neutrophils.

In comparison, none of the total cell recoveries in animals treated with any of the composites was statistically different from cell recoveries in NaCl- and Al_2O_3-treated control animals. Samples #4 and 5 caused the largest increase in airway cells, but these were minor compared to increases in the quartz-treated animals. The percentage of airway neutrophils in the sample #5-treated animals was significantly greater than that in the Al_2O_3-treated animals ($P < 0.01$). The increase in neutrophils in the sample #4-treated animals was marginal ($P = 0.09$).

Particles were visible in AM from all of the animals, indicating persistence of the minerals in alveolar tissue and phagocytosis. The greatest numbers of particles were found in macrophages recovered from animals treated with Al_2O_3, quartz, and sample #6. Few particles were seen in AM lavaged from animals treated with composite #3. Thus the numbers of particles in AM did not correlate well with the profile of responses determined from cells in lavage fluids.

The results of the AM cytotoxicity studies are shown in Figure 15. As expected, the quartz produced marked cytotoxicity (72.55 ± 4.19% ^{51}Cr release by 48 hours), whereas cytotoxicity resulting from Al_2O_3 exposure (47.2 ± 3.2%) was similar to that of culture medium only (42.9 ± 4.0 release by 48 hours). These differences were highly significant ($P < 0.0001$ by one-way analysis of variance for medium alone, quartz, and Al_2O_3).

At each time point examined, macrophages exposed to composites released ^{51}Cr in amounts that were between those released by cells exposed to quartz or Al_2O_3. Of the composites, #5 released the most ^{51}Cr at each time point ($P < 0.01$, compared with Al_2O_3 and quartz). These findings were very consistent within and between experiments. In comparison, samples #3, 4, and 1 released similar amounts of ^{51}Cr, all of which were significantly greater than that released by Al_2O_3 at 48 hours ($P < 0.01$). Composites #6 and 2 released the least ^{51}Cr, an amount similar to that released by Al_2O_3. No significant differences were found with respect to the ability of rabbit AM to phagocytize the different types of dusts.

DISCUSSION

Due to their remarkable mechanical properties, the uses of carbon/graphite fiber-composites are rapidly expanding. Thus it is important to characterize these environmentally and industrially derived particulate materials and to determine the respirability, chemistry, and potential toxicity of carbon and graphite dusts in order to recommend controls of workplace exposures, if indicated.

Our combined data on the aerodynamic diameters of the redispersed, segregated dusts showed the presence of particles between 0.8 and 2.0 μm in all the materials tested. Particles of this size can be deposited in the upper and lower respiratory tract by impaction and sedimentation, respectively. Thus, such dusts may produce both short- and long-term effects in the respiratory system. However, the proportion of particles with these dimensions in our study was only a few percent of the bulk dust.

The range of dimensions of the bulk material in our study was similar to the size range of airborne composite dusts collected in industrial settings by Jones et al. (1982) and by Gieseke et al. (1983). In our study, fiber diameter appeared not to be significantly affected by any individual operation. Constancy in fiber diameter is probably the result of fracturing these fibers crosswise rather than longitudinally, as occurs when asbestos fibers are machined.

Reported concentrations of airborne carbon/graphite composite dusts in various manufacturing plants vary somewhat (e.g., 0.4 mg/m^3, Jones et al., 1982; $<$1 mg/m^3, Saracco et al., 1981; 1.5 to 81 mg/m^3, Fedyakina, 1984). Presumably, the concentration levels depend on the processes involved and the ventilation and sampling procedures used. For dusts in the studies listed above, the respirable fractions varied from 40 to 70% by weight. In our study, the respirable fractions derived from dusts collected at the tool face were only 3 to 4% by weight. However, this low fraction of respirable particles may not be representative of concentrations in the breathing zone of the machine operators in our study. The difference may be due to our method of sampling, which collected all airborne material at the tool face. This might have included large particles that would settle rapidly and would not normally reach the breathing zone.

The chemical and thermal analyses indicate that the material sampled was well cured, was thermally quite stable, and did not contain much desorbable material. Specifically, the low percentage of mass loss, particularly at temperatures comparable to those observed during machining, and the absence of detectable prepolymers or catalysts in the chemical analysis support these conclusions. Among the detected agents are compounds widely used as plastic modifiers (phthalate ester, hexadecanoic acid, phosphate esters). Other components are probably degradation or conversion products of plastic components (alkylphosphine oxides, diphenyl hydrazine).

The histopathology results of this study, derived from a single intratracheal instillation of respirable particulates in rats that were examined 1 month after initiation of exposure, show that none of the composite preparations had effects as severe as those following quartz instillation. Of the six composite samples, #4 (graphite-polyacrylonitrile) and #2 (fiberglass) caused the greatest pathological response. Although samples #2 and 3 as well as #4 and 5 had a similar epoxy composition (Table 1), their graphite/fabric type and trimming operations were different, as were their pathology scores. We do not know which component or mixture of components in the composite groups caused the tissue responses. Both dark and clear, refractile types of particulates were seen in most of the fibrotic lesions.

The lavage studies suggest that none of the composite dusts caused a lasting cellular response in rat lungs that parallels that caused by quartz, an agent with known cytotoxicity in the lung. Two of the composites, #4 and 5, caused minor but significant neutrophilic response, whereas the inert Al_2O_3 did not, suggesting that these two composites may not be completely inert in the lung.

Their place on the spectrum from highly toxic (quartz) to inert (Al_2O_3) appears to be much closer to that of Al_2O_3 than to that of quartz, however.

The *in vitro* studies using rabbit AM suggest that the composites are intermediate in their cytotoxicity between that of quartz and Al_2O_3; composite #5 appeared to be most cytotoxic in these experiments (67% of the difference between Al_2O_3 and quartz at 48 hours). The results of these *in vitro* studies cannot be extrapolated directly to whole animals or to humans, but they serve to rank the potential cytotoxicity of these materials in relation to known toxic (quartz) and inert minerals (Al_2O_3).

The histopathology and cellular (lavage and cytotoxicity) studies are in general if not perfect agreement. Both indicate that the composite dusts have intermediate cellular and pulmonary toxicity. Histopathologic results indicate that composites #4 and 2 are the most toxic, followed by #5. The cellular studies point to composites #5 and 4 as the most toxic and implicate these two as the most likely to have biological effects in the whole animal.

Materials that generate the lowest fraction of respirable particles under actual manufacturing conditions and those with the least hazardous overall chemical releases would be preferable for manufacturing products. However, if potentially more hazardous materials offer significant technical advantages, appropriate dust-control measures and, possibly, other precautions will have to be taken. Toxicological characterization early in the materials development process will help to determine the proper course of action.

Our studies of the dusts sampled at the source indicate that the respirable portion is largely particulate in nature; comprises only a few percent of the total amount of dust; and that the fibrous component is, typically, of large diameter. Based on this information, hazard evaluation of work operations might include gravimetric analysis of respirable fractions of graphite-epoxy material rather than chemical analysis or fiber-counting.

Future experimentation will undoubtedly focus on characterizing the chemistry, morphology and potential toxicity of yet newer composite materials of diverse composition.

ACKNOWLEDGMENTS

We thank Michael Stewart, Dr. Barry Dunphy, Dr. Denis Bourcier and Nicholas Novak for their cooperation and supply of dust samples; Dr. David Kalman and Dr. David Covert for characterization and preparation of the respirable dust fractions; and Steve Meyer and Dr. Gilbert Omenn for suggestions and encouragement.

REFERENCES

Boatman, ES, D Covert, D Kalman, D Luchtel, and GS Omenn. **1988.** Physical, morphological and chemical studies of dusts derived from the machining of composite-epoxy materials. Environ Res 45:242-255.

Chou, TW, RL McCullough, and RB Pipes. **1986.** Composites. Sci Am 255:192-203.

Conner, WD. **1981.** *Monitoring Techniques for Carbon Fiber Emissions: Evaluation A,* EPA-600/S2-81-048. U.S. Environmental Protection Agency, Research Triangle Park, NC.

Fedyakina, RP. **1984.** Experimental study of the biological effects of the dust of carbon fibrous materials on the organism (in Russian). Gig Tr Prof Zabol 7:30-32.

Gieseke, JA, RB Reif, and EW Schmidt. **1983.** *Characterization of Carbon Fiber Emissions from Current and Projected Activities for the Manufacture and Disposal of Carbon Fiber Products,* Contract EPA-68-02-3230. U.S. Environmental Protection Agency, Research Triangle Park, NC.

Jones, HD, TR Jones, and WH Lyle. **1982.** Carbon fibre: Results of a survey of process workers and their environment in a factory producing continuous filament. Ann Occup Hyg 26:861-868.

Kalman, DA. **1986.** Survey analysis of volatile organics released from plastics under thermal stress. Am Ind Hyg Assoc J 47:270-275.

Kowalska, M. **1982.** Carbon fibre reinforced epoxy prepregs and composites - Health risks aspects. SAMPE Q (January):13-19.

Luchtel, DL, TR Martin, and ES Boatman. Histopathologic response of the rat lung to respirable fractions of fiber-epoxy composite materials. Environ Res (**in press**).

Mazumder, MK, RJ Chang, and RL Bond. **1982.** Aerodynamic and morphological properties of carbon-fiber aerosols. Aerosol Sci Technol 1:427-440.

Owen, PE, JR Glaister, B Ballantyne, and J Clarry. **1986.** Subchronic inhalation toxicology of carbon fibers. J Occup Med 28:373-376.

Peters, ET, KT Mengies, EJ Cook, and M Rossetti. **1981.** *Monitoring Techniques for Carbon Fiber Emissions: Evaluation B,* EPA-600/S2-81-145. U.S. Environmental Protection Agency, Research Triangle Park, NC.

Saracco, GB, M Scolaris, GF Rubino, and G Scansetti. **1981.** Manufacturing of articles with carbon fiber reinforced plastics (C.F.R.P.) within the aerospace industry. G Ital Med Lav 3:141-147.

Troickaja, NA, BT Velickovskij, FM Kogan, and LN El'vicnyh. **1984.** Comparative fibrogenicity of carbon fibre and asbestos (in Russian). Gig Sanit 6:18-20.

Zumwalde, RD and LT Harmison. **1980.** *Carbon/Graphite Fibers: Environmental Exposure and Potential Health Implications.* U.S. DHHS, NIOSH, Cincinnati, OH.

A Study of the Biological Activity of Erionite in Relation to its Chemical and Structural Characteristics

David L. Coffin,[1] S. E. Peters,[2] Lalita D. Palekar,[3] and E. P. Stahel[2]

[1]Health Effects Research Laboratory, U.S. Environmental Protection Agency, Research Triangle Park, NC 27711

[2]Department of Chemical Engineering, North Carolina State University, Raleigh, NC 27695-7905

[3]Northrop Services, Inc., P. O. Box 12313, Research Triangle Park, NC 27709

KEY WORDS: erionite, biological effects, physicochemical characteristics

---

ABSTRACT

Fibrous erionite appears to have many times greater potential for mesothelioma induction than asbestos. A member of a class of minerals termed zeolites, it differs markedly from asbestos in many physicochemical characteristics. Zeolites are uniquely powerful in ion exchange, adsorption of small molecules, and catalytic activity. The hallmark of the zeolites is the presence of spaces or voids in the internal structure that communicate with the exterior by means of minute pores with effective diameters of only a few angströms. The critical kinetic diameter of these pores for erionite is 3.6 x 5.2 Å; the interior spaces are larger. These voids in the structure arise from the stacking of the aluminum and silica tetrahedra with shared oxygen atoms, which differ in the various zeolites. Additionally, cations associated with the zeolite structure, most commonly Na^+, K^+, and Mg^{2+} and Ca^{2+}, may occlude the entrance to the pores. Another characteristic of zeolites is the very large surface area (chiefly internal). Erionite, for example, has an internal surface area of approximately 200 m^2/g, which contrasts with a total surface area for chrysotile and crocidolite of 24 m^2/g and 8 to 10 m^2/g, respectively. For preliminary biological studies, our experiments were based on the hypothesis that the active surface sites within the internal voids contribute to the unusual activity of this mineral. Two approaches were followed: encapsulation of isopentane in the internal spaces, and exchange of cations Cr^{2+} and Ca^{2+}. Preliminary data suggest that toxicity to V79 cells was altered by these processes. The implication of the intense tumorigenesis of erionite may be of great basic importance in contributing data for mechanistic studies, such as the identification of a second variable in tumor induction (in addition to the length-width phenomenon). Experiments with erionite should also be of great interest in conjunction with other carcinogens. Strong interaction would be expected, for instance, with small molecular compounds present in gases and vapors from tobacco smoke. Thus erionite (or other zeolites) might have either positive or negative effects on the biological activity of these substances.

INTRODUCTION

The notable observations of Baris, of Ankara, Turkey (1987), recognized that the silicate mineral erionite, like asbestos, induces mesothelial tumors. These observations were made, over a number of years, in certain small Turkish villages in the province of Cappodocia, where there was an extremely high incidence of mesothelioma in the absence of obvious contact with commercial asbestos (Baris et al., 1980). Dr. Baris drew international attention to this phenomenon, and mineralogical studies were carried out. Pooley noted that the mineral erionite was ubiquitous in certain of these villages, its source being volcanic tuff (Pooley, 1979; Sebastien et al., 1981). Other studies, however, detected the presence of small amounts of tremolite and chrysotile asbestos (Rohl et al., 1982). Soon after these observations, experimental animal studies demonstrated that fibrous erionite from Turkish and North American sources was more tumorigenic on a mass basis than asbestos from intrapleural inoculation (Wagner, 1982). When similar material was used in inhalation experiments in rats, only mesotheliomas were induced. This was in striking contrast to all the previous experiments using asbestos, where mesotheliomas were of minor importance compared to pulmonary carcinomas (Wagner et al., 1985).

A similar predominance of mesotheliomas had previously been noted in the Turkish data (Figure 1, Table 1; Artvinli and Baris, 1982). Intrapleural inoculation data from our laboratory strongly corroborate the vastly more potent mesothelioma induction attributable to erionite, compared to asbestos, when the dose was computed by the number of categorized fibers inoculated (Coffin et al., unpublished data from work in progress). Preliminary analysis of data from an intratracheal study underway in our laboratory (Table 2) also demonstrates a similar preponderance of mesothelioma induction by erionite (Coffin et al., this volume). It thus appears that the disease reported from Turkey was due to exposure to erionite. It also seems clear that this mineral has a greater potency to induce mesotheliomas, in both human beings and rats, than does asbestos. Despite these findings, negative results from experiments with nonfibrous erionite indicate that, even with this mineral, a fibrous structure appears essential for mesothelioma induction (Wagner, 1982). The fascinating resolution of the Turkish endemic focus has recently been reviewed by Baris (1987).

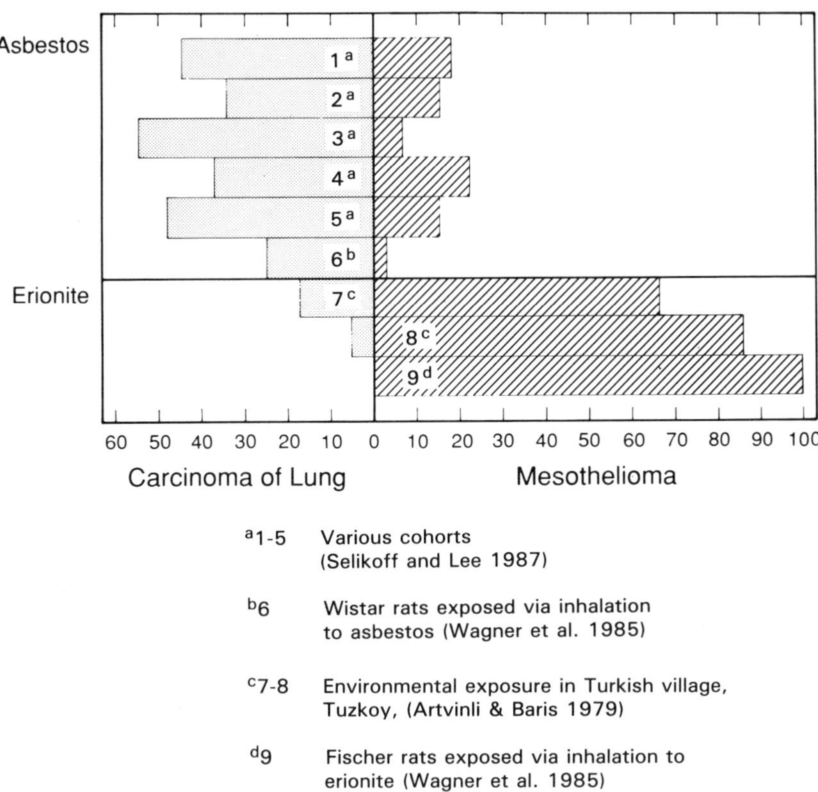

Figure 1. Incidence of lung cancer and mesothelioma in humans and rats following exposure to asbestos and erionite. 1-5 = cohorts industrially exposed to unspecified asbestos; 6 = rats exposed by inhalation to various asbestos species; 7 = human exposures to erionite in Turkish village; 8 = same but females only; 9 = inhalation exposure of rats. See Table 1 for numerical data.

Table 1. Comparative cancer induction in rats by intratracheally administered erionite and asbestos.

	Asbestos						Erionite		
	Cohort[a]	Cohort[a]	Cohort[a]	Cohort[a]	Cohort[a]	Rats[b]	Total[c]	Female[c]	Rats[b]
% Cancer of all deaths	46.6	42.3	31.1	36.0	39.9	NA	61.1	69.2	96.4
% Lung cancer of all cancers	44.9	47.8	51.5	37.5	47.1	21.1	19.5	5.5	0
% Mesotheliomas of all cancers	17.7	16.0	6.7	20.8	15.2	2.1	65.8	88.9	100
Lung cancer/ mesotheliomas	2.54	2.99	7.69	1.80	3.10	10.05	0.30	0.62	0/100

[a]Various cohorts (Selikoff and Lee, 1978)
[b]Wagner et al., 1985
[c]Artvinli and Baris, 1979

Table 2. Lung cancers and mesotheliomas induced by erionite compared to those from asbestos after intratracheal administration.

Mineral Fiber	Tumors (%) Lung Cancer	Mesothelioma	$\leq 8\ \mu m\ \bar{x} \geq 0.25\ \mu m$ per Unit Mass
Crocidolite	13	3.8	8.6
Chrysotile	32	7	1090
Erionite	4	48	3.3

MINERALOGY OF ERIONITE

In view of the high potency of erionite for mesothelioma induction, examination of its special physical and chemical properties indicates that they appear to be responsible for this phenomenon. As noted above, experiments with fibrous and nonfibrous erionite indicate that, despite its mineral peculiarities, a fibrous shape is a prerequisite for mesothelioma induction. (No biological studies appear in the available literature on the only other fibrous zeolite, mordenite.) Although it is also a silicate, other aspects of erionite differ greatly from those of asbestos, because it belongs to a class of minerals (zeolites) that are unique, crystalline, hydrated aluminosilicates. Structurally, zeolites consist of a "framework" that is based on an infinitely extending three-dimensional network of AlO_4 and SiO_4 tetrahedra linked by sharing all the oxygen molecules. This framework contains channels and interconnecting voids ("cages") that are occupied by cations and water molecules. The cations are commonly Na^+, K^+, Mg^{2+} and Ca^{2+}, but many other cations may be exchanged or held. The interconnected internal voids communicate with the surface via minute pores that have effective diameters of only a few angströms (Breck, 1974).

By virtue of these internal channels and cages, zeolites contain an enormous surface area per unit mass. For instance, erionite has a surface area of 200 m^2/g, compared to 10 m^2/g for crocidolite asbestos. Importantly, nearly all the surface area for zeolite is internal, while for asbestos it is external. The large internal surface furnishes a great number of sequestered active sites and void spaces of defined size that gives zeolites (including erionite) uniquely active properties for ion exchange, adsorption of small molecules, and strong catalytic properties. Thirty-four natural zeolites have been reported, and more than 100 have been synthesized from silica gel. These unique physicochemical properties of zeolite have been exploited widely for chemosorption of small molecules, ion exchange, and catalysis. Naturally occurring zeolites are mined for use as soil amendments for agriculture; are used in the removal of radioactive wastes; administered as additives to stock feed; used as adsorbents for wastewater treatment and oxygen enrichment, and for many other purposes (Breck, 1974; Zeo-Agriculture, 1984). Zeolites have been synthesized with special properties for specific purposes, such as the refining of petroleum, where adsorption of specific hydrocarbons in specially tailored synthetic zeolites enables catalytic cracking of the smaller compounds, with enhanced production of gasoline that has higher octane ratings. From the standpoint of tumorigenesis, fibrous erionite (and, possibly, fibrous mordenite) are of interest for two reasons: (1) the possibility that human health effects similar to those observed in the Turkish villages may occur in other countries; and (2) identifying the mechanisms responsible for induction of tumors might elucidate, in general, the mechanisms by which the mineral fibers cause tumors.

POSSIBLE EPIDEMIOLOGY CONSIDERATIONS

What are the possibilities for health risks from exposure to erionite in the United States? In the Turkish locations, the mineral is widely dispersed in nearly every niche in the environment: rocks, soil, etc. Coupled with the close-to-the-earth lifestyle of the population (ensuring exposure from the cradle to the grave), this strongly favors tumor induction. In the United States, 40 natural zeolites are known, many in the western part of the country, and in scattered locations elsewhere. Erionite occurs, in a rather pure form, in a number of arid sites in the Great Basin and Rocky Mountain area (South Dakota, Oregon, Nevada, and Arizona) in sedimentary volcanic rock, chiefly tuff (Figure 2). It has also been reported in similar sites as a contaminant with other zeolites, clinoptilolite, for instance. Fibrous mordenite has been reported in 13 locations. It is likely that a detailed geological survey would reveal other sources in deposits of tuff throughout the western United States (Shedd et al., 1982).

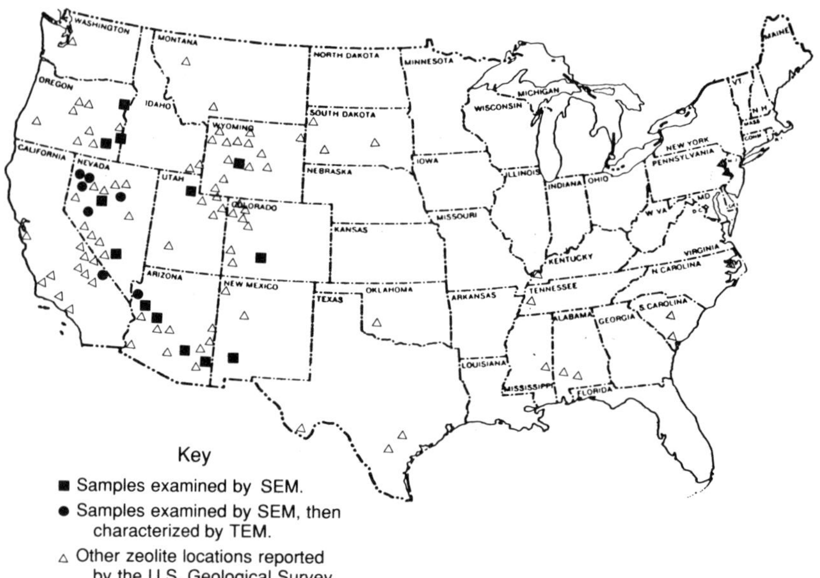

Figure 2. Occurrence of zeolite in the United States (adapted from Sheppard, 1971).

It may be fortunate, as far as human risks are concerned, that these areas in the United States are sparsely populated, resulting in few possibilities for human contact. By the same token, the sparse population makes epidemiological studies difficult. Although mesotheliomas have been reported in people from the Rocky Mountain region, where asbestos contact would be expected to be minimal (Enterline and Henderson, 1987), no case-control studies have been conducted to associate such cases with erionite deposits or contact with asbestos.

Another source of contact with erionite must be considered: accidental exposure to contaminating erionite fibers in other natural zeolites (such as clinoptilolite), which are mined for use in various agricultural or pollution-control activities. Therefore, such zeolites should be carefully analyzed for possible contaminating fibrous erionite (or mordenite) before their widespread commercial application.

VALUE OF ERIONITE FOR MECHANISM STUDIES

The most obvious difference between erionite and asbestos is the presence of the internal voids in the zeolite. Thus it appears reasonable to postulate that some mechanism associated with these voids might contribute to its potency. Possible mechanisms might be increased radical emission from interaction with the numerous enclosed oxygen sites; exchange of an ion required as a building block for a compound necessary for cellular defense against a carcinogen; or, possibly, a catalytic activity similar to that used for petroleum-cracking (Robson et al., 1971). Gates et al. (1979) speculated that, in petroleum, the superior activity of zeolite, in comparison to that of aluminosilica, is due to a combination of three effects: (1) greater concentrations of active sites; (2) greater concentration of hydrocarbons near active sites; and (3) the electric field within the zeolite voids might polarize C-H bonds and amplify the carbonium ion mechanism (Peters, 1988). Most of these conditions are reported in petroleum-cracking; it may be that similar conditions occur in animals through interaction with NH^{4+}. Regardless of the validity of such theories, the pores in zeolite are usually thought to play an essential role in its unusual chemical activity.

MATERIALS AND METHODS

The hypothesis described above was investigated by the following methods:

(1) blockage of the pores and void spaces by encapsulation of isopentane and exchange of Cr^{2+} and Ca^{2+} (Eberly, 1964), and measuring the biological effect by *in vitro* cytotoxicity testing of V79 cells. Palekar et al. (1985) have shown a statistical correlation with mesothelial tumor induction in the V79 system.

(2) determination of ion exchange by implantation of the mineral, contained in sealed diffusion tubes, in the peritoneal cavity of rats;

(3) measurement, via spin magnetic resonance, of radical emission after treatment of the mineral with various substrates present in animal tissues; and

(4) determination of radical emission by reaction with V79 cells *in vitro* when the mineral was contained in sealed tubes as described by Pooley (1979) and discussed above.

In all instances, these reactions would be compared with similar treatments with crocidolite, chrysotile, asbestos, and attapulgite (Peters, 1988).

Briefly, the encapsulation process was carried out as follows: known amounts of the mineral to be encapsulated were introduced into a closed system (Peters, 1988) and subjected to a high vacuum (less than 10^{-5} torr) and heated to 350 to 400°C for 12 hours to remove residual gases, surface impurities, and water of hydration. Subsequently, encapsulation of purified isopentane was accomplished by introducing it into the same system and exposing it to a pressure of 2000 torr and a temperature of 400°C for 2 hours. Isopentane was chosen for encapsulation because, at room temperature, its critical kinetic diameter is slightly larger than the pore size of the erionite, but it can be forced through the pores by high pressure and temperature. Successful encapsulation was demonstrated via infrared spectroscopy. The isopentane did not de-encapsulate when immersed in water. Peters (1988) described details of these procedures. Ion exchange was carried out by exposing the purified fibers to chromium or calcium chloride.

RESULTS

Experiments are still in progress, but preliminary results of the encapsulation and ion exchange studies are shown in Table 3. The data for reducing the biological effects of erionite by encapsulation of isopentane and augmenting biological effects by exchange of Ca^{+} ions are statistically significant. However, these studies should be considered preliminary and should be repeated and compared with similar studies on other minerals, such as asbestos and attapulgite, before attributing significance to the findings.

DISCUSSION AND CONCLUSIONS

Mesothelioma induction by erionite differs from that of asbestos in at least three aspects; the former has: (1) a greater degree of tumorigenesis per unit mass or number of fibers; (2) a shorter induction period; and (3) a greater tendency to induce pleural mesotheliomas, rather than lung tumors, when exposed by inhalation or intratracheal instillation (Table 2). Because the size and the shape of erionite fibers are not very different from those of asbestos, it appears that some other factor or factors (in addition to the length and width of the fibers) must play a determining role in erionite tumorigenesis. The zeolites (including erionite) have unique physicochemical properties (exchange of cations and cation complexes, and adsorption of small molecules) because of the void spaces within the crystalline lattice, which provide opportunities for intense interactions with chemical compounds. Under certain conditions, zeolites interact with NH^{4+}, probably by chain reactions via active sites within the voids, thus promoting protonation, or electron transfer, or the ability to donate or accept protons. Although we do not know whether these mechanisms foster carcinogenesis, extension of our preliminary encapsulation and cation exchange studies seems to indicate it. It might also be fruitful to investigate potential ion exchange and/or molecular adsorption after implanting erionite fibers in animal tissues. Using hollow-fiber membranes to contain the mineral fibers would allow recovery and, possibly, analysis of the fibers after *in vivo* exposure. These tubes allow free passage of materials that have molecular weights of up to 300,000, while cell migration is blocked. This is the first method that allows recovery of fibers after *in vivo* implantation.

Table 3. Effect (cell survival, % of control) of encapsulation of isopentane and ion exchange with Ca^{2+} and Cr^{3+} on survival of V79 hamster lung cells *in vitro*. Control in each instance was dehydrated, degassed erionite.

Sample	Plate Number	Number of Colonies	Average	Percent of Control
Control	1	82		
	2	73	76	
	3	73		
Degassed Erionite	1	30		
	2	26	28	36.8
	3	28		
Ca^{2+} Exchanged Erionite	1	5		
	2	7	7	9.2
	3	9		
Cr^{3+} Exchanged Erionite	1	20		
	2	25	23.33	30.7
	3	25		
Encapsulated Erionite	1	45		
	2	33	45	59.2
	3	57		

It would be interesting to study the interaction of zeolite with tobacco smoke, where exchange with nitric oxide and ammonia, and possible adsorption of small molecules present in the gas phase, might be expected to alter the biological activity of the smoke, either positively or negatively.

Further research on physicochemical interactions should be carried out with both carcinogenic and noncarcinogenic materials. Hypotheses other than those we have suggested may have some merit. Examining the scale of these events on a molecular level raises serious questions as to our understanding of the mechanism. We know that fibers in the micrometer size range must have a certain aspect ratio to induce tumors. Because internal zeolite pore sizes are orders of magnitude smaller than single organic molecules of higher molecular weight, biomolecules cannot penetrate the internal pores. However, we might speculate that the following mechanism occurs: A regular array of biological molecules might be held in juxtaposition to the fiber surfaces via adsorption of their pendent groups into the pore sites. Thus, the regularity and specificity of the zeolite structure would provide a mandrel, with binding sites leading to an ordered array of biological reaction candidates in apposition to an active third-party energy donor. In the case of erionite, such a phenomenon would be of much greater magnitude than for asbestos, which would have little or no potential for molecular bonding.

The study of erionite in conjunction with asbestos, using physicochemical and molecular biological methods, might open avenues for determining the basic mechanism of tumorigenesis by mineral fibers. Additionally, careful epidemiological observation in selected areas where human contact with the mineral is possible might reveal mesotheliomas or cases of pleural disease in other areas where deposits of this mineral occur.

REFERENCES

Artvinli, M and YI Baris. **1979.** Malignant mesotheliomas in a small village in the Anatolian region of Turkey: An epidemiologic study. J Natl Cancer Inst 63:17-22.

Artvinli, M and YI Baris. **1982.** Environmental fiber-induced pleuropulmonary diseases in an Anatolian village. An epidemiologic study. Arch Environ Health 37: 177-181.

Baris, YI. **1987.** *Asbestos and Erionite Related Chest Diseases.* Department of Chest Diseases, Hacettepe University School of Medicine, Ankara, Turkey.

Baris, YI, M Artvinli, and AA Sahin. **1980.** Environmental mesothelioma in Turkey. Ann NY Acad Sci 330:423.

Breck, DW. **1974.** *Zeolite Molecular Sieves, Structure, Chemistry, and Use.* Wiley-Interscience Publication, John Wiley and Sons, New York, NY.

Eberly, PE, Jr. **1964.** Adsorption properties of naturally occurring erionite and its cationic-exchanged forms. Am Mineral 49:30.

Enterline, PE and VL Henderson. **1987.** Geographic patterns for pleural mesothelioma deaths in the United States, 1968-81. J Natl Cancer Inst 79:31.

Gates, BC, JR Katzer, and GCA Schuit. **1979.** *Chemistry of Catalytic Processes.* McGraw-Hill, New York, NY.

Palekar, LD, BG Brown, and DL Coffin. **1985.** Correlation between *in vivo* tumorigenesis and *in vivo* cytotoxicity in CHO and V79 cells after exposure to mineral fibers, p. 155. In: *Short Term Bioassays for Analysis of Complex Environmental Mixtures,* MD Waters et al. (eds.). Plenum Publishing Co., New York, NY.

Peters, SE. **1988.** Thesis, in partial fulfillment of master's degree, North Carolina State University, Department of Chemical Engineering, Raleigh, NC.

Pooley, FD. **1979.** Evaluation of fiber samples taken from the vicinity of two villages in Turkey, p. 41. In: *Dust and Disease,* R Demen and JH Dement (eds.). Pathotox Publication, Park Forest South, IL.

Robson, HE, JP Hamner, and WR Arey, Jr. **1971.** Synthetic erionite and selective hydrocracking. In: *Advances in Chemistry,* Series No. 102, Molecular Sieve Zeolites. American Chemical Society, Washington, DC.

Rohl, AN, AM Langer, G Moncure, IJ Selikoff, and A Fischbein. **1982.** Endemic pleural disease associated with exposure to mixed fibrous dust in Turkey. Science 216:518.

Sebastien, P, A Gaudichet, J Bignon, and YI Baris. **1981.** Zeolite bodies in human lungs from Turkey. Lab Invest 44:420.

Selikoff, IJ and DHK Lee. **1978.** *Asbestos and Disease. Environmental Sciences.* Academic Press, New York, NY.

Shedd, KB, RL Virta, and AG Wylie. **1982.** *Size and Shape Characteristics of Fibrous Zeolites by Electron Microscopy,* United States Bureau of Mines, Document No. 1.28.23 8674. U.S. Government Printing Office, Washington, DC.

Sheppard, RA. **1971.** In: *Advances in Chemistry,* Series No. 101, *Molecular Sieve Zeolites,* ER Gould (ed.), p. 279. American Chemical Society, Washington, DC.

Wagner, JC. **1982.** Health hazards of substitutes, p. 244. In: *Asbestos Health and Safety.* Canadian Asbestos Information Center, Montreal, Canada.

Wagner, JC, JW Skidmore, RJ Hill, and DM Griffiths. **1985.** Erionite exposure and mesothelioma in rats. Br J Cancer 51:727.

Zeo-Agriculture. 1984. *Use of Natural Zeolites in Agriculture and Aquaculture,* WG Pond and FA Mumptons (eds.). Westview Press, Boulder, CO.

Effect of Erionite Inhalation on the Lungs of Rats

Neil F. Johnson[1] and J. Christopher Wagner[2]

[1]Inhalation Toxicology Research Institute, Lovelace Biomedical and Environmental Research Institute, Albuquerque, NM 87185*

[2]Medical Research Council RC External Staff, Team on Occupational Lung Diseases, Llandough Hospital, Penarth, Glamorgan, UK

KEY WORDS: erionite, inhalation exposure, mesothelioma, lung, rat

ABSTRACT

Until recently, mesothelioma was generally considered pathognomonic for asbestos exposure. However, the recently recognized intense and localized occurrence of these tumors in the Anatolian region of Turkey links erionite, a fibrous zeolite, as an additional causative agent for mesothelioma. These human data have been confirmed in rats by inhalation studies in which exposure to an atmosphere of 10 mg/m^3 for 1 year produced a mesothelioma incidence of 96% (Wagner et al., 1985). Crocidolite, under similar conditions, produced a tumor incidence of 1 to 2%. The erionite-induced tumors also appeared more rapidly than their crocidolite-induced counterparts. The rapid and high rate of tumor induction may provide the means to effectively study the mechanisms of induction of pleural tumors and also parenchymal changes in the lung following dust inhalation.

To determine whether erionite acts in a fashion similar to crocidolite, small groups of animals (three to four Fischer-344 rats) were exposed by whole-body inhalation exposure to either erionite or crocidolite (10 mg/m^3) for 6 hours/day, 5 days/week for 1, 2, 4, 8, 12, 26, and 52 weeks. An additional group of animals was exposed for 12 weeks and allowed to recover for a 12-month period. A control group

*Former address: Medical Research Council Toxicology Unit, Woodmansterns Rd., Carshalton, Surrey, UK.

was treated similarly except that they were exposed only to fresh air. The animals were sacrificed, and the lungs were infused with buffered glutaraldehyde. Tissue was taken from the left lung for conventional light microscopy and electron microscopy.

Parenchymal changes were similar in the two dust-exposed groups with the exception of those observed after short periods of erionite exposure, when there was a marked perivascular inflammatory response. Dust particles and fibers were associated with both alveolar and interstitial macrophages. The former were frequently aggregated at the alveolar duct/terminal bronchiolar region, where there appeared to be a limited increase in the amount of collagen present and increased cellularity. The longer periods of exposure were also associated with ferruginous body formation with both fiber types. The most marked difference between the two dust exposures was in the pleural response. Erionite was associated with pleural thickening, which was evident after 26 weeks of exposure and was more marked on the parenchymal side of the subpleural space. Two of the three animals in the 12-month recovery group after 12 weeks of exposure had mesotheliomas.

The results confirm the pathogenic potential of erionite and its potential usefulness for the study of fiber-induced lung and pleural changes.

INTRODUCTION

Exposure to fibrous materials, notably asbestos, can result in primary lung cancer, interstitial pulmonary fibrosis, mesotheliomas and pleural plaques (Dunnill, 1982). Exposures can occur in the general environment or in the workplace and are frequently associated with exposure to other air pollutants, such as radiation or cigarette smoke. Cigarette-smoking in association with asbestos exposure has been shown to increase the risk of developing lung cancer to a greater extent than the additive effects of the agents alone (Selikoff et al., 1968). A similar effect has not been demonstrated for the risk of developing mesotheliomas. The reason for this divergent effect is unknown.

Animal experiments suggest a significant link between fiber size and the potential to induce mesotheliomas (Stanton et al., 1977). The fiber dimensions considered pathogenic are diameters less than 0.20 μm combined with lengths greater than 8.0 μm. Such a link between fiber size and lung cancer or pulmonary fibrosis is more tenuous. Mesothelioma induction is also linked with fiber type; however, this is dependent upon the relative number of fibers of each mineral type within the size range considered pathogenic. The biological durability of the fiber is also important. The more durable materials remain within the lung to exert their effects for extended periods. In addition, prolonged intrapulmonary residence times allow preferential clearance of short fibers from the lung (Johnson et al., 1982), which increases the relative numbers of longer fibers associated with pleural tumor formation. Focal accumulations of such fibers can occur following prolonged exposure, because fibrous and other inorganic materials are known to collect at lymphatic drainage points in the subpleural region. This creates a high focal concentration of particles (Morgan et al., 1977) adjacent to potential tumor-forming cells.

The mechanisms of fiber-induced lung disease remain to be elucidated. Appropriate animal models for the induction of lung carcinoma and mesothelioma via physiological exposure routes can only be obtained by lengthy and costly inhalation studies. These types of investigations rarely result in the induction of mesothelioma (Wagner et al., 1974). However, mesotheliomas can be readily induced by intrapleural or intraperitoneal inoculation of fibrous materials, while lung carcinomas can be similarly induced following intratracheal administration of the dusts. These methods are not physiological, and the two types of tumors cannot be induced concurrently by either method.

The limitation of the inhalation route for the induction of mesotheliomas has been overcome in a recent study using fibrous erionite (Wagner, 1982), which showed a high rate (95%) of pleural tumor induction. Erionite had been previously implicated as the causative agent in the high incidence of mesotheliomas in the Anatolian region in Turkey (Baris et al., 1978). This is an important observation because, until this result, crocidolite asbestos has been considered the only fibrous mineral associated with mesotheliomas in humans.

The results reported here represent a pilot investigation to determine the feasibility of using erionite in short-term inhalation studies (up to 3 months) to delineate factors important in the induction of mesothelioma and to determine whether the parenchymal response was similar to that for crocidolite asbestos. The presence of mesotheliomas is often considered pathognomonic for crocidolite, is associated with interstitial fibrosis and primary lung cancer, and behaves synergistically with cigarette smoke for the induction of lung cancer. The disease caused by crocidolite in man is similar to that experimentally induced in rats (Wagner et al., 1974).

MATERIALS AND METHODS

The SPF Fischer-344 rats were exposed at age 6 weeks to an atmosphere of UICC crocidolite, fibrous erionite (from Rome, OR; supplier: Minerals Research, Clarkston, NY), or filtered room air. The animals were maintained in the inhalation chambers for the entire exposure period. Thereafter, they were either sacrificed or transferred to clean cages and maintained under standard laboratory conditions. The details of the aerosol generation, exposure chambers and aerosol monitoring have been published previously (Wagner et al., 1974). In brief, groups of three rats were exposed to a dust atmosphere of 10 mg/m^3 for 7 hours/day, 5 days/week for 1, 2, 4, 8 and 12 weeks, then sacrificed. Another group of three animals was exposed for 12 weeks and allowed to recover for 12 months before sacrifice. An equal number of unexposed control rats were used at each exposure period. The animals received whole-body exposures in a Timbrell chamber. The dust was generated by a Timbrell generator, and the respirable dust concentration was measured using size-selective gravimetric dust samples (Casella type 113A).

Following the selected exposure period, the animals were sacrificed by inhalation of ether. The chest wall was opened, and the trachea exposed and ligated caudal to the larynx. A fine-gauge needle was inserted below the ligature, and the lungs gently infused with fixative (3% glutaraldehyde buffered in Sorensen's phosphate buffer; pH, 7.2 to 7.4) at a hydrostatic pressure of 30 cm. While still infused, the trachea was ligated below the needle entry point, and then cut between the two ligatures. The lungs were removed and immersed in fixative at room temperature for at least 4 hours. Tissue was collected from the same location in the left lung of all animals (Figure 1). Transverse sections from upper, middle, and lower lung were processed for conventional paraffin-wax histology. Adjacent lung sections were collected, processed for electron microscopy, and embedded in Spurr's resin (Spurr, 1969). The paraffin-embedded tissues were sectioned and stained with hematoxylin and eosin or Masson's trichrome. Following sectioning, the sample of tissue from the middle region of the lung was removed from selected paraffin blocks. The wax was removed with xylene, and the tissue washed with three changes of absolute ethyl alcohol, and allowed to dry to a constant weight. The dried, weighed tissue was dissolved in 5.25% sodium hypochlorite (Sigma, St. Louis, MO), centrifuged (1000 x g for 20 minutes), the supernatant removed, and the residue suspended in 30% hydrogen peroxide (Sigma, St. Louis, MO), and left overnight at room temperature. The solution was centrifuged, the supernatant removed, and the residue washed twice with distilled water. The washed residue was resuspended in 50 μl absolute ethyl alcohol and transferred to a carbon stub for scanning electron microscopy and X-ray microprobe analysis.

Tissue from the electron miscroscopy block (Figure 1) was used to count the various cell types present in the lung parenchyma of animals exposed for 1 and 12 weeks, those exposed for 12 weeks followed by 12 months of recovery, and from the appropriate controls. Sections from at least three depths (separated by at least 30 μm) in each animal were examined; they contained no major airways or blood vessels. Cells were counted only on grid squares containing structures distal to the terminal bronchiole/alveolar duct region. In such areas, all nucleated cell cross-sections were counted until at least 100 nucleated endothelial cells had been identified. The same sections were used to obtain an estimate of the alveolar free-cell population by counting all recognizable cell cross-sections encountered in the air spaces of the entire section. The numbers of nucleated endothelial cell profiles were counted in 25 grid squares from at least three different sections from each animal. The data were evaluated with an analysis of variance, and the test groups were analyzed against the pooled control data. Sections from all animals were examined for any ultrastructural abnormalities.

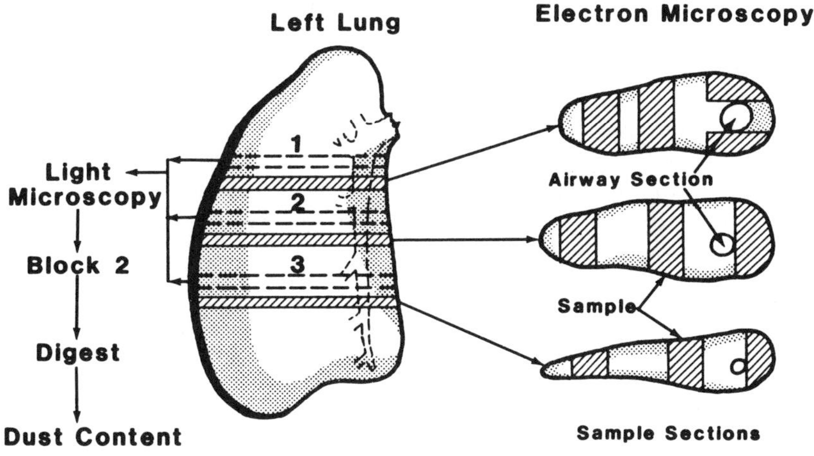

Figure 1. Schematic diagram showing the locations of tissue samples collected for light and electron microscopy and fiber recovery.

RESULTS

The characteristics of the inhaled dust clouds are given in Table 1. The UICC crocidolite contained a greater number of fibers than the erionite sample. While erionite had a greater percentage of potentially pathogenic fibers (i.e., percent respirable fraction), crocidolite possessed more per unit mass. Detailed fiber-size analysis of these particular materials have been previously published (Wagner et al., 1974, 1985). X-ray microprobe analysis showed the major elemental constituents of crocidolite to be sodium, aluminum, silica and iron; for the erionite, they were silicon, aluminum and calcium. Fibers were recovered from all the exposed animals examined (Figure 2). X-ray microprobe analysis of the recovered fibers showed an elemental composition similar to that of the original dust sample (Figure 3), except for an occasional additional calcium peak in the recovered crocidolite samples.

Table 1. Characteristics of respirable crocidolite and erionite aerosols used in inhalation exposures of rats.

	Crocidolite	Erionite
Source	UICC	Rome, OR
Mean Concentration	10 mg/m^3	10 mg/m^3
Exposure Period	7 hr/day 5 days/wk	7 hr/day 5 days/wk
Fibers/ml > 5 μm Length	1630	354
Fibers/ml > 5 μm Length Percent Respirable Fraction	52.7	44.0
Fibers/ml > 5 μm Length < 0.2 μm Diameter	78	51
Fibers/ml > 5 μm Length < 0.2 μm Diameter Percent Respirable Fraction	4.8	14.3

The controls' lungs displayed no apparent ultrastructural abnormalities. The distribution of the various cell types in the lung parenchyma is shown in Table 2. One control animal for the 12-week exposure period, after 12 months of recovery, showed a mild focal perivascular lymphocytic cuffing.

The earliest exposure periods (1 and 2 weeks) were associated with a focal perivascular and alveolar lymphocytic infilitration. This response was most marked in the erionite-exposed animals (Figure 4) and was not evident in the animals exposed for 40 or 60 days. Apart from these changes, the lung parenchyma was unremarkable until 12 months after 12 weeks of exposure. Alveolar macrophages contained variable numbers of dust particles

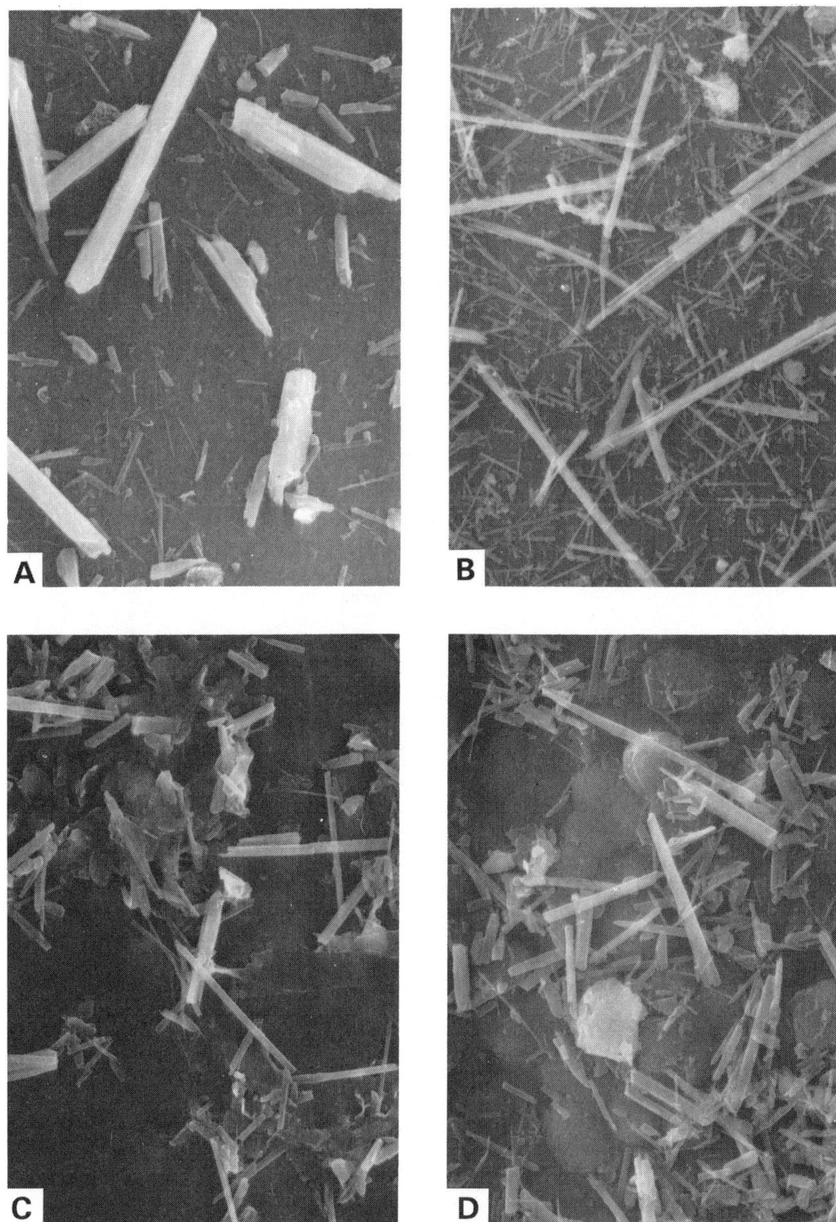

Figure 2. Scanning electron micrographs of the original samples of erionite (A) and crocidolite (B) and fibers recovered from animals exposed to erionite (C) or crocidolite (D) for 12 weeks, followed by 12 months of recovery. Fibers were recovered from all exposed animals examined. Magnification, 1500X.

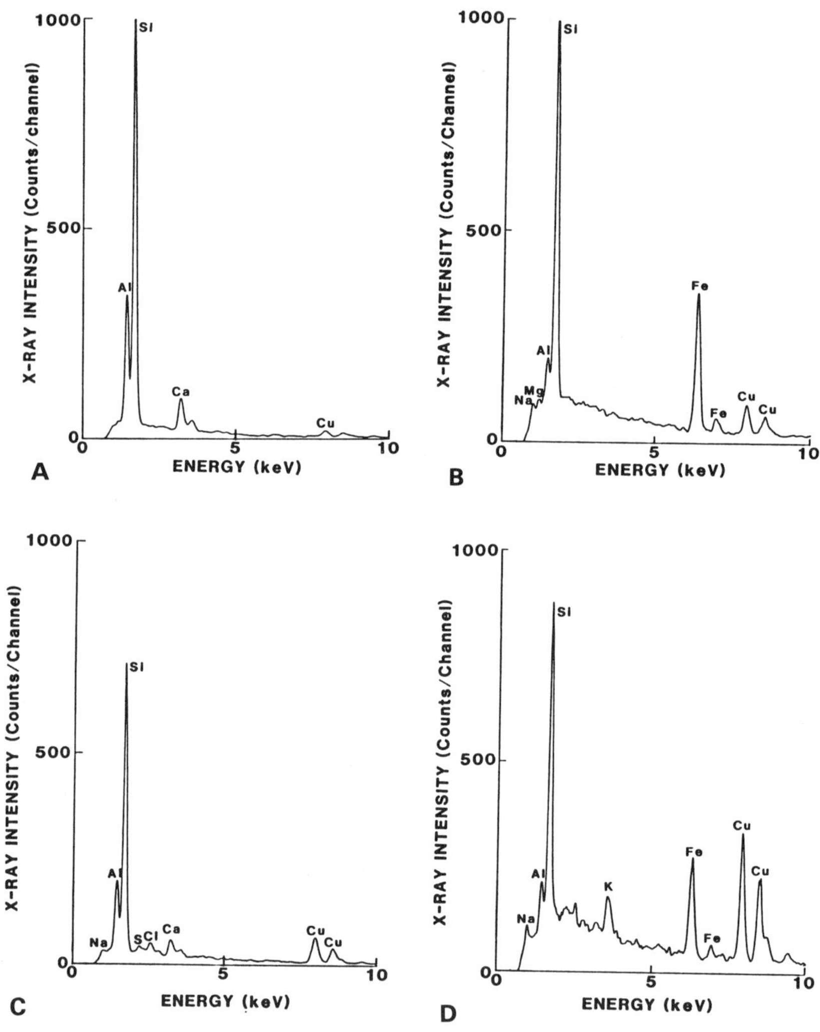

Figure 3. X-ray energy-dispersive histograms showing the major elemental peaks for the original samples of erionite (A) and crocidolite (B) and for samples of erionite (C) and crocidolite (D) recovered from animals exposed for 12 weeks, followed by 12 months of recovery. There is no apparent difference between the original samples and those recovered from tissue with the exception of an occasional additional calcium peak in the recovered crocidolite samples. Al = aluminum, Ca = calcium, Cu = copper, Fe = iron, Mg = magnesium, Na = sodium, K = potassium.

throughout all exposure periods. Dust-laden macrophages were largely confined to the air spaces; a few such cells were found in the interstitium after 12 weeks of exposure. Following 12 months of recovery from the latter exposure period, accumulations of dust-laden macrophages were found at the alveolar duct/terminal bronchiolar region. This region was also associated with the presence of interstitial dust-laden cells, polymorphonuclear leukocytes, and fibroblasts. This area of increased cellularity was also associated with increased amounts of collagen, evident by both light and electron microscopy. Type II cell hyperplasia was also seen after all exposure periods; however, this was evident only by detailed numerical evaluation (Table 2). The increase in Type II cells was not accompanied by any reduction in the number of Type I cells. This numerical response also revealed a significant increase in the absolute number of alveolar macrophages present after 12 weeks of exposure and after the recovery period. However, no significant change was noted in the differential cell count of alveolar free cells.

Table 2. Distribution of cell types in rats following exposure to crocidolite or erionite for 1 and 12 weeks and for a 12-week exposure followed by 12 months of recovery[a]

	Exposure Duration						
	1 Week		12 Weeks		60 Days plus 12 Months of Recovery		
	Erionite	Crocidolite	Erionite	Crocidolite	Erionite	Crocidolite	Control
Macrophages							
Alveolar	9.5 ± 2.1	10.3 ± 1.8	18.0 ± 3.0	21.2 ± 1.9	15.5 ± 3.7	18.7 ± 2.4	8.7 ± 0.9
Interstitial	1.5 ± 1.2	1.7 ± 1.3	3.0 ± 1.7	2.4 ± 1.8	5.3 ± 1.8	4.9 ± 2.3	1.3 ± 1.1
Cell Type							
Type I Cell	27.3 ± 3.0	32.1 ± 3.1	24.4 ± 2.6	28.5 ± 1.4	31.0 ± 2.5	27.5 ± 3.0	29.0 ± 2.6
Type II Cell	38.6 ± 4.4	42.6 ± 4.0	41.3 ± 3.7	37.0 ± 2.9	45.8 ± 2.9	48.6 ± 6.2	34.4 ± 1.3
Endothelial[b]	81.8 ± 2.0	73.3 ± 5.1	76.9 ± 3.2	75.4 ± 6.0	69.4 ± 4.6	73.6 ± 5.9	74.2 ± 4.1

[a]Number of cells ± SEM compared to 100 endothelial cells

[b]Number of nucleated cell cross-sections/25 grid squares

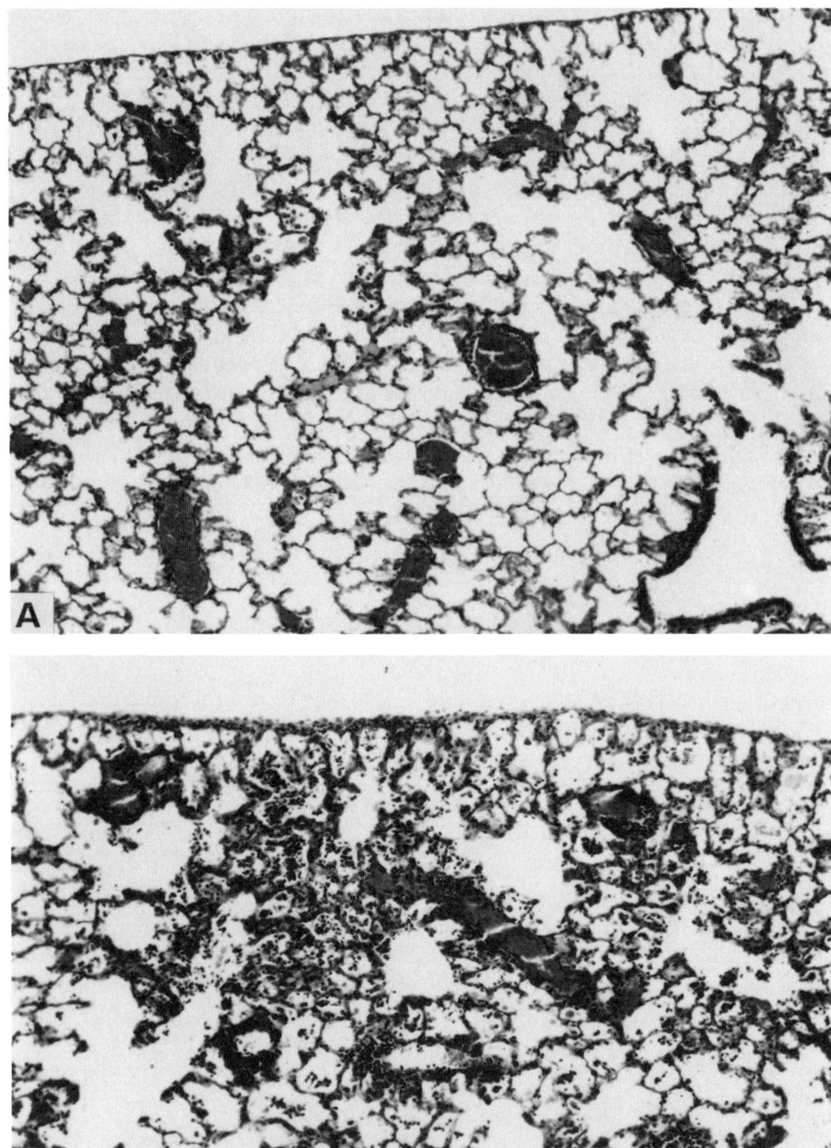

Figure 4. Light micrographs of lung tissue from a rat exposed to crocidolite for 1 week (A) and a rat exposed to erionite for 2 weeks (B). The tissue is typified by a perivascular and alveolar lymphocytic infiltration, which was mild in crocidolite-exposed animals (A) but marked with erionite exposures (B). Magnification, 50X.

In all cases, the percentage of alveolar macrophages was in excess of 96%; the remainder of the cells were polymorphonuclear leukocytes and lymphocytes. This analysis failed to reveal the lymphocytic infiltration noted in early exposure periods because the areas selected were distant from major blood vessels.

In addition to the hyperplastic changes in the Type II alveolar cells, there were areas of bronchiolar/alveolar hyperplasia associated with the recovery period from 12 weeks of exposure (Figure 5). This occurred, to some extent, in all six exposed animals.

Pleural changes were evident by light microscopy after 12 weeks of exposure to erionite but not following exposure to crocidolite. This change involved collagen deposition adjacent to the alveolar wall side of the submesothelial connective-tissue layer. Similar changes could be seen by electron microscopy after 8 weeks of exposure. With both fiber types, 12 weeks of exposure, followed by 12 months of recovery, was associated with further changes.

Crocidolite exposure produced mild changes, typified by collagen deposition adjacent to the alveolar wall of the subpleural connective tissue zone. In one of the crocidolite-exposed animals, a focal fibrotic plaque was seen (Figure 6). In contrast, erionite-exposed animals displayed a spectrum of marked pleural changes. Pleural fibrosis was widespread, and the fibrotic lesions were covered either by squamoid or hyperplastic mesothelial cells (Figure 6). In the milder lesions, the collagen was associated with the alveolar side of the subpleural connective tissue (Figure 7); with the more extensive fibrosis, the lesion was more cellular, with bundles of collagen distributed throughout (Figure 8).

All of the crocidolite- and erionite-exposed animals had multiple focal mesotheliomas. In one exposed animal, the tumor had spread to involve the pericardium. The focal tumors were either more diffuse and mainly composed of sarcomatous cells (Figure 9A) or were well-described and composed largely of epithelium-like cells (Figure 9B). These tumors were frequently associated with a thickened subpleural connective tissue layer, distended lymphatic channels containing lymphocytes and other mononuclear cells, and a loose connective-tissue zone overlying the thickened collagenous layer adjacent to the alveolar wall. The tumors were covered with a complete layer of normal squamoid or hyperplastic mesothelial cells.

Electron microscopy confirmed the light microscopic findings of both epithelial and sarcomatous tumor cells. In addition, it showed the deposition of apatite-like spicules in the subcellular matrix (Figure 10).

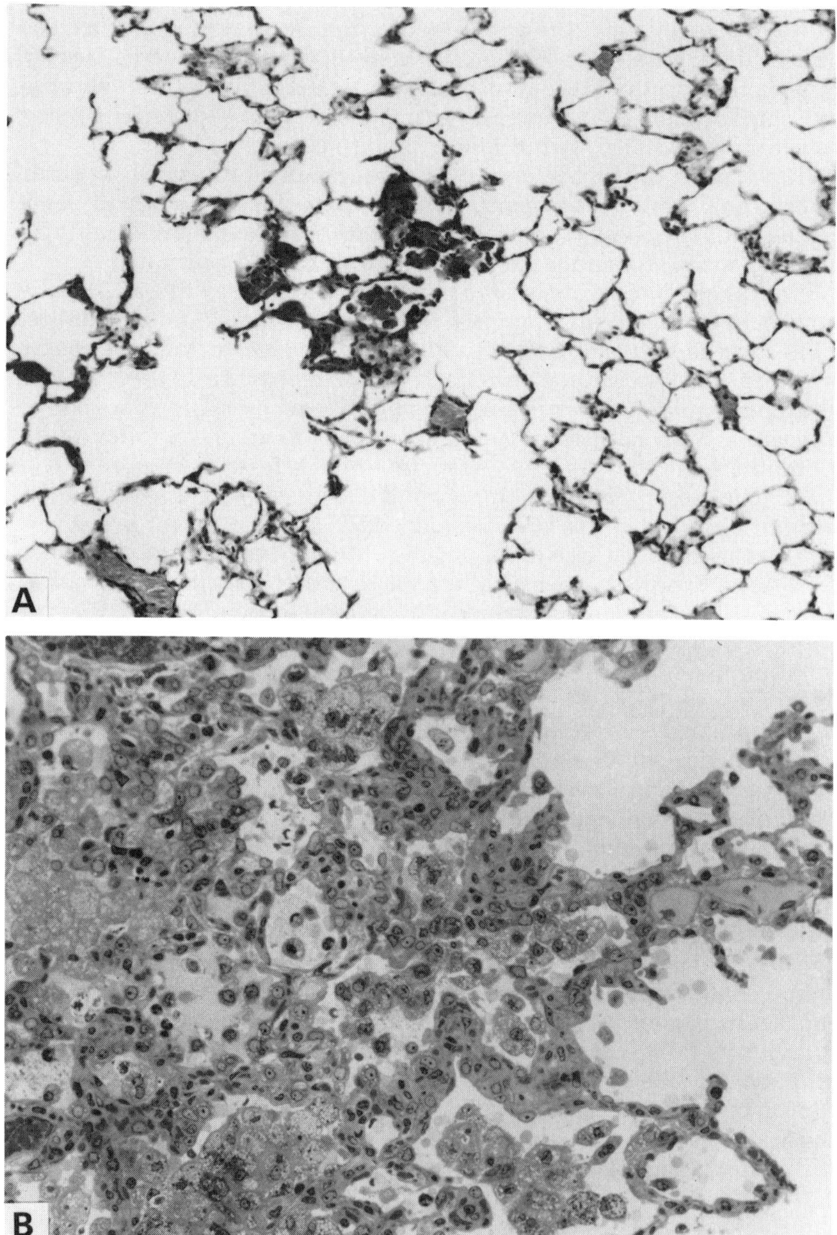

Figure 5. Light micrographs of lung parenchyma, displaying (A) accumulations of dust-laden macrophages at the level of the alveolar duct; (B) bronchiolar/alveolar hyperplasia after 12 weeks of exposure to erionite, followed by 12 months of recovery. Magnification, (A) 125X, (B) 225X.

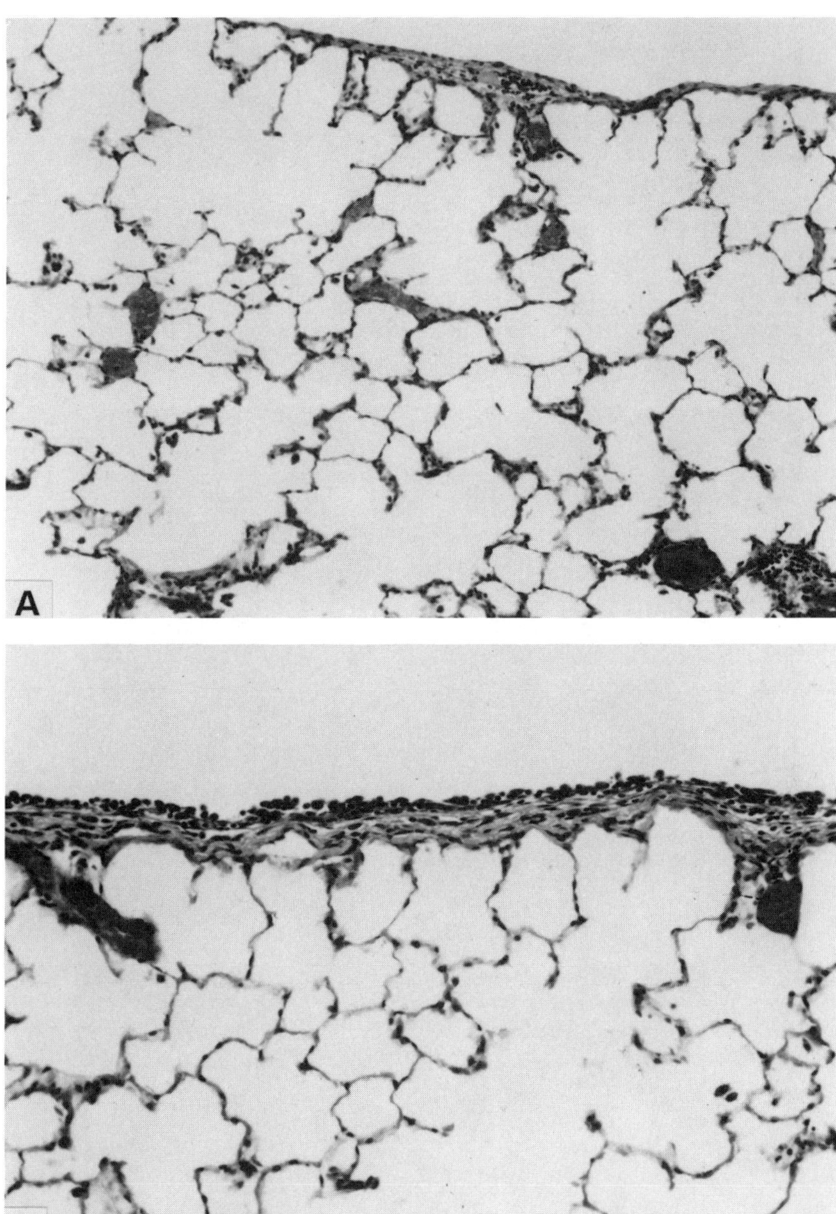

Figure 6. Light micrographs of the single fibrotic lesion identified in the crocidolite-exposed animals (A) and a pleural fibrotic lesion covered by hyperplastic mesothelial cells (B). The latter example was from an animal exposed to erionite for 12 weeks, followed by 12 months of recovery. Magnification, 125X.

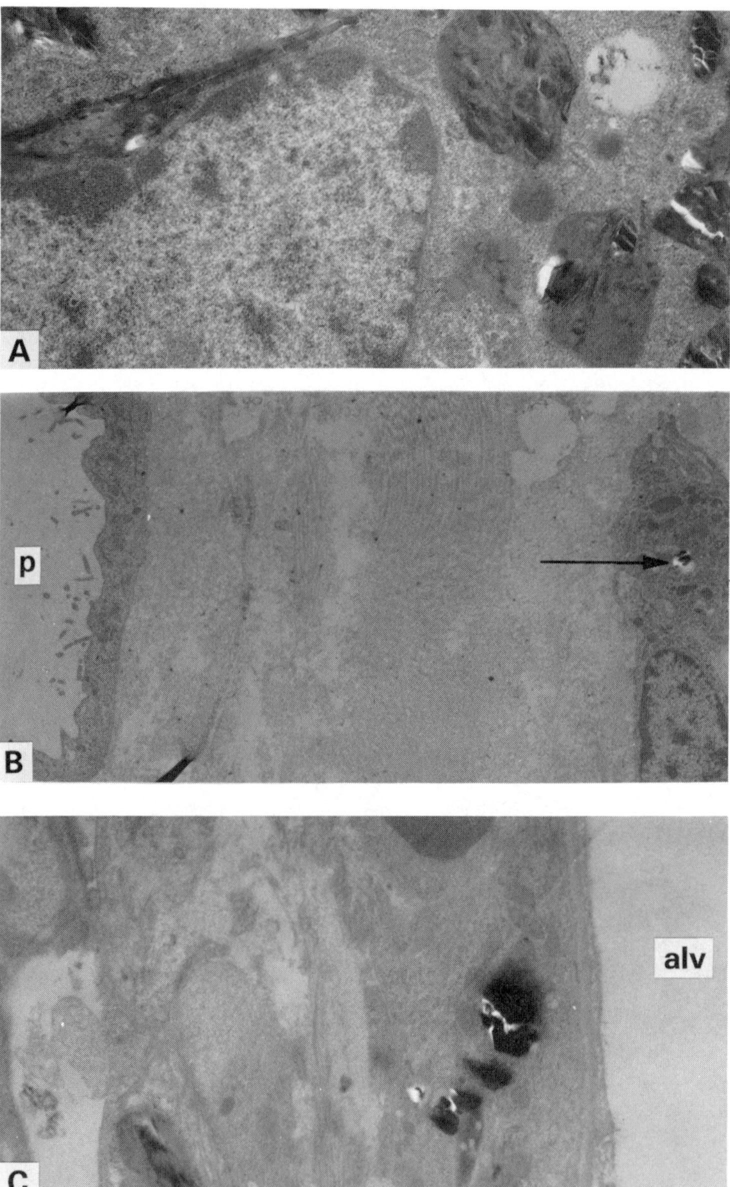

Figure 7. Electron micrographs of cell-bound erionite fibers within an alveolar macrophage (A), within a fibroblast-like cell lying in the subpleural connective tissue (B). Fiber particle is marked by an arrow; p = pleural space. In (C) fibers are within a fibroblast-like cell lying immediately beneath the alveolar epithelium (alv). Magnification, (A) 15,000X, (B) 4500X, (C) 21,000X.

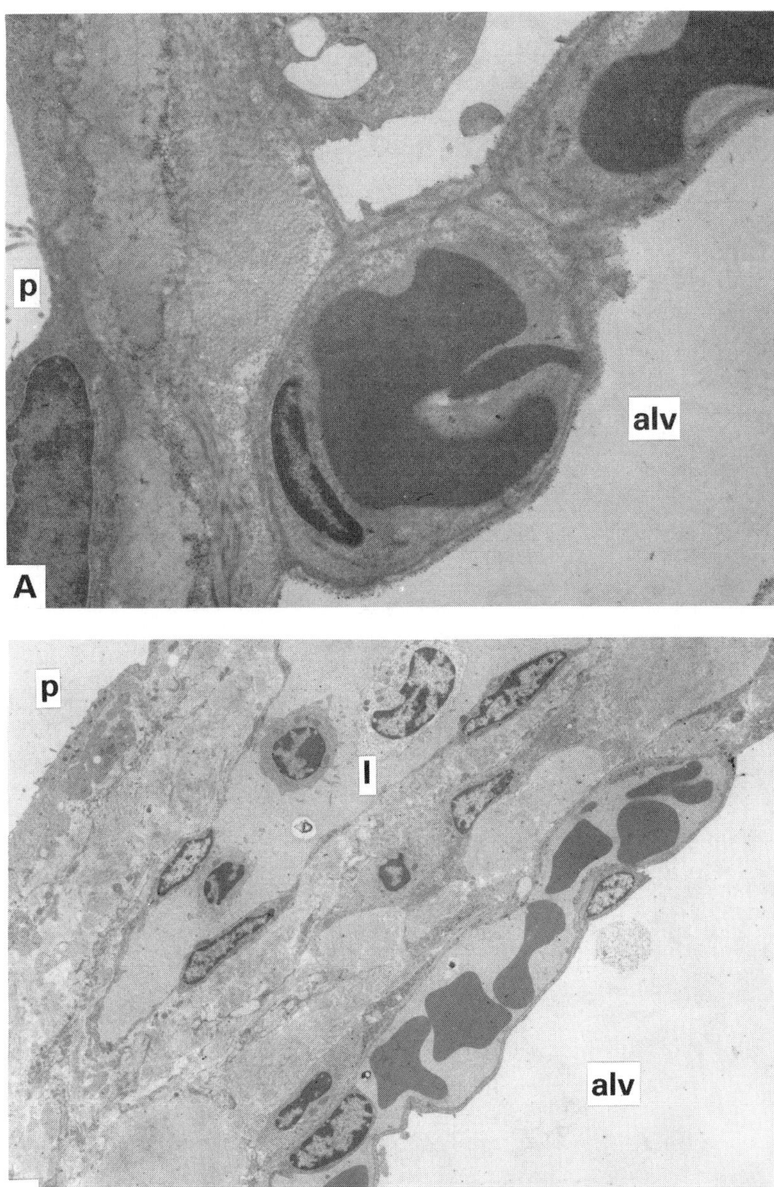

Figure 8. Electron micrographs of subpleural connective tissue after 12 weeks of erionite exposure, followed by 12 months of recovery. (A) shows deposition of collagen adjacent to the alveolar wall; (B) shows deposition of collagen throughout, and a distended lymphatic vessel. p = pleural space, alv = alveolar air space, l = lymphatic vessel. Magnification, (A) 7500X, (B) 2000X.

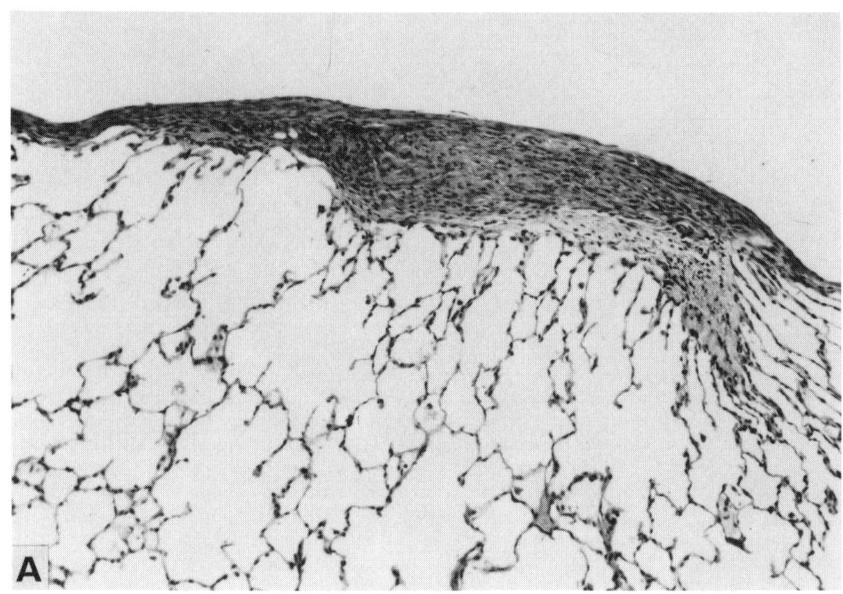

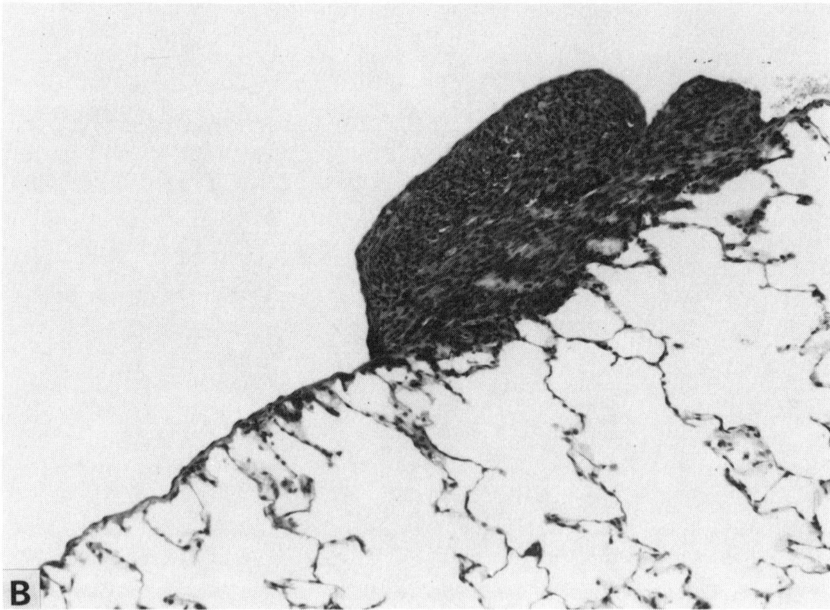

Figure 9. Light micrographs of induced focal mesothelioma following 60 days of erionite expoure and 12 months of recovery. (A) Sarcomatous tumor overlying thickened pleura, (B) epithelial tumor. Magnification, 150X.

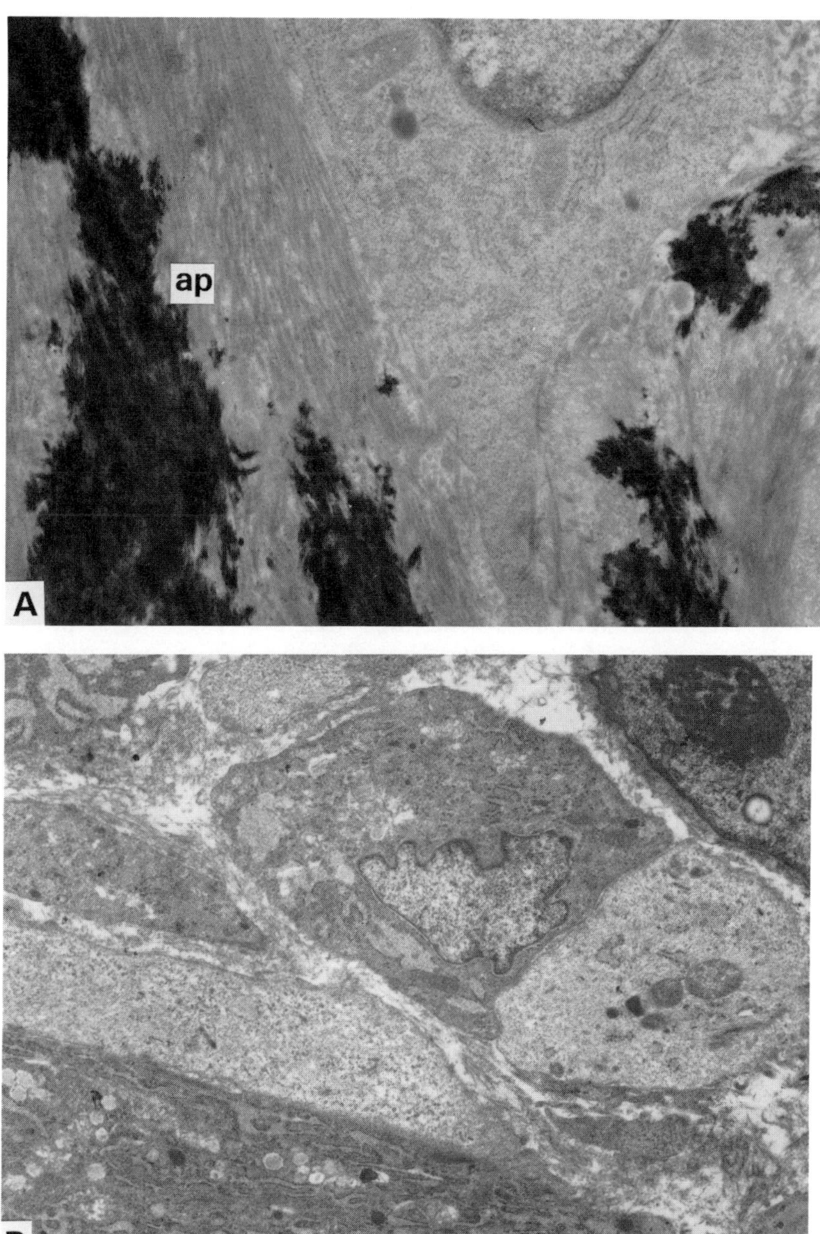

Figure 10. Electron micrographs of erionite-induced mesothelioma. (A) Tumor cell associated with extracellular matrix containing apatite-like spicules (ap); (B) sarcomatous tumor cells. Magnification, (A) 15,000X, (B) 4500X.

Electron microscopy revealed the cellular location of the inhaled dust particles. The majority was found within predominantly alveolar macrophages at all exposure periods. Following 60 days of exposure, dust-laden macrophages were seen within the interstitium at bifurcations within the airways. This feature was more marked following 12 months of recovery, when, in addition, fibroblast-like cells occasionally contained dust particles. While the parenchymal location of the two dust types appeared similar, erionite exposure was associated with dust-containing fibroblast-like cells within the subpleural connective tissue zone (Figure 7). In the crocidolite-exposed animals, nine ferruginous bodies were identified; only one such body was encountered in the erionite-exposed animals.

DISCUSSION

The results of this pilot investigation confirm those of Wagner (1982) and demonstrate the highly pathogenic nature of this sample of fibrous erionite from Rome, OR. This biological activity could not have been predicted from the fiber-size data. The respirable erionite dust cloud contained fewer fibers than the crocidolite sample within the pathogenic size range postulated by Stanton et al. (1977). Inhalation of crocidolite under conditions similar to those for erionite resulted in four mesotheliomas in 124 exposed animals, whereas erionite produced tumors in 28 of 29 exposed animals (Wagner et al., 1985). Those studies involved a 12-month exposure regime. In our study, 12 weeks of erionite inhalation followed by 12 months of recovery resulted in three of three animals presenting with mesotheliomas. The appearance of these epithelial and sarcomatous tumors was similar to those previously described following erionite inhalation for 12 months (Johnson et al., 1984) and following intrapleural inoculation (Suzuki, 1982). The focal tumors found in our study were completely covered with normal or hyperplastic mesothelial cells. The tumor masses were generally confined to the mesothelial aspect of the subpleural connective tissue zone and were not seen to penetrate the basement membrane of the alveolar wall. The origin of the progenitor cells for these tumors is uncertain, but it may have been a multipotential stem cell lying within the mesothelial cell layer or immediately adjacent to it.

Dust accumulation at the pleural surface is a known feature of occupational exposure to dusts (Dunnill, 1982) and can be experimentally demonstrated in animals following asbestos exposure (Morgan et al., 1977). The pleural effects of erionite may be exerted through a greater accumulation of fibers than those of crocidolite. This deposition may be enhanced by the fibrotic reaction associated with erionite exposure. The accumulation of fibers will, in part, be governed by lymphatic drainage of the material. Lymphatic drainage may be impaired by pleural fibrosis, which, in the case of erionite, would result in a high focal concentration of pathogenic fibers. Inhalation of fibrous and nonfibrous dusts are known to result in a variety of fibrotic pleural lesions. For example, crystalline silica (Figure 11) and anthophyllite can result in pleural thickening that is not associated with mesothelioma induction. Crystalline silica has well-documented *in vivo* and *in vitro* cytotoxic effects leading to pulmonary fibrosis (Heppleston, 1982). The limited amount of *in vitro* work conducted on erionite reveals no unusual cytotoxic activity (Brown et al., 1980). However, Poole et al. (1983) demonstrated that erionite is the only fibrous mineral to give reproducible and unequivocal positive results in *in vitro* tests to determine genotoxicity.

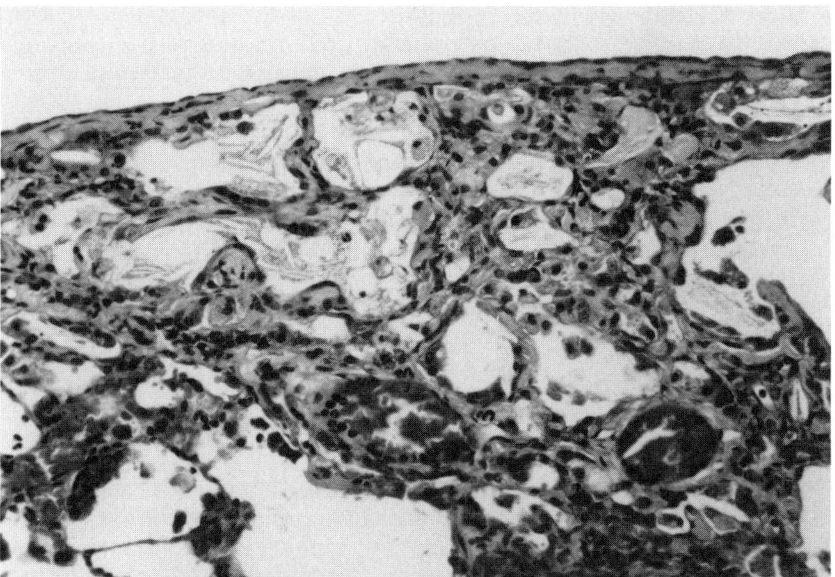

Figure 11. Light micrograph of crystalline-silica-induced pleural fibrosis. Animals were exposed under conditions similar to those described here for 60 days, followed by 12 months of recovery. Magnification, 125X.

The association between the occurrence of pleural fibrosis and mesotheliomas in humans is controversial. Our results indicate a close association between the two lesions. The ability of a dust such as erionite to induce both pleural fibrosis and mesothelioma will result in the rapid appearance of the latter, while a fibrogenic material such as silica produces only fibrosis. The action of crocidolite could be explained by its lack of fibrogenic activity, which, combined with its potential to cause mesotheliomas, results in a delayed appearance of pleural tumors.

The parenchymal changes induced by the two dust types were similar. The quantitative changes observed in the crocidolite-exposed animals were similar to those described in a previous experiment (Johnson, 1987). The cellular deposition of the fibers was also similar, although more ferruginous bodies were seen following crocidolite exposure. However, because of the small sample this may be artifactual. Ferruginous bodies have been described (Sebastien et al., 1981) in association with erionite exposure in humans.

The elemental composition of the original and recovered erionite fibers was similar, indicating that erionite is resistant to degradation following prolonged residence in the lung. This situation is similar to that seen with crocidolite. This durability allows the minerals to exert their biological effect over extended periods and subjects them to biological influences such as preferential clearance of small fibers by macrophages.

Our study indicates that erionite readily induces mesotheliomas and pleural fibrosis in animals exposed by inhalation to the dust. Because these changes are similar to those seen in humans, erionite inhalation in animals would be a good model for studying these important pulmonary diseases. The similarity in the parenchymal responses of exposed humans and animals may also indicate that erionite may be a suitable model for general lung changes following dust inhalation.

ACKNOWLEDGMENTS

Part of this work was sponsored by the U. S. Department of Energy, Office of Health and Environmental Research under Contract No. DE-AC04-76EV01013 and part by the United Kingdom's Medical Research Council.

The help of RJ Hill of the MRC Toxicology Unit, Carshalton, Surrey, UK, is gratefully acknowledged.

REFERENCES

Baris, YU, AA Sahin, M Ozemi, E Kerse, B Ozen, B Kolacan, M Altinors, and A Goktepeli. **1978.** An outbreak of pleural mesothelioma and chronic fibrosing pleurisy in the village of Karain/Urgup in Anatolia. Thorax 33:811-192.

Brown, RC, M Chamberlain, R Davies, and GT Sutton. **1980.** The *in vitro* activities of pathogenic mineral dusts. Toxicology 17:143-147.

Dunnill, MS. **1982.** *Pulmonary Pathology,* Churchill Livingstone, London, England.

Heppleston, AG. **1982.** Silicotic fibrogenesis: A concept of pulmonary fibrosis. Ann Occup Hyg 26:446-449.

Johnson, NF. **1987.** Asbestos-induced changes in rat lung parenchyma. J Toxicol Environ Health 21:193-203.

Johnson, NF, DM Griffiths, and RJ Hill. **1982.** Size distributions following long-term inhalation of MMMF, pp. 102-125. In: *Biological Effects of Man-Made Mineral Fibers,* Vol 2, Proceedings of a WHO/IARC Conference, Copenhagen, Denmark. World Health Organization, Geneva, Switzerland.

Johnson, NF, RE Edwards, DE Munday, N Rowe, and JC Wagner. **1984.** Pluripotential nature of mesothelioma induced by inhalation of erionite in rats. Br J Exp Pathol 65:377-388.

Morgan, A, JC Evans, and A Holmes. **1977.** Deposition and clearance of inhaled fibrous minerals in the rat. Studies using radioactive tracer techniques, pp. 259-272. In: *Inhaled Particles,* Vol. 4, HH Walton (ed.). Pergamon, Oxford, England.

Poole, A, RC Brown, CJ Turver, JW Skidmore, and DM Griffiths. **1983.** *In vitro* genotoxic activities of fibrous erionite. Br J Cancer 47:697-705.

Sebastien, P, A Gaudichet, J Bignon, and YI Baris. **1981.** Zeolite bodies in human lungs from Turkey. Lab Invest 44:420-425.

Selikoff, IJ, CE Hammond, and I Churg. **1968.** Asbestos exposure, smoking, and neoplasia. J Am Med Assoc 204:106-110.

Spurr, AR. **1969.** A low viscosity resin embedding medium for electron microscopy. J Ultrastruct Res 26:31-37.

Stanton, MF, M Layard, A Tegeris, E Miller, and E Kent. **1977.** Carcinogenicity of fibrous glass pleural response in relation to fiber dimension. J Natl Cancer Inst 58:587-603.

Suzuki, Y. **1982.** Carcinogenic and fibrogenic effects of zeolites: Preliminary observations. Environ Res 27:433-445.

Wagner, JC. **1982.** Health hazards of substitutes, pp. 244-266. In: *Asbestos, Health and Safety.* Canadian Asbestos Information Center, Montreal, Quebec, Canada.

Wagner, JC, GB Berry, JW Skidmore, and V Timbrell. **1974.** The effects of the inhalation of asbestos in rats. Br J Cancer 29:252-269.

Wagner, JC, JW Skidmore, RJ Hill, and DM Griffiths. **1985.** Erionite exposure and mesotheliomas in rats. Br J Cancer 51:727-730.

Comparison of Mesothelioma Induction in Rats by Asbestos and Nonasbestos Mineral Fibers: Possible Correlation with Human Exposure Data*

David L. Coffin,[1] Lalita D. Palekar,[2] Philip M. Cook,[3] and John P. Creason[1]

[1]U.S. Environmental Protection Agency, Health Effects Research Laboratory, Research Triangle Park, NC 27711

[2]Northrop Services, Inc., P. 0. Box 12313, Research Triangle Park, NC 27695-7905

[3]U.S. Environmental Protection Agency, Environmental Research Laboratory, Duluth, MN 55804

KEY WORDS: intrapleural injection, mesothelioma, asbestos, non-asbestos fibers, correlation with human data

---

ABSTRACT

Fischer-344 rats were injected intrapleurally with chrysotile or crocidolite asbestos, erionite or attapulgite and observed for their life spans. Fibers of the various size categories for each mineral species were determined in terms of number per unit mass. The dose was also computed in terms of number of fibers. Data for survival time and number of tumors induced suggest that, in addition to the aspect ratio, an additional unknown property may play a role in the potential of fibers for tumor induction. Analysis of the available data from the literature for populations known to have been exposed to pure mineral

*These studies were supported by funds provided by the U.S. Environmental Protection Agency under the aegis of the Health Effects Research Laboratory Durable Fibers Program (Contract #68-02-4032). The contents of this paper do not necessarily reflect the views and policies of the U.S. Environmental Protection Agency, nor does the mention of trade names or commercial products constitute endorsement or recommendation for use.

fibers indicates that ranking the different types of fibers for their ability to induce mesotheliomas yields similar results in both humans and rats.

INTRODUCTION

Since the intrapleural implantation experiments of Stanton et al. (1981), there has been a growing body of evidence that the length and width of mineral fibers play a determinant role in the induction of mesothelial tumors in the pleural or peritoneal cavities (Stanton et al., 1981). Stanton's evidence appears quite clear, and it is generally assumed that his data show an optimal effect at length $\geqq 8\ \mu m$ and width $\leqq 0.25\ \mu m$. These data were obtained mainly from vitreous synthetic fibers of various types where length/width characteristics could be fairly well defined. Therefore, two questions have arisen: (1) Do the same parameters hold for asbestos or asbestiform minerals, which are crystalline and infinitely variable in size? (2) Is there a cut-off in length or width beyond which these parameters are no longer effective? Experiments with asbestos indicate that when animals are exposed to short or long fibers of the same mineral species, tumors more frequently result from the longer fibers (Wagner et al., 1980). These experiments are confounded, however, by the considerable overlap in the length of such fibers. Recent experiments using amosite, where length was controlled by ball-milling, showed a distinct reduction of tumorigenesis when the length of the fibers did not exceed 5 μm (Davis et al., 1986).

Despite the strong evidence that aspect ratios are the tumorigenic factor for mineral fibers, there has been a suspicion that persons exposed to crocidolite are more prone to develop mesotheliomas than those exposed to chrysotile (McDonald and McDonald, 1980; Wagner et al., 1960). A recent review of data from certain human exposure to pure fibers has shown that mesotheliomas were induced, in decreasing order, by crocidolite, amosite and chrysotile (Hughes and Weill, 1986). Furthermore, a striking preponderance of mesothelioma induction has been attributed to an erionite fiber of the zeolite family (Artvinli and Baris, 1982). The greater propensity for this zeolite to induce mesotheliomas, compared to asbestos, has been confirmed by intrapleural, inhalation and intratracheal studies in rats (Wagner, 1982; Wagner et al., 1985; Coffin et al., this volume).

These findings suggest that some factor other than length/width may influence the degree of risk for mesothelioma induction. Identifying such a nongeometric factor and elucidating its mechanism would be important in estimating human risk of environmental exposure to various asbestos and nonasbestos natural fibers. In addition, such information would be important in evaluating the hazards of new species of fibers proposed as asbestos substitutes. In the latter category, striking differences in the induction of pleural or peritoneal tumors have already been demonstrated in animal experiments (Smith et al., 1988). To test the hypothesis of tumorigenic factors other than fiber aspect ratios, a series of experiments were undertaken with natural mineral fibers of widely varying tumorigenic potential.

MATERIALS AND METHODS

A very thorough mineralogical characterization was essential for our purpose. In it, the number of size and shape categories of mineral fibers were computed per unit mass of the minerals. The following fibers were chosen: UICC chrysotile asbestos; UICC crocidolite asbestos; erionite, a fibrous silicate of the zeolite class; Georgia/ Florida attapulgite, a fibrous clay mineral.

Two preparations of erionite from the same source (Rome, OR), supplied by Minerals Research, Clarkson, New York, were used in this study. They were prepared by air elutriation (erionite W) and water sedimentation (erionite C) after very brief milling.

Table 1 indicates the number of mineral fibers of three size categories per unit mass: (a) all structures classed as fibers, i.e., having an aspect ratio of > 3; (b) a short, fine fiber of less than 5 μm by 0.1 μm, or smaller; and (c) a fiber $\geqq 8$ μm long and $\leqq 0.25$ μm wide. The latter class of fibers has generally been considered the most tumorigenic (Stanton et al., 1981). The ranking in the number of fibers per unit mass is from left to right. For example, in the 8 x 0.25-μm category, there are 330X more fibers for chrysotile than for erionite W and 126X more than for crocidolite. Also included in the table are mean and median values for length, width and aspect ratios.

Fischer-344 rats, approximately 3 weeks of age, were inoculated through the chest wall at the midpoint of the right side of the thorax according to the protocol shown in Table 2, then barrier-maintained until natural death.

RESULTS

For this preliminary report, only descriptive statistical data are presented. Data for dose effect and lesion considerations will be presented later, after review and statistical analysis are completed.

Table 1. Analysis of mineral fiber parameters by means of transmission electron microscopy[a]

Parameter	Erionite (W)	Erionite (C)	Crocidolite (UICC)	Chrysotile (UICC)
Number of Fibers x 10^6/mg, $A \geq 3$[b]	850	1080	3360	21,000
Number of Fibers x 10^6/mg, $L \geq 8$ μm $W \leq 0.25$ μm[c]	3.3	2.1	8.6	1,090
Number of Fibers x 10^6/mg, $L \geq 5$ μm, $W \leq 0.1$ μm	152	390	983	13,300
Mean Length (μm)	2.22	1.41	1.30	2.38
Median Length (μm)	1.60	0.99	0.82	1.08
Mean Width (μm)	0.25	0.17	0.16	0.10
Median Width (μm)	0.28	0.13	0.14	0.08
Mean Aspect Ratio (L/W)	10.76	10.27	7.95	29.55
Median Aspect Ratio (L/W)	8.00	7.31	5.94	11.53

[a]Analyzed by Dr. Philip Cook
[b]A = aspect ratio (L/W)
[c]L = length, W = width

Table 2. Experimental treatment protocol for intrapleural injection of Fischer-344 rats with various mineral fibers.

	Number of Animals Exposed							Controls		
Dose (mg):	0.5	2	4	8	16	32	Total	Untreated	Sham	Total
Chrysotile	50	50	50	50	50	50	300	20	20	40
Crocidolite	50	50	50	50	50	50	300	20	20	40
Erionite W	50	50	50	50	50	50	300	20	20	40
Erionite C	50	50	50	50	50	50	300	20	20	40
Attapulgite	50	50	50	50	50	50	300	20	20	40

Data for survival time following treatment, determined by the Kaplan-Meier method, show a ranking, for survival, from erionite W (shortest) to attapulgite (longest). A summary of the data by mean and median survival time shows that the effect of the respective treatments differs widely (Table 3). Median values ranged from 369 days for erionite W to 789 days for crocidolite; results for attapulgite did not differ from those of pooled controls.

Table 3. Survival time (days after injection) of rats intrapleurally injected with various mineral fibers.

	Treated			Untreated Controls			Saline Controls		
	N	Mean	Median	N	Mean	Median	N	Mean	Median
Erionite W	299	372	369	20	818	843	20	887	878
Erionite C	299	482	462	20	820	848	20	879	913
Chrysotile	299	617	625	20	839	834	20	870	845
Crocidolite	299	769	789	20	812	801	20	801	829
Attapulgite	299	821	839	20	720	729	20	790	796
Totals				**100**	**801**	**811**	**120**	**845**	**852**

Tumor induction was generally congruent with survival time, ranging from 95% incidence of mesotheliomas for erionite to 1.4% for attapulgite; the latter was similar to that in controls (Table 4). The relationship of survival time to percentage of tumors is shown in Figure 1.

Table 4. Incidence of mesotheliomas in mineral-fiber-treated rats[a]

Test Substance	N	No. Tumors	% Tumors
Erionite W	144	137	95
Erionite C	144	123	85
Chrysotile	142	118	83
Crocidolite	144	65	45
Attapulgite	140	2	1.4
Controls (Sham and Untreated)	79	1	1.3

[a]Based on pooled results of randomly selected (24) animals from each concentration of fibers injected. Data represent animals that died as a result of tumor.

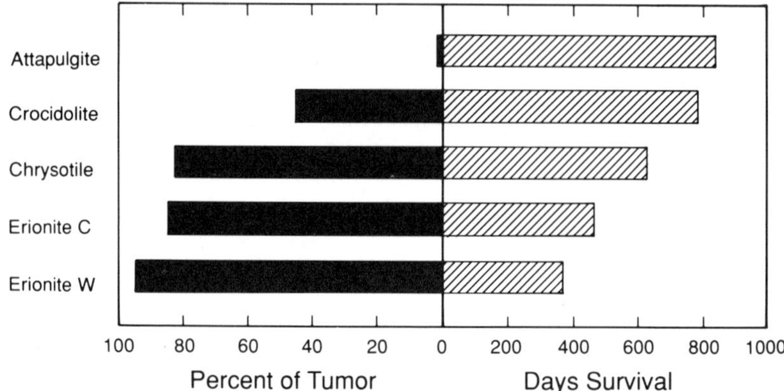

Figure 1. Comparison of percentage of rats with tumor to median survival (both parameters pooled across dose range) after intrapleural injection of various mineral fibers.

DISCUSSION AND CONCLUSIONS

The number of fibrous particles in our samples differed markedly (Table 1). If the prevailing view is correct (that long, narrow fibers are required to induce mesotheliomas [Stanton et al., 1981]), tumor induction should increase and survival time should decrease if a large number of such fibers were injected.

In our study, the opposite was true: the smaller number of fibers (erionite) resulted in more tumor deaths and shorter survival time than either type of asbestos. In fact, there is an inverse relationship between tumorigenesis/life span and the number of mineral fibers. When compared on the basis of number of fibers of $L \geqq 8\ \mu m$, $W \leqq 0.25\ \mu m$ that were injected, the rank order for survival time and tumorigenesis is: erionite, crocidolite, chrysotile.

A striking difference is evident in the apparent tumorigenic potential of the mineral fibers per unit number when the relationship is expressed as reduction in life span or percent tumor induction. Compared to data in the literature for relative frequency of human mesotheliomas from exposure to these same mineral fibers, there is a remarkable similarity (Table 5). Table 6 shows the close ranking of our data with the data for human exposure to pure fibers, when compared either as percent mortality from mesotheliomas or ratio of mesotheliomas to lung cancer (after the latter has been corrected for standardized mortality ratio.

Table 5. Comparative incidence of mesotheliomas and lung cancer in human populations exposed to various mineral fibers.

	Deaths from Lung Cancer				Deaths from Mesothelioma		
	Total Deaths Observed	Observed No.	Excess over Predicted No.	% Excess over Predicted No.	Observed No. of Deaths	% of Total Deaths	% of Excess over Predicted No.
Chrysotile[a]	5500	407	99.0	1.8	12	0.22	12.1
Amosite[a]	861	144	85.5	9.9	19	2.2	22.2
Mixed Fibers	6751	960	485.3	7.2	320	4.7	65.9
Crocidolite[a]	735	80	31.5	4.2	52	7.1	165.1
Erionite[b,c]	67	8	5.0	7.4	27	40.0	540.0

[a]Data for asbestos from Hughes and Weill, Am Rev Respir Dis 133:5-13, 1986.
[b]Data for erionite from Artvinli and Baris, Arch Environ Health 37:177-181, 1982.
[c]Data for age-adjusted standardized mortality ratio for lung cancers in Turks kindly furnished by Dr. Artvinli.

Table 6. Relative potency of mineral fibers in mesothelioma induction and other parameters expressed as an index (erionite = 100)[a]

	A	B[b]	C[c]	D[c]	E[c]
Erionite	100	100	100	100	100
Crocidolite	7.7	23.5	11.8	33	17
Chrysotile	0.2	0.3	2.5	2	5.5

[a]KEY: A = Life-shortening in rats (U.S. EPA data); Dose: mineral fibers $\geq 8\ \mu m$ long and $\leq 0.25\ \mu m$ wide
B = Tumorigenesis (U.S. EPA data); Dose: mineral fibers $\geq 8\ \mu m$ long and $\leq 0.25\ \mu m$ wide
C = % difference from lung cancer (U.S. EPA, 1985)
D = % difference from lung cancer (Hughes and Weill, 1986)
E = % mortality (Hughes and Weill, 1986)
[b]Ratio, number tumors/number fibers $> 8.0\ \mu m \times < 0.25\ \mu m$
[c]Data for erionite (C through E) (Artvinli and Baris, 1982)

These comparisons suggest the presence of another chemical or physical agent (in addition to length and width) as a factor in mesothelioma induction. Characterization of this factor may be important in evaluating the potential hazards of asbestos exposure. Furthermore, it may contribute significantly to understanding the striking differences observed in mesothelioma induction among certain synthetic fiber species.

ACKNOWLEDGMENT

The authors express their appreciation to Dr. Christopher Wagner, Penarth, Wales, United Kingdom, who kindly furnished the sample of erionite W.

REFERENCES

Artvinli, M and YI Baris. **1982.** Environmental fiber-induced pleuropulmonary diseases in an Anatolian village: An epidemiologic study. Arch Environ Health 37:177-181.

Davis, JMG, I Addison, RE Allen, K Donaldson, MD Jones and T Smith. **1986.** Pathogenicity of long versus short fiber samples of amosite asbestos administered to rats by inhalation and intraperitoneal injection. Br J Exp Pathol 67:2415-2430.

Hughes, JM and H Weill. **1986.** Asbestos exposure--quantitative assessment of risk. Am Rev Respir Dis 133:5-13.

McDonald, AD and CJ McDonald. **1980.** Malignant mesothelioma in North America. Cancer 46:1650-1656.

Smith, DM, LW Ortz, RT Archuleta, and NF Johnson. **1988.** Long-term health effects in hamsters and rats exposed chronically to manmade mineral fibers. Ann Occup Hyg 31:731-742.

Stanton, MF, M Layard, et al. **1981.** Relation of particle dimension to carcinogenicity in amphibole asbestos and other fibrous materials. J Natl Cancer lnst 67:965-975.

U.S. (EPA) Environmental Protection Agency. 1985. Airborne Asbestos Health Assessment Update, EPA 600/8-84-003F. Office of Health Assessment, Environmental Criteria Assessment Office, Research Triangle Park, NC.

Wagner, JC, **1982.** Health hazards of substitute, p. 244. In: *Asbestos Health and Safety.* Canadian Asbestos Information Center, Montreal, Canada.

Wagner, JC, GB Berry, JW Skidmore, and FC Pooley. **1980.** The comparative effects of three chrysotiles by injection and inhalation in rats, pp. 363-372. In: *Biological Effects of Mineral Fibers,* JC Wagner (ed.). IARC, Lyon, France.

Wagner, JC, JW Skidmore, RJ Hill, and DM Griffiths. **1985.** Erionite exposure and mesothelioma in rats. Br J Cancer 51:727.

Wagner, JD, CA Sleggs, and P Marchand. **1960.** Diffuse pleural mesotheliomas and asbestos exposure in the North Western Cape Province. Br J Ind Med 17:260-271.

Chromosomal Changes Associated with Tumorigenic Mineral Fibers*

Lalita D. Palekar,[1] John F. Eyre,[1] and David L. Coffin[2]

[1]Northrop Services, Inc., Environmental Sciences, P. O. Box 12313, Research Triangle Park, NC 27709

[2]U.S. Environmental Protection Agency, Health Effects Research Laboratory, Research Triangle Park, NC 27711

KEY WORDS: chromosomal changes, rat pleural mesothelioma cells, mineral fibers, V79 cells

---

ABSTRACT

Mineral fibers such as asbestos and erionite (a fibrous zeolite) induce mesotheliomas in humans and animals. A chromosomal involvement is strongly implicated in the production of these tumors because of the deleterious cytogenetic effects of tumorigenic mineral fibers in mammalian cells *in vitro,* and because mineral-fiber-induced tumors possess chromosome abnormalities.

Our earlier cytogenetic studies (Palekar et al., 1987) with the tumorigenic mineral fibers crocidolite, chrysotile and erionite in V79 Chinese hamster lung cells demonstrated their ability to induce chromosome breakage and to induce a significant reduction in diploid cells with an accompanying increase in aneuploid and polyploid cells. Additionally, chrysotile and crocidolite induced chromosome mis-segregation at anaphase, while fewer cells entered anaphase when treated with erionite. Although these tumorigenic mineral fibers have demonstrated deleterious cytogenetic effects, the specific

*These studies were supported by funds provided by the U.S. Environmental Protection Agency under the aegis of the Health Effects Research Laboratory Durable Fibers Program (Contract #68-02-4032). The contents of this paper do not necessarily reflect the views and policies of the U.S. Environmental Protection Agency, nor does the mention of trade names or commercial products constitute endorsement or recommendation for use.

chromosome(s) involved in the induction of mesotheliomas have not been identified. The purpose of the current study is to investigate the cytogenetic characteristics of mineral-fiber-induced pleural mesotheliomas in the rat in an attempt to identify specific chromosomal events associated with either the action of specific tumorigenic mineral fibers or with the pathogenesis of pleural mesotheliomas. Cell lines were established *in vitro* from six chrysotile- and seven erionite-induced pleural mesotheliomas in rats. Each cell line was composed of several cell populations that were heterogeneous in their chromosome make-up but had a readily recognizable predominant cell population in each cell line, based on chromosome number. The cell lines were characterized by either aneuploid or pseudodiploid cells with chromosome modal numbers ranging from 40 to 92. Karyotype analyses revealed a heterogeneous display of chromosome rearrangements. Each cell line had unique abnormalities: e.g., the characteristic chromosome abnormalities of a pseudodiploid cell line were -5, t(7;11), 10q-, and one marker; while a cell line with 43 chromosomes had 1q+, t(10;13), and +20. No recurrent abnormality can as yet be associated with either chrysotile- or erionite-induced mesothelioma cells. However, anomalies of chromosome No. 1 (10/13 tumor cell lines) were frequently observed, suggesting chromosome No. 1 involvement in the pathogenesis of rat pleural mesotheliomas.

INTRODUCTION

There is considerable interest in identifying mechanisms of mineral-fiber-induced tumorigenesis. Various viewpoints have been expressed by investigators, however none are conclusive. We have explored the possibility of chromosomal involvement in mineral-fiber-induced tumorigenesis, selecting three fibers (erionite, crocidolite asbestos and chrysotile asbestos) whose tumorigenic potencies are in decreasing order. Chromosomal abnormalities induced with short-term exposure to these mineral fibers in V79 Chinese hamster lung cells were determined. In addition, we have analyzed chromosomal changes in the cell lines derived from rat pleural mesotheliomas induced with mineral fibers.

MATERIALS AND METHODS

Mineral Samples

The test samples selected for these studies were erionite, UICC crocidolite asbestos and UICC chrysotile asbestos. Erionite (Rome, OR) was prepared with the use of a Teflon-coated ball mill, and the sample was analyzed by selected area electron diffraction pattern and identified as aluminosilicate with traces of Ca, Mg, K and Na. The size-distribution analysis was performed by transmission electron microscopy.

Cell Culture

The V79 Chinese hamster lung cells were maintained in Williams' Medium E (GIBCO), supplemented with 5% fetal bovine serum (GIBCO), 300 μg/ml L-glutamine (GIBCO), 2.5 μg/ml fungizone (GIBCO), and 30 μg/ml gentamicin (GIBCO) at 37°C in a humidified 5% CO_2 atmosphere. Exponentially growing cells were seeded in T25 Corning plastic flasks containing 2 ml of culture medium. Two-milliliter suspensions of test minerals were added to the cell cultures to achieve concentrations of 10, 40, 60, and 100 μg/ml. Control cultures contained cells and medium only. Duplicate flasks were treated for 24 hours at 37°C in a humidified 5% CO_2 atmosphere.

Chromosomal Preparations for Metaphase Analysis

During the final 2 hours of treatment, colcemid at a concentration of 0.10 μg/ml was added to arrest mitotic figures. For chromosomal preparations, the cells were then trypsinized and centrifuged at 200 x g for 10 minutes and treated with a hypotonic solution of 0.075M KCl. Cells were then fixed with methanol/acetic acid (3:1). Slide preparations were made by using conventional air-drying methods and staining with 1:50 diluted Gurr's R66 Giemsa stain (Gurr). A minimum of 100 metaphases per data point were examined for chromosome number and chromosome breaks. Aberrations were classified into chromatid type and chromosome type according to Evans and O'Riordan (1975).

Chromosomal Preparation for Anaphase Analysis

Exponentially growing 2 x 10^5 cells were seeded in 2 ml of culture medium in 60-mm petri dishes containing glass coverslips. The cells were exposed to mineral fibers in a total volume of 4 ml and incubated as described earlier. After 24-hour exposure, the cells were treated as described by Nichols et al. (1979) for anaphase analysis. Briefly, the cells were fixed with methanol, stained with Giemsa and dehydrated, using several acetone/xylene rinses. One hundred anaphases were examined (when possible) for acentric fragments, bridges, side-arm bridges, lagging chromosomes, and multipolar configurations.

Induction of Tumors

Six- to eight-week-old male Fischer-344 rats were given intrapleural injections of 20 mg of either erionite or UICC chrysotile. The animals were maintained in a barrier facility and given food and water *ad libitum.*

Preparation of Cell Lines from Pleural Mesothelial Tumors in the Rat

Immediately after death the animal was necropsied aseptically, and the pleural tumor was removed and cut into two pieces. One piece was preserved in 10% buffered formalin for pathological evaluations; the second piece was rinsed aseptically in sterile physiological saline for preparation of a cell culture.

The tissue was then rinsed in Dulbecco's phosphate-buffered saline (DPBS), placed in a petri dish with 0.25% trypsin (GIBCO), and minced with two scalpel blades. The supernatant was discarded to remove blood cells and debris. The remaining pieces were incubated in 0.25% trypsin and again incubated at 37°C with 5% CO_2 for 15 minutes. The supernatant containing tumor cells was incubated in a 4-cm^2 microwell dish (Costar) containing Dulbecco's modified Eagle's medium (DMEM; GIBCO), 20% v/v fetal bovine serum (GIBCO), 2.5 μg/ml fungizone, and 50 μg/ml of gentamicin. The trypsin treatment and the establishment of tumor cells in the culture medium was repeated two more times. The microwells were incubated at 37°C, in 10% CO_2 in a humidified chamber. When colonies of cells were visible in the microwells, they were trypsinized and transferred to 25-cm^2 culture flasks (Corning), and incubated.

Chromosomal Preparations of Tumor Cells

Cell cultures of early passage were selected. Chromosomal preparations were made for conventional Giemsa staining or for G-banding. For conventional Giemsa staining, 40 to 60% confluent cell cultures were treated with colcemid (0.10 μg/ml) to arrest mitotic cells. Chromosome preparations were made as described earlier.

For G-banding chromosomes, 0.06 μg colcemid was added 1 to 1½ hours before harvesting. The cells were treated with hypotonic solutions and fixatives as described earlier. G-bands were elicited by immersing slides for from 20 seconds to 3 minutes in a 1:10 dilution of 0.25% trypsin (GIBCO) in DPBS without Ca^{++} and Mg^{++}. The slides were then rinsed with DPBS and quickly passed through two changes of absolute alcohol. The slides were air-dried and stained with 1:50 dilution of Gurr's R66 Giemsa (Gurr).

RESULTS

Chromosomal Analysis of V79 Chinese Hamster Lung Cells

The selection of the doses for this study was based on an earlier cytotoxicity study, where we found that the dose range between 10 and 100 μg/ml produced cytotoxicity (Palekar et al., 1985a, 1988). In addition, the examination of mitotic indices of the cultures treated with erionite, UICC crocidolite and UICC chrysotile showed a reduction in dividing cells at all dose levels, further indicating that an appropriate range was being studied (Table 1).

Table 1. Effects of mineral fibers on chromosome number in V79 Chinese hamster lung cells[a]

Treatment Group	Mass Dose (μg/ml)	Mitotic Index (%)[b]	Hypo-diploid Cells (%)	Diploid Cells (%)	Hyper-diploid Cells (%)	Total Aneu-ploid Cells (%)[c]	Poly-ploid Cells (%)[d]
Control	0	8.7	0.3	89.7	9.7	10	0.3
Erionite	10	7.9	1.0	79.0[e]	16.0	17	4.0[e]
	40	6.1	2.0	77.0[e]	19.0[e]	21[e]	2.0
	60	4.0	4.0[e]	77.0[e]	13.0	17	6.0[e]
	100	2.7	8.0[e]	69.0[e]	19.0[e]	27[e]	4.0[e]
Crocidolite	10	8.2	2.0	83.0	9.0	11	6.0[e]
	40	6.1	0.0	68.0[e]	23.0[e]	23[e]	9.0[e]
	60	3.4	6.0[e]	60.0[e]	16.0	22[e]	18.0[e]
	100	3.9	5.0[e]	75.0[e]	14.0	19	6.0[e]
Chrysotile	10	6.9	0.0	82.0	9.0	9	9.0[e]
	40	2.4	1.0	68.0[e]	20.0[e]	21[e]	11.0[e]
	60	4.0	3.0	76.0[e]	18.0	21[e]	3.0
	100	2.0	7.0[e]	55.0[e]	32.0[e]	39[e]	6.0[e]

[a]A total of 600 metaphases were scored from control cultures and 100 metaphases from treated cultures at each dose.

[b]1000 cells were counted for mitotic index.

[c]Includes hypodiploid (20 to 21 chromosomes) and hyperdiploid (23 to 29 chromosomes) cells.

[d]Includes cells with 30 to 44 chromosomes.

[e]Denotes statistically significant values at overall $P < 0.05$, as determined by chi-squared statistics or Fisher's Exact Test.

Metaphase Analysis. Six hundred metaphases from untreated control cultures and 100 from cultures treated with each mineral fiber at each dose were scored to determine the effect on chromosome number and structure. Three categories of chromosome numbers were considered: diploid (22 chromosomes), aneuploid (20 to 21 or 23 to 29 chromosomes), and polyploid (30 to 44 chromosomes). Compared to the untreated controls, all three mineral fibers induced a significant decrease in diploid cells, which was accompanied by an increase in aneuploid and polyploid cells. The results are shown in Table 1. When the number of diploid, aneuploid and polyploid cells were compared among the three treated groups, no significant difference was observed. Erionite, which is more tumorigenic than asbestos, showed a similar degree of chromosomal abnormalities as that observed in the UICC crocidolite and UICC chrysotile cultures at the mass dose range between 10 and 100 μg/ml. It is, however, well recognized that fiber dimension is an important factor during biological interactions (Stanton, 1973; Stanton et al., 1977). The mass dose was therefore converted into the number of fibers in three most commonly used categories: aspect ratio (A) > 3; length (L) $> 8\ \mu$m, width (W) $< 0.25\ \mu$m; and L $\leqq 5\ \mu$m, W $\leqq 0.1\ \mu$m. Table 2 shows the dose, in number of fibers per category, and corresponding numbers of aneuploid and diploid cells. These data clearly indicate that fewer fibers of erionite (represented by a decrease in diploid cells) than of asbestos were required to produce a similar effect. The results were more pronounced in the UICC chrysotile treatment, where the numbers of fibers were severalfold greater than those of erionite in the categories A $\geqq 3$; L $\geqq 8\ \mu$m, W $\leqq$ 0.25 μm; L $\leqq 5\ \mu$m, W $\leqq 0.1\ \mu$m. These results correlate with the tumorigenic potential of the fibers, which shows that erionite fibers are more tumorigenic than asbestos.

Clastogenic Effect. One hundred metaphases from each sample at each dose, and 600 from untreated controls, were examined for chromosomal and chromatid aberrations (Table 3). There were a significantly greater number of chromatid aberrations in cell cultures treated with UICC chrysotile at 100-μg/ml concentrations. In the cultures treated with UICC crocidolite, erionite and lower concentrations of UICC chrysotile, the effect was moderate. These data are not surprising considering the difference in the number of fibers in the erionite and in the UICC crocidolite samples and those in the UICC chrysotile sample.

Anaphase Analysis. The types of anaphase abnormalities observed were: (1) lagging chromosomes; (2) fragments; (3) bridges; (4) detached chromosomes; (5) tripolar anaphase; and (6) multipolar anaphase (Figure 1). In most cases, fibers were observed either in

Table 2. Comparison between mass and number of fibers of mineral samples with respect to their effects on chromosome numbers in V79 Chinese hamster lung cells

Treatment Group	Aneuploid Cells (%)	Diploid Cells (%)	Mass Dose (μg/ml)	Dose in Number of Fibers x 10^6/ml[a]		
				A ≥ 3	L ≥ 8 μm, W ≤ 0.25 μm	L ≤ 5 μm W ≤ 0.1 μm
Control	10	89.7	0	0	0	0
Erionite	17	79.0	10	10.8	0.021	3.9
	21[b]	77.0[b]	40	43.2	0.084	15.6
	17	77.0[b]	60	64.8	0.126	23.4
	27[b]	69.0[b]	100	108.0	0.210	39.0
Crocidolite	11	83.0	10	33.6	0.086	9.85
	23[b]	68.0[b]	40	134.0	0.344	39.40
	22[b]	60.0[b]	60	202.0	0.516	59.10
	19	75.0[b]	100	336.0	0.860	98.50
Chrysotile	9	82.0	10	210.0	10.9	133.00
	21[b]	68.0[b]	40	840.0	43.6	532.00
	21[b]	76.0[b]	60	1260.0	65.4	798.00
	39[b]	55.0[b]	100	2100.0	109.0	1330.00

[a]A = Aspect ratio, L = length, W = width

[b]Denotes statistically significant values at overall $P < 0.05$, determined by chi-squared statistics or Fisher's Exact Test

Table 3. Clastogenic effects of mineral fibers in V79 Chinese hamster lung cells[a]

Treatment Group	Mass Dose (μg/ml)	Cells with Aberrations (%)	Aberrations	
			Chromatid (%)	Chromosome (%)
Control	0	0.83	0.83	0
Erionite	10	0	0	0
	40	4	4	0
	60	2	2	0
	100	5[b]	5	0
Crocidolite	10	0	0	0
	40	6[b]	9	0
	60	6[b]	6	0
	100	2	2	0
Chrysotile	10	4[b]	5	0
	40	3	3	1
	60	5[b]	1	4
	100	15[b]	18	2

[a]For controls, 600 cells were scored; for treated cultures, 100 cells were scored at each dose.

[b]Denotes statistically significant values at overall $P < 0.05$.

close proximity to anaphases or appeared to be directly penetrating the chromosomes. Actual anaphase counts are shown in Table 4. The number of cells in anaphase decreased after 24-hour treatment with mineral fibers; the decrease was more pronounced at higher concentrations. There were considerably more abnormal anaphases in the chrysotile-treated cultures than in those treated with crocidolite. The erionite-treated cultures showed relatively fewer cells in anaphase and, consequently, fewer cells with abnormal anaphases.

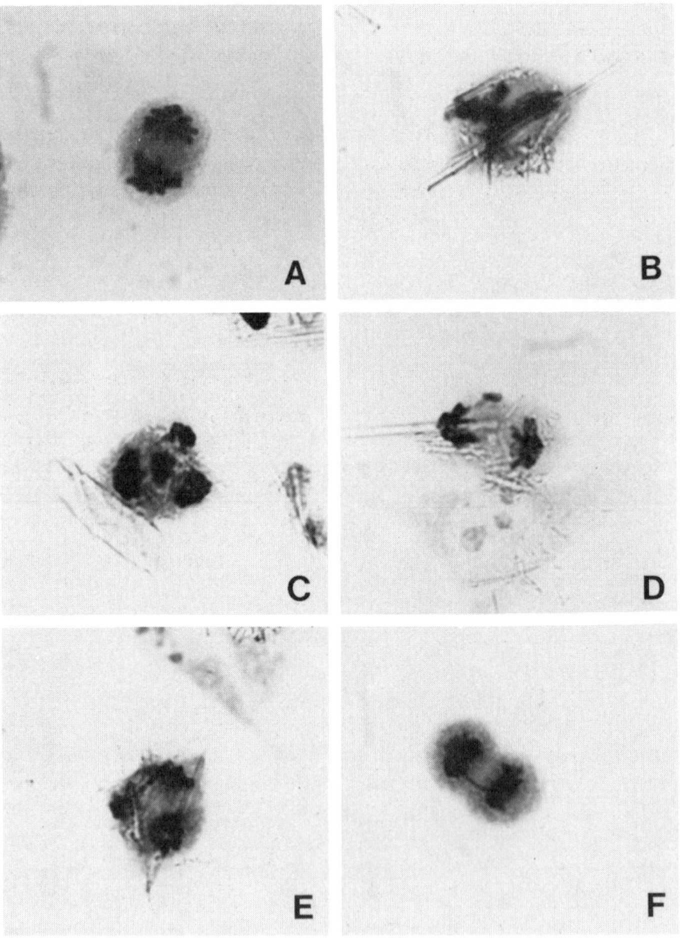

Figure 1. Types of anaphases in V79 cells treated with mineral fibers: A, normal; B, mineral fibers entangled with anaphases; C, multipolar; D, lagging chromosome or large fragments; E, tripolar; and F, bridges. Note mineral fibers in the vicinity.

Table 4. Anaphase analysis of V79 Chinese hamster lung cells exposed to mineral fibers.

Treatment Group	Mass Dose (μg/ml)	Cells in Anaphase[a] (%)	Number of Anaphases Scored	Acentric Fragments (%)	Mis-segregations[b] (%)
Control	0	4.2	303	1.0	2.3
Erionite	10	2.2	101	1.0	2.0
	40	0.4	48	2.1	0.0
	60	0.1	55	0.0	0.0
	100	0.1	4	0.0	0.0
Crocidolite	10	2.6	103	2.9	4.9
	40	1.5	100	1.0	6.0
	60	0.8	74	1.4	8.2
	100	0.4	31	0.0	9.7
Chrysotile	10	2.4	100	3.0	16.0[c]
	40	0.7	92	5.4	23.9[c]
	60	0.4	16	0.0	18.8[c]
	100	0.2	1	0.0	0.0

[a]1000 cells were counted.
[b]Denotes bridges, multipolar configurations, detached and lagging chromosomes
[c]Denotes statistically significant values at overall $P < 0.05$, as determined by chi-squared statistics or Fisher's Exact Test.

Morphological and Cytogenetic Analysis of Pleural Mesothelial Tumors Induced in Rats with Either Erionite or UICC Chrysotile Asbestos

Morphology of the Tumor Cell Lines. Seven cell lines from chrysotile-induced and six from erionite-induced rat pleural mesothelial tumors were studied. The morphologies of the cells in culture resembled those of the pleural tumors. Epithelial-type tumors produced cell lines which were predominantly epithelial (Figures 2A and B), while fibrosarcomatous tumors produced predominantly fibroblastic cell lines (Figures 3A and B). Tumors which appeared to be mixed (showing both epithelial and fibroblastic patterns) had both types of cells in the culture.

Cytogenetic Analysis of the Tumor Cell Lines. Metaphase preparations were made from early passage tumor cell lines. One hundred metaphases were examined from 13 cell lines for chromosomal number and structure. The numbers of chromosomes in each

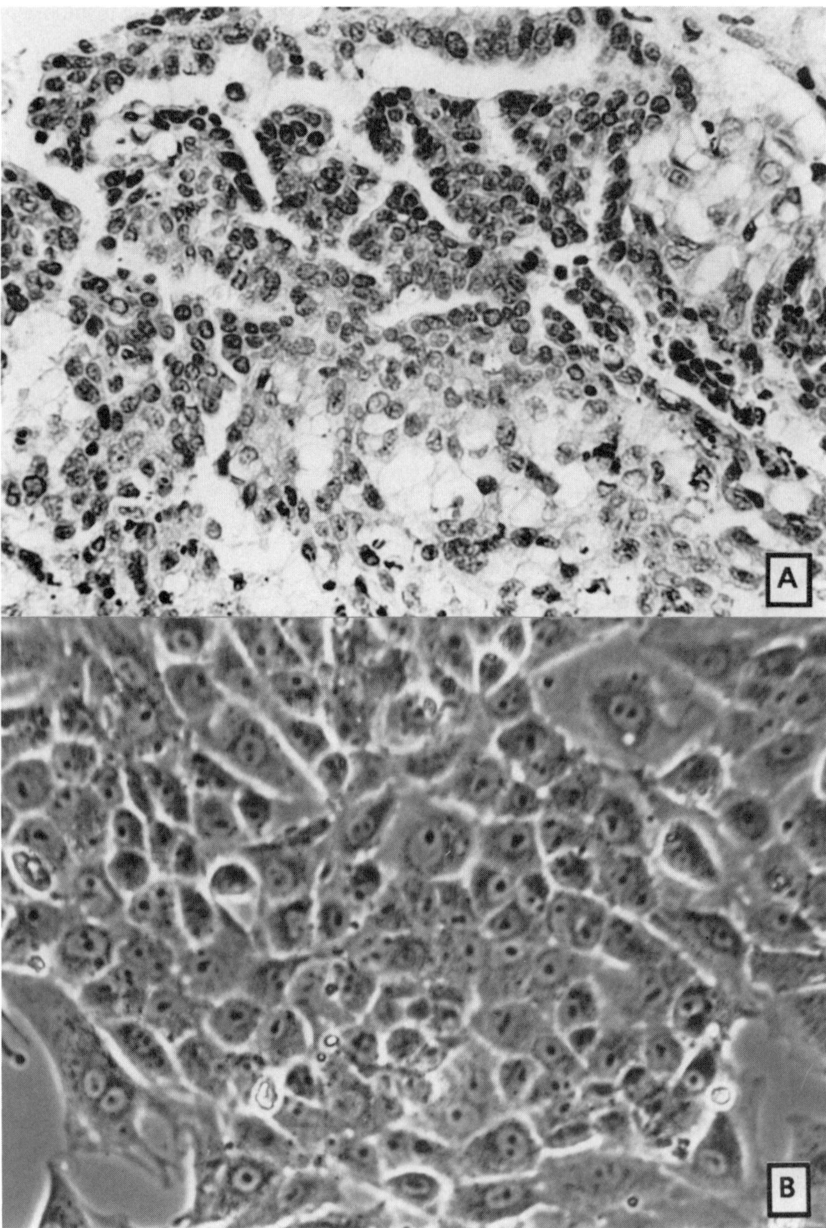

Figure 2. A, Tubulopapillary-type pleural tumor induced in a rat with erionite; predominantly epithelial cells; B, Cell culture derived from the tumor, showing cobblestone-shaped epithelial cells.

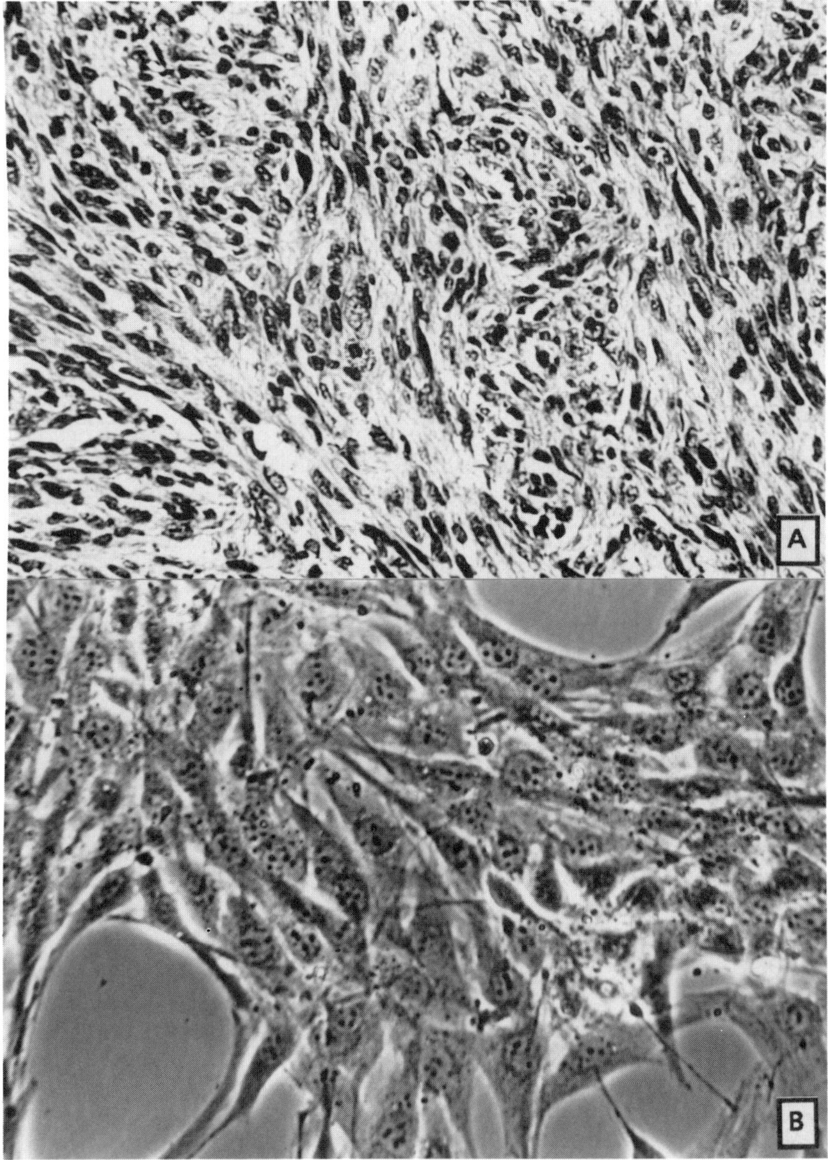

Figure 3. A, Fibrosarcomatous-type pleural tumor induced in a rat with UICC chrysotile; predominantly elongated, fibroblast-like cells. B, Cell cultures derived from the tumor, showing spindle-shaped fibroblasts.

metaphase were recorded, and the modal number (the most common chromosome number in a tumor cell population) was determined. In general, the 13 tumor cell lines had numerous chromosomal abnormalities. None were identifiable as unique to the test substances (erionite or chrysotile asbestos). Some of the chromosomal peculiarities of these cell lines are summarized in Table 5. For the chrysotile-induced tumor cell lines T1 through T6, the modal numbers were 40 (hypodiploid), 42, 42 (pseudodiploid), 55, 76, and 92, respectively. In the erionite-induced tumor cells, lines T7 through T13, T7 and T10 had two distinct modal numbers, 42 and 84, and 63 and 66, respectively. The modal numbers of T8, T9, T11, T12 and T13 were 43, 48, 72, 74 and 84, respectively.

Table 5. Chromosomal analysis of rat pleural mesothelial tumor cell lines[a]

Tumor-Inducing Agent	Tumor Cell Lines	Modal Number[b]	Abnormal Chromosome No. 1[c]	Marker Chromosomes[d]
Chrysotile	T1	40	+	+
	T2	42	+	+
	T3	42	–	+[e]
	T4	55	+	+
	T5	76	–	+
	T6	92	+	+
Erionite	T7	42,84	+	+
	T8	43	+	–[e]
	T9	48	+	+
	T10	63,66	+	+
	T11	72	+	+
	T12	74	–	+
	T13	84	+	+

[a]Chromosomal analysis was made by using conventional methods of Giemsa-staining unless stated otherwise.

[b]Modal number is the most common chromosome number in a tumor cell population. The cell lines also possessed a wide variety of cells with different numbers of chromosomes.

[c]The types of chromosome No. 1 abnormalities observed were: (1) monosomy, (2) deletions, (3) insertions and (4) trisomy.

[d]Marker chromosomes represent unidentifiable chromosomes, indicative of chromosomal breaks and rearrangements.

[e]G-banded chromosomal analysis demonstrated a variety of chromosomal abnormalities, including breaks and chromosomal rearrangements.

Karyotyping the tumor cell lines was difficult, as each cell line possessed numerous chromosomal abnormalities, including monosomy, trisomy, pentasomy and various marker chromosomes. Examples of a normal rat karyotype and karyotypes from a few tumor cell lines are shown in Figures 4A, B and C, respectively.

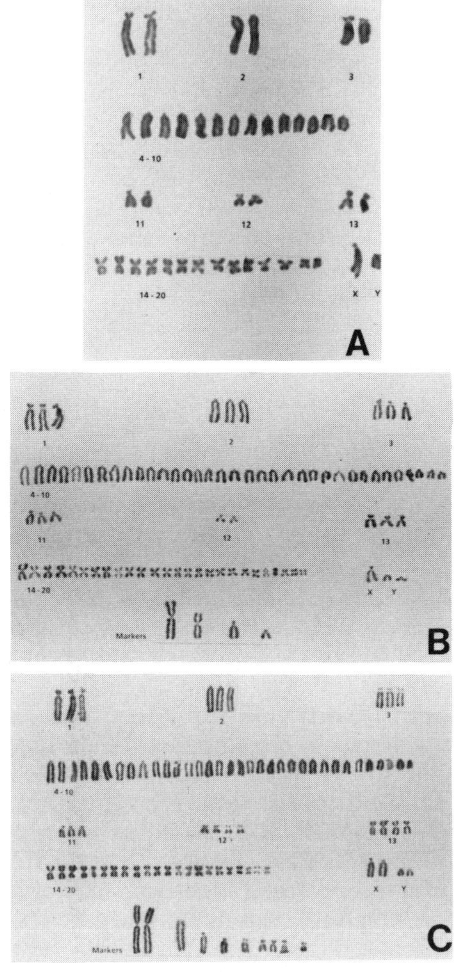

Figure 4. A, Normal karyotype of male Fischer-344 rat; B, karyotype of a cell line derived from a pleural mesothelial tumor induced in a rat with erionite; and C, karyotype of a cell line derived from a rat pleural mesothelial tumor induced with UICC chrysotile.

Among the 13 cell lines, T3 and T8 appeared to have relatively fewer chromosomal abnormalities, based on their diploid (42) and near-diploid (43) modal numbers, and they were selected for karyotyping using G-banded chromosomes.

The G-banded analysis of T3 and T8 found numerous chromosomal abnormalities, such as breaks, deletions, insertions and translocations. In T3, seven different chromosomes were abnormal, while in T8 five different chromosomes were abnormal. Both cell lines showed abnormalities of chromosome No. 10 at the vicinity of 10q31 band. A deletion at 10q26 and translocation of chromosome No. 13 at band 10q32 were observed in T3 and T8 cell lines, respectively. Chromosome No. 10 was the only chromosome which was abnormal in both cell lines.

Ten of the 13 cell lines studied had various abnormalities of chromosome No. 1. These abnormalities included monosomy, deletions, insertions, and trisomy. *H-ras* oncogene has been identified on rat chromosome No. 1, and therefore this observation may be of special significance in understanding mineral-fiber-induced tumorigenesis.

DISCUSSION

It has been proposed that chromosomal imbalance plays an important role in neoplastic development (Yunis, 1983). Chromosomal imbalance can be caused by the gain or loss of a whole chromosome (aneuploidy) or by chromosome deletions, breaks and rearrangements.

In this investigation we have demonstrated various chromosomal abnormalities in V79 Chinese hamster lung cells exposed for 24 hours to mineral fibers. Additionally, numerous chromosomal abnormalities were observed in the cells derived from rat pleural mesothelial tumors induced with mineral fibers. It was our intention to correlate the degree of chromosomal damage with the tumorigenic potencies of the three mineral-fiber samples. Erionite is known to be more tumorigenic than chrysotile and crocidolite in humans (Artvinli and Baris, 1979, 1982) and in animals (Wagner et al., 1985; Palekar et al., 1985b). The results presented here indicate that, when the cytogenetic effect is measured in mass dose, it does not correlate with the tumorigenic potentials of mineral fiber. Although a significant degree of aneuploidy was observed in the cells treated with the three mineral samples (within the dose range of 10 to 100 μg/ml), the degree of aneuploidy in the erionite-treated cells was similar to those observed in the asbestos-treated cells. Interestingly, when the mass dose was converted to numbers of fibers, appropriate ranking was established. Fewer fibers of erionite, compared to those of crocidolite or chrysotile, were required to produce similar degrees of aneuploidy.

The clastogenic response of chrysotile was significantly higher than those of erionite or crocidolite. However, considering that the number of fibers in the chrysotile samples was severalfold higher than in the other samples, it appears that the number of fibers plays an important role in such abnormalities.

These data also support our earlier findings, which showed that the degree of cytotoxicity to V79 Chinese hamster lung cells correlated with the tumorigenic potentials of mineral fibers when the dose was converted into numbers of fibers (Palekar et al., 1988).

Although the mechanism of asbestos-induced tumorigenesis is unclear, the biological effects of asbestos are being elucidated. Asbestos is inactive in gene mutation assays (Chamberlain and Tarmy, 1977; Kenne et al., 1986; Jaurand, 1985; Barrett et al., 1983), yet it produces clastogenic and/or numerical chromosome changes in mammalian cells (Palekar et al., 1987; Jaurand et al., 1986; Kelsey et al., 1986) and in human mesothelial cells (Lechner et al., 1985).

Direct physical interaction of mineral fibers with chromosomes is a plausible mechanism for explaining the genotoxicity of mineral fibers at the chromosome level rather than at the gene level. We have found a significant increase in aneuploidy and polyploidy in the V79 cells treated with asbestos and erionite. Chromosomal effects of asbestos are also manifested at anaphase as missegregation of chromosomes, and the consequence of missegregation is aneuploidy. Indeed, we have found various types of abnormal anaphases, such as bridges, lagging chromosomes, and multipolar configurations, in V79 cells treated with chrysotile asbestos and crocidolite asbestos; with erionite treatment, fewer cells entered anaphase. In some cases, fibers were observed in close contact with chromosomes. Similar observations have been made in Syrian hamster embryo cells treated with crocidolite asbestos (Hesterberg and Barrett, 1985).

These observations strongly implicate a chromosomal mechanism in mineral-fiber-induced tumorigenesis. This is further supported by a scanning electron microscopy study which found that metaphase chromosomes were damaged by direct physical contact with chrysotile or crocidolite fibers (Wang et al., 1987).

The pleural mesotheliomal tumors in rats selected for cytogenetic analysis were malignant and highly proliferative. Various chromosomal abnormalities in human mesotheliomas (Gibas et al., 1986) and in other solid human and animal tumors have been reported by other investigators (Sandberg and Turc-Carel, 1987). Our results with rat mesotheliomas are like those in humans. The cell lines derived from both erionite- and chrysotile-induced tumors possessed various numerical and structural chromosomal changes. The modal number of these tumors varied from 40 to 92, and all cell lines showed chromosomal rearrangements. There was, however, no obvious difference between the cytogenetic changes in the cell lines derived from the erionite-induced and the chrysotile-induced tumors.

The most interesting finding from the analysis of the 13 tumor cell lines was that 10 of 13 had a chromosome No. 1 abnormality. This may be of great importance in understanding the mechanism of mineral-fiber-induced tumorigenesis, because the *H-ras* oncogene is identified on rat chromosome No. 1 (Szpirer et al., 1985).

The data presented here confirm that it is more appropriate to define dose in number of fibers rather than in mass when comparing the biological activities of mineral fibers. The data also suggest that rat chromosome No. 1 may be involved in mineral-fiber tumorigenesis. The extent to which chromosome No. 1 and/or the *H-ras* oncogene is involved in mineral-fiber tumorigenesis is unknown. Furthermore, the presence of abnormal anaphases in close contact with mineral fibers and the increase of aneuploidy as well as polyploidy in the treated cells suggest that the mechanism may be partially due to their physical interference with normal cell division.

ACKNOWLEDGMENTS

We thank Professor Mumpton, of Mineral Research, Clarkson, NY, for providing the erionite sample and Dr. P. M. Cook of the U.S. Environmental Protection Agency, Duluth, MN, for preparing and analyzing the mineral samples.

REFERENCES

Artvinli, M and YI Baris. **1979.** Malignant mesotheliomas in a small village in the Anatolian region of Turkey: An epidemiologic study. J Natl Cancer Inst 63:17-22.

Artvinli, M and YI Baris. **1982.** Environmental fiber-induced pleuropulmonary diseases in an Anatolian village. An epidemiologic study. Arch Environ Health 37: 177-181.

Barrett, JC, DG Thomassen, and TW Hesterberg. **1983.** Role of gene and chromosomal mutations in cell transformation. NY Acad Sci 407:291-300.

Chamberlain, M and EM Tarmy. **1977.** Asbestos and glass fibers in bacterial mutation tests. Mutat Res 43:159-164.

Evans, HJ and ML O'Riordan. **1975.** Human peripheral blood lymphocytes for the analysis of chromosome aberrations in mutagen tests. Mutat Res 31:135-148.

Gibas, Z, FP Li, KH Antman, S Bernal, R Stahel, and AA Sandberg. **1986.** Chromosome changes in malignant mesothelioma cancer. Genet Cytogenet 20:191-201.

Hesterberg, TW and JC Barrett. **1985.** Induction by asbestos fibers of anaphase abnormalities: Mechanism for aneuploidy induction and possibly carcinogenesis. Carcinogenesis 6:473-475.

Jaurand, MC. **1985.** Comparative responses of cultured cells to asbestos fibers in relation to carcinogenicity. NATO Adv Study Inst Ser G 3:215-220.

Jaurand, MC, L Kheuang, L Magne, and J Bignon. **1986.** Chromosomal changes induced by chrysotile fibers or benzo-3-4-pyrene in rat pleural mesothelial cells. Mutat Res 169:141-148.

Kelsey, KT, E Yano, HL Liber, and JB Little. **1986.** The *in vitro* genetic effects of fibrous erionite and crocidolite asbestos. Br J Cancer 54:107-114.

Kenne, K, S Ljungquist, and NR Ringertz. **1986.** Effects of asbestos fibers on cell division, cell survival, and formation of thioguanine-resistant mutants in Chinese hamster ovary cells. Environ Res 39:448-464.

Lechner, JF, T Tokiwa, M LaVeck, WF Benedict, S Banks-Schlegel, H Yeager, Jr., A Beneijee, and CC Harris. **1985.** Asbestos-associated chromosomal changes in human mesothelial cells. Proc Natl Acad Sci USA 82:3884-3888.

Nichols, WW, RC Miller, and C Bradt. **1979.** *In vitro* anaphase and metaphase preparations in mutation testing, pp. 225-233. In: *Handbook of Mutagenicity Test Procedures,* BJ Kilbey, MS Legator, W Nichols, and C Ramal (eds.). Elsevier, Amsterdam, The Netherlands.

Palekar, LD, BG Brown, and DL Coffin. **1985a.** Correlation between *in vivo* tumorigenesis and *in vitro* cytotoxicity in CHO and V79 cells after exposure to mineral fibers, pp. 155-169. In: *Short-Term Genetic Bioassays in the Analysis of the Complex Environmental Mixtures,* MD Waters, SF Sandu, J Lewtas, L Claxton, G Strauss, and S Nesnow (eds.). Plenum Publishing Corporation, New York, NY.

Palekar, LD, JF Eyre, HC Price, BG Brown, and DL Coffin. **1985b.** Biological activities of zeolite (erionite) in comparison with asbestos. The Toxicologist 5:38.

Palekar, LD, JF Eyre, BM Most, and DL Coffin. **1987.** Metaphase and anaphase analysis of V79 cells exposed to erionite, UICC chrysotile and UICC crocidolite. Carcinogenesis 8:553-560.

Palekar, LD, BM Most, and DL Coffin. **1988.** Significance of mineral fibers in the determination of V79 cytotoxicity. Environ Res 46:142-152.

Sandberg, AA and C Turc-Carel. **1987.** The cytogenetics of solid tumors. Cancer 59: 387-395.

Stanton, MF. **1973.** Some etiological considerations of fiber carcinogenesis, pp. 289-294. In: *Biological Effects of Asbestos,* P Bogovski, JC Gilson, V Timbrell, and JC Wagner (eds.). International Agency for Research on Cancer, Lyon, France.

Stanton, MF, M Layard, A Tegeris, E Miller, M May, and E Kent. **1977.** Carcinogenicity of fibrous glass: Pleural response in the rat in relation to fiber dimension. J Natl Cancer Inst 58:587-603.

Szpirer, J, D Defio-Jones, RW Ellis, G Levan, and C Szpirer. **1985.** Assignment of three rat cellular *ras* oncogenes to chromosomes 1, 4, and X. Somat Cell Genet 11: 93-97.

Wagner, JC, JW Skidmore, RJ Hill, and MD Griffiths. **1985.** Erionite exposure and mesotheliomas in rats. Br J Cancer 51:727-730.

Wang, NS, MC Jaurand, L Magne, L Knevang, MC Pinchon, and J Bignon. **1987.** The interactions between asbestos fibers and metaphase chromosomes of rat pleural mesothelial cells in culture. Am J Pathol 126:343-349.

Yunis, JJ. **1983.** The chromosomal basis of human neoplasia. Science 221:227-236.

MISCELLANEOUS RELATED PRESENTATIONS

A Possible Influence of Mineral Fibers on Cigarette-Smoking-Induced Changes in Lipids and Lipid-Metabolizing Enzymes

Ching-Hong Chen

Northwest Lipid Research Clinic, Department of Medicine, University of Washington, Harborview Medical Center, Seattle, WA 98104

KEY WORDS: serum lipids, enzymes, cigarette smoke

ABSTRACT

Cigarette-smoking and serum lipid concentrations have been shown to be independently related to cancer incidence. To examine the relationship between them, studies were carried out by measuring cholesterol (CH), triglycerides (TG), apolipoprotein A-1 (apo A-1), apolipoprotein B (apo B), and lecithin-cholesterol acyltransferase (LCAT) in serum samples from an adult population, ages 26 to 54 years, in the city of Taipei, Taiwan. Men and women who smoked cigarettes had significantly lower concentrations of high-density lipoprotein (HDL)-CH, apo A-1, and LCAT than men and women who did not smoke cigarettes. However, no significant differences between smokers and nonsmokers were observed in serum TG and apo B. The smokers' serum HDL-CH was approximately 83%, apo A-1 was 86%, and LCAT was 85% of the corresponding components in the serum of nonsmokers. These results indicated that, in human subjects, cigarette-smoking may either affect the synthesis of HDL components, including CH, apo A-1, and LCAT, or the transport of HDL from the site of synthesis (liver) to the circulation. Furthermore, the reduction in HDL may be a predisposing factor for cancer development. The possible influence of mineral fibers on cigarette-smoking-induced changes in lipids and lipoproteins can be ascertained by examining subjects who were exposed to both mineral fibers and cigarette smoke.

INTRODUCTION

Cigarette-smoking has been shown to be an important risk factor for both cancer (Farber, 1981; Schatzkin et al., 1988) and coronary heart diseases (CHD; Criqui et al., 1987; Doyle et al., 1962). Similarly, serum lipids, especially cholesterol (CH), have also been shown to be closely associated with cancer (Kark et al., 1980; Schatzkin et al., 1988; Stubbe et al., 1982; Williams et al., 1981) and CHD (Castell et al., 1983; Levy, 1981). Low concentrations of serum CH are believed to be related to increased cancer incidence (Kark et al., 1980; Schatzkin et al., 1988; Williams et al., 1981), whereas high concentrations of serum CH are known to be strongly linked to CHD (Castell et al., 1983; Levy, 1981). Because of their relationship to both cancer and CHD, cigarette-smoking and serum lipid concentrations, including those of lipoproteins, would be expected to correlate with one other. Recently, several reports have indicated that cigarette-smoking decreases the mass of high-density lipoprotein (HDL)-CH (Carrison et al., 1978; Haffner et al., 1985; Stubbe et al., 1982), HDL-apolipoproteins (Berg et al., 1978; Haffner et al., 1985; Stubbe et al., 1982), and lecithin-cholesterol acyltransferase (LCAT; Albers et al., 1982; Haffner et al., 1985) in human plasma. Until now, there has been no systematic study on the effect of cigarette-smoking on the concentrations of serum lipids and lipoproteins, and on the activity of lipid-metabolizing enzymes in human subjects.

This study was designed to investigate, in human subjects, the influence of cigarette-smoking on concentrations of serum CH and triglycerides (TG), HDL-CH and TG, serum apo A-1 and apo B, and serum LCAT activity. We hope that the results will provide information for a better understanding of the relationship of smoking and serum lipid concentrations to the risk of cancer and CHD.

METHODS

Human Subject Selection

The study population consisted of 143 volunteers from northern Taiwan. Subjects were between 26 and 54 years old, had no signs of renal, hepatic, heart, or metabolic disorders and were otherwise healthy. Seventy-nine subjects were male (37 nonsmokers and 42 smokers) and 64 were female (34 nonsmokers and 30 smokers). They consumed a normal diet and drank little or no alcohol. At the time of the study, smokers had been smoking for at least 8 years, at a rate of more than 20 cigarettes per day. In order to more clearly determine the effects of smoking on serum lipids, subjects were selected so that their average age was about 40 years (middle age).

Serum Sample Preparation

Blood samples were collected into tubes, under standard conditions, after an overnight fast of 12 to 14 hours (Chen and Albers, 1982a, 1986). Serum samples were obtained by centrifugation at 1500 x g for 30 minutes at 4°C. Samples were then stored at 4°C and analyzed without unnecessary delay, usually within 30 minutes.

Lipid Analysis

The HDL fraction was obtained by the dextran sulfate magnesium precipitation method (Chen and Albers, 1982b). Total serum CH, HDL-CH, total serum TG, and HDL-TG were determined by the enzyme procedure described by Albers et al. (1986) and Chen and Albers (1982b).

Apolipoprotein Measurement

Serum apo A-1 and apo B were measured by radial immunodiffusion, as previously described by Albers et al. (1986) and Chen and Albers (1986); coefficients of variation were <5 and <6%, for apo A-1 and apo B, respectively.

Lecithin-Cholesterol Acyltransferase (LCAT) Activity Assay

LCAT activity was determined by a precise common substrate method (Albers et al., 1986; Chen and Albers, 1982a); coefficient of variation was <5%.

Statistical Analysis

Results were expressed as mean ± standard deviation. The Wilcoxon rank sum test (Armitage, 1971) was used to determine significant differences between men and women, and between smokers and nonsmokers. Correlations between variables were analyzed by linear regression analysis.

RESULTS AND DISCUSSION

In this study, the effect of cigarette-smoking on total serum lipids (CH and TG), HDL lipids (CH and TG), apolipoproteins (A-1 and B), and LCAT activity were examined in 79 healthy men (37 nonsmokers and 42 smokers) and 64 healthy women (34 nonsmokers and 30 smokers) between the ages of 26 and 54 years. The smoking histories of all subjects were completely documented. The average

age and body mass index of these subjects were comparable between nonsmokers and smokers of both gender groups (Table 1).

Table 1. Mean (± SD) for age and body mass index (BMI) of nonsmokers and smokers examined.

Group	Number	Age (Years)	BMI (kg/m^2)
Nonsmokers			
Men	37	42.4 ± 11.2	23.5 ± 1.6
Women	34	38.2 ± 15.3	21.8 ± 1.4
Smokers			
Men	42	40.6 ± 12.4	22.1 ± 1.3
Women	30	39.5 ± 13.0	23.7 ± 1.7

When lipids were compared between males and females in this selected population, men had slightly higher total serum CH concentrations than women in both nonsmoking and smoking groups (Table 2). In contrast, men tended to have lower total serum TG concentrations than women in both nonsmoking and smoking groups (Table 2). These relationships have been found repeatedly in healthy populations of various races (Haffner et al., 1985).

Table 2. Effect of cigarette-smoking on lipid concentrations in serum and on the high-density lipoprotein (HDL) fraction in subjects examined.

Group	Number	Serum Cholesterol (mg/dl)	HDL Cholesterol (mg/dl)	Serum Triglycerides (mg/dl)	HDL Triglycerides (mg/dl)
Nonsmokers					
Men	37	176 ± 24	42.5 ± 9.4	88.7 ± 34	7.5 ± 2.4
Women	34	172 ± 21	43.6 ± 8.7	97.8 ± 32	8.6 ± 3.2
Smokers					
Men	42	180 ± 27	35.2 ± 7.3	87.5 ± 41	7.2 ± 2.8
Women	30	175 ± 20	37.5 ± 6.4	101.4 ± 43	9.0 ± 3.0

When lipids were compared between smokers and nonsmokers, male smokers had slightly higher total serum CH concentrations than male nonsmokers (180 versus 176 mg/dl), and female smokers also had slightly higher total serum CH concentrations than female nonsmokers (175 versus 172 mg/dl); neither difference reached statistical significance. However, it is important that smokers' serum had significantly lower HDL-CH concentrations than nonsmokers' serum, both in men (35.2 versus 42.5 mg/dl) and women (37.5 versus 43.6 mg/dl; Table 2). An average reduction in HDL-CH of approximately 17 and 13% was observed for male and female smokers, respectively. On the other hand, no significant difference in HDL-TG was found between smoking and nonsmoking groups of either gender (Table 2). These results indicated that smoking did not cause a significant change in total serum CH, total serum TG or HDL-TG, but it did cause a significant reduction in HDL-CH, as was also shown recently by other investigators (Carrison et al., 1978; Haffner et al., 1985; Stubbe et al., 1982). The decrease in HDL-CH caused by smoking may be related to the risk of CHD, because HDL is believed to be a protective factor against CHD. Whether the reduction in HDL-CH is also a predisposing factor for cancer development needs further investigation.

As in the effect of smoking on HDL-CH, 16 and 14% reductions in serum apo A-1 concentrations were observed for male and female smokers, respectively, compared to their corresponding nonsmoking groups. Mean apo A-1 concentrations were 102.0 and 121.5 mg/dl, respectively, for male smokers and male nonsmokers, and 110.5 and 128.6 mg/dl, respectively, for female smokers and nonsmokers. Because apo A-1 is a major protein component of HDL, a reduction in apo A-1 was accompanied by a decrease in HDL-CH (Table 3). It appears that apo A-1 may be a better indicator than HDL-CH for the effect of smoking on lipoproteins, because proteins are generally known to be less responsive than lipids to dietary changes. The effect of smoking on apo B, which is a major protein component of low-density lipoprotein (LDL), was not statistically significant; a slight increase in serum apo B concentration was observed in the serum of smokers of both sexes (Table 3). These results also indicate that smoking affected mostly the HDL fraction.

In human serum, most of the LCAT enzyme has been found to be associated with the HDL fraction (Chen and Albers, 1982b). Therefore, one would expect a cigarette-smoke-mediated decrease in HDL to be accompanied by a decrease in LCAT enzyme; a comparison of Tables 2 and 3 bears this out. A decrease of approximately 13% in LCAT activity has been reported in both men and women smokers by others (Albers et al., 1982; Haffner et al., 1985). LCAT is believed to play a key role in removing CH from circulation and peripheral tissues. The decrease in LCAT enzyme, together with the reduction in HDL-CH (LCAT substrate) and apo A-1 (LCAT cofactor) that was caused by cigarette-smoking, may alter lipoprotein metabolism in serum and aggravate the risk of atherosclerosis and cancer. The mechanism by which cigarette-smoking decreases the serum HDL fraction is not known; it may be due to decreased biosynthesis of HDL components or to a reduction in the transport of HDL from cells to the circulation, or both.

Table 3. Effect of cigarette-smoking on serum apolipoprotein A-1 (apo A-1) and apolipoprotein B (apo B) concentrations and lecithin-cholesterol acyltransferase (LCAT) activity in subjects examined.

Group	Number	Serum Apo A-1 (mg/dl)	Serum Apo B (mg/dl)	Serum LCAT Activity (nmol/hr/ml)
Nonsmokers				
Men	37	121.5 ± 22.0	98.7 ± 23.6	95.7 ± 16.2
Women	34	128.6 ± 25.8	97.4 ± 20.2	98.6 ± 18.0
Smokers				
Men	42	102.0 ± 18.2	102.3 ± 22.5	81.5 ± 13.6
Women	30	110.5 ± 20.7	99.2 ± 24.3	83.8 ± 14.7

Recently, mineral fibers and cigarette-smoking have been shown to synergistically increase DNA damage, thereby increasing the incidence of cancer (Jackson et al., 1988; Kao-Shan et al., 1987). We do not yet know whether mineral fibers have a similar effect on cigarette-smoking-induced changes in serum lipids and lipoproteins. However, investigations are in progress to answer this question by exposing animals individually or simultaneously to mineral fibers and cigarette smoke.

REFERENCES

Albers, JJ, RO Bergelin, JL Adolphson, and PW Wahl. **1982.** Population-based reference values for lecithin-cholesterol acyltransferase. Atherosclerosis 43:369-379.

Albers, JJ, C-H Chen, and AG Lacko. **1986.** Isolation, characterization, and assay of lecithin-cholesterol acyltransferase. Meth Enzymol 129:763-783.

Armitage, P. **1971.** *Statistical Methods in Medical Research.* John Wiley Press, New York, NY.

Berg, K, AL Borresen, and G Dahlen. **1978.** Effect of smoking on serum levels of HDL apoproteins. Atherosclerosis 30:17-25.

Carrison, RJ, WR Kannel, M Feinleib, WP Castell, PM McNamara, and SJ Padgett. **1978.** Cigarette smoking and HDL cholesterol. Atherosclerosis 30:17-25

Castell, WP, RD Abbott, and PM McNamara. **1983.** Summary estimates of cholesterol used to predict coronary heart disease. Circulation 67:730-734.

Chen, C-H and JJ Albers. **1982a.** Characterization of proteoliposomes containing apoprotein A-1: A new substrate for the measurement of lecithin-cholesterol acyltransferase activity. J Lipid Res 23:680-691.

Chen, C-H and JJ Albers. **1982b.** Distribution of lecithin-cholesterol acyltransferase (LCAT) in human plasma lipoprotein fractions. Biochem Biophys Res Commun 107: 1091-1096.

Chen, C-H and JJ Albers. **1986.** Stimulation of lecithin-cholesterol acyltransferase activity by apolipoprotein A-II in the presence of apolipoprotein A-I. Eur J Biochem 155:589-594.

Criqui, MH, LD Cowan, HA Tyroler, S Bangdiwala, G Heiss, RB Wallace, and R Cohn. **1987.** Lipoproteins as mediators for the effects of alcohol consumption and cigarette smoking on cardiovascular mortality. Am J Epidemiol 126:629-637.

Doyle, JT, TR Dawber, WB Kannel, AS Heslin, and HA Kahn. **1962.** Cigarette smoking and coronary heart disease. N Engl J Med 266:796-801.

Farber, E. **1981.** Chemical carcinogenesis. N Engl J Med 305:1379-1389.

Haffner, SM, D Applebaum-Bowden, PW Wahl, JJ Hoover, GR Warnick, JJ Albers, and WR Hazzard. **1985.** Epidemiological correlates of high density lipoprotein subfractions, apolipoproteins A-I, A-II, and D, and lecithin cholesterol acyltransferase: Effect of smoking, alcohol, and adiposity. Arteriosclerosis 5:169-177.

Jackson, JH, IU Schraufstatter, PA Hyslop, K Vosbeck, R Sauerheber, SA Weitzman, and CG Cochrane. **1988.** Role of oxidants in DNA damage: Hydroxyl radical mediates the synergistic DNA damaging effects of asbestos and cigarette smoke. J Clin Invest 80:1090-1095.

Kao-Shan, CS, RL Fine, J Whang-Peng, EC Lee, and BA Chabner. **1987.** Increased fragile sites and sister chromatid exchanges in bone marrow and peripheral blood of young cigarette smokers. Cancer Res 47:6278-6282

Kark, JD, AH Smith, and CG Hames. **1980.** The relationship of serum cholesterol to the incidence of cancer in Evans County, Georgia. J Chronic Dis 33:311-322.

Levy, RI. **1981.** Cholesterol, lipoproteins, apoproteins and heart diseases: Present status and future prospects. Clin Chem 27:653-662.

Schatzkin, A, RN Hoover, PR Taylor, RG Ziegler, CL Carter, D Albanes, DB Larson, and LM Licitra. **1988.** Site-specific analysis of total serum cholesterol and incident cancer in the National Health and Nutrition Examination Survey. 1. Epidemiologic follow-up study. Cancer Res 48:452-458.

Stubbe, I, J Eskilsson, and P Nilsson-Ehle. **1982.** High-density lipoprotein concentrations increase after stopping smoking. Br Med J 284:1511-1513.

Williams, RR, PD Sorlie, M Feinleib, PM McNamara, WB Kannel, and TR Dawber. **1981.** Cancer incidence by levels of cholesterol. J Am Med Assoc 245:247-252.

A Novel Culture System for Maintaining Differentiated Respiratory Epithelial Cells Between Air and Liquid Phases: A Possible Model for Studying Interactions Between Mineral Fibers, Gases, and Airway Epithelium*

Kenneth B. Adler,[1] Nancey J. Akley,[1] Gail Ayers,[1] Wendy J. Holden-Stauffer,[1] Jody B. Khosla,[1] and Kwang C. Kim[2]

[1]Department of Anatomy, Physiological Sciences and Radiology, College of Veterinary Medicine, North Carolina State University, Raleigh, NC 27606

[2]Pulmonary Center, School of Medicine, Boston University, Boston, MA 02118

KEY WORDS: airway, epithelium, culture, mucus

ABSTRACT

In this report we describe a unique cell culture system in which the pseudostratified columnar epithelium of guinea pig airways, containing normal-appearing ciliated, secretory and basal cells, is reproduced in primary culture. Quantitative electron microscopic morphometric analysis of the cell cultures versus intact segments of guinea pig airways revealed almost identical values for several parameters, including frequency of cell types (goblet, secretory and basal); cells per unit length of basement membrane, epithelial height, and volume density of mucus granules per goblet cell. The cultures incorporate radiolabeled precursors of mucus into the secretory cells, and synthesize and release mucus with the same biochemical properties as

*Supported by Grants HL-37B36 and HL-3B982 from the National Institutes of Health, and a grant from the State of North Carolina. Dr. Adler is an Established Investigator of The American Heart Association.

mucus collected from animals *in vivo* or from airway tissue explants. The cultured cells metabolize arachidonic acid via both cyclo-oxygenase and lipoxygenase pathways, and release mucus in response to exposure to a number of environmentally related substances, such as oxygen radicals.

INTRODUCTION

Interactions between inhaled particulates and gases, and epithelial cells of the respiratory mucosa (the first cells with which these substances come in contact upon inhalation) necessarily play a major role in the pathogenesis of many neoplastic and obstructive pulmonary disorders. Despite the obvious importance of these interactions, cellular mechanisms involved have not been fully elucidated. This is due, in large part, to the lack of an appropriate model system with which to study these biological phenomena.

For several decades, researchers have used explants of mammalian airways maintained in organ culture to study epithelial-cell function under normal and pathologic conditions. (For a review, see Adler, 1986.) However, organ cultures have the inherent problem of containing many different cell types. For example, an explant of mammalian airway contains, along with epithelium, connective tissue cells, mast cells, muscle cells, endothelium, and blood elements such as platelets and leukocytes. All of these can release bioactive components that can secondarily affect epithelial function, confounding attempts to elucidate, in detail, intracellular mechanisms governing epithelial cell responses and actions.

Recently, attention has turned to development of monolayer cell cultures of respiratory epithelium. Although these systems generally present a relatively homogeneous population of epithelial cells for studies of mechanisms, the cells maintained in monolayer culture generally have little, if any, resemblance to airway epithelium *in situ,* often displaying minimal differentiated characteristics. Recently, we have described a monolayer cell-culture system in which the pseudostratified columnar cells of the guinea pig tracheobronchial epithelium is essentially reproduced *in vitro* (Adler et al., 1987a; Whitcutt et al., in press). The cells are maintained on a collagen gel atop a permeable filter, and are fed from beneath only; they are exposed to an air interface on top. In this report we describe experiments further characterizing cells maintained in this system.

METHODS AND MATERIALS

Cell Cultures

Primary cultures of respiratory epithelial cells from the guinea pig were established as described previously (Whitcutt et al., in press;

Adler et al., 1987a). Briefly, the trachea and mainstem bronchi are dissected free from male, Hartley-strain guinea pigs, weighing approximately 250 g, opened longitudinally, and incubated in sterile 0.1% pronase for 1 hour at 37°C. The epithelial layer is removed, and the cell clumps tritiated before centrifugation at 800 rpm for 8 minutes at 4°C. The cell pellet is resuspended in 5 ml complete PC-1 medium (Ventrex Corp., Portland, ME) containing 10% fetal calf serum. After a second centrifugation, the cell pellet is resuspended in PC-1 medium, and the cells seeded onto the collagen-coated culture chamber (see below) at approximately 1×10^5 cells per chamber. After the fourth day, the cells are fed with serumless Ventrex PC-1 medium and are fed every 2 to 3 days thereafter. Optimal growth, differentiation and polarity occurs between 7 and 14 days.

The chamber system for maintaining these cells consists of commercially purchased inserts (Millipore Corp., Bedford, MA) coated with Matrigel® (Collaborative Research, Boston, MA). In this system, all the medium added to the cells is added from beneath; the cells are exposed only to an air interface (95% air/5% CO_2/100% humidity). A complete description of this system is provided in Adler et al. (1987a).

Morphometric Analysis of Cultures

After 8 days in culture, six separate culture wells were fixed in 2.5% glutaraldehyde in 0.2 M cacodylate buffer, pH 7.4, at 340 mosm, for 2 hours at room temperature. The cells were postfixed in 1% OsO_4, dehydrated through a graded series of alcohols and propylene oxide, and embedded in Spurr's medium for morphometric studies.

Sections of the cell cultures (approximately 2 x 2 mm) were mounted randomly on plastic blocks and step-sectioned as follows: Five thick (1-μm) sections were cut and discarded, then six thin (600-to 800-Å) sections were cut and mounted on a 200-mesh copper grid. The block was then thick-sectioned through an additional 10 μm before being thin-sectioned, and the thin sections were mounted on another 200-mesh grid. The process was repeated to allow for at least 30 separate transverse sections through the eight separate cultures.

To compare the cellular population of the cultures to that in actual airways, sections of guinea pig trachea were cut and fixed immediately in the glutaraldehyde fixative described above. The sections were osmicated, embedded, and sectioned as described for the cell cultures, with care taken to section transversely. Approximately 30 sections were examined for each of two animals.

All sections were photographed in a Philips 410 transmission electron microscope at 900X magnification, and the prints further magnified to 2,400X. The micrographs then were analyzed for the following morphometric parameters: percentage of cell types (e.g., ciliated, goblet, basal) identified on the basis of morphological criteria; cell frequency (cells per unit length of "basement membrane"); cell size; average epithelial height; and volume density of mucin granules per goblet cell.

Biochemical Analysis of Mucin Secreted by Cultures

Spent media from seven separate cultures were pooled and lyophilized after measurement of pH. The lyophilized samples were redissolved in double-distilled water, and applied to a Sepharose CL-4B chromatography column (1.0 x 60 cm) eluted with phosphate-buffered saline (PBS). Void volume fractions (#22 through #25, total 2.2 ml, 52 cpm/10 lambda) were treated with *Streptomyces* hyaluronidase (Sigma Chemical Co., St, Louis, MO). Five hundred microliters of sample were then treated with 30 lambda of enzyme (10 units) at 37°C for 16 hours, then rechromatographed on Sepharose CL-4B columns eluted with PBS plus 0.1% sodium dodecyl sulfate (SDS). The sample then was treated with heparinase (Sigma: 30 lambda enzyme; 10 units) followed by chromatography on Sepharose CL-4B eluted with PBS plus 0.1% SDS. The last step was digestion of 500 lambda of sample with 20 lambda chondroitinase ABC (0.5 units; Sigma) plus 5 lambda 0.2 M $CaCl_2$ at 37°C for 6 hours.

Effects of Environmentally Related Substances on Mucin Secretion

Oxidant Exposure. Inhalation of a variety of toxic agents is known to stimulate production of oxygen-free radicals by a number of cell types within the respiratory system. As oxygen-free radicals are often associated with pulmonary lesions related to airway obstruction, we investigated the effects of oxidants on secretion of mucin by cell cultures. Superoxide anion was generated chemically by addition of xanthine oxidase (0.02 U/ml) to purine (0.2 mM) in the culture medium, and hydrogen peroxide (H_20_2) was generated by addition of glucose oxidase to β-D-glucose. Secretion of mucin was measured after 1-hour exposure of the cells to the oxidants (see below).

Platelet-Activating Factor (PAF). PAF is a low-molecular-weight lipid immunological and inflammatory mediator known to cause a variety of deleterious effects in the lung, including bronchoconstriction and edema (Morley et al., 1985). Concentrations of PAF may be increased in the lung in response to inhalation of particulate or gaseous pollutants as part of an inflammatory response. We have previously demonstrated that high concentrations of PAF stimulate secretion of mucin by explant cultures of guinea pig airways (Adler et al., 1987b). We therefore wished to determine the effects of PAF on secretion of mucin by the cultures. The PAF was tested in concentrations of 10^{-6} M to 10^{-10} M.

Assay for Mucin Secretion

Mucin secretion was measured by incubating the cells with the mucin precursor tritiated glucosamine (10 μCi/ml) for 18 hours, allowing for its incorporation into intracellular granules. Secreted radiolabeled mucin was separated by chromatography on Sepharose CL-4B columns, and the void volume peak containing the high-molecular-weight mucins was counted by liquid scintillation. The amount of secretion for a 1- or 2-hour period after exposure to the test substances was expressed as a percentage of a 1- or 2-hour baseline secretion before addition of the agent. Media without the added agents were controls.

Metabolism of Arachidonic Acid

Exposure to pollutant particulates and gases is associated with production of metabolites of arachidonic acid in the lung (Adler et al., 1985). We investigated the ability of these cell cultures to metabolize arachidonic acid by exposing them to the calcium ionophore A-23187, known to stimulate arachidonic acid metabolism, then measuring the release of immunoreactive thromboxane B2 and leukotrienes by radioimmunoassay (RIA). Since the cell cultures were exposed to a liquid phase beneath and only air on top, accumulation of eicosinoids could be measured separately from the tops and bottoms of the cultures, reflecting apical or basal release. Accumulation of immunoreactive thromboxane B2, and leukotrienes LTC_4 and LTB_4 was measured by using RIA kits purchased from New England Nuclear (Boston, MA) or Amersham Corp. (Arlington Heights, IL).

RESULTS

Morphometric Analysis of Cultures

Results of the morphometric studies are illustrated in Table 1. The frequencies, sizes and intracellular granule populations of the goblet cells were quite similar to those values in intact segments of guinea pig airways.

Table 1. Morphometric analysis of cell cultures.

	Percent in Cell Cultures	Percent in Intact Airways
Cells		
Ciliated	27.6	28.9
Secretory	31.7	26.4
Basal	28.2	39.9
Other	12.5	5.4
Number of cells/10 μm basement membrane length	2.4	3.0
Epithelial height (μm)	18.4	26.8
Volume density of mucin granules/ secretory cell	37.7	38.2

Biochemical Analysis of Mucin Secreted by Cultures

Ninety-six percent of the hyaluronidase-resistant large-molecular-weight material eluting in the void volume was resistant to chondroitinase ABC and to heparinase, as was consistent with the properties of authentic mucin.

Effects of Environmentally Related Substances on Mucin Secretion

Oxidant Exposure. As illustrated in Table 2, purine plus xanthine oxidase stimulated secretion of mucin by the cell cultures, whereas glucose plus glucose oxidase, which generated hydrogen peroxide, was ineffective.

Platelet-Activating Factor (PAF). The effects of PAF on secretion of mucin by the cultures are illustrated in Table 2. The maximal response was to a PAF concentration of 10^{-9} M.

Arachidonic Acid Metabolism

As illustrated in Table 3, the cells released prostaglandins, thromboxane and leukotrienes, both basally and apically. Release was augmented by exposure to calcium ionophore.

Table 2. Effects of oxidants and platelet-activating factor (PAF) on secretion of mucin by cell cultures.

Agent/Concentration	Number of Cultures	Mucin Secretion Expressed as Percent of Control
Purine (0.2 mM) plus xanthine oxidase (0.02 U/ml)	22	179 ± 21[a]
β-D-Glucose (1%) plus glucose oxidase (3.5 U/ml)	12	108 ± 13
β-D-Glucose (1%) plus glucose oxidase (0.35 U/ml)	12	103 ± 5
PAF (M)		
10^{-6}	10	111 ± 7
10^{-7}	10	126 ± 7
10^{-8}	10	145 ± 9[a]
10^{-9}	10	208 ± 24[a]
10^{-10}	10	119 ± 11

[a]$P < 0.05$ compared to controls

Table 3. Accumulation of arachidonate metabolites by cell cultures[a]

	Control	Ca Ionophore A-23817 (10 μM)
Thromboxane (pg/ml)		
Top	49.0 ± 12.4	133.8 ± 6.7
Bottom	91.2 ± 21.2	240.5 ± 9.4
LTB_4 (pg/ml)		
Top	17.6 ± 11.7	13.2 ± 3.2
Bottom	13.1 ± 12.9	193.5 ± 21.6
LTC_4 (pg/ml)		
Top	22.0 ± 14.0	34.6 ± 12.5
Bottom	26.0 ± 21.2	63.3 ± 26.5

[a]N = 6 for each experiment

DISCUSSION

The culture system described in this report combines many advantages of cell culture (a homogeneous population of mucosal epithelium with which to study mechanisms) while maintaining epithelial cells in near-normal orientation. This system also allows for cell-cell interactions, which undoubtedly influence responses *in vivo* and *in situ* to exogenous particulate and gaseous materials, as well as to endogenous immunological and inflammatory mediators. Because these cultures are fed only from beneath, and are exposed to an air interface above, the system is ideal for studying interactions between respiratory epithelium and inhaled fibers and gases.

Many of the studies described in this report were undertaken to investigate similarities and differences between cells maintained in this system and those *in situ* in airway epithelium, or maintained in explant cultures. With regard to morphology, the morphometric studies revealed a dramatically similar structure in both the cultured epithelial cells and in guinea pig airway epithelium *in situ*. Of special interest with regard to studies of mucin secretion was the similarity in the relative frequency of goblet cells and the mucous granule content within the cells. These similarities carried through to the biochemical characteristics of the secreted mucin. The mucin released by the cell cultures which originated from the intracellular granules was almost identical to mucin released by explant cultures of rodent airways. In both, 96% of the hyaluronidase-resistant macromolecules were also resistant to chondroitinase ABC and heparinase.

The response to agents that have been shown to stimulate secretion by explant cultures was also similar. In previous studies, we demonstrated that purine plus xanthine oxidase, which generates superoxide anion, stimulated mucin secretion by explants of rodent airways, while hydrogen peroxide, generated by β-D-glucose and glucose oxidase, did not affect secretion (Adler and Repine, 1987). The cell cultures responded to purine plus xanthine oxidase, but not to β-D-glucose, paralleling the response of the explants.

A difference was noted, however, in the response to PAF. Previously, we have demonstrated that PAF stimulated secretion of mucin by explant cultures, but only at relatively high ($>10^{-5}$ M) concentrations (Adler et al., 1987b). The cell cultures, however, responded maximally to lower concentrations of PAF, those in the nanomolar range. Interestingly enough, this is the same concentration at which PAF exerts its maximal bronchoconstrictor effect (Vargaftig et al., 1981; Morley et al., 1985), raising interesting possibilities for a generalized PAF-induced response in the lung related to generation of an asthmatic response.

Results of studies on arachidonic acid metabolites produced by these cell cultures suggest that airway epithelial cells may release these products in a directional manner (e.g., apically versus basally or basolaterally). As illustrated in Table 2, generation of thromboxane was about two times greater basally than apically, while LTB_4 was released at a 10:1 ratio (basal:apical). Because eicosinoids produced by airway epithelium are known to modulate the responsiveness of airway-associated smooth muscle (Butler et al., 1987), these results may have important implications for elucidating mechanisms of airway hyper-reactivity in relation to epithelial damage caused by a variety of inhaled or infectious agents.

REFERENCES

Adler, KB. **1986.** Mucin secretion by respiratory tract tissue *in vitro,* pp. 27-50. In: *In Vitro Models of Respiratory Epithelium,* LJ Schiff (ed.). CRC Press, Boca Raton, FL.

Adler, KB, GB Butler, DR Hemenway, JE Schwarz, PO Banks, and JN Evans. **1985.** Exposure of small airways to cristobalite *in vitro,* pp. 293-301. In: *In Vitro Effects of Mineral Dusts,* Vol G-3, E Beck and J Bignon (eds.), NATO ASI Series. Springer-Verlag, Heidelberg, Federal Republic of Germany.

Adler, KB and JE Repine. **1987.** Superoxide anion stimulates arachidonic acid-dependent secretion of mucin by explant and cell cultures of rodent respiratory epithelium. Am Rev Respir Dis 135:A164.

Adler, KB, JE Schwarz, MJ Whitcutt, and R Wu. **1987a.** A new chamber system for maintaining differentiated guinea pig respiratory epithelial cells between air and liquid phases. Biotechniques 5:462-467.

Adler, KB, JE Schwarz, WH Anderson, and AF Welton. **1987b.** Platelet-activating factor stimulates secretion of mucin by explants of rodent airways in organ culture. Exp Lung Res 13:25-43.

Butler, GB, KB Adler, JN Evans, and J Szarek J. **1987.** Modulation of rabbit airways smooth muscle responsiveness by respiratory epithelium: Involvement of an inhibitory metabolite of arachidonic acid. Am Rev Respir Dis 135:1099-1104.

Morley, J, CP Page, and S Sanjar. **1985.** Pulmonary responses to platelet activating factor. Progr Respir Res 19:117-123.

Vargaftig, BB, M Chignard, J Benveniste, J Lefort, and F Wal. **1981.** Background and present status of research on platelet-activating factor (PAF-acether). Ann NY Acad Sci 370:119-137.

Whitcutt, JM, KB Adler, and R Wu. A biphasic chamber system for maintaining polarity of differentiation of cultured respiratory tract epithelial cells. In Vitro (**in press**).

Physicochemical Properties and Membranolytic Activities of the Titanium Dioxide Polymorphs Compared with those of Quartz

Robert P. Nolan,* Arthur M. Langer,* and George B. Herson

Center for Polypeptide and Membrane Research, Mount Sinai School of Medicine, New York, NY 10029

KEY WORDS: titania, rutile, anatase, quartz, membranolytic activity, erythrocytes

ABSTRACT

Due to the variations in the surface properties of the titanium dioxide polymorphs rutile and anatase, some specimens were found to be membranolytic to erythrocytes, and others were inactive. The membranolytic activity of five TiO_2 specimens was compared with that of quartz. Three rutile samples and the quartz were active; one rutile specimen and one anatase specimen were inactive. For each of the six specimens, the structure was verified by continuous-scan X-ray diffraction, the particle-size distribution was determined, and energy-dispersive X-ray analysis was used to further characterize the chemistry. The surface properties of each specimen were characterized by their ability to hydrogen-bond polymers, the effect of heating, and the mechanism for erythrocyte lysis. The properties of the six specimens were compared to determine their relationship with membranolytic activity.

INTRODUCTION

The physicochemical properties and membranolytic activity of two titanium dioxide polymorphs, rutile and anatase, were compared

*Present address: Environmental Sciences Laboratory, Applied Science Institute of the City University of New York at Brooklyn College, Flatbush Avenue, Brooklyn, NY 11210.

with those of quartz. Both polymorphs are widely used commercially, ubiquitous in the environment, and commonly found in the human lung. Although these minerals occur naturally, the commercially available specimens are usually synthesized, using the sulfate or, more recently, the chloride reduction process. Virtually 100% of the particles made synthetically are in the respirable size range. In the past, TiO_2 was considered to have no irreversible effects on the lung after inhalation and, on that basis, was identified as a nuisance dust. It was commonly used as a negative control for inhalation studies and as an inert particle in lung-clearance studies (Ferin and Oberdörster, 1985). Then, in 1985, Lee et al. (1985a,b) reported that a synthetic rutile caused lung cancer in rats exposed to it by inhalation.

The TiO_2 used in the inhalation and clearance studies was seldom characterized in enough detail to allow comparison with the specimen used by Lee et al. (1985a,b). Besides the crystallographically distinct rutile and anatase, the synthetic titanium dioxides have particle surfaces that have been industrially altered to enhance their performance in various applications. As an example of the diversity of rutiles available, one major manufacturer markets four rutile slurries and at least seven different synthetic rutiles, for use in various industrial applications.

We have posed the questions: Do all the TiO_2 specimens used experimentally have the same low biological activity, or could some of the specimens have different surface properties that have enhanced biological activity? An initial study of 16 TiO_2 specimens demonstrated that the naturally occurring specimens of rutile and anatase lacked many of the characteristics associated with biologically active minerals (Nolan et al., 1987b). Of the remaining 11 synthetic rutile and anatase specimens studied, only two rutiles had properties consistent with biologically active minerals. The industrial source of only one of these rutiles was known with certainty; it was the same as the source of the specimen used in the inhalation experiments by Lee et al. (1985a,b). The chloride reduction process was used in their manufacture.

Three synthetic rutiles manufactured by the chloride reduction process were selected for further study (Table 1). They were compared with a rutile, an anatase and three quartz specimens used experimentally (as either positive or negative controls) in pneumoconiosis research. Each specimen was mineralogically characterized, and its membranolytic activity was determined.

Table 1. Characteristics of rutile, Du Pont R-100, R-900 and R-960.

Grade	Density (g/cm^3)	Typical Analysis	Principal Paint Pigment Application
R-100	4.2	97% TiO_2, 1.7% Al_2O_3	Interior glass finishes; trade sale and industrial
R-900	4.0	94% TiO_2, 4.5% Al_2O_3	General purposes; high-gloss and semi-gloss finishes
R-960	3.9	89% TiO_2, 3.5% Al_2O_3, 6.5% SiO_2	Exterior finishes requiring outstanding gloss, tint-retention, and chalk-resistance

MATERIALS AND METHODS

Materials

R-100 and R-900 (manufactured in Delisle, MS), and R-960 (manufactured in New Johnsonville, TN)—three rutile specimens obtained from E.I. Du Pont de Nemours & Company, Wilmington, DE 19896

Titanium Dioxide, Rutile—obtained from Central Research and Development Department, E.I. Du Pont de Nemours & Company, Haskell Laboratory for Toxicology and Industrial Medicine, Haskell No. 11, 564, P. 0. Box 50, Elkton Road, Newark, DE 19714

Titanium Dioxide No. 10082—a rutile specimen obtained from N. Wotherspoon, Mount Sinai School of Medicine (reportedly made by Du Pont)

IOM-1—a rutile specimen obtained from K. Donaldson, Institute of Occupational Medicine, Edinburgh, Scotland (for size distribution and X-ray characterization, see Nolan et al., 1987a)

Anatase P25—an anatase specimen obtained from Prof. F. Pott, University of Düsseldorf, Federal Republic of Germany (reportedly made by Degussa, FRG).

Min-U-Sil 15—a fine industrial quartz powder obtained from Pennsylvania Glass and Sand Company, Pittsburgh, PA. The "15" denotes that 98% of the particles are less than 15 μm in diameter. This specimen was studied both as an unfractionated powder and after fractionation into different size splits. The 1-, 2- and >2-μm Stokes' diameter fractions were separated. (For description of method, see Nolan and Langer, 1983.) The Min-U-Sil 15 size distributions therefore contains four sets of measurements. (For X-ray characterization, see Nolan et al., 1987a)

Quartz, Dorentrup, Mehlug, **DQ12,** and Quartz Frenchen, Sikron, **F600**—obtained from Prof. F. Pott, University of Düsseldorf, Federal Republic of Germany.

2-PVPNO [2-poly (vinylpyridine-N-oxide)]—obtained from Polyscience, Inc., Warrington, PA. The average molecular weight of the 2-PVPNO polymer, determined by light-scattering photometry, was 276,000 (Nolan and Langer, unpublished data).

DIDS (4,4′-diisothiocyanostilbene-2,2′-disulfonic acid disodium salt trihydrate); molecular weight, 552.5—obtained from Pierce Chemical Company, Rockford, IL.

Characterization of Particles

Optical Microscopy. Approximately 1-mg aliquots were withdrawn from each of the specimens, placed on a glass slide, immersed in mounting oil (N = 1.515), dispersed in the oil by means of gentle rotation with a second slide, coverslipped, and then examined with a polarizing microscope.

The industrially synthesized TiO_2 powders were observed to be optically pure, uniformly small in diameter (100% <2 μm), and homogeneous. The powders were indistinguishable by optical microscopy characterization.

Size-Distribution Measurements. Each specimen was photographed by transmission electron microscopy at 2000X direct magnification. The photographic plates were enlarged 2.5X to yield a final magnification of 5000X. However, the >2-μm Stokes' diameter fraction of Min-U-Sil 15 was photographed at 1000X direct magnification and enlarged to a final 2500X print magnification. The greatest dimensional aspect of each individual particle was measured; the results are therefore skewed toward larger particle-size values (Tables 2 and 3). Figures 1 through 4 are light and electron photomicrographs of the specimens.

X-Ray Diffraction Analysis. All specimens were examined by the continuous-scan powder diffraction technique, with instrument settings and conditions of analysis as described by Nolan et al. (1981). Powders were subjected to diffraction analysis in their received condition; they were not subjected to further pulverization. Scans were made between 5 and 85° 2-theta, corresponding to d-spacings between 17.7 and 1.14 Å.

Table 2. Particle-size distribution of titanium dioxide specimens.

	N	<0.20 μm (%)	0.0–0.50 μm (%)	0.21–0.50 μm (%)	0.51–0.75 μm (%)	>0.75 μm
Rutile, R-100	652	11.4		76.2	12.4	0
Anatase, P25	207	45.9		54.1	—	0
Rutile, R-900	434		90.1		9.9	
Rutile, R-960	430		90.0		10.0	

Table 3. Particle-size distributions measured on photographic prints (5000X magnification) obtained by electron microscopy.

Particle Size (μm):		<1.0	1.1-3.0	3.1-5.0	5.1-10.0	10.1-15.0	15.1-20.0	>20.0
	N[a]	Percentage						
Min-U-Sil 15								
Unfractionated	718	52.7	37.3	6.4	2.6	0.7	0.3	—
1-μm Stokes' diameter	770	60.9	34.6	3.8	0.8	—	—	—
2-μm Stokes' diameter	690	71.0	9.6	12.8	6.4	0.1	—	0.1
>2-μm Stokes' diameter[b]	581	45.7	19.1	4.0	18.3	11.0	1.4	0.5
DQ12	932	76.3	23.4	0.2	0.1	—	—	—
F600	719	38.3	40.5	14.1	6.7	0.6	—	—

[a]N = number of particles sized
[b]2,500X magnification

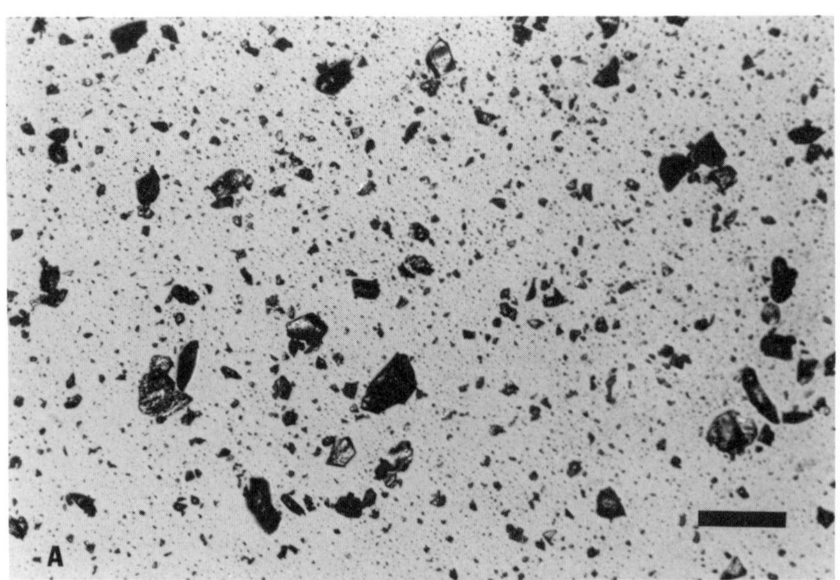

Figure 1. Light photomicrographs of three titanium dioxide specimens: A, naturally occurring rutile, Graves Mountain, GA; B, synthetic rutile, R-900; C, synthetic anatase P25. Bar represents 100 μm.

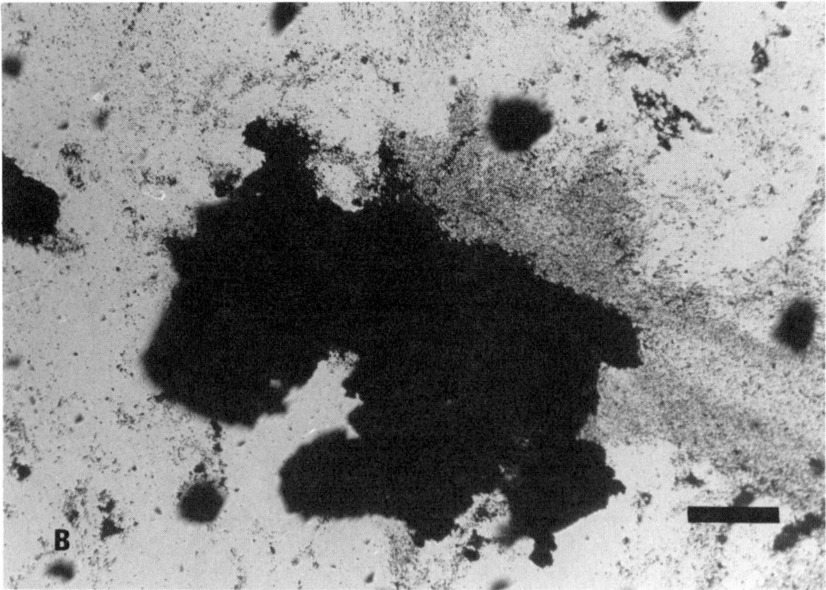

Figure 1B.

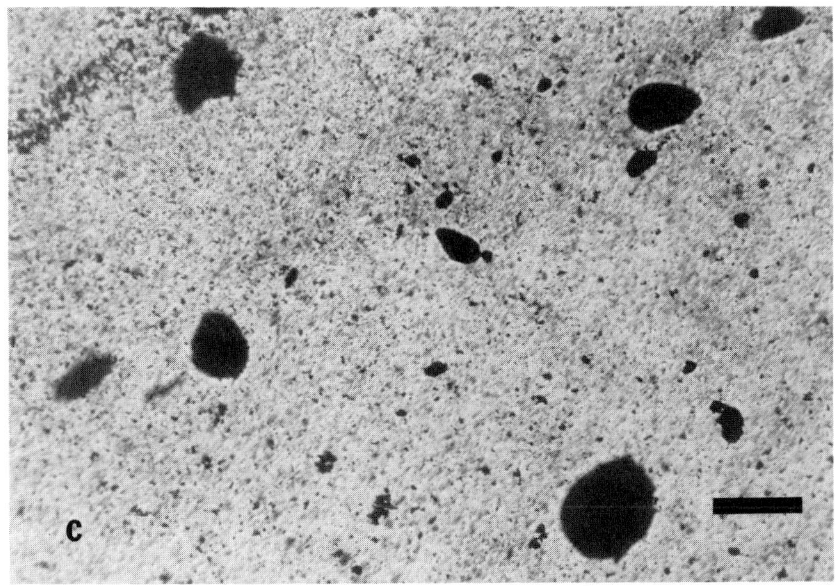

Figure 1C.

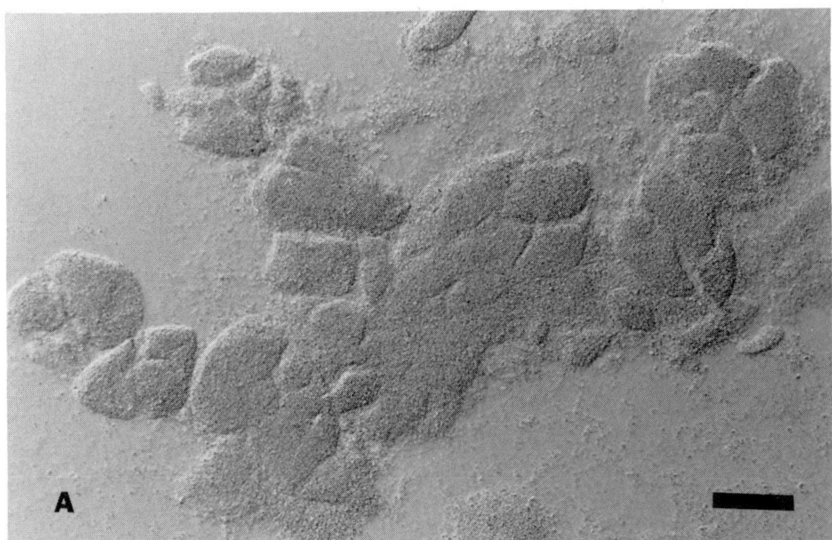

Figure 2. Light photomicrographs of three quartz specimens: A, DQ12; B, 1-μm Stokes' diameter Min-U-Sil 15; C, >2-μm Stokes' diameter Min-U-Sil 15. Bar represents 100 μm.

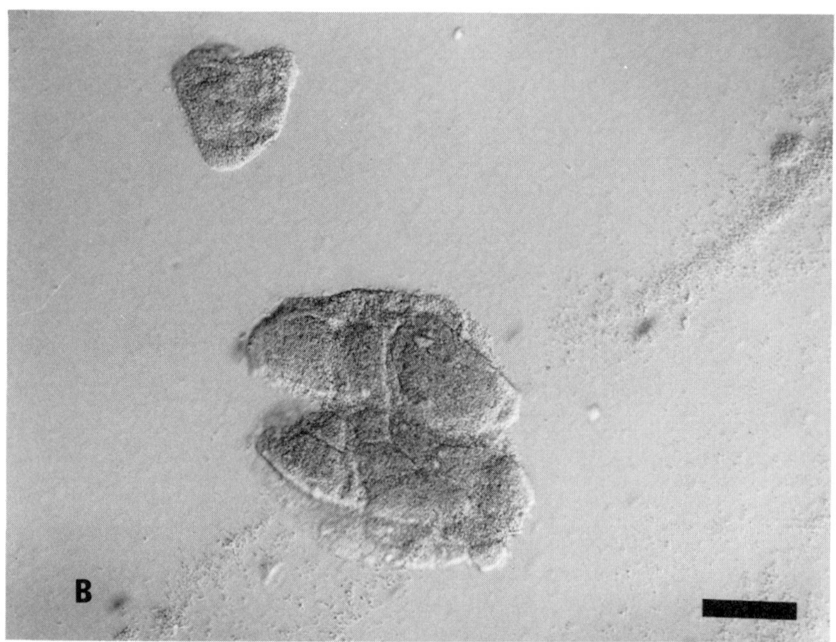

Figure 2B.

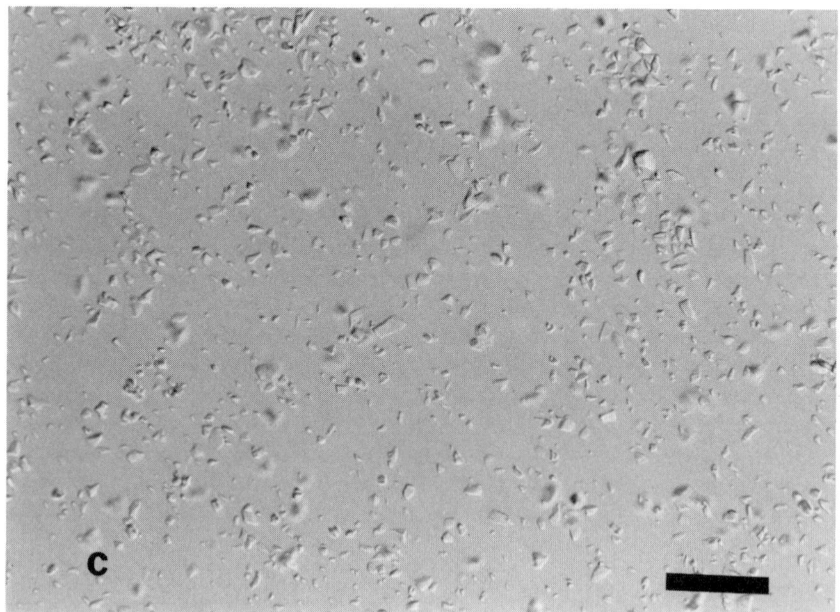

Figure 2C.

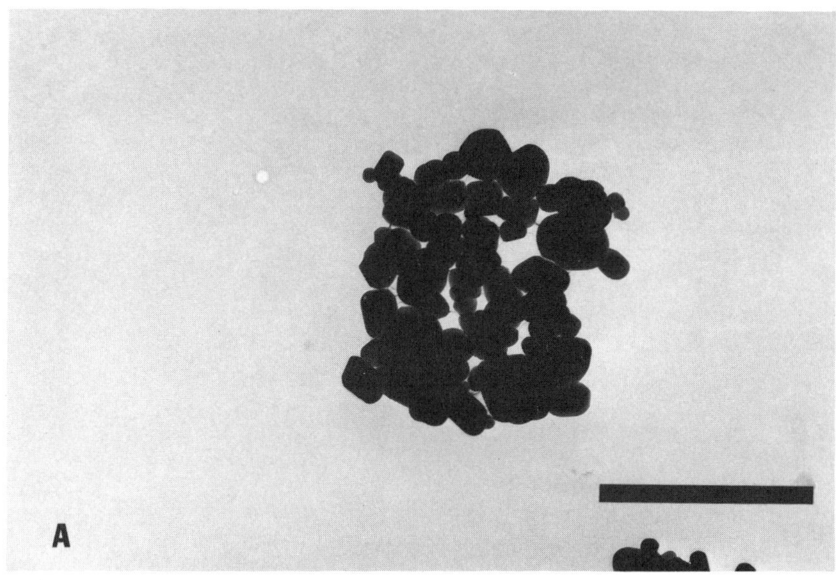

Figure 3. Electron photomicrographs of four synthetic titanium dioxides: A, anatase P25; B, rutile, R-100; C, rutile, R-900; D, rutile, R-960. Bar represents 1 μm.

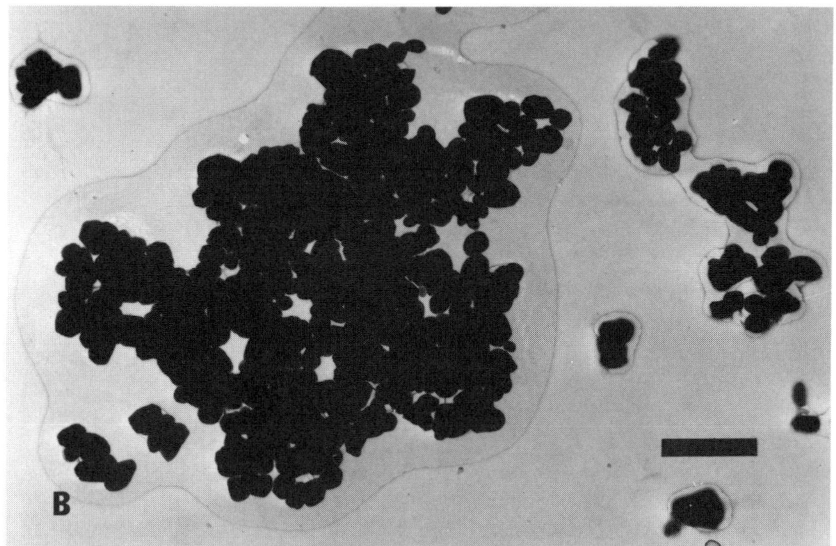

Figure 3B.

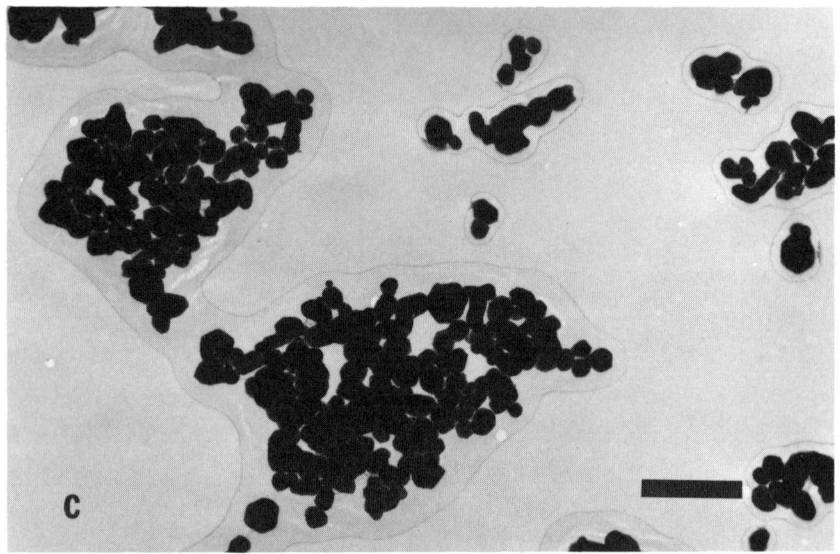

Figure 3C.

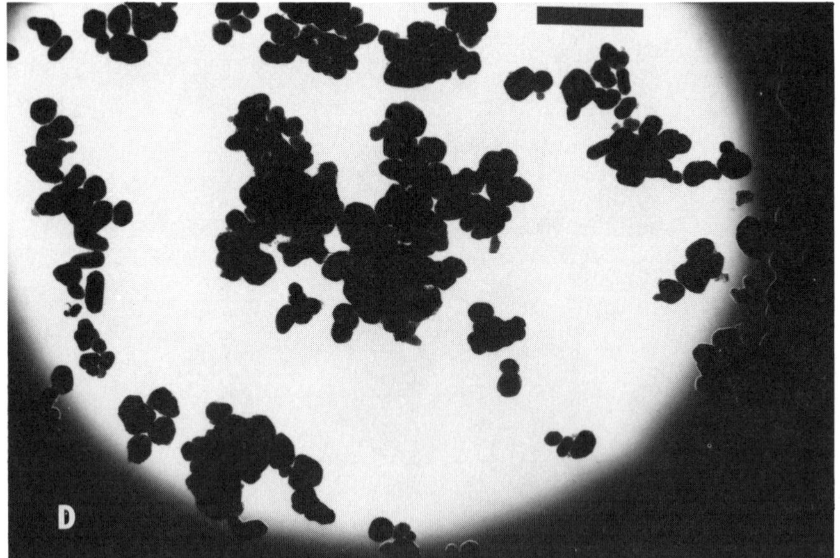

Figure 3D.

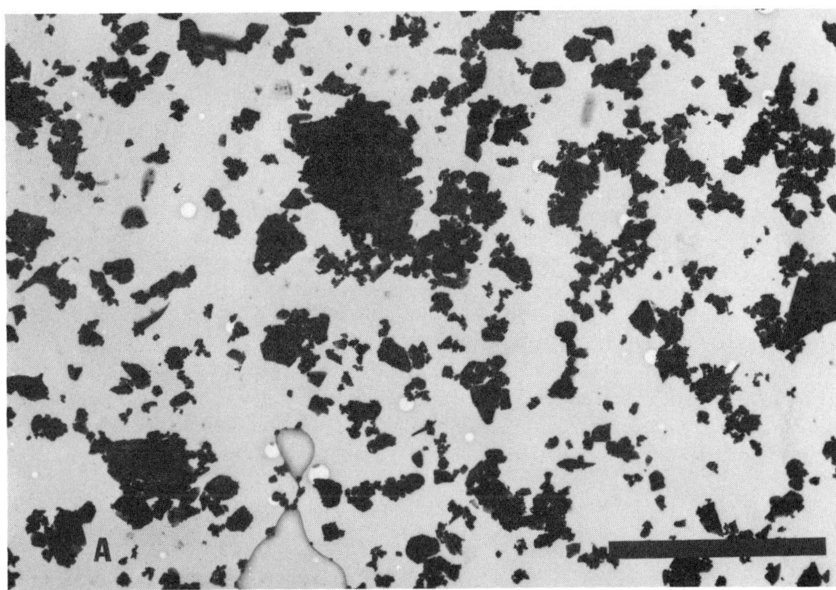

Figure 4. Electron photomicrographs of five quartz specimens used in pneumoconiosis research: A, DQ12; B, F600; C, 1-μm Stokes' diameter Min-U-Sil 15; D, 2-μm Stokes' diameter Min-U-Sil 15; E, >2-μm Stokes' diameter Min-U-Sil 15. Bar represents 10 μm.

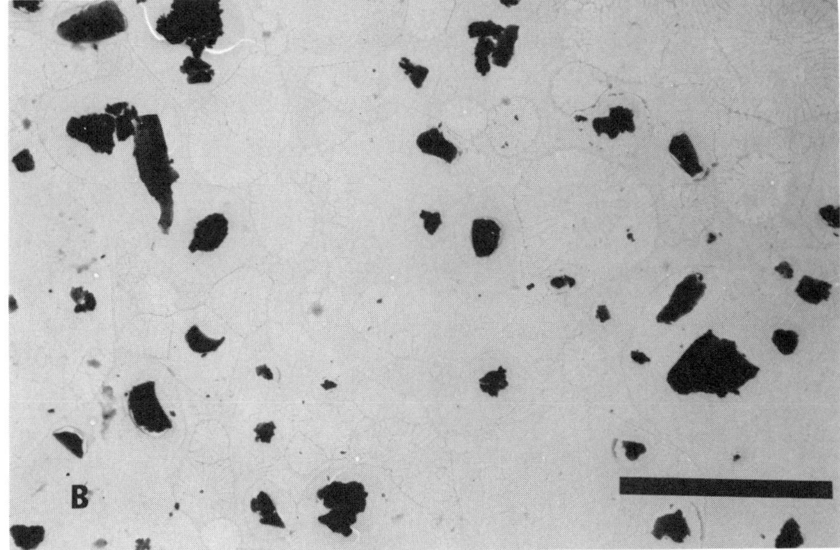

Figure 4B.

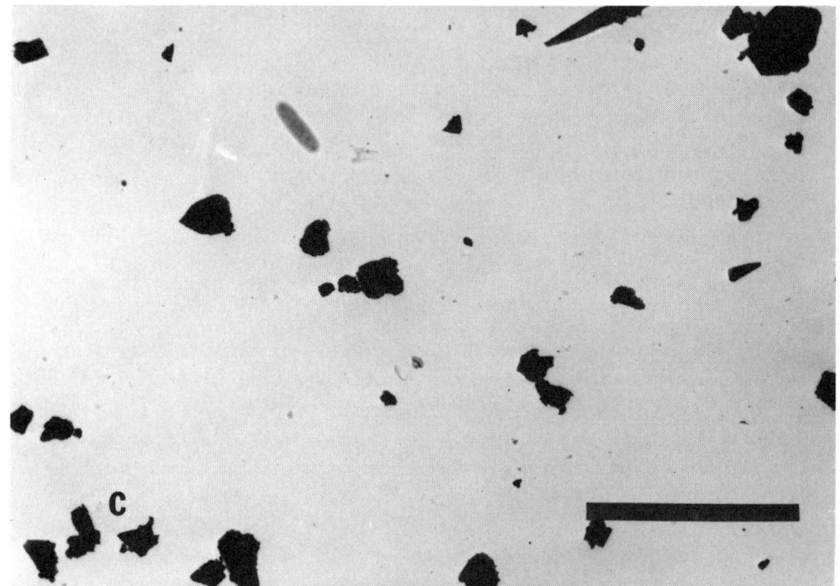

Figure 4C.

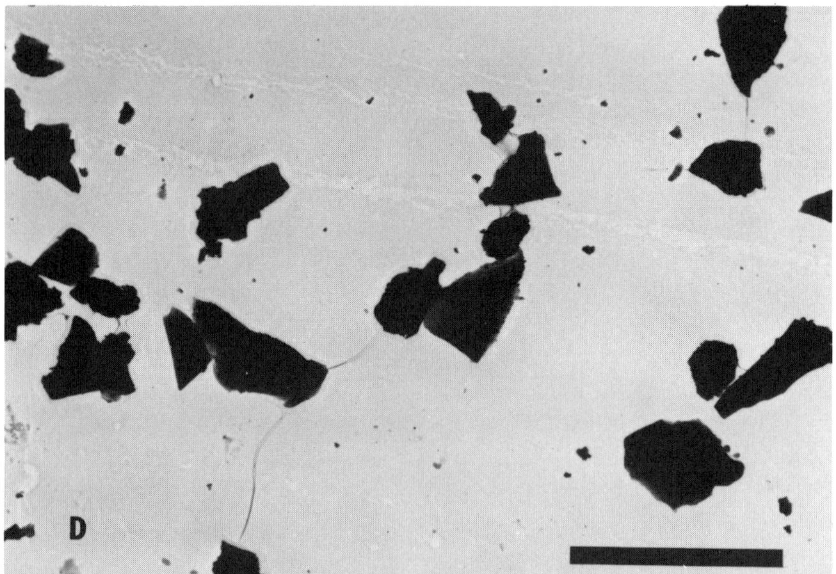

Figure 4D.

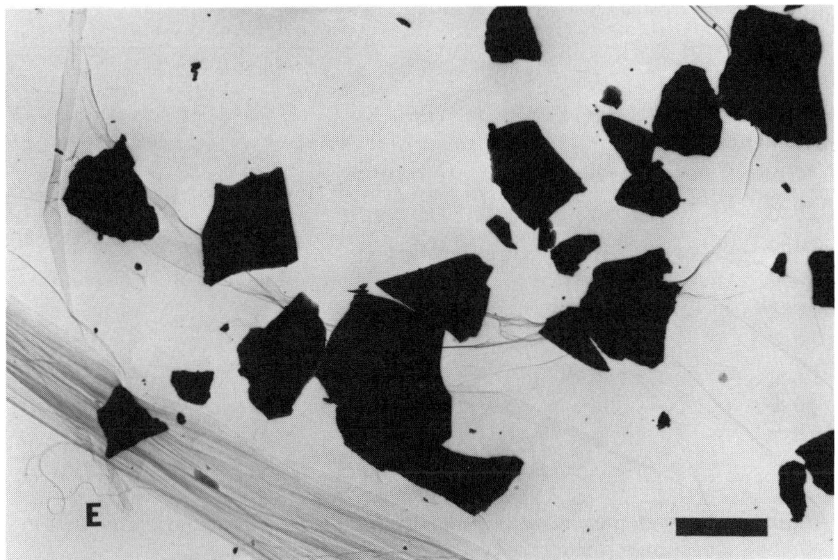

Figure 4E.

Rutile Manufactured by Du Pont (R-100, R-900, and R-960), and the Haskell Specimen. The three rutile powders were crystalline and produced sharp, well-defined X-ray patterns when analyzed in the continuous-scan diffraction mode. The patterns matched the standard for rutile in both reflection positions and intensities. These powders are pure rutile and are indistinguishable by X-ray diffraction analysis (Table 4). See Nolan et al. (1987b) for X-ray characterization of the Haskell specimen.

Anatase, Degussa P25. The Degussa specimen was crystalline and produced a sharp, well-defined X-ray pattern when analyzed in the continuous-scan diffraction mode. After the first reflection (d-spacing, 3.52 Å), the following eight (d-spacings, 2.431 to 1.481 Å) matched the standard anatase pattern within ±0.003 Å, and the intensities of the reflections were virtually identical. The two major rutile peaks, at 3.24 and 2.48 Å, were recognizable on the baseline and indicated a rutile concentration estimated as less than 1% of the total specimen mass (Table 5).

Table 4. Continuous-scan X-ray diffraction data for rutile, Du Pont R-100, R-900 and R-960.

R-100		R-900		R-960		Standard Rutile (ASTM Card 21-1276)		Miller Index[a]
d(Å)	I	d(Å)	I	d(Å)	I	d(Å)	I	hkl
3.230	74	3.230	64	3.230	67	3.250	100	(110)
2.480	38	2.480	31	2.480	31	2.487	50	(101)
2.290	5	2.291	4	2.290	4	2.297	8	(200)
2.182	18	2.183	15	2.182	16	2.188	25	(111)
2.048	7	2.051	5	2.049	5	2.054	10	(210)
1.686	52	1.686	42	1.684	46	1.687	60	(211)
1.622	15	1.623	14	1.621	15	1.624	20	(220)
1.477	8	1.479	6	1.478	7	1.479	10	(002)
1.451	7	1.453	5	1.451	6	1.453	10	(310)

[a]Standard mineralogical notation for planes within minerals (axial intercepts and ratios); measure of distance along a, b and c axes.

Table 5. Continuous-scan X-ray diffraction data for anatase, Degussa P25.

Degussa P25		Standard Anatase (ASTM Card 21-1272)		Miller Index[a]	
d(Å)	I	d(Å)	I	(hkl)	Other Phases
3.560	100	3.520	100	(101)	
3.240	1-2	(3.250)	—	—	Rutile[b]
2.480	1	(2.487)	—	—	Rutile
2.428	7	2.431	10	(103)	
2.379	24	2.378	20	(004)	
2.332	7	2.332	10	(112)	
1.893	31	1.892	35	(200)	
1.699	23	1.699	20	(105)	
1.669	23	1.667	20	(210)	
1.493	4	1.493	4	(213)	
1.483	18	1.481	14	(204)	

[a]Standard mineralogical notation for planes within minerals (axial intercepts and ratios); measure of distance along a, b and c axes.
[b]Rutile forms because the anatase process is imperfect; the stability fields are juxtaposed, and lowering pressure and temperature allows formation of rutile.

Quartz. The 25 reflections for low (alpha) quartz that occurred in the region between 5 and 85° 2-theta, the standard quartz patterns in the literature (Frondel, 1962; American Society for Testing and Materials; ASTM Card No. 5-040, 1974), were compared with the patterns obtained for F600 and DQ12. Both the F600 and DQ12 specimens yielded high-quality, diagnostic diffraction patterns characteristic of alpha quartz. The F600 pattern, however, produced a more intense series of reflections than DQ12 under identical conditions of analysis and showed two weak reflections (0003 and 21$\bar{3}$0), which were not resolved in DQ12 (Table 6). Peak resolution beyond 50° 2-theta ($\kappa\bar{\alpha}$ to $\kappa\alpha_1$) was better in the F600 compared to DQ12, as the DQ12 quartz peaks tended to be ragged, requiring visual judgment for assigning a precise 2-theta value. On-scale peaks were within ± 0.001 Å of the diagnostic standard reflections. The reflection peaks yielded by DQ12 suggest line-broadening characteristics of particles approximately 1,000 Å in diameter.

Table 6. Continuous-scan X-ray diffraction data for quartz, DQ12 and F600.

DQ12		F600		Frondel (1962)		Standard Quartz (ASTM Card 5-0490)	
d(Å)	I	d(Å)	I	d(Å)	hkl Form[a]	d(Å)	I
4.27	100	4.27	100	4.255	10$\bar{1}$0 (m_1)	4.26	35
3.36	100	3.35	100	3.343	10$\bar{1}$1 (r_1)	3.343	100
2.46	88	2.46	100	2.457	11$\bar{2}$1	2.458	12
2.29	79	2.28	100	2.281	10$\bar{1}$2	2.282	12
2.24	40	2.238	55	2.236	11$\bar{2}$1 (s_1)	2.237	6
2.13	60	2.131	85	2.128	20$\bar{2}$0 (m_2)	2.128	9
1.98	39	1.983	51	1.980	20$\bar{2}$1	1.980	6
1.821	100	1.819	100	1.818	11$\bar{2}$2 (a_1)	1.817	17
—	—	1.806	8	1.802	00$\bar{0}$3 (c_3)	1.801	1
1.672	39	1.674	61	1.672	20$\bar{2}$2 (r_2)	1.672	7
1.660	18	1.660	21	1.659	10$\bar{1}$3	1.659	3
—	—	1.609	5	1.608	21$\bar{3}$0	1.608	1
1.543	91	1.542	100	1.541	21$\bar{3}$1	1.541	15
1.454	18	1.454	23	1.453	11$\bar{2}$3	1.453	3
1.419	3	1.420	7	1.418	30$\bar{3}$0 (m_3)	1.418	1
1.383	58	1.383	77	1.382	21$\bar{3}$2	1.382	7
1.376	80	1.376	92	1.375	20$\bar{2}$3	1.375	11
1.373	76	1.374	100	1.372	30$\bar{3}$1	1.372	9
1.289	20	1.288	22	1.288	10$\bar{1}$4	1.288	3
1.257	25	1.257	33	1.256	30$\bar{3}$2	1.256	4
1.229	11	1.229	16	1.228	22$\bar{4}$0	1.228	2
1.200	29	1.200	33	1.200	21$\bar{3}$3	1.9997	6
1.198	21	1.199	26	1.198	22$\bar{4}$1	1.198	2
1.185	21	1.185	23	1.184	11$\bar{2}$4	1.184	4
1.181	31	1.181	42	1.180	31$\bar{4}$0	1.180	4

[a]Miller Index, based on hexagonal cell; crystal form given in parentheses.

Planes of failure in the quartz, although generally poorly expressed, followed the common facial forms (i.e., m, r, s), the Brazilian twin plane (a), and the basal pinicoid (c). Both specimens contained trace mineral impurities (<0.5%).

Analytical Electron Microscopy. Approximately 0.1-mg aliquots of each specimen were dispersed in 10 ml of distilled water by sonication at 70 W power for 2 to 3 seconds. A 10-μl aliquot of each suspension was placed on carbon-coated Formvar®-support, 200-mesh copper locator grids, and allowed to dry before being examined using analytical electron microscopy (Langer and Nolan, in press).

The chemical analyses were obtained on single particles, with X-rays accumulated for 100 seconds between 0 and 10,240 eV. The cursor was placed on the titanium $\kappa\alpha_{1,2}$ peak at 4.51 KeV and, after signal-smoothing, the total counts were compared with aluminum $\kappa\alpha_{1,2}$ at 1.49 KeV and silicon $\kappa\alpha_{1,2}$ at 1.74 KeV. These values were integrated as a single chemical system, and ratios were calculated to yield a rough "first-order approximation" of elemental content:

$$\frac{C_{Al}}{C_{Si}} \approx \frac{X_{Al}}{X_{Si}} \quad ,$$

where C = concentration of the element, X = its X-ray emission.

	Al, $\kappa\alpha_{1,2}$	Si, $\kappa\alpha_{1,2}$	Ti, $\kappa\alpha_{1,2}$
Rutile, R-100	148	—	2,103
Rutile, R-900	517	—	10,756
Rutile, R-960	179	315	3,729

The anatase specimen and the rutile specimen (with the exception of the R series) are pure TiO_2, as assayed by this X-ray fluorescence method. The R series of TiO_2, 100, 900, 960, show detectable Al, Al>Si and Si>Al, respectively. These values are close to the maxima reported for these materials by the manufacturer (Table 1).

Human Erythrocyte Hemolytic Model. The abilities of the TiO_2 and quartz specimens to alter the permeability of human erythrocytes were determined quantitatively. The erythrocytes were obtained from peripheral blood (50 ml) obtained by venipuncture in a plastic syringe containing 15 U/ml preservative-free heparin. Ficoll-Hypaque gradient centrifugation was used to separate the peripheral blood lymphocytes and plasma proteins from the erythrocytes. A 50-ml blood sample was diluted with an equal volume of saline, overlaid onto a 25-ml Ficoll-Hypaque gradient, and centrifuged at F = 850 g at 20°C for 45 minutes. The lymphocytes and plasma proteins were removed, and the erythrocytes were stored at 4°C and used within a week.

Before the stored erythrocytes were used, about 5 ml of packed human erythrocytes were diluted to 50 ml with pH 7.4 Veronal buffered saline (VBS; 2.4 mM sodium barbital and 145 mM sodium chloride) in a plastic centrifuge tube and spun at F ≅ 800 g, at room temperature, for 30 minutes. The erythrocyte wash was repeated twice (a total of three washes). Using visible spectroscopy, the washed human erythrocytes were made into a standard suspension of about 3.6 x 10^8 cells/ml (Nolan et al., 1981).

A single stock suspension of each specimen was also made in VBS. To disperse the suspensions, each was sonicated, using a sonifier cell disrupter (Heat Systems; Ultrasonics, Inc.), at 50 W power for several minutes until the suspension was visibly homogeneous. Each of the stock mineral suspensions was diluted to at least four different concentrations (mg/ml) in duplicate. Each of the four dilutions was adjusted to 4 ml, to which 4 ml of the standard erythrocyte suspension was added, making the final volume at each concentration 8 ml. The erythrocytes were then incubated at 37° for 120 minutes while being shaken continuously with a gyrating motion.

The plotted relationship (mg/ml) of mineral:hemolysis (%H) is generally linear up to about 40% hemolysis. The duplicate determinations were averaged, and the values are shown in the tables, with their means. A linear regression analysis was made for each set of points, and the equation of the line was calculated and used to compute the HC50 (Table 7), the concentration of powder (in mg/ml) required to lyse half the erythrocytes in the suspension.

Determination of 2-PVPNO Binding. The amount of 2-PVPNO that bound to several specimens was determined quantitatively. Various amounts of the mineral powders were weighed into glass centrifuge tubes and to each was added 30 ml of 50-μg/ml 2-PVPNO in distilled water. Each tube was sonicated at 50 W power until the suspension appeared uniformly dispersed. The tubes were allowed to stand at room temperature for 30 minutes. The tubes were centrifuged at F ≅ 8000 g, at room temperature, for 40 minutes, which pelleted the powder at the bottom of the tubes. The amount of polymer able to bind to each concentration of powder was thereby removed from the supernatant. This amount was calculated using the 2-PVPNO polymer's known molar absorptivity (E) of 5031 at

260 nm (which had, in turn, been calculated, using the molecular weight of the monomer, 121.1). The absorbance of the supernatant was measured at 260 nm, and the concentration of 2-PVPNO thereby determined to be missing from the supernatant was assumed to be bound to the particle surface. The data were plotted graphically as mineral powder (mg/ml) versus 2-PVPNO (μg/ml). The technique has been used previously for both quartz (Nolan et al., 1981; Nolan and Langer, 1985) and TiO_2 (Nolan et al., 1987b).

Table 7. Determination of HC50 of rutiles (R-100, R-900, R-960, Haskell, and IOM-1), anatase (Degussa), and quartz (Min-U-Sil 15).

Specimen	HC50 (mg/ml)[a]
Rutile, R-100	1.54 ± 0.17
Rutile, R-900	0.58 ± 0.03
Rutile, R-960	1.13 ± 0.09
Rutile, Haskell	2.15 ± 0.40
Rutile, IOM-1	Inactive
Anatase, Degussa	Inactive
Quartz, Min-U-Sil 15 (Sonicated)	1.54 ± 0.17
Quartz, Min-U-Sil 15 (Unsonicated)	2.59 ± 0.75

[a]HC50 determined using three different erythrocyte donors. Mean value is shown with standard deviation.

RESULTS

Membranolytic Activity of the TiO_2 Specimens

All TiO_2 specimens obtained from Du Pont were membranolytically active (Figure 5). The HC50* of these specimens were determined using at least three different erythrocyte donors; those of the least active (Haskell) and most active (R-900) rutile specimens differed by more than 3.5-fold (Table 7). The membranolytic activity of rutile specimens R-100, R-900 and R-960 was inhibited by 2-PVPNO (data not shown). The anatase (Degussa) and the rutile IOM-1 were also examined for membranolytic activity, using three different erythrocyte donors, and were found to be inert (Table 7; Figure 6).

*Concentration of powder (mg/ml) required to lyse 50% of the erythrocytes in suspension.

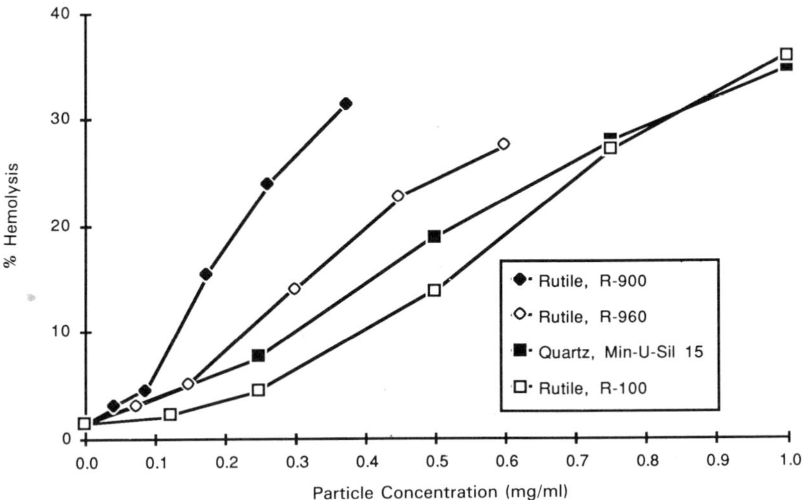

Figure 5. Membranolytic activity of three rutiles made synthetically using the chloride reduction process, and of quartz.

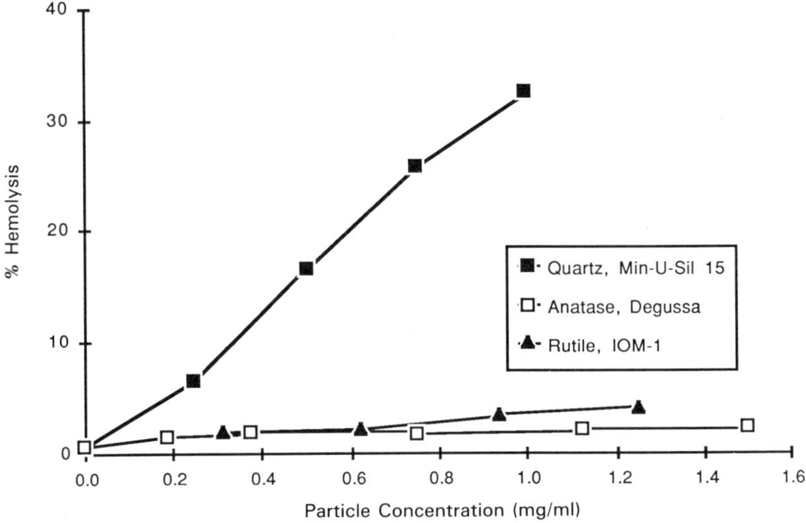

Figure 6. Comparison of the membranolytic activity of a synthetic anatase and rutile used in pneumoconiosis research with that of quartz.

Effect of Heating on the Membranolytic and Hydrogen Bonding Activity of the TiO_2 Surface

The activity of rutile (#10082), which was shown to be membranolytic (Nolan et al., 1987b), was markedly reduced by heating (Figure 7). Another rutile specimen, IOM-1, which was membranolytically inactive, remained so after heating. The rutile specimens R-100, R-900 and R-960 lost the ability to lyse erythrocytes after heating (Table 8). The ability of both heated and unheated R-100 to bind 2-PVPNO was similar (Figure 8).

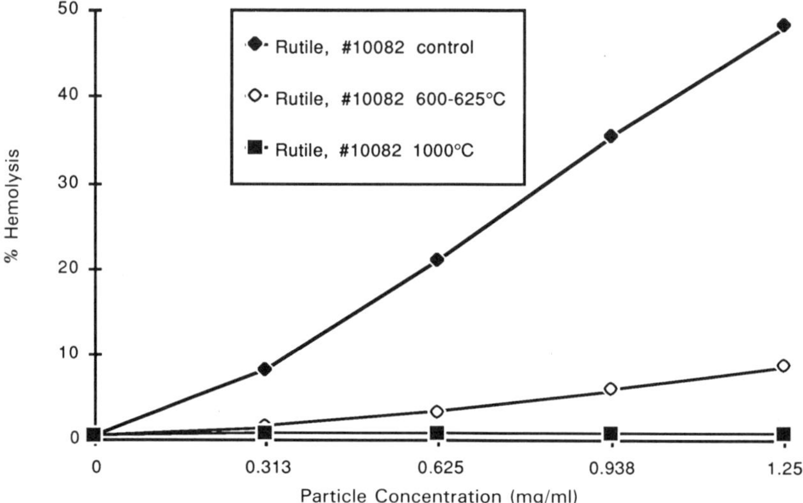

Figure 7. Effect of heating (for 6 hours) on the membranolytic activity of rutile (#10082) at two temperatures.

Table 8. Effect of heating on membranolytic activity of rutile R-100, R-900, and R-960. Each specimen was heated to 600 to 800°C for 6 hours.

Rutile R-100 (mg/ml)	% Hemolysis Heated	% Hemolysis Unheated[a]	Rutile R-900 (mg/ml)	% Hemolysis Heated	% Hemolysis Unheated[a]
—	0.8 ± 0.0	—	—	0.8 ± 0.0	—
0.125	0.9 ± 0.0	0.4 ± 0.4	0.044	1.1 ± 0.1	2.4 ± 0.1
0.250	1.4 ± 0.1	4.8 ± 0.7	0.088	1.1 ± 0.0	6.4 ± 0.2
0.500	3.3 ± 0.3	13.7 ± 1.8	0.175	1.2 ± 0.2	14.3 ± 0.5
0.750	6.2 ± 0.1	22.5 ± 2.8	0.263	1.5 ± 0.2	22.3 ± 0.8
1.000	7.0 ± 0.0	31.4 ± 3.9	0.350	1.9 ± 0.1	30.2 ± 1.1

Rutile R-960 (mg/ml)	% Hemolysis Heated	% Hemolysis Unheated[a]	Min-U-Sil (mg/ml)	% Hemolysis Unheated
—	0.8 ± 0.0	—	—	0.8 ± 0.0
0.075	1.9 ± 0.1	2.1 ± 0.5	0.25	4.2 ± 0.1
0.150	1.9 ± 0.0	5.5 ± 0.8	0.50	10.6 ± 0.0
0.300	2.9 ± 0.4	11.9 ± 0.9	0.75	16.9 ± 0.1
0.450	4.7 ± 0.0	18.9 ± 1.9	1.00	21.2 ± 0.3
0.600	6.9 ± 0.2	25.5 ± 2.5		

[a]For each concentration, % hemolysis was calculated three times, using equations of the line of the three different erythrocyte suspensions. Their means and standard deviations are shown.

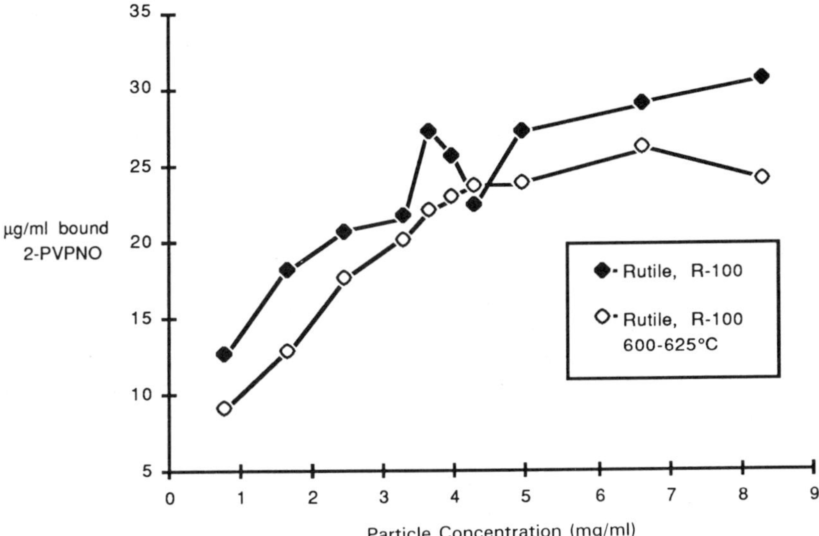

Figure 8. Effect of heating on the hydrogen-bonding ability of rutile.

Inhibition of the Membranolytic Activity of Rutile

The membranolytic activity of all active rutiles was inhibited by 2-PVPNO. Neither Al^{3+} nor Fe^{2+} had any inhibitory effect on rutile membranolytic activity under the conditions studied. The anion transport inhibitor DIDS was an effective inhibitor of rutile membranolytic activity (Figure 9).

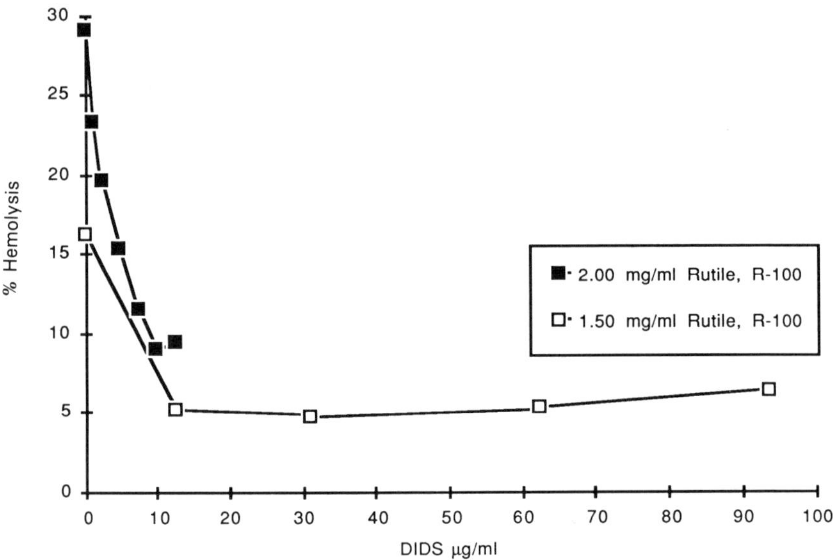

Figure 9. Effect of the anion transport inhibitor DIDS on the membranolytic activity of rutile.

Determination of HC50 of the Quartz Specimens

The HC50 of the unfractionated Min-U-Sil 15 and the three size-fractionated specimens of DQ12 and F600 are shown in Table 9. The need to disperse the very fine DQ12 to determine the HC50 accurately is shown by the data in Figure 10; the HC50 decreased, by almost one order of magnitude, as a function of sonication time. The DQ12, F600 and the Min-U-Sil 15 were sonicated at 50 W for 5 minutes, were diluted, and exposed to erythrocytes as described in the Materials and Methods section. After sonication, the three quartz suspensions remained undisturbed for 2 hours, were diluted, and the HC50 of each suspension was again determined. The amount of powder required for achieving the HC50 for DQ12, F600 and Min-U-Sil 15 increased by 179, 157 and 103%, respectively. Significant reaggregation had occurred in the very-fine-particle-size quartz specimens over the 2-hour time interval and had effectively reduced their available surface.

Table 9. HC50[a] of six quartz specimens, determined by using at least three different erythrocyte donors.

	HC50 (mg/ml)
Min-U-Sil 15	
Unfractionated	2.74 ± 0.38
1-μm Stokes' diameter	0.46 ± 0.25
2-μm Stokes' diameter	1.82 ± 0.59
>2-μm Stokes' diameter	8.04 ± 0.84
DQ12	0.12 ± 0.04
F600	0.90 ± 0.36

[a]Concentration of powder (mg/ml) required to lyse 50% of the erythrocytes in suspension.

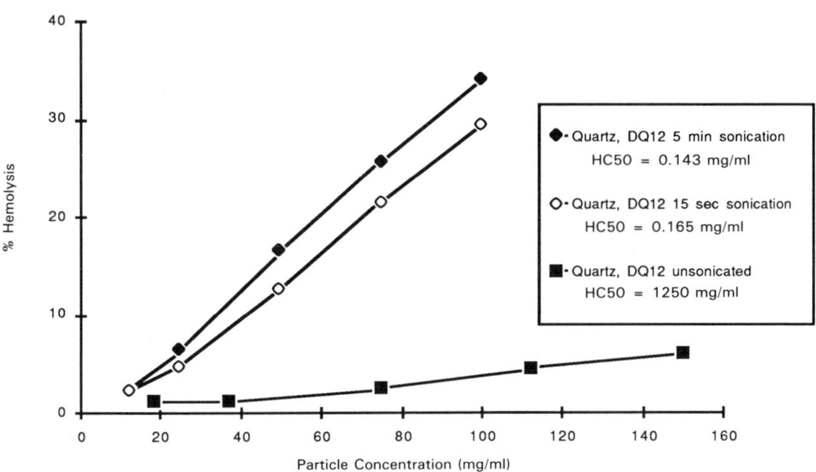

Figure 10. Effect of sonication on the membranolytic activity of an aggregated, fine-particle-size quartz such as DQ12.

The surfaces of the three quartz specimens were further characterized by the ability of each specimen's surface to hydrogen-bond 2-PVPNO. The quartz with the finer size distribution bound more 2-PVPNO; the order of decreasing binding ability was DQ12, F600, Min-U-Sil 15 (Figure 11). The tendency of the quartz particles in DQ12 and F600 to aggregate required that each be sonicated for maximal binding of 2-PVPNO to occur. The membranolytic activity of all three specimens was inhibited by the polymer (Figure 12).

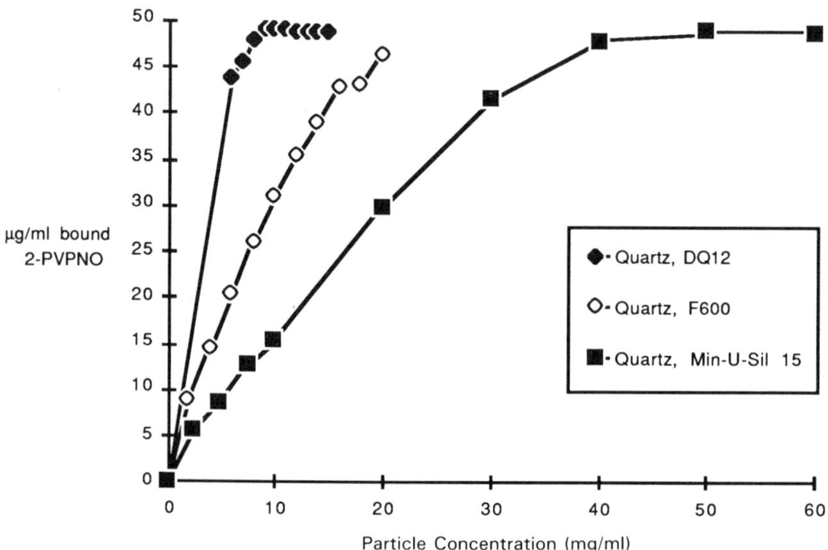

Figure 11. Comparison of the hydrogen-bonding ability of quartz specimens DQ12, F600, and Min-U-Sil 15.

Effect of Heating on the Membranolytic Activity of the Quartz Surface

The effect of heating on the DQ12 and F600 specimens was determined. Five hundred mg of each specimen were heated to approximately 500°C for 7 hours, then allowed to gradually cool overnight. Heating reduced the membranolytic activity of each specimen slightly (Figure 13). This loss of activity could be explained if a slight fusion of particles occurred during heating.

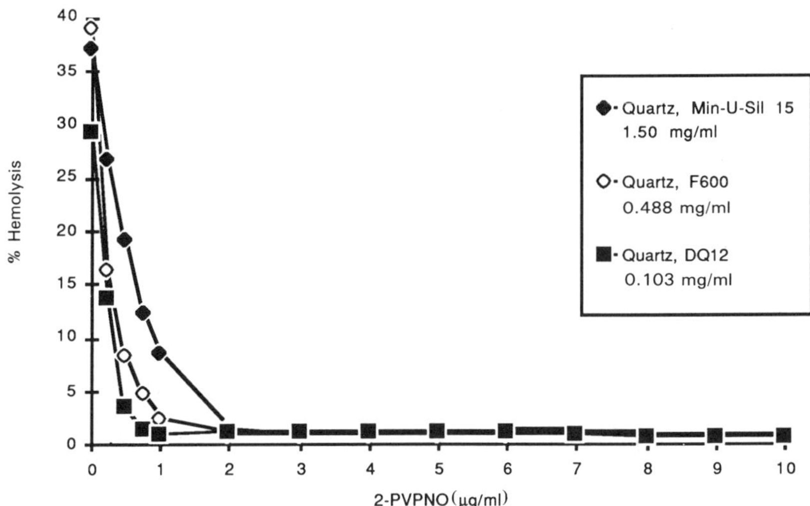

Figure 12. The hydrogen-bonding polymer 2-PVPNO inhibits the membranolytic activity of all three quartz specimens.

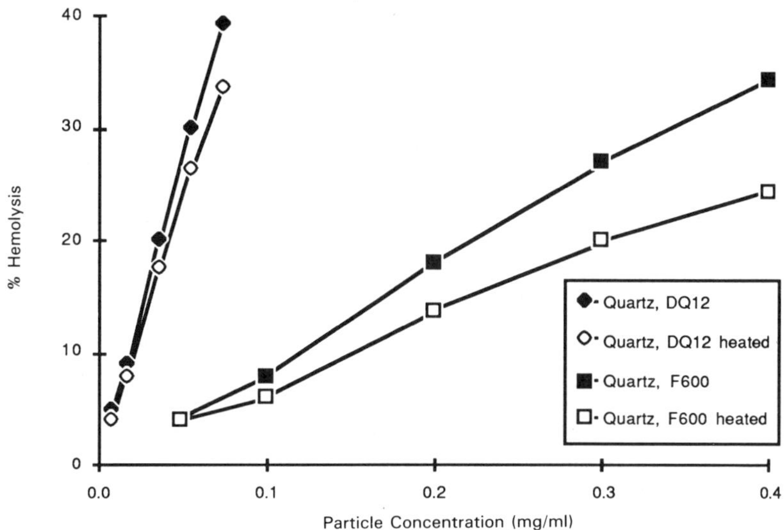

Figure 13. Effect of heating on the membranolytic activity of two quartz specimens.

DISCUSSION AND CONCLUSIONS

Hazard-evaluation of inorganic particulates in aerosol form must take into consideration the potential variability of their physicochemical state, i.e., state of aggregation and surface properties. These properties have recently become of interest in the analysis of the data concerning the TiO_2 polymorphs rutile and anatase. For regulatory purposes, both of the titania polymorphs have been considered a single substance having no permanent irreversible biological effect on the human lung after inhalation. The permissible exposure limit to these polymorphs has been set at 15 mg/m^3 (NIOSH, 1980). Each of the polymorphs has been used as an inert control in experimental pneumoconiosis research, where it has been common practice not to identify the specific polymorph used, much less its physicochemical properties.

The induction of lung tumors in rats by inhalation of high concentrations of TiO_2 was unexpected (Lee et al., 1985a,b); tumors occurred only in the female rats that were exposed to the highest concentration of particulates. From the evidence available, it seemed likely that the tumors were an artifact produced by the extremely high concentration of aerosol dust. Furthermore, the TiO_2 used in the inhalation studies, a synthetic rutile, had unique physicochemical properties; possibly both factors played a role. A comparison of the properties and membranolytic activity of the rutile used in the inhalation study with other inactive titanium dioxides and active quartz and titania specimens would help in evaluating the results of the positive inhalation study. Such a study might even explain such disparate test results and shed light on the fundamental mechanisms of interaction between particles and biological systems.

The particle-size distributions of all synthetic titanium dioxides we examined were in the respirable size range. Therefore, synthetically produced rutile and anatase require no further size reduction or size fractionation to become respirable (Nolan et al., 1987a,b).

All four of the synthetic rutile specimens made by Du Pont, using the chloride reduction process, were membranolytically active. The rutile (IOM-1) and anatase (Degussa) used experimentally in pneumoconiosis research were both inactive. All naturally occurring rutile and anatase, as well as the synthetic anatase specimens studied thus far, are also inactive. Only one report in the literature states that synthetic anatase is membranolytic (Zitting and Skytta, 1979). The activity of the synthetic rutile specimens appears to depend on the process of synthesis and superimposed surface modifications.

The synthetic rutiles that were membranolytically active lost activity after heating. The lowest temperature required to inactivate the surface was not determined, although heating to 600°C proved effective. The inactive rutiles remained so after heating, thus differing from quartz, which retained activity after heating to such temperatures. Surface-modified quartz that lost membranolytic activity was reactivated by heating (Nolan et al., 1987a). Physical methods, such as heating, could now be used to vary the membranolytic activity of synthetic rutile, with the particle size remaining unchanged. The chemical information on the surfaces of these specimens must be different. It has been reported that the hydrogen-bonding properties of quartz impart the mineral's pathogenic activity (Nash et al., 1966). However, the hydrogen-bonding characteristics of the membranolytically active rutiles shown below, before and after inactivation by heating, were indistinguishable from one another (Figure 8).

	Membranolytic Activity	Hydrogen-Bonding Ability*
Rutile, R-100	+	+
Rutile, R-100, heated	–	+
Rutile, White Mountain, CA	–	+
Rutile, IOM-1	–	–
Rutile, PRU, Wales	–	–

*Selected data from Nolan et al., 1987b for comparison.

The polymer 2-PVPNO was an effective inhibitor of the membranolytic rutile specimens. The hydrogen-bonding ability of rutile was variable and does not correlate with membranolytic activity. The surface charge of quartz has been correlated with its membranolytic activity (Nolan et al., 1981). The ionizable silanol group on quartz is analogous to the ionizable titanol group on the surface of rutile. This functional group imparts a net negative surface charge on quartz. The chemistry of the titanol and silanol groups differs, so that the cations, which may be used to block the negative charge on the quartz, were not very effective on rutile. The anion transport inhibitor DIDS, which binds to the receptor site of the transport protein, band 3, effectively inhibited the membranolytic activity of rutile (Branton, 1983; Cabantchik et al., 1978). The inhibition of the membranolytic activity of quartz by anion transport inhibitors has been reported (Nolan et al., 1984; unpublished data). Quartz and rutile appear to lyse erythrocyte membranes by the same mechanism.

ACKNOWLEDGMENTS

This study was made possible by support from NIOSH and the Société Nationale de L'Amiante, Canada. R. P. Nolan wishes to acknowledge support as a Fellow of the Stony Wold-Herbert Fund, Inc. The authors thank Ms. Barbara Mensch for the photographic work.

REFERENCES

Branton, D. **1983.** Erythrocyte membrane protein associations and erythrocyte shape. Harvey Lect 77:23-42.

Cabantchik, ZI, PA Knauf, and A Rothstein. **1978.** The anion transport system of the red blood cell. The role of membrane protein evaluated by the use of probes. Biochim Biophys Acta 515:239-302.

Ferin, J and G. Oberdörster. **1985.** Biological effects and toxic assessment of titanium dioxides: Anatase and rutile. Am Ind Hyg Assoc J 46:69-72.

Frondel, C. **1962.** Systems of mineralogy. In: *Silica Minerals,* Vol. III. Wiley, New York, NY.

Langer, AM and RP Nolan. Fiber type and burden found in parenchymal tissues of workers occupationally exposed to asbestos in the United States. Implications for assessment of risk in the general population. In: *Mineral Fibers in the Non-Occupational Environment,* International Agency for Research on Cancer, September, 1987, Lyon, France (**in press**).

Lee, KP, HJ Trochimowicz, and CF Reinhardt. **1985a.** Pulmonary response of rats exposed to titanium dioxide (TiO_2) by inhalation for two years. Toxicol Appl Pharmacol 79:179-192.

Lee, KP, HJ Trochimowicz, and CF Reinhardt. **1985b.** Transmigration of titanium dioxide (TiO_2) particles in rats after inhalation exposure. Exp Mol Pathol 42:331-343.

Nash, T, AC Allison, JS Harington. **1966.** Physio-chemical properties of silica in relation to its toxicity. Nature 210:259-261.

NIOSH. 1980. *Pocket Guide to Chemical Hazards,* NIOSH/OSHA. U.S. Government Printing Office, Washington, DC, 180 p.

Nolan, RP and AM Langer. **1983.** Quartz hemolysis: Physicochemical factors controlling membrane activity, pp. 63-81. In: *Health Issues Related to Mining and Minerals,* W Wagner, J Merchant, and W Rom (eds.). Ann Arbor Press, Ann Arbor, MI.

Nolan, RP and AM Langer. **1985.** Particle size and chemically-induced variability in the membranolytic activity of quartz. Preliminary observations, pp. 39-50. In: *In Vitro Effects of Mineral Dusts,* EG Beck, and J Bignon (eds.), Third International Workshop. Springer-Verlag, Berlin.

Nolan, RP, AM Langer, JS Harington, G Oster, and IJ Selikoff. **1981.** Quartz hemolysis related to its surface functionalities. Environ Res 26:503-520.

Nolan, RP, AM Langer, and KW Foster. **1984.** Recognition of quartz by erythrocyte membranes, Abstract 198. In: *VIth International Pneumoconiosis Conference 1983,* Vol. 2, September 20-23, 1983, Bergbau-Berufsgenossenschaft, Bochum, Federal Republic of Germany. Wirtschaftsverlag, Verlag für neue Wissenschaft, Bremerhaven, Federal Republic of Germany.

Nolan, RP, AM Langer, RA Eskenazi, GB Herson, and KW Foster. **1987a.** Membranolytic activities of quartz standards. Toxicol In Vitro 1:239-245.

Nolan, RP, AM Langer, I Weisman, and GB Herson. **1987b.** Surface character and membranolytic activity of rutile and anatase—Two titanium dioxide polymorphs. Br J Ind Med 44:687-698.

Zitting, A and E Skytta. **1979.** Biological activity of titanium dioxide. Int Arch Occup Environ Health 43:93-97.

Inorganic Particles Found in Cigarette Tobacco, Cigarette Ash, and Cigarette Smoke

Arthur M. Langer,[1] Robert P. Nolan,[1] D. R. Bowes,[2] and S. B. Shirey[3]

[1]Environmental Sciences Laboratory, Applied Sciences Institute of The City University of New York at Brooklyn College, Brooklyn, NY

[2]Department of Geology, University of Glasgow, United Kingdom

[3]Department of Terrestrial Magnetism Geophysical Laboratory, Washington, DC

KEY WORDS: cigarette smoke, cigarete ash, inorganic particles

---

ABSTRACT

Major brands of cigarettes, purchased in New York City, were selected and studied on the basis of length, filtered and nonfiltered types, imported and domestic brands, and nicotine and tar contents. Cigarette tobacco fillers were ashed at 550° C to determine their ash residues. Each ash residue was examined by polarized light microscopy, X-ray diffraction, transmission electron microscopy, selected area electron diffraction, and electron microprobe analysis. Particles in mainstream cigarette smoke were captured on Millipore® filters, using a smoking-machine "puff." These materials were prepared for transmission electron microscopy, and the inorganic constituents of the cigarette smoke were determined.

All cigarettes produced an amount of ash related to cigarette size, amounting to approximately 15% of the original tobacco weight. The following major compounds in cigarette ash were identified: calcite ($CaCO_3$), sylvite (KCl), fairchildite $K_2Ca(CO_3)_2$, arcanite (K_2SO_4, quartz (SiO_2), and buetschliite ($3K_2CO_3 \times 2CaCO_3 \times 6H_2O$, K_2CO_3, $K_2CO_3 \times 1.5\ H_2O$). These phases occurred in approximately the following percentages: 37, 29, 24, 8, and 2. Quartz, probably a contaminant from soil, occurred frequently.

Microchemical analysis of particles in the cigarette smoke showed them to be sintered mixtures of minerals rather than discrete compounds. Mixtures of inorganics, as opposed to single minerals, appeared to be supported by complex, selected-area, electron diffraction patterns and chemistry. Mineral particles were recovered from unfiltered cigarettes only and constituted but a small fraction of mainstream smoke. None of the noxious compounds listed in reconstituted tobacco sheet patents were identified in cigarette ash or smoke. We conclude that the inorganic minerals and compounds in cigarette tobacco, ash, and smoke are either adventitious soil particles or crystallization compounds formed during tobacco combustion.

INTRODUCTION

This project, the study of inorganic components of cigarette tobacco, ash, and smoke had its conceptual origin in about 1970. At that time our laboratory was focusing on several very different lines of inquiry which appeared to converge at a single point:

- Since the 1950s The American Cancer Society had been following more than one million people in a survey which explored the role of life style in cancer outcome. Most notable was the role of cigarette-smoking in the etiology of lung cancer. Although a statistical association was evident, some questions remained concerning the relative importance of each of the many chemical carcinogens identified in cigarette smoke, e.g., the nitroso compounds, the polycyclic aromatic hydrocarbons (PAH), etc. These agents were shown to be present in smoke in minute quantities, and it was thought that other agents, as yet unidentified, might amplify their carcinogenic effects.

- In 1968, Selikoff et al. showed that cigarette-smoking, asbestos-exposed insulation workers incurred a risk of developing lung cancer which was greater than the sum of the individual risks associated with exposure to each of these agents individually. The total risk of lung cancer was about equal to the product of the risks associated with each agent singularly. This synergism appeared biologically plausible, and it was thought that if such a particle-smoke relationship existed for asbestos-exposed workers, it was possible that a similar synergy might explain the potency of cigarette smoke to induce malignant bronchial tumors in humans exposed to particles other than asbestos.

- In the late 1960s, observations were made that the parenchymal tissues of "heavy" cigarette smokers often displayed a diffuse interstitial scarring. The development of scar tissue in the alveolar interstitium of the lung is a typical lesion following exposure to mineral fibers, e.g., asbestos (in all its forms), and also for nonfibrous mineral dusts of fine particle size, e.g., crushed quartz of less than 0.5 μm diameter. This heightened interest in inorganic dusts as possible co-agents in the etiology of cigarette-induced pulmonary disease.

- In 1970, we learned that the tobacco industry held patents on the use of minerals and man-made vitreous fibers in making small cigars and cigarettes (Table 1). A series of reconstituted tobacco sheet formulations were specifically designed for combustion control and ash quality, and some patents specifically stipulated the use of chrysotile and/or crocidolite asbestos as a property modifier (as a sorbent) for PAH in mainstream smoke.

Table 1. U.S. patents pertaining to mineral and inorganic tobacco additives for cigarette manufacture[a]

Patent No.	Date	Inorganic Additives Cited in Patent	Use, as Cited in Patent
1 518 944 1 581 619 2 020 646 2 733 720	09/13/20 08/18/21 11/12/35 02/07/56	Chrysotile asbestos	In cigarette paper to control ash character; to control temperature of smoke
3 022 863	10/03/61	Asbestos, carbon in form of charcoal, glass, silica fibers	To induce pyrolysis of organics in cigarette smoke, to accelerate combustion process
3 125 098	03/17/64	Asbestos, glass, fibers, diatomaceous earth	To improve character and strength of ash
3 255 760	06/14/66	Chrysotile asbestos, glass fiber	To control tar
3 410 276	11/12/68	Chrysotile, crocidolite, glass wool, Fiberfrax,™ talc, kaolin, other minerals, e.g., clays[b]	To filter smoke, control temperature, and filter radioactive particles, i.e., ^{210}Po
3 419 013	12/31/68	Glass fiber, glass shards	To reduce tars and nicotine in smoke
3 477 865	11/11/69	Chrysotile, crocidolite, glass wool, Fiberfrax,™ talc, kaolin, calcite, titania	To control combustion process, to provide insulation

[a]Patents which pertain to cigarette paper and to small cigars are reviewed in Langer et al., 1971.

[b]Fiberfrax™ is the trademark of a man-made aluminum silicate ceramic fiber manufactured by the Carborundum Company.

- The contribution of inorganics had not been studied, for the most part, with regard to tobacco carcinogenesis. This area of study had been confined largely to particles as passive vehicles: particles which acted as condensation nuclei for the organic vapor phase of cigarette smoke. However, rather than containing simple "soot," the tobacco plants were shown to contain elements and compounds which suggested that a complex combination of crystalline particles might be present. For example, bulk chemical analyses of tobacco plants showed the presence of SiO_2. The latter oxide, silica, was not assigned to a specific compound or mineral, e.g., quartz, as SiO_2, or as an oxide component contained within a silicate mineral. However, these data suggested the possibility that silicate minerals were present in tobacco.

These separate data sets and observations converged in a logical set of questions: "Are inorganic particles present in cigarettes? What are their origins? Do they enter mainstream smoke as respirable particles?" "Do they play a role in the etiology of any of the pulmonary diseases observed in cigarette smokers?" These questions were answered for small cigars in 1971 (Langer et al., 1971); cigarette studies remained to be done.

Natural Inorganic Chemistry of Cigarette Tobacco

The overall inorganic chemistry of tobacco, which varies to some degree, has been attributed to many factors (Table 2). Data have been collected on 155 tobacco varieties, grown on virtually every continent and its off-shore islands (Table 3).

Tobacco plant variety and plant parts are the principal factors which control its inorganic chemistry. For example, in one study, analysis of leaf and root from the same plant has shown an Al_2O_3 content of 0.6 to 1.0 ppm for the leaf and 25 to 350 ppm for the root. The suggestion had been made that the Al_2O_3 was derived from an adventitious soil mineral, e.g., kaolin clay, $Al_4Si_4O_{10}(OH)_8$. The variance of all components with plant part is thought to be principally related to botanical properties rather than exogenous factors.

The tobacco leaf is itself a product of soil character, geographical and climatological factors, etc. As an illustration, bright leaf in the United States averages about 4.0% chloride content, whereas imported Turkish leaf contains, on the average, only some 2.0% chloride. These differences have been ascribed to drainage of fields, fertilizers used, etc. Both soil chemistry and mineralogy follow basic geochemical principals: magnesium tends to follow calcium (probably related to soil profile and underlying rock-type, in this case, a carbonate limestone); iron and manganese tend to occur together.

Table 2. Factors found to influence the inorganic chemistry of tobacco plants[a]

Plant Determinants

- Plant type; country of origin
- Plant part: root, stalk, stem, leaf
- Time of planting; absence or occurrence of rain; environmental temperature
- Time of harvest: maturation of plant tissue and its components

Soil, Geographic, and Climatic Factors

- Soil chemistry and mineralogy, major determinants of bulk chemistry and trace metals; alkalinity of tobacco
- Groundwater quality: pH, chemistry (dissolved salts, etc.); movement
- Average rainfall and temperature extremes
- Topography and drainage: moisture saturation of soils

Soil and Plant Modifiers

- Fertilizers used: magnesium-, calcium-, nitrogen-, phosphate-based compounds; associated trace metals

Curing

- Temperature, duration, and humidity

[a]This list is not exhaustive. These factors do not include the contribution of adventitious soil particles. We have found no data on the formation of inorganic compounds in the combustion process.

Table 3. Natural inorganic compounds observed in tobacco plants and shredded tobacco

Constituent Oxide[a]	Percentage of Total Plant at Harvest[b] (range)	Content in American Cigarettes (μg/cigarette)[c]	Percentage in American Cigarettes (500 mg)[d]	Content in American Cigarette Smoke (μg/cigarette)[c]
CaO	1.80 to 6.50	Up to 27,500	5.50	Up to 0.4
K_2O	1.28 to 5.10	Up to 26,800	5.36	Up to 134.0
Chloride	1.15 to 10.10	$\bar{X}$, 19,300	3.89	NDA
MgO	0.60 to 1.04	$\bar{X}$, 5,100	1.02	$\bar{X}$, 0.07
FeO	0.08 to 9.50	$\bar{X}$, 540	0.11	$\bar{X}$, 0.08
SiO_2	1.05 to 3.01	NDA[e]	—	NDA
PO_4	0.09 to 0.26	NDA	—	NDA
MnO	Trace	$\bar{X}$, 190	0.04	Up to 0.04
Al_2O_3	Trace	Up to 930	0.19	Up to 0.02

[a]Oxides generally reported as percent of the entire tobacco plant. Cl- is reported as chloride. No partition between free silica, e.g., quartz, and silicate minerals. Iron occurs in an insoluble form, probably in a mineral; MnO should follow carbonate salts as, e.g., calcite; Al_2O_3 is likely an insoluble form, probably a silicate mineral, e.g., a clay or mica.
[b]Oxide percentages of total tobacco plant. Some data available on individual plant parts. Trace, based on analyses, is (as reported in the literature) less than 0.1%.
[c]"Up to . . ." denotes highest value reported; $\bar{X}$ is average value in literature.
[d]A cigarette that contains 500 mg of tobacco
[e]NDA = no data available

It is widely reported that the use of magnesium-based fertilizers invariably increases the chloride content of the tobacco plant. Any soil supplement is carried directly to the plant when dissolved, and it becomes incorporated in the plant tissue.

Curing tobacco mostly influences the calcium and potassium content of the plant: the greater the cure time and the higher the temperature, the greater the ash content of the plant. It has been shown that the CaO content of tobacco leaf may increase up to threefold during an average "cure."

We have not found in the literature that any systematic studies have been carried out to determine the contribution of shredded, reconstituted tobacco sheet, particles from cigarette paper additives or property modifiers, or compounds which may be created in the combustion process. The main focus in the past has been on the role that inorganics play in the control of tobacco combustion and burning quality. Furthermore, these analyses failed to assign any of the oxides to individual minerals or compounds; they failed to determine where the trace metals were sequestered; and also failed to distinguish whether certain metals and oxides were exogenous or endogenous to the tobaccos.

There have been many studies in the chemical carcinogenesis field which have suggested that *particles* may act as "carriers" of organic carcinogens, and that the agents in cigarette smoke are transported to the lung by means of these vehicles (e.g., Falk et al., 1958; Kotin and Falk, 1963). It is crucial to note that the investigators characterized these particles as "soot," although they discounted any relationship among scarring, particle accumulation, and lung cancer. The characterization of these particulates has been simplistic, frequently limited to color and size rather than to composition or identity. The generic name "soot" commonly appears in the chemical carcinogenesis literature (the particulate phase consists of combusted plant, i.e., charred cellulose). No systematic study of inorganics in cigarettes and cigarette smoke has been carried out.

More recently, a number of studies have been conducted on particles in the pulmonary tissues of cigarette smokers. We will publish an overview of these data in another manuscript (in preparation).

STUDY RATIONALE

Existing patents indicate that some minerals and man-made inorganics have been considered for incorporation in cigarettes as property modifiers. Interest in some of these materials has been great in the medical community, because some (e.g., quartz and the asbestos minerals) are known fibrogenic and carcinogenic agents.

It came to our attention in 1970 that, at one time, cigarette companies may have used reconstituted tobacco sheets in their filler formulations. Our information indicates that these formulas were developed and patented before 1970 and added as fillers to as many as 17% of the tobaccos in experimental formulations. These cigarettes would not have fallen under Federal Trade Commission requirements for labeling, as did small cigars (which carried the label "predominantly tobacco with non-tobacco ingredients added"). The question of whether or not this practice was used in 1974, coupled with the undefined inorganic nature of tobacco, both before and after combustion, motivated us to perform this study.

MATERIALS AND METHODS

Selection of Cigarettes for Study

Cigarettes were selected from among the 65 brands and 230 style varieties marketed in New York City in 1974. These included "popular" brands (based on market share), all style varieties (king, regular, filtered, unfiltered, flavored, e.g, with menthol), and cigarettes with a range of tar and nicotine (T&N) contents (Table 4).* For each of the study brands and styles of cigarettes, we selected a single pack from a carton and gravimetrically determined the tobacco filler content of each of its 20 cigarettes. Each of the 20 determinations was made at ambient temperature and humidity. The 20 determinations were averaged, and the values are given in Table 4.

The individual values per pack varied little. We noted that the low T&N cigarettes contained less tobacco filler than the high T&N cigarettes, but the gravimetric difference in filler (~690 mg, compared with about 900 mg, or ~72% of the filler) could not account for the reduced T&N (<8 mg:>17 mg, or ~47% of the T&N content). We concluded that filler character (tobacco type) accounted for most of the T&N differences, although some contribution may be made by smaller filler quantity.

Examination of Cigarette Filler

We examined chopped cigarette tobacco filler to determine: (1) whether inorganics were directly admixed with tobacco as property modifiers (e.g., aluminum oxide-hydroxide compounds of 25-μm particle size), or (2) whether chopped, reconstituted tobacco sheet was present.

*Tar and nicotine content determined the portion of tax levied by the federal government: > 17 mg, 0.04¢/pack; < 8 mg, 0.00¢/pack; intermediate > 8 and < 17 mg, 0.03¢/pack.

Table 4. American test cigarettes: tobacco contents, ash residues, and burn temperatures.

Cigarette Brand and Type	Amount of Tobacco Filler (mg)[a]	Peak Temperature of Burn (°C)[b]	Amount of Ash Residue (mg)[c]	Ash[d] (%)	N
Low Tar & Nicotine (Filtered)[e]					
Marlboro (Box)	708	570	105	14.8	
Kent (King)	770	572	119	15.5	
Benson & Hedges (Regular)	565	595	86	15.3	
Vantage (Regular)	731	540	101	13.9	
True Blue (Regular)	646	520	103	16.0	
Doral (Regular)	715	595	99	13.8	
Mean	**689 ± 73**	**565 ± 30**	**102 ± 11**	**14.9 ± 0.9**	**6**
Moderate & High Tar and Nicotine (Filtered)					
Marlboro (Soft Pack)	740	620	111	15.0	
Winston (King, Soft)	771	585	111	14.3	
Kent 100's	860	598	129	15.0	
Benson & Hedges (King)	745	600	110	14.8	
Mean	**779 ± 56**	**601 ± 14**	**115 ± 9**	**14.8 ± 0.3**	**4**
Moderate & High Tar and Nicotine (Unfiltered)					
Chesterfield (Regular)	836	580	114	13.6	
Chesterfield (King)	1009	540	142	14.0	
Philip Morris (Regular)	811	520	117	14.4	
Philip Morris (King)	990	550	145	14.6	
Lucky Strike	861	595	116	13.5	
Pall Mall (Regular)	1011	605	137	13.6	
Old Gold	787	585	126	16.0	
Mean	**901 ± 99**	**568 ± 31**	**128 ± 13**	**14.2 ± 0.9**	**7**
Grand Mean	**797 ± 123**	**575 ± 30**	**116 ± 16**	**14.6 ± 0.8**	

[a]$\bar{X}$ tobacco content, based on 20 separate cigarette determinations, one pack.
[b]$\bar{X}$ tobacco ash, combusted at 550° C, based on $\bar{X}$ of 10 separate cigarette determinations (see text)
[c]$\bar{X}$ tobacco ash per cigarette
[d]N = 17; ash content (Y) = 0.12 tobacco (X) + 1.93, r = 0.937; r^2 = 0.878 (see text)
[e]Low tar and nicotine = $\leq$8.0 mg/cigarette; high tar and nicotine = $\geq$17.0 mg/cigarette (1974 tax requirements)

Two representative cigarette varieties were selected from among the three groups of brands studied (Table 4), and the tobacco was removed from several individual cigarettes. The tobacco shreds were examined by light optical, stereoptic microscopy. Shreds were separated by hand-pick on the basis of color. Several slides were made of separated shreds mounted in an immersion oil (n ≅ 1.515), and examined by polarized light microscopy. Additionally, shred mounts were burned in an open furnace at temperatures which produced smoldering and combustion, then cooled and mounted on slides in a similar manner.

We did not find free inorganic particles in the tobacco matrix which would be categorized as additives. The shreds did not show the presence of tobacco sheet with inorganic components, although stalk-leaf composites were present. Burned shreds consisted principally of carbonized remnants of plant. A few inorganic objects were visible between crossed nicols. Identification could not be achieved, although indices of refraction were greater than 1.515. We concluded that these particles were: crystalline; irregular in shape; that they averaged about 1-2 μm in their greatest dimension; that their extinction between crossed nicols was sharp, so that the particles were single crystalline fragments; and that they resembled soil particles, i.e., quartz and feldspar fragments. We classed the particles as adventitious in origin. Their amount per cigarette was small, and they constituted less than 1% of the tobacco ash.

We stress the following observation: we failed to find any of the additives that are described as present in small cigars (Langer et al., 1971), i.e., man-made vitreous fibers or diatom fragments; nor did we find asbestos fiber additives.

Ash Determination and Characterization

Given the chemistry of cigarette tobacco, we considered that the combustion process and the environment of a burning cigarette might be conducive to the formation of inorganic compounds. We first determined the temperature at which cigarette tobacco burned during the smoking process.

Measurement of Cigarette Burn Temperature

The temperatures achieved in a burning cigarette during the normal smoking process were measured in the following manner:
A chromel-alumel thermocouple (15 mil, point-beaded) was inserted to a depth of about 4 mm into the cigarette 1.5 cm from the end to be lighted. The thermocouple signal was amplified as the output on the x-axis of a Moseley XY recorder of a differential thermal analyzer system. The system used was a DuPont 900, equipped with a 1200°C cell, with standard signal processing and amplification electronics and an ice-point reference. The x-axis of the recorder (*temperature*) was zero-shifted along the y-axis (ΔT) after each puff so that the maximal excursion point for each puff peak temperature could be

precisely monitored. The temperature axis was set at 4.0 mV, the equivalent of a 100°C interval per inch. A shift of 1 of 20 divisions on the chart paper was equal to a 5°C change, and measurements of ±2°C were easily distinguished.

Fresh cigarettes were then randomly removed from unopened packages and the thermocouple was inserted. A volunteer cigarette smoker was asked to light the cigarette and smoke it in his/her normal manner. The temperatures were recorded until the combustion zone passed the point of the thermocouple, and it broke through the ash. The maximal temperatures recorded are given in Table 4.

For the American cigarettes studied,* we noted that the ultimate combustion point ranged from 520°C to 620°C, with $\bar{x}$ = 575°C ± 30°C. The thermal history was as follows: after lighting the cigarette, the temperature of the mainstream smoke appears to remain relatively level, between 40°C and 50°C.** After several puffs, the average temperature increased slightly, but puff draw brought the temperature up to about 140°C, as a defined spike. Idling of the cigarette allowed the temperature to drop to 50°C. Additional puffing produced an increase in temperature of mainstream smoke and gases to almost 350°C. Cessation of puffing at this point caused the idling temperature to decrease to only 75°C to 90°C. Resumption of puffing allowed attainment of peak burns at the lighted, oxygenated tip. The ash cooled rapidly to ambient temperatures.

Although the cigarette profiles and maximal temperatures were found to be uniform, smoking style ("puff" size, "puff" time, idling time) controlled the slope of the combustion profile (not unlike the features described in Touey and Mumpower, 1957). All combustion curves were log-normal when plotted as a function of puff number and followed a third-order equation profile. Each cigarette produced a friable ash "clinker" after combustion.

Ash Determination

Ten cigarettes from each of the study brands were used for 10 separate determinations of ash residue. Tobacco from each was placed in a clean porcelain crucible, which was put in a muffle furnace set at 550°C, allowed to burn, then roasted until the ash weight remained constant. At this time, each crucible was weighed, and an average ash content for each cigarette brand was determined. The average tobacco weight, ash residue, and percent residue for each cigarette type are given in Table 4.

---

*An additional five varieties/brands studied displayed temperatures in the same range.

**All statements made on the basis of thermocouple at 1.5 cm from lighted end.

The amount of tobacco and the subsequent amount of ash appeared to be linearly related. A *t*-test comparison of the ashed residue percentages of the different cigarette populations (based on T&N contents) indicates that there are no statistically significant differences among the various ash residues. It appears that the various organic components of the tobacco which exist in a compositional range are unrelated to the incombustible portion of the plant; T&N levels did not influence inorganic ash contents. The ash content of American cigarettes was:

$$\text{Ash} = 0.12\ (\text{tobacco filler}) + 1.93.$$

The intercept (1.93) and the slope (0.12) were estimated by a regression analysis based on 17 observations. Percent of variation of ash, explained by the regression of ash on tobacco filler, was 87.8%.

The ash residues (Table 4) for the different brands and types are statistically identical; although style variety dictates the amount of tobacco per cigarette, the resultant ash is always in the same proportion to the tobacco (~14–15%).

Statistical comparison of ash residue from each group or variety yielded:

Compared Populations	Computed *t*-value	Probability that Population Values Differ
Ash 1–Ash 2	0.43	P > 0.9 (not significant); statistically identical ash values
Ash 1–Ash 3	0.34	P = 0.8–0.9 (not significant); statistically identical ash values
Ash 2–Ash 3	0.16	P = 0.8–0.9 (not significant); statistically identical ash values

Polarized Light Microscopic Examination of Cigarette Ash

Representative aliquots of ash from each of the brands examined were placed on clean glass slides, mounted in an immersion oil (n = 1.512), and examined by means of polarized light microscopy. After an initial examination, in which a number of inorganic, refringent (crystalline) particles were tentatively identified, specific immersion oils (n = 1.490; 1.550; 1.660) were used on duplicate aliquots for verification purposes. These refractive indices were used to grossly distinguish among minerals present.

Several adventitious mineral particles appeared to be associated with each ash: quartz fragments were common in all. The quartz particles were several micrometers in their greatest dimension and appeared consistent with common soil components. Both feldspar fragments and materials resembling clays and/or micas were observed. In addition to these recognizable minerals, all brands contained plant relics. These blackened and charred plant parts obviously constituted the materials commonly referred to as "soot."

Each cigarette ash contained a "background" matrix material which consisted of micrometer-sized refringent particles which create a "ground mass" effect. There were no preferred orientations of these grains as indicated by their range of extinction angles. One of the more unexpected features observed for all the cigarettes was that most of the ash residues appeared to be crystalline rather than amorphous. Matrix particles appeared to possess indices of refraction >1.515.

X-Ray Diffraction Analysis of Cigarette Ash

Cigarette ash from each brand was placed in an agate mortar and lightly ground, by hand, with an agate pestle for approximately 10 to 15 seconds. Little pressure was necessary for grinding because the ashes were friable. Materials so prepared in the mortar produced a fine powder, suitable for X-ray diffraction analysis. Powders were loaded into an aluminum sample holder and scanned, in a continuous mode, in a Philips X-ray diffractometer. Instrumental settings and conditions are stated in Table 5.

The crystalline material of which cigarette ash is composed consists of carbonate, sulphate, and chloride minerals (Table 5). Their reflections are sharp and well defined, and they conform to those of described minerals. The silica and silicate minerals are clearly present, in trace quantities.

Sylvite, arcanite, and fairchildite are potash salts. Although calcite is the predominant carbonate mineral, the potash minerals also incorporate carbonate groups (fairchildite-buetschliite) (Table 5). A comparison of the X-ray data shows that X-ray diffraction patterns which are virtually indistinguishable for all cigarette types (based on T&N content). For example, in the X-ray range of 5.0 Å to 1.54 Å, the patterns were identical. Minerals identified by light microscopy, i.e., quartz, micas, and carbonate minerals, were also found by X-ray.

Transmission Electron Microscopy and Selected Area Electron Diffraction

A 1-mg aliquot was collected from each cigarette ash and dispersed in 5 ml of triple-distilled water. The mixture was sonified with a cell disrupter set at 70 W of power, for approximately 5 seconds, until a

Table 5. Minerals identified in cigarette filler ash and smoke[a]

Mineral[b]	Composition	No. Observed/ No. Studied	Relative Percentage[c]
Sylvite	KCl	17/17	~29
Arcanite	K_2SO_4	17/17	~8
Fairchildite	$K_2CO_3 \cdot CaCO_3$	17/17	~24
Calcite	$CaCO_3$	17/17	~37
Calcium Oxide	CaO	4/17	Trace
Quartz	SiO_2	17/17	~2
Mica(s)	XYZ $Si_4O_{10}(OH)$	9/17	Trace
Buetschliite	$3K_2CO_3 \cdot 2CaCO_3 \cdot 6H_2O$ K_2CO_3 $K_2CO_3 \cdot 1.5H_2O$		Trace

[a]X-ray patterns determined on a Philips diffractometer: Cu target; 45 kV; 20 mA; graphite monochrometer; 1° 2θ min; scintillation counter set at 960 VDC; 1°-006-1° slit openings; 1000 cps = full scale.

[b]Standards (Joint Committee on Powder Diffraction Standards):

Sylvite	ASTM 4-0587
Arcanite	ASTM 5-0613
Fairchildite	ASTM 3-0504; 6-0321
Calcite	ASTM 5-0586
Quartz	ASTM 5-0490

[c]The relative percentage of the five major phases was determined by X-ray reflection, peak summation technique on pure standards. We had to synthesize fairchildite and compare it with the ASTM data file card. Some buetschliite was also formed in the synthesized fairchildite. This co-existence is compatible and reflects the juxtaposition of their respective stability regions on the $CaCO_3 \cdot K_2CO_3 \cdot H_2O$ phase diagram. The buetschliite chemistry is close to that of fairchildite; see under "Composition."

cloudy supernatant was obtained. A 10-μl micropipette was used to withdraw an aliquot from each suspension, which was then pipetted onto the center of a carbon-coated, Formvar®-support, nickel, 200-mesh locator grid. After the suspension dried, another carbon coat was evaporated onto the grid surfaces. These samples were examined by transmission electron microscopy and an electron microprobe technique.

On the basis of morphology, size, and crystallinity, cigarette ash, in all cases, appeared to contain a range of particle types. At relatively low magnifications, a typical cigarette-ash field contained particles which ranged from several hundred ångstroms to tens of micrometers in size. Shapes ranged from irregular to rounded; occasionally, polygonal plates were observed. Cigarette-ash compounds commonly formed clusters of individual particles which appeared to be sintered aggregates with random orientation. Single crystals were observed, as determined by selected area electron diffraction; occasionally, clay minerals were observed. Ash of some brands appeared to contain more crystalline particles than others. We do not know whether this particle population reflected an effect of burn temperature, or whether it was the result of slight compositional differences among different tobacco types.

Most particles examined in cigarette ash appeared to be crystalline, corroborating the light microscopic and X-ray data. The aggregate grains displayed characteristics of both single crystals and polycrystalline aggregates. For the latter, the selected area diffraction patterns displayed Debye-Scherrer rings rather than the single, discrete spot reflections which characterize single crystals.

Microchemical Analysis of Particles in Cigarette Ash

Electron microscope grid preparations used for transmission electron microscopy were also used for microchemical analysis of the particles. Grids were transferred to a field emission scanning electron microscope and examined in the transmitted electron mode. Selected particles and fields of particles were analyzed by the electron microprobe technique, using energy-dispersive X-ray spectroscopy. Ten fields per specimen were analyzed for elemental chemistry. The beam was allowed to survey an entire grid opening and total X-ray count, generated from the entire particle population in the beam field; the signal was integrated over 60 seconds. Each field yielded an analysis of approximately 500 clusters of particles (which probably represented several thousand discrete particles).

Calcium and potassium compounds predominated in the ash. Elemental chlorine was detected in all fields. Silicon was detected in only ~10% of fields, then only as a trace. Iron and manganese were detected in a few fields, also as a trace. Elemental sulfur was also common, but only in selected fields.

Individual particles, selected on the basis of morphology (as observed by transmission electron microscopy), were analyzed in a similar manner. Elongated crystals emitted primarily calcium signals, with minor amounts of potassium and trace amounts of other elements. Small rounded grains appeared to consist primarily of potassium and chlorine (sylvite). Clusters of particles consisted of calcium, potassium, chlorine, and sulfur. Aluminum and silicon signals were detected in small particles which appeared to be a clay mineral (kaolinite).

Investigations of the microchemical nature of particles in the cigarette ash enabled us to determine that the calcium compounds present were not associated with chlorine; only the high-potassium-content compounds were associated with chlorine. This corroborates the X-ray data on the minerals in the ash: sylvite (KCl) was the only chloride mineral identified. Particles were found in which sulfur and potassium were present, correlating with the arcanite (K_2SO_4) found by X-ray analysis.

Transmission electron microscopy and probe examination of the particle population in the cigarette ash confirmed the following: the discrete crystalline phases ranged in size from nonrespirable to several hundred ångstroms. Although individual particles were found, polycrystalline sintered aggregates predominated in the mineral population. Sylvite and arcanite were present as discrete particle types.. Complex chemical signals, and Debye-Scherrer diffraction patterns, reinforced the perception that fairchildite-buetschliite was present as mixtures in sintered aggregate form. We stress the following: clay(s), mica(s), and quartz were found in tobacco ash; the diameter of the particles (quartz, 1 to 2 μm; mica, 1 to 2 μm; clay, <1 μm) suggests that they were soil-derived.

Particles in Smoke

Two brands of cigarettes were selected from each of the three study categories. Selected cigarettes were inserted in a Tygon® tube which allowed passage of cigarette smoke. The tube was inserted into the air inlet of a Casella filter holder cartridge fitted with a Millipore® AA membrane filter. This device was then interfaced with a smoking machine, and "smoking" was mechanically set for a 35-ml puff every 12 to 15 seconds.

Filters were allowed to accumulate cigarette smoke until discoloration was noticeable.* Smoking was then stopped, and the filter was prepared for electron microscopy (EM) by dissolving it in acetone and directly transferring it to EM grids.

The filter preparations were sparse in particles. Those observed on the filter had some tarry residue, evidenced by a "bubbling" action when the electron beam was intensified by means of the condenser lens system. These particles were small (<1 μm in diameter), crystalline (diffracted electrons), and electron-transparent (thin). A few soil particles (e.g., quartz) were also noted. Energy-dispersive spectrometry characterization was achieved on only the

*We noted that heavily laden filters could not be successfully cleared of tars and nicotine. Even when the load on the filter was considered "light" (i.e., electron translucent when examined by TEM), the preparations still contained tarry residues.

largest particles (those resolvable in the optical system), which were found to be calcium and calcium-potash salts. We recovered particles only from unfiltered cigarettes.

DISCUSSION AND CONCLUSIONS

Inorganic minerals have not been studied as components of cigarette smoke as have their gases and organic compounds. The rationale for this is that the 400-odd organic compounds observed in cigarette smoke include such known carcinogens as the polycyclic aromatic hydrocarbons, anthracenes, nitrosamines, etc. These compounds have monopolized the efforts of chemical carcinogenesis investigators for many years. "Particulate" phases have included only "tarry" residues, such as nicotine and alkaloids, non-volatile nitrosamines, naphthalenes, etc. Particulates were often considered only as the "tarry components" which condensed from smoke at room temperature. Additionally, radioactive species, trace metals, and chlorinated compounds (from insecticides) have been described in smoke. Some particles described as "soot" were studied as vehicles and/or condensation nuclei for liquid and gas phases. Interest in these particles was always secondary to the gas and organic phases.

Data from a number of sources, some involving studies in disparate fields, suggest that the inorganic mineral components of cigarette smoke could play a role in tobacco carcinogenesis. The data on cigarette-smoking, asbestos-exposed workers, and their elevated incidence of lung cancer, underscore the potential synergism between mineral particles and components of cigarette smoke. This observation, coupled with other data and the potential use of mineral-based, reconstituted tobacco sheets in cigars and cigarettes, raised interest in the nature of inorganic minerals as components of cigarette smoke.

The natural chemistry of cigarette smoke is strongly influenced by the tobacco types, their properties, the plant parts incorporated into the filler, the age of the plant, the cure history of the leaf, soil chemistry, climatic factors, fertilizers used, etc. Superimposed on these characteristics are secondary additives which influence burn character; e.g., humectants, burn modifiers, flavorings, etc. All these factors affect both bulk chemistry and burn quality.

In the past, various temperature zones of burning cigarettes were studied (see review in Wynder and Hoffmann, 1968; Osdene, 1976). An understanding of how a cigarette burns, how it acquires oxygen, its zones of combustion and oxygen saturation, etc., are important in determining at what temperature a cigarette burns and what inorganic compounds may be created during the burn process.

Chopped and shredded reconstituted tobacco plant parts may have been used in cigarette manufacture. Some of these sheets included a large variety of inorganics; many patents even suggest the use of asbestos in the sheet formulation. If present, they would contribute significantly to the mineral content of cigarette smoke, thereby playing an important role in carcinogenesis.

We have approached the elucidation of the inorganic minerals in cigarette tobacco, cigarette ash, and cigarette smoke as one of mineral analysis. We have therefore used the mineralogical assay tools, determined the combustion temperature of cigarettes, and assayed tobacco filler, tobacco ash, and cigarette smoke for their mineral content. Our observations are as follows:

(1) The tobacco fillers examined did not include chopped reconstituted tobacco sheet containing inorganic additives but, rather, varieties of tobacco and tobacco plant parts.

(2) Occasionally, inorganic particles were detected in the tobacco filler. By size and character, they were found to be adventitious soil particles.

(3) The cigarette combustion temperature may reach the 600°C range, ample heat for converting plant tissue salts into crystalline compounds.

(4) The major minerals and inorganic compounds found in cigarette ash are those which have been described as components of fused wood-ash in the mineralogical literature (Milton and Axelrod, 1947). These include fairchildite ($K_2CO_3 \cdot CaCO_3$), buetschliite ($3K_2CO_3 \cdot 2CaCO_3 \cdot 6H_2O$), which is itself a secondary hydrated phase of fairchildite; calcite ($CaCO_3$), a decomposition product of buetschliite; and, by hydration of fairchildite, lime (CaO), a product of incomplete reaction. We also noted the formation of the sulfate mineral arcanite (K_2SO_4) and the mineral sylvite (KCl). The latter deserves attention. We believe that sylvite is, in part, a byproduct of combustion promotion. The interior of a burning cigarette is an oxygen-depleted environment. Combustion promoters are used to allow the uniform burning of a cigarette as it idles. The use of a perchlorate compound, (2)$KClO_3$, allows breakdown into (2)KCl + (3)O_2. Some quartz and a trace of other soil particles have been observed in ash as well.

(5) The particle diameter of the minerals found ranged from hundreds of ångstroms to tens of micrometers, making them excellent condensation nuclei.

(6) Analysis of cigarette smoke shows very few inorganic particles in the mainstream. Athough the data are too scant to

judge the efficacy of cigarette filters in entraining mineral particles, only unfiltered cigarettes yielded particles. Because particles act as vehicles and condensation nuclei for T&N, we conclude that, as the filter traps these organic-laden compounds, fewer noxious agents will be inhaled.

(7) The ash content produced by cigarette combustion appears to be proportionately constant with the tobacco weight of a cigarette. Although the T&N content of various cigarettes differs, the presence of inorganic mineral constituents appears to be independent of the organic nature of the tobacco.

Inorganic particles may act as passive vehicles and condensation nuclei for gases and organics in cigarette smoke. The minerals we have observed (the sulfate, chloride, and carbonate forms of potash and lime) are likely soluble in human lungs and, if inhaled, will dissolve with time. The respirable adventitious soil particles may be noxious; this may be especially true for quartz.

We have failed to find asbestos of any variety in any of the cigarettes on the basis of several levels of analysis. The cigarettes we studied contained no inorganic reinforced, homogenized tobacco leaf. Inorganic mineral particles created during the combustion process, such as the types described in this report, may be important as vehicles only.

ACKNOWLEDGMENTS

This work was supported by a grant from the National Institute of Enviromental Health Sciences (NIEHS) ES-00797. Dr. Langer wishes to acknowledge additional support on a Career Development Award from the NIEHS ES-44812, and a Center Grant from the NIEHS, ES-00928. Dr. Nolan was supported by a Fellowship from the Stony Wold-Herbert Fund. The writing of this manuscript was made possible through a gift from the R. J. Reynolds Tobacco Company.

The authors wish to acknowledge all of those who aided the project with technical support: R. Ashley, Y. Bystricka, H. Collins, J. Joelson, W. Moranta, J. Nehrer, I. Rubin, L. Shackman, E. Sygman, A. Tordini, and R. Welner, of the Environmental Sciences Laboratory of The Mount Sinai School of Medicine. We also wish to thank several scientists of the Philip Morris Tobacco Company for providing us with a bibliography of tobacco chemistry, valuable discussions concerning the inorganic chemistry of tobacco, and a smoking machine. Our sincere thanks to Drs. Helmut Wakeham, Thomas Osdene, Robert Seligman, and Calhoun Howard.

REFERENCES

Falk, HL, A Miller, and P Kotin. **1958.** Elution of 3-4 benzpyrene and related hydrocarbons from soot by plasma proteins. Science 137:474-475.

Kotin, P and HL Falk. **1963.** Atmosphere factors in the pathogenesis of lung cancer. Adv Cancer Res 7:475-514.

Langer, AM, AD Mackler, I Rubin, EC Hammond, and IJ Selikoff. **1971.** Inorganic particles in cigars and cigar smoke. Science 174:585-587.

Milton, C, and J. Axelrod. **1947.** Fused wood-ash stones: Fairchildite, $K_2CO_3 \cdot CaCO_3$, buetschliite, $3K_2CO_3 \cdot 2CaCO_3 \cdot 6H_2O$, and calcite, $CaCO_3$, their essential components. Am Mineral 32:607-624.

Osdene, TS. **1976.** Reaction mechanisms in the burning cigarette, pp. 42-49. In: *The Recent Chemistry of Natural Products, Including Tobacco,* NJ Fina, ed., 2nd Philip Morris Science Symposium, Richmond, VA. Philip Morris, Inc., New York, NY.

Selikoff, IJ, EC Hammond, and J Churg. **1968.** Asbestos exposure, smoking and neoplasia. J Am Med Assoc 204:104-110.

Touey, GG and RC Mumpower. **1957.** Measurement of the combustion zone temperature of cigarettes. Tobacco Sci 1:33-37.

Wynder, E and D Hoffmann. **1968.** *Tobacco and Tobacco Smoke Studies in Experimental Carcinogenesis,* p. 730. Academic Press, New York, NY.

Characterization of Dusts Collected During the Machining of Epoxy-Reinforced Fibrous Materials*

Edwin S. Boatman, David Covert, David Kalman, Daniel Luchtel, and Gilbert S. Omenn

Department of Environmental Health, School of Public Health, University of Washington, Seattle, WA 98195

KEY WORDS: dust characterization, epoxy-reinforced fibers, machining

---

ABSTRACT

The objective of the work reported here is to determine whether respirable dusts derived from machining composite epoxy materials pose a health risk to machine operators. Dust samples representative of a number of composites and of various structural components were collected at the tool face and aerodynamically sized and fractionated. Bulk and fractionated samples were examined by light and electron microscopy and analyzed chemically by thermogravimetry (TGA), gas chromatography (GC) and mass spectrometry (MS).

By microscopy, bulk particles ranged in diameter from 7 to 11 μm, with mean aspect ratios ranging from 4 to 8:1. Aerodynamic diameters of fractionated particles ranged from 0.8 to 2.0 μm, with a mean diameter of 2.7 μm, as determined by light microscopy. The relative fraction of respirable-to-total mass of the bulk samples ranged from less than 1% to about 3%. By TGA, weight losses of fractionated materials were negligible below 520° C; they were variable but elevated at temperatures up to 860° C. Analysis by GC/MS indicated a variety of compounds in different amounts for each sample.

We conclude that, under presently used machining protocols, dusts generated at the tool face contained few particles of respirable size,

*Editor's Note: This material was presented by Dr. Luchtel. Due to illness, the leading author did not prepare a full paper.

with no evidence of fibers splitting longitudinally. The chemical content of the samples was low in volatility.

Overall, composites were judged to be well-cured and thermally stable. Clearly, composites that generate the fewest respirable particles and have the least hazardous chemical release should be chosen so long as design and performance specifications are met. We are currently evaluating the biologial response(s) to these dusts in order to draw firm conclusions regarding health effects.

WORKSHOP DISCUSSIONS

Editorial Note

As stated in the Preface, the primary objective of this symposium was to develop, rather than merely to present, knowledge and new ideas. Toward that end, reasonable speculation was encouraged.

Discussants were deliberately not identified to encourage forthright discussions, even though the organizers are aware that the anonymity of the speakers has some disadvantages for readers of the Proceedings.

The fragmented nature of the informal discussions, as well as the poor quality of both the transcripts and the audiotapes, necessitated heavy editing of the recorded versions. The text presented here has been reviewed by the chairmen, and certain portions have been reviewed by the discussants involved, to ensure maximal authenticity.

Edited Transcript of the Discussions of Day 1

Chairman: Dr. F. J. C. Roe

Papers by the following authors were discussed in this session: Roe, Wehner, Martonen, Sterling, Pott, Ferin, Davis, Churg, Muhle, Gerde, and Scholander.

DR. ROE: Ladies and gentlemen, I will call the discussion to order. During the first hour or so we will talk about the papers which were presented this morning. I think it is only right to give you an opportunity for questions and comments on each of these talks and, obviously, I gave the first talk, so I must offer you the chance of criticizing and commenting on what I said. Regarding the maximum loading for dust inhalation, I believe we should take into consideration the nature of the dust, especially its density, and not only the mass of the dust. Basically I am saying that the dust quantity, whether it is, say, 2 to 3 mg/m^3 or 16 mg/m^3, would be a function of the density of the dust. Too little attention has been paid to this in the past. In relation to overload, there is a "magic" number for maximal dust loads. The maximum is between 1 and 2 mg, up to 4 mg of dust/g of lung tissue. Knowing the minute volume and the exposure time, and assuming the deposition rate, one can estimate the aerosol concentration. Obviously, one of the basic factors for these estimates is the density.

DISCUSSANT: We have worked with asbestos fibers and titanium dioxide, and found an overloading of lung clearance even with "inert" particles. With cytotoxic particles such as asbestos, of course, this overloading occurs at much lower concentrations.

I will first explain what happens with inert particles with respect to overloading the lung clearance mechanism because we do not have the compounding effect of cytotoxicity here. Macrophages have a limited capacity for phagocytizing particles; you can fill them up to about 50%. This is approximately the point at which alveolar clearance becomes severely retarded, and the movement of the macrophages becomes slower and slower. Also, at this point they start to form clusters, so that aggregated macrophages are seen in tissue slides.

Alveolar clearance can be retarded from a half-time of 80 days to half-times of up to 500 days, even by inert particles, if you fill up the macrophages by more than 50% of their capacity.

DISCUSSANT: One thing I think you should take into consideration, at least based on our observations, when you are making your calculations: We found that there is at least one subpopulation of pulmonary macrophages that does not phagocytize particles, and this subpopulation may contribute from 25 to 35% of the total population. I do not know whether it has to do with receptors or whether the nonphagocytizing macrophages are simply immature or old.

DR. ROE: One very interesting thing that I came across when we were looking at the effects of inhaled cigarette smoke was that, early in the study, we observed macrophages in the lungs, in the region of the terminal bronchioles, which did not stain positively for iron. When we then looked again at a later time in the study, not necessarily after more smoke exposure, many macrophages were found to stain positively for iron. The question is, from where did the iron come? There is, for practical purposes, no iron in cigarette smoke. It is not coming from there—and in any case, even if it were, it does not stain immediately—so it seems that the iron is picked up perhaps as a result of absorption of fluid that is getting into the lung by transudation from the blood, and it is therefore a secondary phenomenon. This suggests that pulmonary macrophages phagocytize particles other than those that stimulate their proliferation. This may be a variable which, perhaps, is relevant to interaction.

DISCUSSANT: Following up on both those comments, the lung should certainly not be regarded as a static organ.

DISCUSSANT: In the case of inert particles, one does not see many new macrophages.

DISCUSSANT: What defines an inert particle?

DISCUSSANT: That is a good question. In our view, there is no such thing as an inert particle. All particles impact on the lung, although not necessarily because they are cytotoxic.

DISCUSSANT: "Inert" is really like "insoluble"; it is a relative concept.

DR. ROE: It is obviously easier to detect inertia amongst colleagues than among particles.

DISCUSSANT: I find this discussion a bit disquieting because it assumes that one can extrapolate from animal studies directly to humans. A review of data on inhalation of dust by human subjects does not lead to any concrete conclusions that smoking interferes with dust inhalation. Some investigators have reported that smoking suppresses particle clearance, and others have reported that it stimulates it.

Cohen used a magnetometric technique to determine the elimination of dust that was *not* labeled radioactively, and I understand that this technique is mostly used with radioactive dust. Cohen's subjects inhaled large quantities of ferric oxide and then were magnetized and the regions of magnetism recorded. I am sure that most of you are familiar with this kind of technique. However, there is a serious difficulty with the interpretation of Cohen's results.

What happened in Cohen's case was that when he subjected smokers who had swallowed or inhaled iron particles to strong magnetic forces, these particles traveled in the mucus stream within the lung and formed large clusters. The reason that smokers in the Cohen study did not eliminate metal dust as quickly as nonsmokers do was because these clusters of metal were too large to be moved.

Cohen's experiment was simulated by Reinstein, and the whole subject was discussed at the meeting of the Magnetometric Society, which was an acrimonious and noisy affair. In my opinion, Cohen's experiment should not be considered as proof that smoking can affect the elimination of dust from the lungs.

Over the years, a number of investigators have measured, by magnetometric techniques, dust elimination from the lungs in smoking and nonsmoking individuals who were occupationally exposed to welding and mining dust. These investigators either found no difference, or refrained from publishing their failure to find any difference, because they believed that such publications would not be of interest to the general population. Everybody assumes that smoking interferes with the elimination of dust, so any study that does not support this assumption is suspect and may not be accepted for publication.

There are other questions that need to be addressed: Are all types of dust eliminated in the same way? Maybe smoking does interfere with elimination of the kind of dust to which asbestos workers are exposed but not with that of other dusts with which it is safer to experiment.

DR. ROE: We seem to be rapidly getting into the field of metal analysis.

DISCUSSANT: I agree. The kind of data I am talking about should rightly be considered in context with metal analysis.

DISCUSSANT: I should like to comment on one thing Dr. Muhle said. He claimed that one does not get macrophage influx in lung tissue following exposure to innocuous dusts. I believe this is largely true over a certain range of doses, but not entirely true. We have looked at the comparison between titanium dioxide as an innocuous dust and asbestos and quartz. With 10 mg/m^3, there was a massive influx of macrophages with asbestos and quartz, and none with titanium dioxide. When we did the same experiment with 50 mg/m^3, there was, after 6 to 8 weeks, quite a large influx of macrophages, even with the titanium dioxide. Fifty mg/m^3 is, of course, a very high dose. Nevertheless, it is important to recognize that even with this otherwise innocuous material, macrophage influx can occur.

DR. ROE: On the subject of anatomical models of the respiratory tree, I remember papers published in the 1950s in which there were models of the respiratory tract, and not just the lower respiratory tract but of the upper respiratory tract as well. As far as I recall, the findings using these models were no different from those which were presented today. Be that as it may, I ask myself: Is it reasonable to expect a silicone surface to be a valid model for a warm, living, moist surface, which is changing all the time with respiration, and which has several specialized layers of surface fluid? Is it reasonable to expect such a simple model to tell one very much of importance?

DR. WEHNER: Not being a specialist in that field, my gut reaction would be that such a model would probably be better than no model at all.

DISCUSSANT: The whole concept of using such a model is to try to develop something that simulates a biological entity. By definition, a model can never be perfect, regardless of what the model intends to simulate. Ideally, I would have conducted my experiments with human replica casts. We still propose to do that. The advantage of human replica casts is that they have anatomical features, such as cartilaginous rings, which simulate realistically the conditions in the human body. However, when we did our experiments, we did not have access to replica casts.

DR. ROE: Could you describe what you mean by a replica cast?

DISCUSSANT: A replica cast is made from the lung of a cadaver. A replica cast is a cast made from a biological organ.

DR. ROE: In terms of the respiratory tree shape, clearly, a replica cast is ideal. However, it is important to ask: With what is it lined?

DISCUSSANT: We make the replica cast from lungs of the cadaver, then we line the inner surface of those replica casts with silicone oil to simulate the mucus lining, so that the particles will be deposited in various locations and will not become re-entrained in the air flow.

In my view, these models are therefore suitable surrogates. The reason for using these models is that if one wishes to identify factors affecting deposition in the human lung, one can do appropriate tests with them.

One never measures deposition; one infers deposition from subsequent clearance data. One can then estimate tracheobronchial deposition by what has been cleared within, say, 20 hours, and subsequently one can measure pulmonary clearance in terms of gross compartmental clearance.

The advantage of latex replica casts is that one can simulate breathing patterns and study microscopic deposition patterns. One will not be able to quantify or even observe microscopic deposition patterns in the human lung, because one will need a high-resolution instrument capable of focusing on a three-dimensional, branching, tree-like network.

I do not advocate, and never have advocated, that deposition experiments be conducted using only models. Modeling should be regarded as complementary to human tests.

In my view, models are an integral part of an inhalation-exposure protocol, and I think they are definitely realistic in the sense that, by coating them appropriately, and by making the walls thin enough so that they can indeed expand and contract on inhalation and expiration when we introduce chrysotile dust, we are engaging surrogate modeling to the state of the art we have today within the limits of practicality.

DR. ROE: You said you used 100% smoke. Did you make allowances for the fact that smokers only inhale the more dilute smoke?

DISCUSSANT: Yes.

DR. ROE: And did you control such variables as humidity and temperature, etc.?

DISCUSSANT: We are doing that. I was educated by a very wise professor, Dr. Werner Stöber, who told me that science is error, error, error. Being an engineer, I try to approach problems very simply and then add complexities, rather than look at an overall problem which is too hopelessly complex for a solution.

In our *first* test we introduced an aerosol into a replica cast that was lined with silicone, but the interior was *not* humidified. I am quite aware of the effects of hygroscopic growth and the effects of aerosols on pulmonary deposition and have published numerous peer-reviewed papers on this subject.

In our *next* generation of models, we have developed a bifurcating, three-dimensional model in which the temperature and relative humidity of the upper human airways *are* simulated. This successful engineering model is the culmination of a 2-year research effort that is described in a 40-page publication.

DR. ROE: I thank you very much. I apologize for attacking you, but it was worth it to get the additional information.

DISCUSSANT: Do you have any information about the deposition patterns in the distal lung, in the alveolar regions, either based on calculations or on what you may have seen? Secondly, based on the hot spots in the airways, and with respect to development of tumors, the first thing I thought of is when particles deposit in the distal lungs, they probably do not go anywhere for a certain period of time, because fluid flows are notoriously slow at the alveolar duct bifurcations. However, at the bifurcations of airways, all sorts of things are going on: ciliary activity, mucus flow, etc. I would think that the particles which deposit there probably do not stay there very long. I would like to hear your comments on this.

DISCUSSANT: I wanted to talk about that in my presentation this morning, but I ran out of time. I have two transparencies which I would like to show or at least enter into a discussion this afternoon. They show a fiber deposition model in which we have compared fiber deposition with experiments described in a recent publication in the *Journal of Aerosol Science* by a Japanese author who has developed a bifurcation unit which simulates other areas of the human bronchial tree. He has quantitated, experimentally, the extent to which enhanced deposition of fibers also occurs in other areas.

Now, that has never been observed in humans *in vivo,* for obvious reasons, but I think that bifurcation enhancement of fibers can occur throughout bronchial and alveolar passages, and the extent to which it happens I think we can explain by the few extra models I am prepared to present at the technical session this afternoon.

DISCUSSANT: There was the issue of clearance.

DISCUSSANT: Professor Hofmann and I were trying to take into account factors affecting clearance in the upper bronchi. There are experimental observations of reduced clearance in areas of bifurcations of cats and dogs, but I am not quite certain whether the extent to which inhibited clearance occurred explains the increased risk in terms of underlying airway cells being exposed longer to carcinogens, thereby experiencing (a higher degree of) toxic effects.

Reduced clearance at bifurcations definitely will increase exposure of those cells relative to other airway cells. My cigarette-smoke experiments indicate that clearance is impaired at bifurcations, and this is a factor that has to be considered. In terms of the cloud-settling effect, I want to introduce something brand-new by saying that submicron particles are actually deposited at bifurcations, rather than in more distal airways and are reaching bifurcations later, after being carried up there in the mucociliary stream.

DR. ROE: The major problem that I have with this model is that it really does not simulate smoking. The human inhales the smoke bolus, holds it in his oral cavity for a moment, during which time the characteristics of the aerosol are changing, and then he inhales a part of that bolus further into the lung. To make the matter even more complex, the depth of inhalation and the speed of inhalation vary from smoker to smoker. The model is more applicable to a passive smoking scenario or an ambient air scenario than to active smoking.

DISCUSSANT: As was pointed out in the instructions to the speakers, the oral presentations had to be limited to 20 minutes, and more detailed descriptions had to be relegated to the manuscripts. But since you brought up this question, let me explain what we did.

We introduced the smoke into the oropharyngeal cavity by means of a standard 35-ml puff, drawn over a 2-second period, and then we simulated that pause. That is the way the smoke was introduced.

Now, there is another issue: when a smoker puffs, it is not a concentrated stream that enters the mouth. There is some leakage or dilution occurring around the lips. Unfortunately, there is no way of quantifying the extent of this dilution. We simply lit the cigarette, loosely placed it in position, and then smoked it, using an electronic smoking device under conditions in which dilution was allowed to occur. We just hoped that the venturi effect would simulate what was happening physiologically. By these means, we tried to simulate actual smoking as closely as possible. We also added that oropharyngeal pause specifically in an attempt to take mixing into account.

With regard to cloud-settling, I believe that this effect only occurs in the upper bronchi, because it is only there that the cigarette bolus has not been diluted sufficiently to have single-particle settling. As that bolus travels further toward the deep lung, the volume of the airways increases dramatically and relatively rapidly. The bolus is therefore going to be diluted so much that a cloud-settling effect will no longer occur.

DISCUSSANT: I want to make a comment on the issue of turbulent versus laminar flow. You didn't mention what impact turbulent flow has on the hypothesis of the cloud-settling effect.

DISCUSSANT: Once again, I didn't have time to talk about that. I have six or seven transparencies here that show the mechanism of how the hodgepodge developed, but I would like to specifically address your question. The issue of laminar versus turbulent flow is, I believe, handled correctly in the sense that we do have mixing of the smoke aerosol in the oropharyngeal compartment, and we do have flow going through the larynx. Therefore, I think we have a reasonable simulation of what's happening in humans. Nevertheless, we have a research project in progress in which we are looking at the effects of turbulent and laminar air flow with a surrogate bifurcation. So we are indeed addressing that issue, and I agree with you 100% that it is important, but that was not really part of my talk.

DISCUSSANT: I have a question for Dr. Sterling. In one of his first slides, he referred to some 25 studies from the past, in occupational settings. I understood that there were people who were exposed to asbestos and to some other occupational hazards, and they were divided into smokers and nonsmokers. What was your conclusion from this slide? Do you believe that there is evidence that smoking increases the risk of lung cancer? Yes, or no?

DISCUSSANT: Certainly smoking increases the risk of lung cancer. There is a strong association. I fear you must have misunderstood what I was saying.

In our studies, we undertook comparisons of dust-exposed smokers with non-dust-exposed smokers, and dust-exposed nonsmokers with non-dust-exposed nonsmokers. This is not what is usually done. Most studies use non-dust-exposed nonsmokers as the standard and then compute the relative risk for smokers.

We searched the literature for all the studies we could find and reanalyzed them in the way I have described. We found 18 studies. Of these 18 studies, 15 showed a slightly to a very much greater risk for nonsmokers who were exposed, as compared to nonexposed nonsmokers, than for smokers who were exposed, as compared to nonexposed smokers.

All of these studies also compare those nonsmokers to the smokers, but the interesting thing that we found was a consistently larger risk for nonsmokers who were exposed, as compared to nonexposed nonsmokers, than for smokers who were exposed, as compared to nonexposed smokers. Now, that phenomenon was consistent: you find it in 15 of 18 studies. And these were not our studies, and these were not our computations, but they were done by good people, such as Cuyler Hammond. There is a curious observation here that needs explanation.

The purpose of data in science is to ask questions, and the question we asked first is: Now why the hell is that? We are not the only ones who made that observation.

The facts are that the risk of nonsmokers—exposed nonsmokers, using nonexposed nonsmokers as a standard—is consistently higher than the risk of exposed smokers, using nonexposed smokers as the standard. It is a relevant risk of these individuals. It measures something about the contribution of cigarette-smoking or the changes of cigarette-smoking in the human lungs and, like all puzzling phenomena, it is an itch that's got to be scratched, and we tried to scratch it. It has nothing to do with whether smoking causes and is associated with lung cancer or not.

DISCUSSANT: Are you saying that in most of these studies you found that nonsmokers exposed to toxic agents, such as arsenic and asbestos, are at higher risk than smokers, and that smoking offers some kind of protection? Is that what you are saying?

DISCUSSANT: Yes and no. I am not comparing smokers to nonsmokers. We are not computing the risk of smokers versus the risk of nonsmokers. What we are computing is the risk of exposure. We are computing the risk of occupational exposure to, let's say, arsenic. In order to compare the non-arsenic-exposed nonsmoker to the arsenic-exposed smoker, you compare the exposed smoker to the nonexposed smoker, and the exposed nonsmoker to the nonexposed nonsmoker. These are two separate comparisons.

The reason should be quite clear: if smoking is independent of the outcome of this relative risk calculation, then half of them should be for the nonsmokers to have the higher relative risk and the other half to the smokers to have the higher relative risk, but we do find that this is not quite the case.

DISCUSSANT: So what is written in your table is incorrect. That means that asbestos plus cigarette-smoking increases the risk by 50 times compared to exposure to neither agent?

DISCUSSANT: The values in my table (*shown below*—Ed.) have nothing to do with being correct or incorrect. These risks have not been computed by us. These are the relative risks which the investigators calculated who published these papers. We merely checked their calculations as best we could.

	Exposed to Asbestos	
Smoking	No	Yes
No	1	5
Yes	11	53

This yields the following relative risks:

Exposed nonsmoker versus nonexposed nonsmoker	5/1	=5
Exposed smoker versus nonexposed smoker	53/11	=4.81

In the example of the Hammond and Selikoff studies of insulation workers, our (or the studies') findings are this: the exposed nonsmokers are 5.2 times more at risk than the nonexposed nonsmokers. And the exposed smokers are at approximately 4.8 times the risk of the nonexposed smokers.

Here we are exploring independent measurements of occupational risk and how that risk is modified by smoking. The evidence seems to show that there is some change in lung tissue due to smoking which results in a difference in risk for workers subjected to some toxic substances that are encountered occupationally.

DISCUSSANT: To what extent are the data in these analyses taking into account the age distribution for evaluating the incidence of disease and mortality in terms of lung cancer in cigarette smokers in their 50s and early 60s?

DISCUSSANT: All the values in our tables are age-adjusted figures. I should stress that the studies were not done by fly-by-night investigators. They are good occupational health studies.

DISCUSSANT: I understand that four of the five patients recorded in that study (referring to the Hammond and Selikoff study) as being nonsmokers were subsequently found to be ex-smokers, and that only one of them was a true nonsmoker.

DISCUSSANT: While that is what some people believe, I do not know whether that has been established.

DISCUSSANT: It was a deposition given in court under oath by one of the members of the faculty.

DISCUSSANT: It is correct that there are very few nonsmokers in the cohort. Whether or not these people were telling the truth when they were interviewed—and this is a retrospective, historical survey—there has been some doubt cast as to whether or not their response means something. But if we were to proceed just a little bit further in Dr. Sterling's presentation, he mentioned something about the risks of mesothelioma and smoking, lung cancer and smoking, and how they are related. Basically, a survivor population is a different group. There are some repetitive risks involved with different diseases, so the pattern changes. The presentation may have oversimplified that.

DISCUSSANT: I tried to provide as much detail as possible in my manuscript. However, in viewing the total problem from the perspective of an occupational health epidemiologist, I focused on occupational health problems. A major problem in occupational health studies is smoking. Insofar as the focus is on occupational risk, it is necessary to include smoking, but as a confounder. Many investigations of smoking and health problems look at smoking as a major variable and ignore occupational exposure. Therefore, the relative risks of comparing smokers with smokers and nonsmokers with nonsmokers are very interesting.

There is also an age difference between smoker and nonsmoker lung-cancer mortality. That may be an important piece of evidence, as far as I am concerned, because it shows that it may be more difficult for a smoker to have a particle embedded in his lungs than for a nonsmoker. However, once a particle has been embedded in a lung, the smoker may not only be exposed to contaminants and carcinogens from the outside, but he is also exposed to toxins manufactured by his own smoking. We can think, therefore, of a complex process in which the mucus flow of the smoker may, to some extent, protect him from occupational exposures while, at the same time, once particles are embedded, cigarette-smoking may have an effect on these particles. So the age difference should not be ignored. Unfortunately, very few studies state the average age of lung cancer in the case of a smoker.

DR. ROE: I think this is a very difficult thing to comprehend. What happens, in fact, is that the number of cancers among occupationally exposed smokers is actually greater than in nonsmokers, and what you really have is a less-than-multiplicative effect.

DISCUSSANT: That may be made more accurate by realizing that there are some studies where the absolute numbers of lung cancers among smokers are actually lower than among nonsmokers.

DISCUSSANT: That is not what you were implying where the relative risks were quite close.

DISCUSSANT: I wasn't talking about that. The main data on which I focus are the many studies that show a much higher risk of lung cancer among occupationally exposed nonsmokers compared to nonexposed nonsmokers than among exposed smokers compared to nonexposed smokers.

DR. ROE: I would just summarize here that we are in an area which is very fragile epidemiologically. Nevertheless, Dr. Sterling raised a very important issue because I believe that most of the people who came to this conference thought that the multiplicative effect of smoking and occupational exposure was unchallengeable. A lot of assumptions have been made based on that premise.

Now, I believe, we are being told that we should not build up huge theories on the assumption that this is, in fact, correct, and that it is possible under certain circumstances that smoking can be somewhat "protective" against some forms of dust, at least that is what I understand from this discussion. Does anybody want to disagree with me?

DISCUSSANT: I think you overstated that, particularly when you bring in words like "protective" in terms of smoking. I personally take offense at that. I could probably build a case that driving race cars is protective of one's dying of cancer.

DISCUSSANT: I do not see how you can be offended by data. The fact of the matter is that smokers have an absolutely lower prevalence of disease than nonsmokers, especially in occupational asthma and in pneumoconiosis. These problems (observations) do show up, and they are real, and one has to deal with them. The fact is that certain occupational lung diseases are more frequent among nonsmokers than among smokers. These are scientific data, and they *have* been ignored but *shouldn't* be ignored.

DISCUSSANT: Regarding the term "protective." We are simplifying greatly, not only in experiments where we are modeling and in experiments where we use animals but, it seems to me, also in experiments where we use human beings, where we come to some simplified conclusions that do not take into account all the variables which are encountered when we do a clinical study like the ones mentioned here.

Here is a small example of what I am trying to say: we know that bronchitis by itself, which is produced by smoking, is in some way protective. When you use usual techniques for determining lung clearance, you will find that the clearance in a bronchitic patient is changed. Why? Because the deposition pattern is changed. When the deposition pattern is changed in bronchitis, those particles which are used to identify clearance will deposit more in ciliated airways than in the alveoli, as they do in a nonbronchitic person. Then the clearance rate of that radioactive tracer will be different.

Now, tell me, what does this mean? Does it mean that the bronchitis produced by cigarette smoke is protective? It is not. That is what you would really assume if you were to look only at the results and say, "Oh, in cigarette smokers in a certain stage of bronchitis, we find that clearance is not effective, or it is faster." You can find these types of results, but they do not mean anything if you do not analyze the whole data correctly and carefully enough to get the correct answer; otherwise, you might even say that bronchitis produced by smoking is protective.

DR. ROE: Let me just make clear that when I said the data are fragile, I meant to include exactly the point that Dr. McClellan has made and that you have made: these data on humans all contain variables which were uncontrollable at the moment and which have to be taken into account. You cannot uncritically rely on these data, particularly when you have only small numbers (e.g., lung cancer rates in non-asbestos-exposed nonsmokers versus asbestos-exposed nonsmokers). So I do not think anybody is going to disagree with you or Dr. McClellan.

DR. WEHNER: Perhaps we should stay away from attaching adjectives to the findings, such as "protective" or "beneficial," and should concentrate on characterizing the phenomena. When we investigate and describe certain phenomena, we do not have to pass value judgments or state whether the phenomena are beneficial or protective or harmful. This is the best way to avoid unnecessary controversies.

DISCUSSANT: I have no difficulty with the use of words such as "more frequent," "less frequent," whatever. I agree with that. When you start to take another step and use adjectives that carry with them values, then I have some problems.

DR. ROE: Let us go on to Dr. Pott's presentation. There are many interesting things which were said, such as that there was no multiplicative effect of combined exposures to asbestos and cigarette smoke on fibrosis. I am sure there are some questions.

DISCUSSANT: Professor Pott, there are two of several conclusions you drew for which I would really like more clarification. Firstly, you said there is no effective difference between experimental exposure by inhalation and intraperitoneal injection. As far as I am concerned, they are very different. I have a hard time understanding, in the case of intratracheal instillation, and much more so in the case of intraperitoneal injections, the role of these methods in elucidating mechanisms of pathogenicity or interaction of *inhaled* substances. Please, would you clarify that.

The second point you made was that asbestos fiber numbers relate more to asbestosis than to lung cancer. I wonder whether you have considered that asbestosis is a chronic inflammatory process and whether that could contribute to the development of tumors, whether through oxygen radicals or other mediators. It would seem to me that they are not mutually exclusive.

DISCUSSANT: First we calculated the effective dose, and I underline the word "effective." We can assume that all injected fibers become effective after intraperitoneal injection, because no processes like lung clearance are involved.

For inhalation exposures the situation is markedly different. We have seen, or other authors have found, that very few tumors developed following heavy inhalation exposure to crocidolite. More than 99% of the inhaled fibers were cleared, and a high percentage of the retained fibers was deposited in the unciliated airways. Therefore, only very few fibers were chronically embedded in the ciliated airways. This is an important point: they have to be embedded in the ciliated airways for a long period.

The other point which you mentioned concerned the number of fibers found in the lung. This number shows us the dose which is effective for asbestosis but does not show us the dose which is effective for lung cancer.

I mentioned that about 95% of all human lung cancers occur in the relatively small area of the ciliated airways and only 5% in the large area of the unciliated airways. For this calculation, at the moment, we can disregard the 5%. We have to find an explanation for the high lung-cancer incidence in the small areas of the ciliated airways. When we count the fibers, we find that the very small number of fibers that are chronically implanted in the ciliated airways are responsible for the tumor incidence, and about 99%—certainly more than 90%—are retained in the unciliated airways. After we have determined the number of fibers in the lung of an asbestos worker who died, we have to decide whether his lung tumor was caused by asbestos or not. (Incidentally, I believe that the number of fibers found in the lung of a deceased worker is not a correct measure for the carcinogenic potency which was active 20 or 30 years before.) In Germany we have to decide, on the basis of the number of fibers in the lungs of the dead asbestos worker, whether the worker's family is entitled to compensation for his lung cancer. I think this is the wrong criterion, especially in view of the low, or the relatively low, durability of chrysotile asbestos in the human lung.

I hope I have answered your questions.

DISCUSSANT: I would like to take issue with you on one of your points. You stated correctly, in general, that 95% of lung cancers occur in the larger airways. However, that is not true in the asbestos situation, where many (if not the majority) of cancers occur peripherally.

Secondly, it is well known that the risk of developing lung cancer in individuals who have asbestosis is twice that of asbestos-exposed individuals who do not have asbestosis. Given that background, I would find it difficult to accept your hypothesis on this fiber contact with the larger ciliated airways and either deposition, impaction or contact, or uptake of fibers by those cells, being the major factor responsible for asbestos-related lung cancer. If we are talking about the question of the synergism of smoking with asbestos, certainly the question of whether products of tobacco smoke may interact with larger airway cells is important, and I accept that this interaction may well occur in this case. But I do not think that this necessarily applies to the asbestos situation. In fact, if fibers are retained in the interstitial compartment of the lung, certainly away from the airways, it is very likely that any interaction that is going on there will occur in an entirely different area from the one you described.

I was wondering what comment you might have on that. I might add that several other speakers have also concentrated on the role of the airways, and I frankly wonder whether this really applies in the asbestos situation.

DR. ROE: Before you answer, I would like to ask Dr. Davis for a comment.

DISCUSSANT: I was, in fact, going to follow this up. We have been debating for years the point of whether asbestos-related lung cancers in humans are peripheral or central, and I do not think there is a definite opinion. Some people say one thing, some people say another. In experiments with animals, however, asbestos-related tumors are always peripheral. I've seen hundreds of them, and not one was in a major bronchial tube.

Because we are discussing so much the deposition in the major bronchial tubes, I think the tendency was to assume that certainly some aspects related to tumors in human beings are central. I was going to ask to discuss a theory as to why this should be so. Why should you have asbestos-related tumors in the main bronchial tubes in humans and not with experimental animals?

DR. ROE: In my written paper I addressed the same issue. Conventional thinking is that the epithelial changes in the main airways are the precursors of smoking-associated cancers. The cancers that are present in excess in smoking asbestos workers, are they really the same type of cancers as those in unexposed smokers, or are they two different populations of cancers?

Now, in a nonsmoking asbestos worker, do you see the epithelial changes in the main airways that have been described in smokers? Interaction has to mean something quite different when you have two different target sites in the respiratory system, from when you have only one target. This is something which we might want to discuss.

Now, the issue is complicated by the misuse of the terms, or the variable use of the terms "central" and "peripheral," because to some people, central means the main bronchus and the next one or two generations. But in airway terms, you can have up to 35 generations of airway and you are still in a reasonably big airway in humans, a much bigger airway than even the trachea of a laboratory rodent. So what does "central" and what does "peripheral" mean?

DISCUSSANT: There are additional questions, not only whether it is main bronchus or peripheral, but also which lobe. Two-thirds of the cigarette-smoke-induced tumors are in the main bronchus; two-thirds of the tumors in asbestos workers are in the lower lobe and "peripheral lung."

DISCUSSANT: Yes, of course, in the older literature, in which asbestosis was quite commonly described, most of these cancers were described as adenocarcinomas.

DISCUSSANT: I think it would be interesting—and possibly this has been done—to look at the difference or similarities between the lung cancers of persons who were exposed to asbestos and who smoke and those who do not. Has this comparison been made?

DISCUSSANT: There were only four or five nonsmokers in that cohort. This is just too low a number.

DISCUSSANT: Dr. Churg has the numbers; he has done the studies.

DISCUSSANT: The only numbers I have come from the literature. The notion that adenocarcinoma is most prevalent in asbestos workers is well ingrained. However, when you go back to the original data which make that claim, it really does not hold up. These data show a slight increase in adenocarcinoma in asbestos workers, but this is statistically no different from the non-asbestos-exposed controls. I went back 2 or 3 years ago to find what I could in the literature concerning cases with controls. I was unable to find any evidence that there is a preferential type of carcinoma seen in those with asbestos exposure.

DISCUSSANT: Firstly, I am very sorry that I am not a pathologist, but my arguments were regarding lung cancer in man and not lung cancer in rats. We do not know anything about the combined effect of cigarette smoke and asbestos in rats because we do not have any experimental data.

There may be more peripheral lung cancer cases than only 5%. It is not so important whether we say we have only 5% or as much as 40%. In relation to the surface area, it is a very small percentage, because only 1%, I believe, of the total surface area is ciliated, and 99% is unciliated, and this 99% is peripherally located. We can assume that, at maximum, 50% of the cancers are located in the unciliated 99% area, and 50% may be in the ciliated 1% area. Thus, there is a large difference between these two areas. The other significant difference is that the large 99% surface area contains the bulk of retained fibers. I think there is no doubt about this fact. This may be different in the case of a short inhalation exposure to a high concentration of fibers, when a high deposition in the upper airways occurs. But what I am discussing is that long-term persistence of fibers in the bronchial walls. When we count the number of fibers in the lung, at least 90% or more of these fibers are from the area of the unciliated airways, and this high number is not a correct measure for the carcinogenic potency of the fibers.

DR. ROE: You have made your point very clearly.

Now, may we go back to Dr. Churg? There is a loose end there. I believe you stated, in effect, and I know there are publications on this, that men were dying from asbestosis before the age of 50. I would suggest that the data do exist for preferential existence of lung cancers in the lower lobes and for adenocarcinoma, unless there have been changes, and pathologists are now using different criteria than in years past.

When exposure to asbestos is reduced and men live longer, then it seems as though the location of the lesion shifts closer to the center, and perhaps the type of lesion changes, too. The data which you examined, perhaps from the United States, probably are fairly recent. So, historically, there may have been a change.

DISCUSSANT: I think "historically" is something different. The question is, how far back are you referring to? You said the data exist, so how far back are you going?

DR. ROE: In the United Kingdom, the data go back at least to the 1930s and 1940s.

DISCUSSANT: I argue that it does not stand up to any kind of sound analysis.

DR. ROE: I still think that some of the questions remain unanswered. If you have the same target tissue, and if you accept the data for bronchial epithelial changes as being the precursors of bronchial carcinoma, do you see these changes in asbestos-exposed people or not? Do you get these metaplastic and dysplastic changes at the sites where the fibers are actually or theoretically lodged in the basement membrane?

DISCUSSANT: I don't have data on human experiments. In our rats, we observed squamous cancers that I am sure were alveolus-derived, because we get squamous metaplasia in the alveolar region.

DISCUSSANT: Certainly. In humans, the cell type provides very little good correlation; currently, anyway.

DISCUSSANT: I would like to ask Professor Pott whether he actually said that intratracheal instillation is a good model for inhalation exposure. If he did, I find that very hard to swallow.

There is evidence that intratracheal instillation results in a very high and localized dose to an area. Is that not unrealistic compared to inhalation?

DISCUSSANT: I wasn't emphasizing intratracheal instillation but, rather, intraperitoneal injection for testing the carcinogenicity of fibers. However, intratracheal instillation of dusts may also be a suitable method for clarifying some questions, e.g., for examining the hypothesis that fibers lodge in increasing numbers in the bronchial mucosa as a consequence of inflammatory lesions. As mentioned, only 10 μg of the fibrous dusts were given per instillation; this is not a large amount. Certainly, this method of administration is unrealistic in principle. However, results observed after exposure by nonphysiological routes are not necessarily irrelevant. We are sometimes forced to use nonphysiological methods to elucidate important biological responses. The carcinogenicity of crocidolite and man-made mineral fibers is a good example of the need to use unrealistic routes of administration.

Although several inhalation experiments were performed with man-made mineral fibers, their results were ambiguous as far as tumor induction is concerned. More to the point, only a few critics took notice of the fact that only four of these inhalation studies contained a positive control group that received appropriate fibers: those which do not split up, thereby multiplying their numbers in the body, as chrysotile does. Crocidolite fibers are suitable for a positive control group because they are generally durable and very carcinogenic in humans. Nevertheless, they did not induce tumors in inhalation experiments as expected.

These findings are remarkable. In two of the four studies, no lung tumor or mesothelioma occurred; in one experiment, two lung tumors and one mesothelioma were found in 57 rats; and in the fourth study, 1 of 50 rats developed a pulmonary adenocarcinoma. These sparse effects show clearly that the test system was not sufficiently sensitive to detect the strong carcinogenicity of crocidolite fibers in humans. Therefore, we cannot expect that the system is more sensitive for man-made mineral fibers, and we must expect false-negative results here, too.

In contrast, the serosal tests—especially the intraperitoneal test—demonstrate a high degree of carcinogenicity and clear dose-response relationships after injection of crocidolite and some other natural and man-made mineral fibers. However, some fiber types were not carcinogenic, or only slightly carcinogenic, after intraperitoneal injection. This leads to the conclusions that negative results from an appropriately conducted intraperitoneal test exclude (reasonably well) an unacceptable cancer risk to humans.

With regard to the carcinogenic risk assessment for humans, we can conclude that nonphysiological intraperitoneal tests with fibers produce more relevant results than inhalation studies. Some people argue that positive results from injection studies with fibers must be confirmed by inhalation studies before serious health concerns are justified. However, our society does not accept a carcinogenic risk from fibers that may equal 50% of the risk of highly carcinogenic crocidolite, but which cannot be reliably detected by inhalation studies.

DR. ROE: We now come to Dr. Ferin's paper. I am calling for comments on Dr. Ferin's paper.

DISCUSSANT: Talking about a multiplicative interaction, it is only Selikoff, in his evaluation of the combined effects of smoking and asbestos exposure, who comes up with numbers which suggest multiplicative interaction. Other data dealt with other dusts and came up with numbers indicative of something between additive and multiplicative effects. In terms of mechanism, there are numerous possible ways in which the effects of particles and smoke might interact additively, and there are also numerous ways in which they might interact multiplicatively.

The question to Dr. Ferin is, at the mechanistic level, would it make any difference—would an effect of cigarette-smoking on clearance make any difference, in your opinion, if it were an additive risk factor rather than a so-called synergistic, multiplicative type? Would cigarettes also be able to act in a way that would appear to be additive and still show some deleterious effect on asbestos lung-cancer outcome?

DISCUSSANT: The simple answer would be, "No." Basically, I started by considering the difference between mesothelioma and asbestosis. Mesothelioma is no additional risk factor in an asbestosis case. It does not matter whether smoke plus asbestos exposures are additive or multiplicative. That was really the basic outcome. I tried to emphasize and again suggested the hypothesis that basically the difference is in the dose.

DR. ROE: Is there anybody who seriously believes that intrapleural injection is of any value for the biological evaluation of dusts for lung-cancer potential or other kinds of health risk?

DISCUSSANT: This is not pertinent to that question, but I want to get something off my chest concerning the supposed interaction between tobacco-smoking and asbestos exposure regarding lung cancer.

We are trying to wrestle with a very complex system, in which all sorts of factors are interacting: clearance, as has been discussed here at length today. It seems to me that no one has tried to determine whether there actually is an interaction using some simpler system, such as intraperitoneal or intrapleural injections. In other words, if you can show the interaction between asbestos fibers and some product of tobacco smoke in a simple system, then maybe you might reasonably hope to demonstrate it in a more complex system.

DR. ROE: I suppose this is a generic problem. However difficult it is to have a model which has a realistic end point, once you have established this end point, you can go back and say, "Well, if we can reproduce the right end point, if we had looked earlier or done the thing more simply, is there a cheaper, earlier marker we can use as a surrogate for the realistic end point?" However, unless one is sure that the end point one uses is really a marker for the realistic end point, there will always be doubt concerning the validity of the work.

In the past, I have been involved with people in the tobacco industry who said, "We do not want to do a long-term study. It costs too much and is too difficult." Instead, they have fiddled away, doing short-term tests, and then when they find that they can distinguish between two different products in a short-term test, they come to the toxicologist and ask, "What does this mean? Which is the safer product?" When I have been in this situation, I have had to say I haven't the remotest idea, because there is no point of reference. I can't relate the end point in the short-term test to any meaningful tobacco-associated disease. Thus, in my view, one must start with a realistic end point and then work backwards to simpler approaches. Trying to proceed in the opposite direction simply does not work.

I should like to ask another question. Do people believe that intrapleural injection is a good model for predicting mesothelioma?

DISCUSSANT: I am sorry. I want to take up the first question first: "What is a good model for lung tumors?," which I do not think we have answered. I would like to suggest that the value there is in a negative outcome rather than in a positive outcome. I suggest that negative results in injection studies may provide reasurrance even though the model is artificial and the end point is not realistic. If one tests a dust sample by injecting it into the body cavity, and it does not produce tumors, I would be very surprised indeed if it would do so in lung tissue. By contrast, it is more difficult to interpret positive results in such tests.

DISCUSSANT: I would like to say that we should not confuse two aspects of experimental testing. One is to determine a mechanism. For example, in this case you would say: "Injection into the intrapleural cavity is so far from what is happening in man, why bother?" For that purpose, obviously this is not a good test. But if you are talking about some really basic question, such as: "Is this compound capable of producing a tumorigenic response or not?

That is a new compound about which we do not know anything yet." In that case, if the test system produces tumors even in this artificial situation, it answers the question it was designed to answer, and therefore it was a good test.

We thus have to determine what we really want to ask of a test. If, for example, you were to say, "Oh, injection into the pleural cavity produced tumors; that means the same will happen by inhalation," that, of course, would be absolute nonsense. But we could say: "Maybe the results warrant additional experimentation," if the findings are relevant to a more realistic situation.

DR. ROE: I imagine there is general agreement on this.

DISCUSSANT: I would like to ask an open question. Certainly we have some ideas of where the dust particles or fibers go. Can anybody tell me where intraperitoneally injected fibers go? Do they land at the bottom of the peritoneum?

DISCUSSANT: What is the bottom of the peritoneum?

DISCUSSANT: Do we know what happens to them?

DISCUSSANT: They end up in aggregates or granulomas that can be located anywhere within the peritoneal cavity.

DISCUSSANT: You are talking about an intraperitoneal injection, not intrapleural?

DISCUSSANT: Yes, but I believe that roughly the same thing happens in the pleural cavity.

DISCUSSANT: But the macrophages pick up very small particles, and they go to the lymph nodes.

DISCUSSANT: That is right, but macrophages which pick up larger fibers tend to form aggregates and to end up as granulomas. We have found that a large number of short fibers get in the lymph nodes, but I believe that the longer fibers do not go in the lymph nodes; the bulk of the longer fibers go to the omentum, and also to the liver and the diaphragm, and so on.

I believe, in principle, we have a good analogy between the carcinogenicity of some dusts after intraperitoneal injection and after administration into the lungs. There are positive effects in both locations for all types of asbestos and for erionite. Perhaps there is sufficient evidence for carcinogenicity following bronchial and intraperitoneal administrations. We have two positive studies, and there is limited evidence in epidemiological studies. There are positive results after both intraperitoneal injection and after intratracheal instillation of cadmium and nickel compounds.

DISCUSSANT: I believe that this is a very controversial area, if you do not mind my saying so. We recently reviewed the epidemiological evidence for man-made mineral fibers and found some positive associations, but there is also a lot of negative evidence. You believe that the positive result in an intrapleural or intraperitoneal study is telling you something important about the hazard of a given test agent to which humans are exposed by inhalation, and I personally am very doubtful about this.

DISCUSSANT: We were having a little discussion yesterday. We do not own an inhalation facility, and therefore we see this problem a little differently from others. I believe that everything that you test in some intact animal has some biological relevance. I refer to the experiments that Chris Wagner's group conducted and the number of tumors produced by inhalation of asbestos minerals.

DISCUSSANT: Have you ever produced a mesothelioma by inhalation of asbestos?

DISCUSSANT: Yes.

DISCUSSANT: It is extremely rare. It is a very difficult experiment. If we had left the resolution of the asbestos problem to the results of inhalation studies, we would still be scratching our heads. It is nice to have an inhalation facility, and it is nice to do these inhalation experiments, but they are time-consuming and they are expensive, and there is only a finite number of facilities where individuals with the proper expertise are capable of conducting them appropriately. They may all be here in this room.

DISCUSSANT: Has anybody actually compared a washed fiber with a fiber on which polycyclic aromatic hydrocarbons (PAH) have been adsorbed.

DISCUSSANT: Yes.

DISCUSSANT: What happened?

DISCUSSANT: Absolutely the same outcome. Dr. Nolan had done this with his crocidolites. He showed that, whether a fiber is contaminated with trace metals or contaminated with PAH, it produced the same number of tumors.

DISCUSSANT: So why should one be so interested in adsorption when it comes to the lungs?

DISCUSSANT: Because it is a nice, simple model. It is a nice, simplistic approach to a complex problem. It is nice to have a passive carrier that transports PAH. It is a very attractive hypothesis. Why not?

DISCUSSANT: I believe that we ought to be very careful about your interpretation of intrapleural injection studies and, perhaps, even more about intraperitoneal studies, because there are several differences between the two injection studies with erionite, and erionite in intrapleural studies is not showing nearly the toxicity that chrysotile showed by inhalation. Inhalation of erionite produced almost 100% mesotheliomas. In intrapleural studies, it produced marginally more than crocidolite. In fact, when you inject it intraperitoneally, as I understand it, you got less—

DISCUSSANT: No.

DISCUSSANT: No, you get 95% with erionite.

DISCUSSANT: One of the points that I did not mention in my presentation this morning, simply because of insufficient time, was that we have recently completed a dose-response study using erionite. I did not receive the data in time to include them in my slides, but now I have the analyzed data. We observed exactly the same dose response, and erionite was somewhat more carcinogenic than chrysotile. In other words, erionite was the most carcinogenic dust, but only by a relatively small amount.

You have this complete anomaly: here is a dust (erionite) that is capable of producing mesotheliomas following inhalation but that is only slightly better than anything else at producing mesotheliomas following injection. This is one of the great mysteries. What is it about erionite that makes it particularly able to produce mesotheliomas by inhalation?

DISCUSSANT: The dose response to which you are referring is by which route of administration?

DISCUSSANT: Intraperitoneal injection.

DISCUSSANT: How did you compare your dose, by mass?

DISCUSSANT: By mass, but we also have fiber number data.

DISCUSSANT: Because we have used fiber numbers, it appears to us that, based on fiber numbers as the criterion, injected fibers are much more inclined to induce mesothelioma in the pleura, and certainly in much shorter time. There seems to be the following ranking order: chrysotile, crocidolite, and erionite.

DISCUSSANT: I think you are right there. Our data are not yet ready for presentation, but the erionite sample was very similar in fiber size and fiber number to UICC crocidolite.

DISCUSSANT: We used fibers/unit mass for crocidolite, but both crocidolite and erionite fibers were far fewer than chrysotile fibers, fewer by several orders of magnitude.

DISCUSSANT: From where did Chris Wagner get that erionite specimen?

DISCUSSANT: I believe from Rome in Oregon.

DISCUSSANT: Rome in Oregon, yes.

DISCUSSANT: He had two samples: one from Rome and one from somewhere else, and he had very similar results with them.

DISCUSSANT: I want to get back to Dr. Ferin's hypothesis that cancer is caused by increased asbestos exposure on account of decreased airway clearance, and the emphasis in Dr. Pott's presentation on the local effect of fibers on the airways and, of course, to the problem for the clinician: the fact that we only seem to see carcinomas in patients with asbestosis. A recent paper from Mt. Sinai describes about 130 patients with pulmonary carcinomas following asbestos exposure; every one of them had some degree of asbestosis. That is 100% of 130 patients—

DISCUSSANT: That is based on pathologic examination?

DISCUSSANT: On pathologic examination, right. These findings are quite convincing regarding the association between asbestosis and lung cancer. So the issue is really: How does asbestosis affect the incidence of lung cancer? How does it affect the carcinogenicity of fibers? How does it affect the development of cancer in the central airways? (And most tumors do develop in the central airways and not in the parenchyma.) If these data are true, why does this happen? Is it because there is concurrent fiber deposition in central airways? Why does asbestosis show such a strong association with lung cancer in the central airways? What is the mechanism here? If it were simply one of fiber deposition in the central airways, one wouldn't expect to see such a strong association with peripheral airway disease and asbestosis.

DISCUSSANT: I do not remember the details of this Mt. Sinai paper, but I doubt that it said that fibrosis was confirmed pathologically. Were these 130 tumors all centrally located? What portion was peripheral?

DISCUSSANT: I do not remember.

DISCUSSANT: I do not think it is central.

DISCUSSANT: That seems to be a rather significant issue.

DISCUSSANT: One of the things with which I am a little uncomfortable: you are really talking about the numerator, because you are talking about pathologic diagnosis and you really do not have a population control with which to compare your results. I am sure most of us in this room appreciate that a pathologic diagnosis and a clinical diagnosis are based on X rays, which oftentimes can be at variance. We really do not have anything with which to compare these findings to determine whether or not many of those patients had clinical asbestosis. I believe that this is an important point.

DISCUSSANT: Take, for instance, the population of patients with asbestosis in the studies from Great Britain, in which the dose causing pneumoconiosis was certified by fiber count in all of those patients. The incidence of lung cancer in the certified asbestosis patients was extremely high, about 25 to 30%. Thus, the incidence of lung cancer in patients with asbestosis is extremely high as opposed to the incidence of lung cancer in a comparable population of workers who have the same asbestos fiber counts in their lungs, but who do not have asbestosis. We all agree that there is a population of workers with identical exposure who have very high fiber counts; some of them have asbestosis, and some do not. It is the ones who have asbestosis who seem to get the lung cancer, and the longer they have had asbestosis, the greater the incidence of lung cancer in that population. Therefore, fiber count does not seem to me to be the issue. The issue is asbestosis.

DR. ROE: I am coming back to Dr. Pott now.

DISCUSSANT: I only wanted to add that we, too, did not find any difference in the carcinogenicity of erionite and crocidolite after intraperitoneal injection. Up to now I do not have any explanation for the high mesothelioma rate in rats following erionite inhalation, as reported by Wagner et al. Did you see the slides? There should be some carcinomas too, because we have heard that, in Turkey, the lung-cancer incidence was high, too, not only the incidence of mesothelioma.

DISCUSSANT: I am not saying we should have seen lung cancers following our injection studies. We certainly didn't. I never saw Dr. Wagner's slides. I wish I had seen them.

DISCUSSANT: I have seen them. The animals died too soon to get lung carcinomas. They were exposed to the dust for a year, and most of them died within 14 months. That is only 2 months after termination of the dust exposures and too soon for lung carcinomas to develop.

DISCUSSANT: The Turkish data show an appreciable incidence of lung cancer in males. There were, of course, a lot of mesotheliomas, many more than one would expect with asbestosis. If these data are representative, erionite can be expected to produce more mesotheliomas than lung cancers. It could be, I agree, that we sometimes get deaths from mesothelioma in intrapleurally inoculated animals within approximately 370 days. However, we certainly never see lung cancer in a rat at that age following asbestos exposure. It could be that erionite is peculiarly different from asbestos in that it is much more mesotheliogenic than it is carcinogenic for the lung.

DISCUSSANT: Most of us here would agree with this statement. The challenge is to find out why.

DISCUSSANT: We do not have many data, but we have some ideas and some preliminary experiments with erionite, because it is a fiber constructed so very differently from asbestos.

DISCUSSANT: I would like to comment on the question of fibrosis in relation to asbestosis and lung cancer. In experimental animals, we oftentimes see fibrosis. Animals—for example, dogs exposed to plutonium—develop pulmonary fibrosis, radiation pneumonitis, or a variety of nonstochastic changes that influence the incidence of lung cancer. This merely reinforces what Dr. Roe said earlier. Many factors influence the incidence of lung cancer. We have seen lung cancer in rats following chronic silica inhalation. Admittedly, it was a high dose of silica, but the lesions were epidermoid carcinomas, and at least one of them was metastasizing.

So, yes, I believe that there is an association between fibrosis and lung cancer in laboratory animals. We have at least some evidence to suggest that. You can see this broad association of fibrosis with that wide variety of nonstochastic changes that affect the incidence of lung cancer.

DISCUSSANT: The point I was making is that the risk of lung cancer in a population of people who do not have asbestosis may be relatively low compared to that in people with the same number of fibers who do have asbestosis. The fiber counts would be the same in both populations, but the risk would be much different because fibrosis predisposes to cancer development.

DISCUSSANT: Do we have definite data to support this conclusion? It is conceivable that the individuals who do not have asbestosis have a lower fiber count.

DISCUSSANT: We see people who do not have asbestosis with fiber counts that are equivalent to those with asbestosis, is that correct?

DISCUSSANT: Yes, but that is very hard to approach. The best data are from Dr. Wagner.

DISCUSSANT: How was the fiber count done? Was it done from a sample of the lung?

DISCUSSANT: Yes.

DISCUSSANT: So here we have that problem which Dr. Martonen already mentioned. If you analyze a sample of lung tissue and extrapolate from that sample to the total lung, your conclusions may be correct, depending on the size of the sample. But we are emphasizing now the local aspects of the events which happened, from deposition up to the local changes. Therefore, when I mentioned that dose would be the important factor, I meant the dose at certain local spots.

For example, if there are changes in the ciliary epithelium of the airways which focally affect the function of the ciliary escalator, it is possible that the total clearance may not be so much affected as it is affected in some spots. In that case, the dose becomes much larger in these spots.

You can then also ask the question: "Why is it so rare that lung carcinoma after asbestos exposure usually occurs on only one side? Why on that one side? Why, if lung cancer is such a common thing, why doesn't it occur suddenly in 10 places in the lung?"

DR. ROE: Everybody is aware of the diagnostic problems with asbestosis and of the fact that it is usually just a clinical diagnosis, made using radiology. It is insensitive and often misleading, compared with diagnosis based on pathology. The pathologic evalution must be performed appropriately and is more reliable when based on an autopsy rather than on a small tissue sample. But I perceive in the published literature that experimentalists sometimes are very glib in using the term "asbestosis," when, in fact, all they have seen is a lesion in the vicinity of the terminal bronchioles that I call cuboidal metaplasia of the alveolar epithelium. And without any serious evidence, even of fibrois, some people publish papers and illustrate lesions which they call "asbestosis." They use the term simply because the animal happens to have been exposed to asbestos, and not because the lesion suits pathological criteria for the diagnosis of asbestosis. The literature is polluted by this sort of misleading thing. In fact, you can produce exactly the same lesion by exposing animals, for example, to nitrogen dioxide.

Am I correct, or do people disagree with me as to the use of the term?

DISCUSSANT: I do not believe that you produce the same lesion with nitrogen dioxide as you do with asbestos. You do get an alveolar change in the acini with nitrogen dioxide, and you eventually get emphysema, beautiful emphysema, from it, but I do not think it mimics what you see in asbestosis; you don't see the fibrosis there.

DR. ROE: I am not disagreeing with you. I am saying that the literature is polluted by papers where the lesion illustrated does not really include fibrosis, and yet, because the animals have been exposed to asbestos and have some sort of lesion, people put the term "asbestosis" underneath.

DISCUSSANT: I agree with you entirely. I think that in order to use the term asbestosis, you do need evidence of excess fibrosis, particularly in the alveolar walls. Many experimentally induced lesions do justify using the term asbestosis, but in many other papers the term is used for trivial lesions.

DISCUSSANT: Is it necessary to have asbestos fibers within the fibrous tissue in order to call the lesion asbestosis?

DISCUSSANT: Philosophically, I am not sure whether this is necessary. However, in reality, you almost invariably do find fibers.

DISCUSSANT: With respect to your comment, I think one really has to define the terms. In our case, in 1984 we were looking at the earliest lesions of asbestosis, and we demonstrated that the earliest lesions begin 48 hours after just a 1-hour exposure, using a technique called ultrastructural morphometry.

Clearly, that isn't asbestosis, and we didn't mean to imply that it was. However, it is a lesion that is irreversible, because 1 month later, after the 1-hour exposure, that lesion has expanded, and we are presuming that ultimately it progresses, particularly with continuing exposure.

We called it "the earliest form of asbestosis," but we did not mean to imply that it met the textbook criteria for fully developed asbestosis. As a matter of fact, if you looked at those bifurcations, you wouldn't be able to recognize any changes unless you did an ultrastructural morphometric study, using transmission electron microscopy. It thus really depends on whether it is mechanistic, or whether someone just exposed some animals and subsequently tried to diagnose or label what was going on. I therefore believe that the intent is as important as the label.

DR. ROE: When people define their terms, I have less of a problem, but there are some papers in which the terms are not defined. The experiment has been conducted by a nonpathologist, and the slides were subsequently shown to a pathologist, who hears that there has been exposure to asbestos, and he labels it asbestosis because he sees a lesion there. It is a very poor use of terminology. I am not criticizing work where terms have been properly defined.

DISCUSSANT: I would like to respond to the question of whether there is inconsistency in the proposed hypothesis regarding the dose. If the clinical evidence shows that there is asbestosis in almost all cases of carcinoma after asbestos exposure, I do not think there is an inconsistency there; quite the opposite.

If this hypothesis should be proven, then a depressed clearance mechanism will result in more fibers, and if the dose has an effect on asbestosis, which I believe it has, then one shouldn't be surprised to also find asbestosis and cancer.

Of course, as I emphasized, this is only the first step in a sequence of events. Even identical exposures and focally identical fiber retention do not mean an identical pathological response. There is an additional chance to develop a cancer in that spot.

As for the fiber numbers, I have already responded. I believe that a tissue sample—even a small sample—gives some indication of exposure, but it is not necessarily indicative of focal changes where either asbestosis or scar changes occur, or cancer starts.

DISCUSSANT: One more point. You can expose two animals or two humans to high concentrations of asbestos. Very little fibrosis may develop in one of them, while the other may respond with severe fibrosis. This is, I suppose, a genetically determined difference. The point is, one has to recognize that, in announcing theories on dose-response relationships, there are also other factors involved, perhaps genetic factors.

DISCUSSANT: If the effects of asbestos on the airways are local, one would anticipate a greater concentration of asbestos fibers in the central airways where these tumors develop. I do not think that is where you find most of the fibers; you find them in the respiratory bronchioles and not in the central airways.

I am just being a devil's advocate—I am saying: "Look, if your hypothesis postulates that cancer development is due to a direct effect on the central airways, show me that data that demonstrate that the fibers that caused it are there." There are other explanations for why patients with asbestosis develop central tumors, but as far as data are concerned that show that there are more fibers, I do not know of any.

DR. ROE: I think the weakness of what you are saying is that within any part of the lung there are perhaps 30 different types of cells, and unless you know which is the target cell or cells, I do not think it is realistic to say: "This cubic centimeter of lung contains so many fibers, therefore the risk is so much." You have to look at the structure of the cells, and you have to know more than we know now.

DISCUSSANT: Sure; absolutely. But I think that needs to be pointed out.

DISCUSSANT: From what I hear, fiber count appears to emerge as an important variable. Is there a standardized way, a protocol, by which fiber count is determined which says something about sampling procedure and counting procedure, so that you can compare fiber counts from one study with fiber counts from another study?

DISCUSSANT: We can study the fibers in the whole lung in the rat, but you can't do that in humans.

DISCUSSANT: Even if you can, it does not help. There was a meeting in Oxford, I suppose 3 years ago, which resulted in the creation of standard samples that were sent to various laboratories for analysis. All participating laboratories in the study did reasonably well in identifying samples as having high or low fiber counts; however the absolute numbers ranged all over hell.

DISCUSSANT: You have to get the appropriate materials. Pathologists select materials that interest them—usually lesions of various kinds. So, in terms of some statistical sampling of the pulmonary structure, that is out to begin with; secondly, people use light microscopes. We saw a lot of photographs, photomicrographs, light microscopic analyses, and pulmonary tissues with fibers. It is archaic. You only see the tip of the iceberg, depending on fiber type and other factors. Generally, fibers observed by light microscopy can vary in length over four orders of magnitude.

In terms of the instrumentation, we prefer using transmission units, analytical electron microscopes, and diffraction chemistry by one of the energy-dispersive spectrometry methods. You can go along and count, and you can count very well, and you come up with numbers, and the numbers represent a great range, and the ranges reflect low, moderate, or heavy exposure concentrations, and we have some numbers to support that. It is not as bad as some people would have it.

DR. ROE: Anybody who has been there knows that you are right.

I have to go on now and ask specifically for any questions on Dr. Davis's presentation.

DISCUSSANT: There are various studies that show that chrysotile has relatively fast clearance. You have also pointed them out. Do you have any idea why chrysotile is so different from other fibers, especially with respect to fast clearance?

DISCUSSANT: Well, I was speculating this morning that, when we use the term "clearance," we simply mean it disappears from the lung tissue. I was suggesting, in the case of chrysotile, that a lot of it actually dissolves in the lung tissue, in addition to the mechanical clearance. Certainly you can show that chrysotile dissolves very easily in a number of very mild chemical solutions. At the present time, we and, I think, a lot of other people, are trying to get general data on the rate of chrysoltile dissolution in lung tissue, but results are not yet available.

DISCUSSANT: We, too, have a lot of problems. We have seen that fibers split in the lungs, and therefore the number of fibers increases. Over a period of 1 to 2 years, you will get many more fibers at the end than at the beginning, but they are very thin. We have subjected them to analytical transmission electron microscopy.

DISCUSSANT: We found that almost no chrysotile remained in the lungs of 3-year-old rats. We have not done the same detailed studies at 2 years. We looked at 18 months and, in that case, not much chrysotile had cleared. There was about 20 or 30 μg of chrysotile in the whole rat lung, which can still amount to a lot of fibers. But I agree with you, you get a separation of chrysotile fibers into fibrils, so the first effect is an increased number of fibers.

DISCUSSANT: I wonder whether that is not the so-called "healthy-rat" effect. Rats on study that survive for 3 years usually are the ones that did not develop asbestosis and no longer have any chrysotile fibers in their lungs. You are therefore looking at a very skewed population of animals. They are survivors.

DISCUSSANT: To a certain extent that is true, but the fact that they have survived does not mean that they have nice, clean, healthy lungs. They very often have the most severe degree of asbestosis that you have ever seen.

DR. ROE: I would like to comment on this because the terms "healthy-rat effect" and "healthy-worker effect" have been misused today. Let us be perfectly clear. The healthy-worker effect refers to a population of people who are fit to work and are, therefore, fitter than a population that is unfit to work. Consequently, the former population tends to experience a lower incidence of certain diseases than the latter.

The term "healthy-rat effect" has been used in a totally different sense and also wrongly, in my view. If you want rats or hamsters to live longer, you restrict their feed intake. They not only live longer, they get less cancers of all sorts, including cancer of the lung. Hypocalorically maintained rats also develop fewer endocrine dysfunctions and fewer endocrine tumors.

Now, if you want to use the term "healthy-rat effect," that is the sort of thing you ought to be talking about. If you are not age-standardizing the data in your studies, then you should do so. To undertake a study and end up with different incidences of this or that, and then to say it might have been because the animals lived longer than the controls is a position in which you should not be caught. You should conduct your study in such a way that your data are age-standardized, using the appropriate statistics for fatal lesions and incidental lesions. However, it is not always possible to do this.

DISCUSSANT: Can I come back and say, quite simply, that of course we have control populations that usually live slightly longer than the asbestosis population. Sometimes there is no difference. But it is never the other way around. The controls never die first.

DISCUSSANT: I have a question regarding intraperitoneally injected rats. Were those mesotheliomas fatal or nonfatal? Did the rats die and did you then find the mesotheliomas incidentally, or were they diagnosed before the animals died?

DISCUSSANT: Do you mean, were they actually fatal or potentially fatal? They were potentially fatal 100%, yes, but we try to diagnose mesotheliomas in the animals when they are still alive. This can be readily done because peritoneal mesotheliomas are associated with ascites, which results in abdominal distension.

DISCUSSANT: Did you have to euthanize them?

DISCUSSANT: That is right. That does not affect the diagnosis.

DISCUSSANT: Did only your animals with parenchymal tumors have asbestosis or did all animals have asbestosis?

DISCUSSANT: By and large, yes. There is a very good correlation between what I think you can genuinely call asbestosis and the presence of pulmonary tumors, usually in the same animals, but certainly in the same population. We have just discussed that there is very good evidence that lung cancer in asbestos workers is associated with the presence of asbestosis. We can therefore say, yes, that is scar cancer.

Now, asbestosis is always, by definition, parenchymal or peripheral; it does not occur in the main bronchial tubes. So if the statement about a close relationship with scar cancers is correct, all asbestos tumors in human beings ought to be peripheral. The discussion earlier indicated that this certainly was not the case. So we have a lot of anomalies to tie up.

DISCUSSANT: Diffuse interstitial fibrosis increases the incidence of lung cancers in a fair number of people. Then you get both central and peripheral tumors, and maybe it has nothing to do with this, or there may be a common mechanism.

DISCUSSANT: And any cause of fibrosis increases—

DISCUSSANT: Any diffuse fibrosis; collagen disease, for example. There was a good article in *Thorax,* I suppose about 5 years ago, showing this. The author was mostly looking at fibrosis, alveolitis, and collagen disease. They all were associated with an increased incidence of all types of tumors. My recollection is about a ninefold increase, and there were both central and peripheral tumors.

DISCUSSANT: We do not know, but I do not believe that the number of tumors associated with interstitial fibrosis is quite as great as the ones with asbestosis. I see a lot of these patients, and we certainly see an inordinate increase in lung cancer, but I think the ones with significant asbestosis have a greater increase of lung cancer.

DISCUSSANT: My point is that diffuse scarring predisposes for lung cancer, peripheral and central, and that predisposition is not specific to asbestos.

DISCUSSANT: Right. We can conclude from your statement that just diffuse fibrosis alone would not explain the carcinogenicity of asbestosis, and I think it is more than that. I think we all agree on that.

DISCUSSANT: In your study, such concepts as fiber length and fiber diameter appear as quite variable. Is there a standardized way in which one samples fibers to determine length and diameter?

DISCUSSANT: Well, there is a recommended way for industrial use. In our studies, we followed this procedure fairly closely. We collect fibers on Nuclepore® filters, but otherwise the procedure we use is the same as that recommended. The procedure for counting fibers, of course, is also standardized.

DISCUSSANT: So, if somebody else repeats the study, his numbers should be comparable to your numbers.

DISCUSSANT: Provided that he uses the same collection techniques, deposition techniques, and the same initial dust count. It is losing these variables that people forget to allow for. They tend to talk about a cloud of chrysotile or a cloud of crocidolite, assuming that they are identical and, of course, they are not. It depends on how you generate the aerosols. They are tremendously variable from two different origins. If the fibers are properly counted and sized, you should see no difference; but differences will always be there.

DISCUSSANT: You may have noticed that there was a discrepancy between your amosite clearance data and those of Dr. Churg.

I believe you reported that for both the uncut and the cut amosite, there was very little clearance from the lung compared to that for chrysotile. Dr. Churg's data seemed to show that amosite clearance was fairly nominal compared to that for the other types of asbestos. I was wondering whether you might comment or have any idea why there might be a difference.

DISCUSSANT: No, I have not. We were simply comparing four dust samples, and our data did seem consistent. We observed much greater clearance in this period of 6 months with both chrysotile samples, but both the long-fiber samples cleared more quickly than the short-fiber samples. As far as other reports on amosite clearance are concerned, one is often in this position. We just cannot explain these discrepancies.

DR. ROE: Are there specific comments on Dr. Churg's paper?

DISCUSSANT: I have one comment regarding the fibers that are retained in the alveolar wall. How sure were you that you did not scrape off the epithelium during the administration procedure and that the epithelium just grew back over the inoculated dust? There is good evidence that this has happened in the case of chrysotile.

DISCUSSANT: That is a difficult problem. A number of people have said, and I think it is probably true, that one does get some ulceration. They are convinced that this is the major mechanism for penetration of fibers into the interstitium. It may be true. We did not look at each epithelial specimen.

Of course, the smoke is still augmenting the necrosis.

DR. WEHNER: I am surprised by your low carboxyhemoglobin values, 5%. Normally one reads about 10, up to 40, even 50%. In our animals we have observed anywhere from 10 to 40%, depending on the smoke concentration. I wonder, do you have an explanation for your low COHb values? Are they perhaps typical of the guinea pig?

DISCUSSANT: I do not know whether it is particular to the guinea pig. You realize, of course, that anytime you change the geometry in the smoke administration you are going to change what's going into the animal.

All I can tell you is, we did run this against a set of nonexposed controls.

DR. ROE: When were the blood samples collected?

DISCUSSANT: Immediately after exposure. They smoke their 10 cigarettes, and then the animals are sacrificed, following collection of the blood samples.

DISCUSSANT: I was wondering whether you would clarify a point that I thought I heard earlier. It was said that smoking increases the penetration of the asbestos particles, and some of the speakers have discussed impaired clearance caused by cigarette-smoking. I am just not clear on this. When you say "increased penetration," do you find that smoking causes the particles to deposit further down the airways, down the smaller airways, or do you mean that more fibers find their way through the epithelial layer?

DISCUSSANT: I am referring to literal penetration into tissue rather than distal penetration into the lung. The material goes from the airways into the interstitial space.

We have not looked at distribution. Because we were using intratracheal instillation, that may be a bit treacherous. Two things are really separate: one is clearance, or bulk removed, whichever way you want to measure it; the other is penetration of the epithelium as seen under the microscope. This penetration is increased in the smoker's lung samples that are collected from the same area of the respiratory tree.

DISCUSSANT: I wanted to hear Dr. Churg's comments on the macrophage storage phenomenon. You showed some photomicrographs of macrophages in which amosite was nicely stored. Was that observed by light microscopy?

DISCUSSANT: No. We simply took a macrophage pellet, dissolved it, and processed it just as if it were a tissue sample.

DISCUSSANT: I see. So it is not actually quantified by TEM.

DISCUSSANT: Well, the quantification comes from the dissolved pellet. We are not looking at individual macrophages.

DR. ROE: Incidentally, one part of the so-called overloading phenomenon is associated with the alveolar macrophages which aggregate in some alveoli. The storage of particles in these macrophages constitutes a part of the lung burden of particles. For some reason, these macrophages lose the capability to move normally and start to aggregate in alveoli, usually in alveolar ducts near the terminal bronchioles. These macrophages obviously are, in some way, functionally impaired. They may have phagocytized some fibers and really act as depots, staying in the alveoli for long periods.

DISCUSSANT: One could argue that we happened to pick just the right combination of smoke and asbestos dust to kick the animal into overload, but I would rather not believe that. I think overload is very real.

DR. ROE: Smoke particles also contribute to the overload. If you have a combination of asbestos and cigarette smoke and measure only the asbestos in the lung, you do not reach that magic overload number of 2 mg/g of lung tissue because you are analyzing only for asbestos, but there is also some contribution from the cigarette smoke.

Are there specific questions for Dr. Muhle?

DISCUSSANT: I believe one of your results was that the clearance of crocidolite was impaired twofold, and that chrysotile was unaffected, is that right? I am really intrigued by possible mechanisms that may be operative. Normally, I would think that cigarette smoke might have an impact on macrophage mobility or phagocytosis, but that this should differ for different forms of asbestosis is very interesting. Do you have any explanation?

DISCUSSANT: I speculate about this in my paper, but I do not really know whether my speculation is correct. I am referring to the results of Dr. Wagner, who also found, after exposing rats to chrysotile, a steady state after 3 months. According to the same study, during a 24-month exposure to crocidolite, an almost linear increase in retained fibers was observed. Possibly, the deposition mechanism may be different in the upper airways for both fibers. For chrysotile, it is more the clearance in the upper airways, and this may not be impaired by the cigarette smoke. Whereas with crocidolite, we may have higher deposition in the deep lung. That is one possible explanation.

DISCUSSANT: I wonder whether there is not another explanation, namely that cigarette smoke can impair mechanical clearance of both types of asbestos. In addition, chrysotile undergoes simple chemical dissolution, which is not affected by cigarette smoke. I wonder whether that is partly the explanation.

DISCUSSANT: It is possible.

DISCUSSANT: I would like to take that one step further. What if the rate of dissolution is sufficiently high that a two- or threefold increase in, let us say, macrophage retention is simply trivial by comparison? One is then dealing with a situation in which the retention of crocidolite is effectively doubled. Let us assume that the retention of chrysotile is also doubled. If special mechanisms operate, the rate of those mechanisms may be so fast that one cannot get above that baseline except by an extraordinary increase in retention. In other words, if smoking were to lead to retention of 100 times as much chrysotile, one might detect it. But if smoking leads to the retention of only two or three times as much chrysotile in smoke-exposed subjects as in nonsmokers, one would not be able to see it, because its rate of dissolution in the lung is too rapid.

DISCUSSANT: If the dissolution is very high, then, obviously, the pathological response is completely different. There are examples for materials other than asbestos: one is zinc oxide, and another is silica. Experiments with silica—silica in a form which had very small particles—produced inflammation, edema, and so on, that led to the death of most rats. But those which survived no longer had any silica in the lungs, because it had translocated from the lungs to other tissues, which means clearance was complete. On the other hand, most of the rats died!

Zinc oxide is relatively soluble in the lung and will be cleared extremely fast, not through macrophages but probably by dissolution.

Permeability is an additional factor. Say that some substance increases the permeability of the originally tight epithelium; it may, in this way, enter the interstitial space. In those circumstances, obviously, the pathological response would be different.

DR. ROE: Surely the gaps between some cells are not that large. The chance of an asbestos fiber actually hitting a gap is not going to be that great.

DISCUSSANT: It can go through the cell. It does not have to go through the gap.

DISCUSSANT: Exactly. So the gaps are irrelevant.

DISCUSSANT: Not in asbestos penetration. I said there was increased penetration. Some substances change the permeability of the otherwise tight epithelium by either increasing the gap or affecting the epithelial cells themselves so that the penetration is increased. This means that the permeability and the absorption are increased. In that case, the compounds disappear from the lung; they are cleared, but not by the type of clearance that we are discussing mostly: namely, clearance by alveolar macrophages.

DISCUSSANT: Am I missing something? If I were going to attack something with the intention of creating a penetrating wound, I would choose a straight thing for a weapon. How does the penetration theory account for chrysotile, a wiggly thing?

DISCUSSANT: With chrysotile?

DISCUSSANT: Yes. Some people have proposed that penetration is an important factor. How is it going to happen with chrysotile, which is wiggly?

DISCUSSANT: It does not need to penetrate. As Dr. Brody has shown, and as we have shown, if a chrysotile fiber lands on the surface of the alveolus, of which 95% is covered by Type I epithelium, if a macrophage does not phagocytize that fiber, there will be cytoplasmic extensions of the Type I cell.

DISCUSSANT: That is fine, but what about in the main airways? We were shown photographs of long, straight fibers sticking straight into the epithelium. How is that going to happen with chrysotile?

DISCUSSANT: My view is that it would not happen.

DISCUSSANT: That is my view, too.

DISCUSSANT: Why would it not happen?

DISCUSSANT: Because the upper airways are lined with cuboidal epithelium.

DISCUSSANT: That may be so, but we know that there are some changes going on. A fiber may end up in an area that is no longer covered by cuboidal epithelium. The epithelium might have been lost completely.

DISCUSSANT: I believe Dr. Churg's work emphasizes that point: when cigarette smoke is followed by a bolus of asbestos fibers, there will probably be, in the presence of inflammation, enhanced movement of fibers across the epithelium or directly onto a basement membrane that has no epithelium covering it.

DISCUSSANT: Has anybody seen a photograph of a chrysotile fiber sitting deeply in the epithelium of the main airways?

DISCUSSANT: I have never seen that.

DR. ROE: Has anybody seen that? If not, does that not tell us something about mechanisms?

DISCUSSANT: I am not sure many people have looked for it.

DISCUSSANT: That is the problem, those of us working with chrysotile are all looking at the peripheral areas of the lung.

DISCUSSANT: I suspect that one would only have a chance of seeing chrysotile fibers deep in the epithelium if one gave a walloping dose by intratracheal instillation.

DISCUSSANT: Yes, following intratracheal injection, it wouldn't surprise me at all, because then you have got a wire-brush effect.

DISCUSSANT: In that type of study, you get fibers sticking out the anus, or so it has been said!

DISCUSSANT: We certainly have a problem here. I have no difficulty in accepting that direct penetration can occur where epithelia have lost their protective covering, including a deep layer of mucus. I am quite sure you would never get direct penetration—straight into a cell—where these coverings are intact. However, if the epithelium has undergone a metaplastic change, or something like that, then asbestos might possibly have a better chance for a more direct penetration.

DISCUSSANT: As Dr. Pott has pointed out, you have to assume that there are spots in this large surface where something has happened: an injury, temporarily sloughed-off ciliary epithelium, etc. It takes times until this spot heals. During that time, some fibers may land there. That is Dr. Pott's suggestion. If this is true, there may be a possibility that some fibers may end up in the deeper layers of the normal epithelium.

DR. WEHNER: Injured spots also may not be absolutely flat on a cellular level. There may be miniature lesions in the form of minute knolls, depressions or fissures, microscopic protrusions, and/or patches of epithelium not covered by protective mucus. It is conceivable, perhaps even probable, that a fiber could lodge in such a spot like a spear, whether it is chrysotile or crocidolite.

DISCUSSANT: I just want to ask Dr. Muhle a question. Why did you use the Rhodesian chrysotile?

DISCUSSANT: We just had the sample readily available.

DR. ROE: Let's go on to the last two papers, by Drs. Scholander and Gerde; we will discuss these two papers together. Are there any questions?

DISCUSSANT: I have one question. Yours is a nice mathematical approach, but how does it reflect reality in terms of the lipid layer? There is evidence of the lipid layer in the upper airways, and the antomical distribution of mucus is very patchy. How would your model account for these possibilities?

DISCUSSANT: The existence of a surfactant layer in the upper airways has been described in a few articles. I mentioned the article by Ueda. They collected samples from the upper bronchial airways, cooled them very rapidly in liquid nitrogen, and then prepared them for electron microscopy. And there is an article by Schlimmer et al., who blocked off part of the upper airways and washed out the mucus cover. Then they analyzed the surfactant content and found some three to five promille of surfactant lipids there.

The distribution, of course, is not clear from that article, but the authors also tried to redistribute this three to five promille of surfactant lipids within the mucus layer and found that the rate of penetration of highly lipophilic substances does not differ that much. These substances will get trapped within the lipids as soon as they hit a lipid phase. Of course the model is highly dependent on the existence of a continuous mucus layer and its lipid content. On the other hand, the consequences of a missing lipid-aqueous mucus layer are implicitly predicted by the model and should be as interesting. This should result in more localized and considerably higher cellular doses of lipophilic substances at places in the epithelium that are not covered by mucus.

DISCUSSANT: The list of carcinogens which have been identified in tobacco smoke is quite long. Do you think it is justifiable to confine interest in the adsorption theory to polycyclic aromatic hydrocarbons? Do you think some of the other classes of substances ought to be looked at? And is it just a matter of time, is it just a matter of habit, or is there some other justification for selecting PAH?

DISCUSSANT: Well, not being a pathologist, I cannot judge whether PAH is a good choice, but our model should apply to essentially any highly lipophilic substances. Most lipophilic substances of higher molecular weight would probably behave rather similarly. If they have a partition coefficient of, say 10^6 or 10^7, they should behave roughly in the same manner.

DISCUSSANT: Some people would think that nitrosamines are important. How would they behave?

DISCUSSANT: I guess their average molecular weights are smaller, and their lipid-aqueous partition coefficients also are lower. Probably the model is not as applicable to those substances, or, rather, to the assumption that a major resistance to mass transfer of genotoxic substances lies within the mucus layer. But again, this limitation is as interesting. The lower the lipid-aqueous partition coefficient, the more rapid the uptake by the epithelium will be. The mechanism for this is the same as that for the accumulation of lipophilic substances in body fat, known to all toxicologists.

DISCUSSANT: Your model depends on a fiber nosing down into a thick—I believe it is a thick—mucus layer. Have you had any data or done any modeling on how fibers orient themselves in a cilia-driven mucus layer?

DISCUSSANT: I think it was Woodworth et al. who took biopsies of the upper bronchial tree and found fibers—I think even chrysotile fibers—that were partly phagocytized also by the epithelial cells. I believe many of these cells were squamous metaplasia cells. Fibers started to become phagocytized even by the epithelial cells themselves, but whether this is sufficient to account for fibers really penetrating the mucus layer in this fashion, I suppose no one could tell today.

DISCUSSANT: I was trying to get a picture of how the fiber could begin penetration. When the fiber is floating on the mucus, how could it nose in?

My other question: Did you measure the specific surface area of your fibers? I think it would be very interesting to see your graphs normalized to specific surface area.

DISCUSSANT: You mean in the adsorption of PAH?

DISCUSSANT: Just the total available surface area of your glass fibers and of your asbestos fibers, using nitrogen adsorption or a similar technique.

DISCUSSANT: I believe the average specific surface areas differ, roughly, by a factor of 100 between the rock wool samples and the asbestos fibers.

DISCUSSANT: And that was the difference between the surface areas of your two fiber types?

DISCUSSANT: Roughly, yes.

DISCUSSANT: So, what you are saying is, when you added water vapor, the water molecules were filling the cracks in the asbestos fiber and reducing the available surface area.

DISCUSSANT: Well, I think this desorption started even before there was a complete monomolecular layer of water on the fiber surfaces. Water molecules seemed to compete for roughly the same active sites on the fiber surface as the hydrocarbons.

DISCUSSANT: One of the things that cigarette smoke is known to do is to disrupt pulmonary surfactant or a phospholipid mucous membrane. To what extent would that action of cigarette smoke sort of blow a hole in your theory? Is the functional integrity of that phospholipid membrane very important for your hypothesis to work, or could it be that it would work even for a partial injury?

DISCUSSANT: I think if you translate the lipid content of the central airways into a number of monomolecular layers, you would obtain some seven or eight monolayers, continuous layers of lipids, even in the central airways. Of course, if you go below one continuous layer, then the fiber hypothesis would run into trouble, but not the model for the protective properties of the undisturbed lipid-aqueous mucus layer.

DISCUSSANT: I would like to know whether we have direct evidence that tumors appear at bifurcation sites. There are some pathologists who say that there are no such data. We have an assumption that this is where they are appearing. I do not take that position.

DISCUSSANT: I will ask you—and perhaps the others will, too—whether you are looking at humans. By the time you first see a lesion, it extends way beyond the small area of the bifurcation site. It would be a bold person who would say exactly where it did arise.

There is even a further problem. When you have tumors which you discover rather late, they spread toward the hilar area of the lung. So, when we were talking earlier about peripheral and central tumors, the fact is that tumors always spread towards the center. For this reason, the first diagnosis of even a peripherally arising tumor may be of a centrally placed shadow seen in the chest X ray.

Now, there are articles in the literature on populations of people with lung cancer of whom a series of X rays had been taken previously—diagnostic X rays, screening X rays—in which no lesions had been discovered. And there are claims that, when these same X rays were re-examined retrospectively by someone who knew the end result, they often found a lesion which was much more peripheral than the one that was eventually discovered. So all the discussion that we had earlier as to whether tumors are peripheral or central is clouded by the difficulty or impossibility of knowing where they arise.

DISCUSSANT: My question is more specific. I am talking about bifurcations versus the bronchial tubes.

DR. ROE: The answer must be that there cannot possibly be any reliable information on that. Auerbach and his colleagues provide information on the distribution of precancerous lesions and, I believe, reported some tendency for tumors to occur near bifurcations. However, that does not prove that "full-blooded" cancers arise perferentially at bifurcations. There is a report, based on the use of a fluorescent technique, on the distribution of epithelial changes that are not detectable by other means. According to those who have used this technique, it seems that many of the early lesions are *not* at bifurcations but in other areas of the airways. There is no big, long study that used that technique in humans, but that technique is going to be the one, I believe, that is going to answer your question.

I think it is very important. I do not think there are enough data yet to warrant any conclusion.

In some rat studies where there has been very heavy exposure to tobacco smoke, the squamous metaplasia has gone all the way down the trachea. There was no special tendency for it to occur at bifurcations.

DISCUSSANT: I have one point. I wanted to take up the statement that was made in the paper by Dr. Mossman on penetration of fibers in areas of squamous metaplasia. Would such an area be covered by a layer of mucus?

DISCUSSANT: I do not know.

DISCUSSANT: Is there any information regarding electrical charges on asbestos fiber? Does the adsorption of certain chemicals produce a charge which affects the orientation, so that this fiber—if it develops a charge—becomes polar? Could it then change its orientation vis-à-vis the airway and penetrate the cell because of a change in charge? Such phenomena—if they exist—may be related to subsurface qualities. Is there anything known about the impact of charges on the orientation of fibers?

DISCUSSANT: Variation in the amount of adsorbed water vapor might significantly affect surface charge.

DR. ROE: Last question, last comment.

DISCUSSANT: We have gone into a considerable degree of detail thinking about the environment in these airways. We envision curly fibers and straight fibers floating placidly along this relatively uniform tube in this warm, moist environment. Something we need to remember in our catalog of factors that can perturb that environment is the fact that mucus layers are, at least partially, discontinuous.

I think it is reasonable to assume that the ciliated surfaces could probably be bare in places. Areas of metaplasia were just mentioned; I think it is reasonable to assume that those could be bare, at least for part of the time. So we can accept the probability that fibers might encounter the cells directly.

But there is one factor that has not been mentioned: one of the characteristics of smokers is that they have a great tendency to cough. The more they smoke, the more they cough; and the longer they smoke, the more they cough. We know quite a bit about the physiology of the cough, and it is an awesome thing to behold on a microscopic level.

During coughing, the glottis is closed, and tremendous pressures are generated. The epithelia of large airways are then exposed to violent bursts of air passing over their surfaces. These are surely potentially damaging. They might even strip off the epithelium.

As you proceed peripherally, these flow-limiting segments go peripherally and stop at some point that is determined by the elastic properties of the lung. But at that point, the number of airways is so large that the mass flow and the shear force must be fairly small.

The reason why we cough is because—I am being teleological, of course—we can develop enough shear force along that epithelium to strip mucus, to shake it loose. I can imagine that if there is a discontinuity in the epithelial surface—e.g., metaplasia, whatever—that this discontinuity would be a focus of shear force too, an irritating focus.

Therefore, I believe that it is useful to crank those factors into our thinking, too, when we are cogitating about forces that are perturbing these airways.

DISCUSSANT: There probably is an orientation effect on the deposition of long, straight fibers at bifurcations. They would deposit like javelins.

DISCUSSANT: It is much more likely during a cough, during exhalation than during inhalation. That is the point I was trying to make. If you envision projectiles going down the airways and attacking, you'd like to think of it happening during inhalation. I am suggesting you might also want to think of it during exhalation. You could make a much better case for it.

DR. ROE: Any further comments? If not, this concludes the discussions for today. Thank you very much.

Edited Transcript of the Discussions of Day 2

Chairman: Dr. R. O. McClellan

Papers by the following authors were discussed in this session: Omenn, Agostoni, Nolan, Chen, Pinkerton, Warheit (two presentations), Oberdörster, and Mauderly.

DR. McCLELLAN: Our goal for this afternoon is twofold: (1) to have the opportunity to discuss each one of the papers that was presented this morning, and (2) at the same time, to see whether there are other issues that come to the surface that bear discussion.

Unfortunately, Dr. Omenn, who presented the first paper this morning on the chemoprevention of lung cancer, is unable to be with us this afternoon because of his duties as Dean of the School of Public Health. I think it would still be of interest to have some discussion of this very important long-term and extensive study that is underway.

Are there any questions or comments on Dr. Omenn's study?

DISCUSSANT: Had Dr. Omenn been here, I would have wanted to hear some further clarification on the nature of the asbestos worker cohort. Was there further stratification of the workers on the basis of their ILO classification, or were there any stratifications on the basis of pleural changes on X rays or were there any other clinical markers used to distinguish among the different subgroups?

DR. McCLELLAN: All right.

Those are some very important points. I don't know whether any of Dr. Omenn's collaborators are here and would be able to address these questions, but certainly these are very important points in terms of the ultimate interpretation of the results.

DISCUSSANT: Dr. Omenn indicated on his chart, in one of his tables, that the asbestos workers represented groups of workers exposed to asbestos in a number of occupational settings, and some of those occupational settings carry different fiber types. It might be of further interest to explore the possibility of fiber-type potency in terms of asbestos disease and fiber retention.

DR. McCLELLAN: That is another good point.

Other comments?

As I heard his presentation, I couldn't help but think of some earlier thoughts and discussions that I have had over the role of diet, using laboratory animal studies in investigating respiratory disease. I would be interested in other peoples' comments on that subject. Perhaps somebody here has been involved in some of those studies in which there were attempts at diet-altering, in terms of vitamin A, to see whether that influenced the outcome.

Dr. Roe, have you been involved in any of those studies?

DISCUSSANT: Yes, I have. There are two important points in working with animals. You are probably not going to get anywhere fast unless you do as I did and start off with animals which are vitamin-A-depleted, because normally they have got such a store of the vitamin in the liver that they are never, in fact, going to be vitamin-A-deficient, even though you put them on a vitamin-A-deficient diet.

We have also been involved in a human study where we were comparing patients with lung cancer who are still alive. We were questioning them on their diet habits and comparing them with a control group of people with rheumatoid diseases. We came to the conclusion that you cannot get reliable dietary information, not even about what people ate yesterday, let alone what they ate last week, or a month ago. To get reliable information on the amounts that people eat as well as on what they eat, is exceedingly difficult.

In our study, when we quantified the amounts of vitamin A that people were getting through various sources, far and away the biggest influence was vitamin tablets. And, again, it is terribly difficult to find out how much vitamin A there is in the various preparations. The same name applies to many different strengths of the compound. So to get accurate information on this is a major task.

Now the other point: there is one dietary source of vitamin A which is overwhelmingly important compared to anything else, and that is liver. Some people do not know whether they eat or don't eat liver, but when they have paté, then they recall that, never mind from where it comes. My own experience is that the diet side is probably the weak part of the study and is very difficult to control.

DR. McCLELLAN: Regarding your difficulties in questionnaire data on dietary habits, we have somewhat the same problem with smokers. It would have been of interest to see whether the investigators had incorporated any markers in terms of exposure, both within "acknowledged" cigarette smokers and in terms of ex-smokers. Recent work by one of our colleagues in New Mexico showed the difficulties in terms of lack of agreement between the questionnaires and more reliable indices of cigarette-smoking.

DISCUSSANT: There have been a lot of independent studies. There is always considerable trouble with questionnaire ascertainment, in particular dealing with recollection. Although you can't get a clear resolution in terms of relative differentials that are statistically significant, you see clear trends.

It appears that people who eat diets that are high in vitamin A do seem to have reduced levels of lung cancer, or cancer of all types. So there is a question as to whether the statistics are really biologically significant. The lack of significance is based on the fact that there is so much "noise" in the questionnaire system. Therefore, it is going to remain almost unresolvable until you conduct a prospective study, but no one has funds to do that yet.

DISCUSSANT: Liver storage of vitamin A may affect whether dietary vitamin A can influence cancer. Perhaps that is why beta-carotene and retinyl palmitate are being administered. Although you may have a large store of vitamin A in the liver, tissue levels and serum levels of retinol are under tight control. Apparently this is not so with beta-carotene and retinyl palmitate. Their dose levels will be reflected immediately in tissue levels and lung blood levels because they don't have homeostatic control. As Dr. Omenn presented, the supplements administered to his subjects do result in significant increases in the serum and, therefore, presumably in tissue levels.

DISCUSSANT: In the studies I have presented here, 15- and 30-mg daily doses of beta-carotene produced 7-fold and 10-fold increases in serum beta-carotene concentrations within 4 months and slightly higher elevations (essentially steady-state) at 12 and 24 months. Beta-carotene is not subject to homeostatic control similar to that which limits the range of circulating retinol concentrations. Orally administered retinyl palmitate is completely cleaved to yield retinol, and follows retinol kinetics. Administration of either retinol or retinyl palimate leads to a readily detected elevation of circulating retinyl palmitate concentrations. In our studies we observed a peak about 6 hours after dosing and a decline toward baseline over the next 6 to 24 hours. In contrast, retinol concentrations remained little changed (a slight upward trend). Regarding the liver storage of retinol, my colleagues and I originally proposed a higher "loading dose" regimen, to be followed by "maintenance" at the 25,000 IU dose we employ. The NCI and FDA preferred a single dose throughout.

DISCUSSANT: Are all of these forms of vitamin A similarly effective?

DISCUSSANT: We believe that retinol (vitamin A) and retinyl esters *per os* are equally active and enter the circulation similarly as retinyl palmitate. Within the intestinal lining cells, retinyl esters are de-esterified to retinol and then re-established to retinyl palmitate. If radiolabeled retinyl palmitate is administered, the label is lost. Certain synthetic retinoids are being tested for anticarcinogenic efficacy in animal studies and a few clinical studies; their potency relative to retinol needs to be established.

Retinol and these related agents act by enhancing the state of differentiation of epithelial cells, thereby probably suppressing the late stages of tumor promotion and tumor progression. Reports late in 1987 from research groups at the Salk Institute and in France have demonstrated that retinoic acid and retinol bind to a pair of specific vitamin-A-binding proteins in the nucleus. These proteins belong to a class of molecules that have a hormone-specific ligand-binding region and a common structure of Zn-containing "fingers" that are thought to reach out to target regions in the DNA and modulate gene expression. Perhaps these proteins and the genes (on chromosomes 3 and 17) which code for them act through tumor-suppressor mechanisms.

Beta-carotene can be cleaved to yield two molecules of retinol. In addition, it is thought to act directly as an electron/free radical scavenger, reducing any role of such intermediates in late stages of tumor development.

DISCUSSANT: How is the matter of alcohol intake handled?

DISCUSSANT: We take a history of drinking behavior and screen SGOT and alkaline phosphatase in determining eligibility. Anyone who reports a diagnosis of cirrhosis of the liver or hepatitis during the previous year is excluded from the study. We have had numerous examples of individual participants in the study whose SGOT or SGPT is elevated after acknowledged drinking bouts. According to our protocol, it has been necessary to consider any such elevations of liver enzymes as possibly due to the study agents. Therefore we discontinue treatment while symptoms are monitored and, if they disappear, the participant is re-challenged with the study vitamins (or placebo) under the double-blind protocol. We have not investigated whether alcohol intake causes significant changes in the pharmacokinetics or pharmacodynamics of vitamin A.

Studies in the rat, in baboons, and in humans, by Charles Lieber and associates, have shown that experimental administration of ethanol with normal or even enriched vitamin-A-containing diets resulted in a depression of hepatic vitamin A that could not be attributed to insufficient vitamin A intake or to malabsorption. Histologic changes include multivesicular lysosomes with a characteristic electron-dense crescent. Plasma vitamin A levels were not changed. Kidney and testis content of vitamin A was increased. Two mechanisms seem to be involved. First, there is increased mobilization of vitamin A from the liver, shifting vitamin A from liver to other organs through lipoprotein-bound retinyl esters. Second, there is increased catabolism of vitamin A to 4-hydroxyretinoic acid and other metabolites. A particular microsomal cytochrome P 450 (P 450f) increased in activity in ethanol-fed rats. With ethanol ingestion, some additional vitamin A may be needed to overcome depeletion of hepatic stores. However, very high levels of vitamin A may be more likely to cause hepatic toxicity in the presence of alcohol, thereby narrowing the therapeutically safe margin.

DR. McCLELLAN: Let us now turn to the paper presented by Dr. John Butler and Dr. Agostoni. Questions or comments?

DISCUSSANT: I think perhaps the key question is the work rate that they had. What does this really mean in terms of asbestos workers' compensation, in view of the fact that half of the individuals had no detectable exercise impairment?

DISCUSSANT: Well, it is an important but really difficult question. For instance, what would you do about compensating for the presence of an asbestos-related plaque regardless of the presence of dyspnea? It might be considered a disability. So it is a very difficult issue, and I think it is not just a medical problem. It is a problem which involves the entire society, not only us.

DISCUSSANT: Has anybody clearly characterized what is meant by breathlessness? I think that patients have a sense of breathlessness—most of them say they "can't take a satisfactory breath," and it has nothing to do with the parameters that you were actually measuring. My question is, are there parameters that could be measured which relate to the sensation of breathlessness?

DISCUSSANT: Well, we do not know the cause of breathlessness. However, we can rate its perceived severity. One of the most commonly used criteria is a self-assessed 0-10 scale. Then you can ask the patient, after a time, whether there is any change. But this is not an absolute scale, it is only value-related to this particular patient. However, I would like to remind you that the 120 patients in our population were complaining of breathlessness, the cause of which we tried to assess for medico-legal reasons. Therefore, this was a particular, very specific population, not asbestos-exposed workers in general, but people claiming compensation. The majority of them already received some compensation money for their condition, but they were asking for more.

DISCUSSANT: But the obvious question is, if you took 100 people without asbestos exposure who are complaining of breathlessness and seeking compensation, what results would you get in that circumstance?

DISCUSSANT: In those people who had a heart or lung problem we would have abnormal results. We have to compare our results to normal people and analyze them. If I understand your question, if they were 100% normal people, you would probably get normal data from all of them.

DISCUSSANT: But that is the wrong control. What I am suggesting is that you need to have two groups of people, both of them complaining of breathlessness. One has been exposed to asbestos and is seeking compensation, and the other group is not. What happens in those circumstances?

DISCUSSANT: There is rather a nice paper by Keith Morgan which answers that question. He shows that, if there is compensation involved, the percentage that do complain of breathlessness is very much higher. (Morgan, WK. Clinical significance of pulmonary function tests: Disability or disinclination—impairment or importuning? *Chest 75:* 6, 1979.)

DISCUSSANT: That is still not the same point. I am saying that if you reach the point where you have people who are complaining of breathlessness, my impression is that first you have to see that they are matched for the degree of breathlessness and then, if you put them through your tests, what happens then?

DISCUSSANT: Keith Morgan found that when he did this, comparing people with the same degree of breathlessness, many of those who were involved in litigation were not impaired according to his tests. But in the others, who were not seeking compensation, there was a much higher percentage with abnormal test results. Referring to the other question that you asked initially, "Is there some other criterion for breathlessness?," the answer is no. We don't really understand what causes it. It can occur with anemia, it can occur with muscle weakness, it can occur with cardiac problems, and it can occur with respiratory problems. The cause of breathlessness has been a favored field for specious speculation over the years.

DISCUSSANT: It can occur with upper nasal blockage?

DISCUSSANT: Yes.

DISCUSSANT: When you are representing a labor union, which you might well do in a case like this, this is what you should say: "Well, my recommendation to the members of the union would be not to take the test." This could be for a very good scientific reason: The test may not be appropriate. I mean, who enlightened you? Did divine wisdom strike you and say that is the right way to measure breathlessness? And, unfortunately, the results we have now could also be used in an antilabor fashion.

DISCUSSANT: You are right insofar as we are not measuring breathlessness. We do not have the means to measure how short of breath a person is. We are measuring physiological impairment, which we think is completely different. Breathlessness is something personal and subjective that is complained about. These heart and lung-function tests are something that one can measure, which is limiting the ability to exercise.

DISCUSSANT: I have two questions. First, did you happen to measure the CO diffusing capacity in this study? And if so, how did that relate to the alveolar-to-arterial (A-a) oxygen difference (A-a) DO_2?

DISCUSSANT: Yes, we measured the diffusing capacity by the single-breath CO method.

DISCUSSANT: How does it compare with the (A-a) DO_2 in terms of sensitivity?

DISCUSSANT: We did recently what you are suggesting. We compared the single-breath diffusing capacity at rest with the (A-a) DO_2/VO_2 during exercise. First, there was a good correlation. Second, I don't think that the sensitivity of the loss of diffusing capacity in relationship to the ILO score, which is what we were really looking at, is any greater than that of widening of the (A-a) DO_2/VO_2. What we were looking for was some method of verifying that these patients have the functional impairment of asbestosis when we think we see asbestosis on the X ray. And we found that.

DISCUSSANT: I thought that you were plotting the (A-a) DO_2, normalized by oxygen uptake during exercise, against the diffusing capacity at rest.

DISCUSSANT: Correct.

DISCUSSANT: I heard that you normalized using maximal oxygen uptake and not oxygen uptake at the time of the (A-a) DO_2 measurement. Which was it?

DISCUSSANT: Well, both are true. It was the measured maximal oxygen uptake, and we measured the (A-a) DO_2 at the maximal oxygen uptake.

DISCUSSANT: In normalizing it that way, is it possible that you might be increasing the sensitivity too much if you have a subject who is already thinking about receiving money and how he is performing, and so forth? Do you think that you get into problems with that normalization?

DISCUSSANT: Well, we hope not, because we know that the greater the blood flow (cardiac output) through an abnormal lung, the greater the (A-a) DO_2, and the greater the discrepancy between ventilation and perfusion. So we divided by the blood flow rate (actually maximal oxygen uptake, which is roughly equivalent), to try to standardize it for just that problem.

DISCUSSANT: The diagnosis of asbestosis is made solely on the basis of occupational history and X ray. Is that correct? There were no other clinical signs?

DISCUSSANT: No. The diagnosis was made according to the ATS 1986 guidelines, which include X-ray change, clinical findings, and pulmonary-function abnormalities. (American Thoracic Society. The diagnosis of nonmalignant disease related to asbestos. *Am Rev Respir Dis 134:* 363-368, 1986).

DISCUSSANT: I would like to address a question on diffusing capacity for carbon monoxide (D_LCO) and (A-a) DO_2. James Hansen and Darryl Sue, from our laboratory, published in *The New England Journal of Medicine,* just about a year ago, a paper which made this correlation in a large group of asbestos workers (Hansen and Sue. *N Engl J Med 316:* 1301-1306, 1987). When the D_LCO was low or normal, the (A-a) DO_2 was high, so the (A-a) DO_2 had a greater sensitivity. But, on the other hand, there were many patients who had a D_LCO in the normal range, which was taken to exclude asbestosis, but had an increase in (A-a) DO_2; therefore, it had a low specificity.

Regarding the issue of breathlessness on exercise in patients seeking compensation, not all of the patients in our population complained of dyspnea. Some complained of exercise limitations due to fatigue, some complained of dizziness, and sometimes there were no complaints at all. If you have someone who has a maximal oxygen uptake below that predicted, and the maximal oxygen uptake is volitionally reduced, you need to seek other objective abnormalities that the subject cannot manipulate. Then you have information that could confirm impairment and be a basis for the subject's exercise limitations. So that is one advantage.

The other advantage is simply in the age range that both groups were studying. We were surprised that such a large number of these patients in our population (which was different from that of the Agostoni study) also had cardiac disease and did not know it. Nonanginal ST segment changes and arrhythmias were ECG changes observed at low levels of work at which no chest pain was felt. This finding, I think, was helpful whether they were asking for compensation or not.

DISCUSSANT: To what sort of asbestos were these folks exposed, and did you ever collect sputum samples? Did they contain asbestos bodies?

DISCUSSANT: I don't really know what sort of asbestos fibers were around 40 years ago. I believe it was chrysotile with which they were mainly working in the shipyards around this area during and after the war. No, we did not collect routine sputum samples to check for asbestos bodies.

DISCUSSANT: So there was no amphibole asbestos used in the shipping industries where they worked?

DISCUSSANT: Perhaps Dr. Churg knows the answer to that. I am afraid I don't.

DISCUSSANT: We have analyzed a lot of lungs here and, in fact, they had heavy chrysotile exposure. However, they also had very significant amphibole exposure. Almost all of them, I would say.

DISCUSSANT: In the data that you presented, the ratio of smokers and ex-smokers to nonsmokers was more than 1, this was flip-flopped, compared with Dr. Omenn's group. I found that somewhat surprising, because I thought his original feasibility study group was also recruited from this area. Am I recalling correctly?

DISCUSSANT: That is true, but the great similarity of the fraction of nonsmokers in our population—which I will be discussing tomorrow—was interesting. The proportion in your (Agostoni et al.) study was 18%, with 72% smokers and ex-smokers. Ours turned out to be about 20% for never-smokers.

DISCUSSANT: So for me, it was just the opposite: I was impressed with the similarity in the never-smoked category in our study and that of Dr. Omenn.

DISCUSSANT: Similar, yes. I think the difference was that we combined the "smokers" with the ex-smokers, so Dr. Omenn had a bigger "nonsmoker" population that consisted really of nonsmokers plus ex-smokers.

DISCUSSANT: This suggests that more people are stopping smoking now when they learn of the problem of smoking and asbestosis. In this study of Agostoni et al., we are talking about data from a couple of years ago.

DISCUSSANT: The other point is whether, when they say they are nonsmokers now, one should try to confirm whether they truly are ex-smokers. Do you routinely measure carboxyhemoglobin in the blood to find out whether they are telling the truth?

DISCUSSANT: Yes, we did this in most but not all of the subjects.

DISCUSSANT: Did you look at total lung capacity (TLC) in the ILO 1/0 group to see whether airway obstructions were complicating the X-ray diagnosis of asbestosis?

DISCUSSANT: Yes, just as in the study recently reported by Scott Barnhart (Barnhart et al., *Chest 93:* 299-302, 1988) from the group at Harborview Hospital in Seattle, who generally would concur that the total lung capacity was not a good indicator when asbestosis, a restrictive disease tending to reduce TLC, is present together with obstructive disease (due to cigarette-smoking), which tends to increase TLC. Part of this problem is that the shrinkage, because of the scarring of asbestosis, is offset by an increase in total lung capacity because of the obstructive alveolar disease and gas-trapping. They tend to cancel out, so the measurement of TLC is no good.

DR. McCLELLAN: Let's move on to the paper presented by Dr. Nolan on the membranolytic activity and binding character of titania.

DISCUSSANT: I think we should focus on the fundamental contributions of our study. One of these contributions is that the standard mineralogical techniques used to characterize mineral dusts may not be adequate for characterizing properties which contribute to the dust's biological potential.

The biological potential of a mineral dust is imparted, to a large extent, by its surface. Therefore, if you are going to commit to a biological dust study, you will have to perform different characterization measurements not routinely carried out in other studies. At least I would advise that.

DISCUSSANT: I was wondering why you are using an archaic biological indicator when you use sophisticated biomedical tools.

DISCUSSANT: You mean the hemolysis of the red cells?

DISCUSSANT: Yes. I don't know whether you would agree with me that it is a nonstarter as an indicator of biological activity.

DISCUSSANT: The model was selected knowing that it has nothing to do with the disease process of fibrosis. But the human red blood cell's cytoskeletal structure is well known, and its receptors are well known. Therefore, it is the receptors which were the target component of the red blood cell system. The model had nothing to do directly with biological potential as related to the specific disease process. Our study had to do with chemical functionalities on surfaces of minerals and their response to receptors on intact, functioning cells. We wished to determine how a mineral surface, with known chemical functionalities, was recognized by, and communicated with, cell membrane receptors.

DISCUSSANT: There seems to be a contradiction in saying that you had to go beyond the usual physicochemical measurements that are relevant to the world of biology, and now you are saying that there is no biology here.

DISCUSSANT: No, no, no. What we are saying is that the death of the red cell has little to do with the overall problem. People think that if you can lyse red cells you can damage the macrophage membranes, so maybe there is some broad relationship between hemolysis and the fibrogenicity. But the main reason we studied human red blood cells was because we wished to explore specific receptor reactions. The only reason we looked at titanium dioxide was because it was reported that it produced tumors in laboratory animals after inhalation experiments. We were interested in this report because we had a broad data base for silica which indicated that different surface-modified forms of a single mineral displayed a wide range in activity. Therefore, we wanted to look at the titania polymorphs, another oxide mineral set, with similar surface functional groups. We looked at the titanias and found that, like silica, they, too, had very different surfaces. The only two materials that were "membrane-active" behaved like active silica. One of these materials had been used in that inhalation study. The cell membranes, and the animals, obviously distinguished between the active and inactive forms. Yet, on the basis of mineralogical characterization, we could not distinguish among these forms. What we are saying is that the surface properties of the minerals themselves were distinguished by the cell membrane surfaces and their receptors.

DISCUSSANT: I think we need to break that discussion into a couple of parts and go back to the Du Pont study with the titanium dioxide. According to my recollection, that is the only chronic study from that or any other laboratory at very high concentrations. I don't think that there is any evidence to say that this material was more or less biologically active in a long-term bioassay.

DISCUSSANT: If you correlate that with surface activity, in that particular study they used 250 mg/m^3.

DISCUSSANT: If it hadn't been for the overload and continual inflammation for 2 years, it is, in my opinion, unlikely that tumors would have developed. It is difficult to make that correlation between surface activity in that particular particle because it has caused the development of tumors.

DISCUSSANT: The point I was making is that, to the best of my knowledge, they have not studied one of the other materials with low surface activity properties to the same degree of detail. So we are left without the opportunity for comparison.

DISCUSSANT: Compared to quartz, titania's activity is still significantly low. You have about 550 times the number of particles and about a 22-fold difference in the surface area per unit mass of dust compared to quartz. But we are saying that this is a potentially important material because industry is using 800,000 tons of this material a year. Du Pont produces titanias with seven different surface modifications. They sell it in four different kinds of slurries. Titania is probably the most common trace particle in the human lung.

The problem is, as we look through the literature, experimentalists very rarely specify the polymorph phase used. Whether or not those industrial differences will turn out to be biologically important in the future is unknown. They certainly are very important if you are making paint. In the biological community, we are at least concerned to see whether or not they have some relevance to what we are looking at.

DISCUSSANT: One of the important points I got from your paper was the fact that there were differences across the range of TiO_2 species. It is unfortunate that we don't have the biological data to draw the same correlation. If we did, it would be very helpful.

DISCUSSANT: Exactly.

DISCUSSANT: Does the specific surface area have an impact on the biological activity?

DISCUSSANT: The activity depends on the nature of the surface. If you don't have the "right" surface properties, you are not going to get anything.

DISCUSSANT: What is the "right" surface?

DISCUSSANT: Well, that is just something that you will have to determine yourself. There are different industrial processes which produce the same mineral. Anatase was principally produced in the sulfate process, which is by sulfate reduction. It has pretty much been phased out in the United States, because of the difficulties in meeting the EPA's SO_2 emission standards. In the United States we have also been using the chloride reduction process to manufacture titania pigment; this usually produces rutile particles. These particles go through a surface treatment toward the end of the processes, and there is where they acquire different surface characteristics, depending on whether you want to make a latex paint or an oil-base paint, or whether you want to use it in white paper.

This surface modification process is not something about which we know all there is to know. It is an industrial feature that we happened to come across. It fits into what we were looking at, and we approached its measurement in a simple way. People have always criticized the hemolysis model. We did not select it because we thought that it was the greatest thing in the galaxy; we selected it because we thought that it would be the simplest of all models, and that it would be the right place to begin to demonstrate some type of molecular recognition of the different surfaces produced industrially.

We know a lot about the structure. So if we could begin to show that minerals and cells actually recognize one another and that it is a physical functional group on the surface of the mineral that is recognized by functional groups on the surface of the membrane, I would think that a red cell would be a very good model to begin with. Whether that holds true for other situations is something that we don't know.

DISCUSSANT: You show that at least we should not think that every titanium dioxide mineral is the same. About 10 years ago in Finland, they found some kind of fibrosis, unusual in these people. They exposed, I believe, two or three people to anatase, and then they said, "Oh, yes, those people are exposed to anatase." They didn't say anything else except anatase, and then they compared it to rutile in an experiment, which I believe was very poorly performed, and came to the conclusion, "Oh, yes, the anatase is the bad guy and the rutile is the good guy."

DISCUSSANT: In our experiment, at about 130 days both the rutile and the anatase behaved identically. And then, in experiments with macrophages, we didn't find any difference between rutile and anatase. So we concluded, as I see now not properly, that rutile and anatase behave the same way. But obviously rutile and anatase do not behave the same way, according to what you are saying.

DISCUSSANT: Yes, that's right. Again, it depends on their specific surface properties. You need to seek out the right observables for biological activity and not necessarily X-ray crystal structure. There are other surface measurements which were not routinely made in the past that we have begun to look at now.

DISCUSSANT: Are you doing that?

DISCUSSANT: Yes. I think that one of the problems is that a lot of people physically characterized the materials, but they never put them into any biological assay to determine their effects. Therefore, we selected a very simple one, so that at least we would have some assay. Otherwise, you really don't see these subtle differences.

DISCUSSANT: Do you have another comment to offer?

DISCUSSANT: In some injection experiments we used anatase as a negative control, and we did not find a carcinogenic effect.

DISCUSSANT: Can you give us any insight at all, at least in terms of surface activity, as to what might be causing it?

DISCUSSANT: Yes. I think it depends on the rutile that is made in the chloride-reduction processes. This process only came on line in the late '50s and the early '60s. It involves a very sophisticated technology, and the synthetic product is not like the naturally grown rutile particle.

When you grow rutile to a certain size that growth is a continuous process. Therefore, the faces that are exposed are not cleavage faces but faces that this material grows by oxidizing $TiCl_4$ into titanium dioxide. When the temperatures and pressure of this process are controlled to grow the particles, the optimal particle size for paint pigments can be achieved. The rutile particles should be a little bit smaller than the anatase particles because of their ability to reflect light.

I therefore believe that the kinetics that control this growth process produce a very irregular, rough surface. This is the kind of physical characteristic that you would want if you use these particles as pigment for paint. If these particles are put in a flask and swirled around in water, they coat the inside of the flask. They are very "sticky" materials. We believe that this is an indicator of surface "roughness." These rutiles have very multidimensional surfaces. There is something about this topographical structure that cells recognize, and it has a different property as compared to "smooth" surfaces. If you heat these materials, you will notice that some of these properties change. I therefore believe that surface roughness is a feature of the process of trying to develop a good paint pigment.

DISCUSSANT: I think that there are two things that are important: you have to have the right functional group on a mineral surface and you have to have the right topography. The particles that they use at the Intitute of Metals (IOM) happen to be as biologically flat as a piece of paper. They do not have the right surface characteristics. IOM has enhanced some of these characteristics. The aspects that are very well understood are those concerning the process of making a paint pigment. These factors must have some effect on pulmonary clearance, and they will have some effect on which proteins the particles pick up in the lung. They may even interact differently with polyaromatic hydrocarbons, depending on their surface properties.

DISCUSSANT: But you can change those surface properties.

DISCUSSANT: Yes, of course.

DISCUSSANT: We have studied the silica polymorphs, especially quartz. The bottom line is that the quartz activity that we measured in our laboratory, with our crude, simple techniques, ranges over several orders of magnitude. Activities related to the geological origin of the material, cations present on the quartz surface and within its structure, particle size distribution, surface area, and particle number. Superimposed on these effects are the effects of the technique by which the mineral was comminuted and crushed, and whether or not the mineral was hydrated, and whether or it was not heated. In other words, there are intrinsic properties of the mineral and superimposed "laboratory properties" which significantly alter the activity of the mineral.

We wished to bring to this meeting some of our experience and knowledge. That is, a mineral may be characterized by very crude mineralogical techniques, but these may not supply the crucial information that you need: What are the properties that affect biological activity? Have you successfully measured these properties?

DISCUSSANT: I don't want to beat this to death, but one implication that I am seeing is that we are running around looking at all kinds of substitutes for asbestos about which we know absolutely nothing toxicologically.

DISCUSSANT: We have to face up to that problem.

DISCUSSANT: Yes.

DISCUSSANT: But is it possible to understand and elucidate properties which render substitute fibers biologically active?

DISCUSSANT: Yes.

DISCUSSANT: Can we treat asbestos in a way that could change its properties so that it would become less toxic?

DISCUSSANT: That is the idea behind the phosphorylation—modification process.

DISCUSSANT: This would be the way to go, to try to exploit differences in the surface properties and yet maintain a lot of the bulk chemical and physical characteristics that would give you the desired industrial properties.

DISCUSSANT: To my knowledge, as much as we have looked around, still we don't have anything quite as good as asbestos in terms of its industrial properties.

DISCUSSANT: We probably never will.

DISCUSSANT: There is even some hope that, by appropriate treatment, we may create a situation in which we can continue to use asbestos which has retained industrially important properties yet lost its harmful biological potential.

DISCUSSANT: Coming back to our inadequacies on the biological side, we can criticize you because of the simplicity of your biological test system, but we don't have a test system off the shelf that is a great predictor of the long-term carcinogenic potency of a given material. I think that is clear to everybody, but I believe it needs to be emphasized again.

We need to keep looking for appropriate techniques to characterize materials. And we have to be very careful in our toxicological investigations to characterize as rigorously as possible the material in all aspects, including its origin.

DISCUSSANT: When you look at something even as simple as the hemolysis assay, the difference between the quartz particles and the rutile is enormous. That is basically what they found in the inhalation studies.

DISCUSSANT: The difference between silica and titania is not only evident in inhalation experiments. It is generally accepted that silica is a toxic agent for macrophages. When you use titanium dioxide, the macrophages remain very much alive; so even in *in vitro* experiments you can see the difference.

DISCUSSANT: I think that what you are really looking at is the surface. I think that there is a certain percentage of the surface that has silica-like characteristics, and because of the dynamics of the hemolysis system, which is really dependent on surface area, you are able to notice that. This is not the case in a macrophage system. I also think that red cells are probably much more sensitive to lysis by quartz than macrophages are.

DISCUSSANT: How about proposing three or four compounds that are intermediate points between silica and titania that we could use to evaluate the system? You seem to be making a great deal out of these two anchor points, the Du Pont long-term bioassay of titania and numerous assays with silica.

How about proposing three or four points in between these anchor points: materials that have surfaces intermediate between the titania and the silica, that we could evaluate biologically in the laboratory? Can you come up with those?

DISCUSSANT: We can probably start with silica and then find minerals with a derivative structure, which takes you from quartz to feldspars. Feldspars are all tektosilicates, which have the same framework structure as quartz but contain different cations. Therefore the surface charge is altered, and the surface functionalities are likewise altered. The feldspars are good intermediate candidates.

DISCUSSANT: Do you have any information on zinc oxide? Do you know anything about it?

DISCUSSANT: No.

DISCUSSANT: The idea that you necessarily improve your tumor yield with polycylic aromatics by adding a particulate vehicle is not universally confirmed by our own experiments. We observed a far better yield of lung tumors with benzpyrene alone than in combination with a particulate vehicle. Dr. Ferin has obtained the same results.

DISCUSSANT: I think if you were to take a mineral like chrysotile asbestos, and you were to mill chrysotile and alter its surface properties profoundly, you would produce less fibrosis and fewer tumors in animals.

DISCUSSANT: Regarding particle surface: leached chrysotile asbestos—that is, its magnesium is leached—loses its tumorigenic potency. There are chemical means of modifying asbestos, as with phosphorus oxychloride. Phosphorylated chrysotile asbestos—the surface layers, with phosphate groups attached to the magnesium—has an altered biological activity, a reduced tumorigenic potency. So there are ways of modifying the asbestos fiber to alter its biological activity.

DISCUSSANT: The body also alters the surface of the minerals, especially when in residence in the lung.

DISCUSSANT: This is the point. Most of you experimentalists deal with organic compounds which metabolize. It doesn't really matter in what state it exists, because it is ultimately metabolized in the biological host. What is it that a mineral dust does when it is in that biological host? That surface is what the cell perceives, or the membranes perceive. And if you modify the surface of that mineral, it behaves differently in the biological host. It does not metabolize.

DISCUSSANT: A quartz particle is inhaled and is coated with a mucin, and then the classic sequence of events begins: engulfment by macrophages; formation of the lysosome pouch; attack by lysosomal enzymes; stripping of the mucins from the particle surface; the surface of the particle reacts with the membrane of the lysosomal pouch; the pouch is lysed; the lysosomal enzymes are released into the macrophage; the macrophage undergoes autolysis, the particles are released, and then the process repeats itself through an infinite number of cycles, which initiates silicosis.

DISCUSSANT: When you leach magnesium from chrysotile to destroy its tumorigenicity, you also destroy its structural integrity. It breaks down its molecular structure.

DISCUSSANT: Well, there are experiments showing that it loses its ability to damage macrophages and to break red blood cells, while the prime crystal structure is still pretty much intact.

DISCUSSANT: You talk about modifying the structure of fibers. I think what you say is truly important, but it is not completely an invariable matter. I think if you have a fiber, say crocidolite, which has a certain structural size, it is almost impossible to destroy the fiber. You could change its surface chemistry and modify its carcinogenicity, but if you have a highly carcinogenic fiber and don't change the fiber size, you never destroy its carcinogenicity; you might push it up or down a bit.

I am among those people who think that there are two factors: particle size, as long as it is durable in the tissue, *and* surface chemistry.

DISCUSSANT: I will accept that.

DISCUSSANT: We will, yes.

DISCUSSANT: We have also modified fibers along the lines which relate to your studies. We used a peritoneal injection model using Canadian chrysotile, which was recommended by NIOSH. In those assays we did not get any tumors or any significant tumor rates. Activity may be related to some impurities, such as tremolite, or a tendency to split apart *in vivo*.

DISCUSSANT: Yes. Both may be factors imparting activity.

DISCUSSANT: This Canadian chrysotile splits very quickly into fibrils, with the surface of each fibril losing its magnesium. This probably can explain why the Canadian chrysotile was not carcinogenic at all.

DISCUSSANT: We used chrysotile, and Dr. Langer analyzed it: it consisted of very short fibers, but they had a relatively large surface area. We injected 100 mg of these fibers into the peritoneum and observed a tumor rate of about 40%. Another group of animals was injected with the same amount of this chrysotile, together with benzo[a]pyrene, but the tumor incidence was the same. The chrysotile had a very large surface area, and it was possible to adsorb the benzo[a]pyrene. We mixed it in acetone, so there was an enhanced adsorption onto the fiber surface. But there was no enhanced tumor incidence.

DISCUSSANT: What you are saying is quite true, but I think it is very important to consider other factors. Injecting 25 mg of long or short fibers into the peritoneal cavity of rats, we observed a tumor incidence of 95 to 98% with both. The interpretation is that they are equally carcinogenic. However, a dose of 0.25 mg of long fibers produced 60% tumors, but the short fibers produced no tumors. Therefore, you do have to think about the dose. High doses amplify the influence of small concentrations of long fibers.

DISCUSSANT: We found a very small amount of longer fibers in most of the tumors and a very large number of very short fibers, and each had an extremely low effect.

DISCUSSANT: That was exactly our conclusion.

DR. McCLELLAN: Let's move on to the paper by Dr. Chen.

What was the degree of correlation between the high-density lipoprotein (HDL) cholesterol level and the level of apolipoprotein A-1 (Apo A-1) and the lecithin-cholesterol acyltransferase (LCAT) activity? You show that these were 17, 14, and 15%, respectively, reduced in the smokers' serum. Now, has an individual who has a low HDL cholesterol level also a high probability of having low Apo A-1 and LCAT levels?

DISCUSSANT: These three components are components of HDL. Therefore, if HDL cholesterol is reduced, the levels of Apo A-1 and LCAT are also reduced. This result was consistent with the observation that when the same group of people (200 or so) who recently smoked, stopped for about 2 months, their serum HDL cholesterol, Apo A-1 and LCAT enzyme levels returned to normal.

DR. McCLELLAN: Any other comments or questions with regard to Dr. Chen's paper?

DISCUSSANT: Is there any effort on your part to relate the sampling time for the analysis of the lipids to the subject's last meal, or diet, or time of day?

DISCUSSANT: All the subjects participating in the study had to be fasting for 12 hours, so each parameter is a basal value. When a subject only eats dinner and not breakfast, we collect and analyze the subject's blood sample on the morning following the last meal. He therefore is fasting for at least 12 hours to ensure that we are measuring the basal level of serum cholesterol.

DISCUSSANT: These HDL, LDL and LCAT measurements are very tricky to make. How many subjects were involved in this study, and did you make the measurements in your own laboratory?

DISCUSSANT: One hundred forty-three subjects were involved in this study. All measurements were performed in my own laboratory. Because chemical methods cannot always differentiate between cholesterol and cholesterol-like compounds, I used a sensitive and selective method for individually determining cholesterol and triglycerides.

For quantification of Apo A-1 and Apo B, we used the radioimmunoassay, which is also very selective and sensitive. I therefore believe that the reduction in the HDL fraction is quite true, because at least three different components of HDL consistently showed the same result.

DISCUSSANT: Has anybody attempted to quantitate changes in relative risk of heart disease as they relate to changes in the percent of difference in either total serum cholesterol or HDL versus low-density lipoprotein (LDL)? I am just trying to understand what these changes mean biologically.

DISCUSSANT: The HDL cholesterol, the so-called "good" cholesterol, is a protective factor, or a negative risk factor, for heart disease. When the serum HDL cholesterol level is high, the frequency of heart disease is low. In contrast, LDL cholesterol, the so-called "bad" cholesterol, is a positive risk factor for heart disease. When the serum LDL cholesterol level is high, there is a high frequency of heart disease. But the ratio of these two types of serum cholesterols (LDL cholesterol: HDL cholesterol) is considered a better predictor for the risk of coronary heart disease.

DISCUSSANT: Some people in this country have expressed more interest in HDL cholesterol concentrations, but still most people have far more interest in LDL cholesterol, because high concentrations of LDL cholesterol are always associated with a high risk of heart disease. However, low serum cholesterol levels have been associated with cancer. This may suggest a different mechanism in terms of the function of cholesterol. For example, the function of HDL cholesterol may be an important factor here, but many people say that it is an enzyme problem with the blood, maybe the primary factor; at least the available cholesterol may be created with the enzyme.

DISCUSSANT: In breast cancer?

DISCUSSANT: I believe it is, there also.

DISCUSSANT: In a negative association?

DISCUSSANT: —in leukemia. The cellular cholesterol content in leukemia is only 50% that of normal cells. Also, the serum cholesterol content of cancer patients is lower than that of normal subjects.

DISCUSSANT: Do I understand you correctly that you do have studies underway looking at individuals exposed to mineral fibers?

DISCUSSANT: Yes. For studies in humans, it is very hard to determine exposure conditions, particularly dose. Exposure conditions in the animal system are much easier to define, and cholesterol and Apo A-1 in animals are very similar to those in human subjects. So our problem is not in our use of animals instead of humans, the problem is to compare human subjects exposed to asbestos and cigarette smoke with normal nonsmoking subjects because the latter are difficult to find in sufficient numbers for a matched control group.

DISCUSSANT: What was the nature of the asbestos-exposed population from which you are drawing your material?

DISCUSSANT: One very good example: wherever people eat talc-polished rice, for example, the Japanese.

DISCUSSANT: They have stopped doing that now.

DISCUSSANT: There was some question as to whether the talcs were contaminated with tremolite, and there was some issue as to whether the tremolite existed as a common rock-formation material or an asbestiform fiber. I don't think it was ever shown to be tremolite asbestos.

DISCUSSANT: That may be so. Talc is also used as a drying agent and to prevent molds.

DISCUSSANT: But they don't use the rice coating in Japan any more, as I understand it.

DISCUSSANT: In some forms, the talc can combine with asbestiform fiber tremolite, can't it?

DISCUSSANT: I won't refute that.

DR. McCLELLAN: Let's move on, then, to the respiratory tract. The paper by Dr. Pinkerton raised some interesting points. It is now open for discussion.

DISCUSSANT: Did you invent the branch point number?

DISCUSSANT: No, that is a binary classification system that was employed by Dr. Phalen at the University of California in Irvine. It is just a simple system if you have a monopodial branching system for classification. It is a very simple process. By using that type of system, you can put down, in a series of ones or zeroes, the unique branching history of every airway that you follow. Each one will be unique.

DISCUSSANT: Yes, I understood the system. I was very much taken with it because, first of all, it is a real number; that is better than assigning a value. It is a very well-defined, simple method of assigning a value. Secondly, it seemed to be just a straight line related to the number of fibers. So, as a number having a property being assigned according to very well-defined rules, it seems to have some functional relationship to something you wish to measure.

It seems like a very interesting number to use and I am surprised that you are the first one here to use it. It should be explored, because it may have some very important properties to describe the pathway and fate of the asbestos fibers as they penetrate the lung.

DISCUSSANT: I have asked Dr. Churg whether he ever has whole lungs available. He confirmed it and told me that they are pursuing those types of studies. I think that is going to be the most fascinating work, to see whether that type of correlation holds up in the human body, which is a dichotomous branching system. It is not like the rodent's, but we believe that the number of bifurcations along the airways is more important, and that number obviously also reflects generation number.

DR. McCLELLAN: That work originated from a lung-modeling project that was conducted at the Lovelace Inhalation Toxicology Research Institute. Dr. Phalen was one of the key participants. The very early stages of the project were done by Al Holbert. He was a "computernick," very actively involved, and I think the idea and use of that number came from Al. Unfortunately, very early in that study, he died. We lost a valuable colleague. That is just a little bit of the background on the origin of this number.

DISCUSSANT: How did you model the effluent in a monopodial rat lung structure? There appears to be a very interesting correlation between the calculated fiber deposition and the observation.

DISCUSSANT: Fiber deposition was determined using the geometric model of the tracheobronchial tree of Schum and Yeh (*Bull Math Biol 42:* 1-15, 1980). Calculations of fiber deposition for each lung region were based on a knowledge of branch point number and total surface area of each airway path followed in this study.

DISCUSSANT: But how do you cope with the asymmetry and ventilation that you get in a monopodial lung structure?

DISCUSSANT: For the rat, the ventilatory patterns for different regions of the lungs are not known and, to my knowledge, have never been measured. Isolation of specific regions of the lung by microdissection of the airways allowed us to characterize each airway path for length, branch point number, and cumulative branch angle. The assymetry of the monopodial lung was clearly demonstrated in these isolation procedures, but these differences between airway paths provided us with the opportunity to better understand why differences in regional lung fiber deposition and retention may be occurring.

DISCUSSANT: I have two questions. First of all, could you please review the relationship between airway pathlength and gravity, and then for independent flow and deposition?

My second question is: Can we generalize the implications from your study? For instance, in a toxicology study with a crystalline material, can we just open the cranial lobe and see whether there are any lesions there after a year, or do we still need to take brand-new sections throughout the lungs?

DISCUSSANT: Airway branch point number and airway pathlength appear to be the most influential factors which determine the degree of fiber deposition in the lung parenchyma. Parenchymal tissues arising from an airway path of short length will contain greater numbers of fibers than tissues arising from an airway path of longer length. Results of our studies suggest that gravitational effects in the lung of the rat influence the size distribution of fibers deposited. We found in the dorsal lung region of the rat that a large proportion of the fibers were of short length ($< 10\ \mu m$) compared to other regions of the lung. For fibers to reach this region, flow in the airways must go against gravity. The highly complex relationship between airway pathlength and gravity cannot be adequately addressed by the simplicity of this study.

In answer to your second question, I think that the findings of our study may have important implications for the deposition of other crystalline materials in the lungs. The tissue response in a specific lung region is likely to show a high degree of correlation with the amount of material deposited. The objective of our study was to demonstrate that airway characteristics play an important role in the number and size distribution of fibers found in the lung parenchyma, which appear to greatly influence the degree of tissue injury and fibrosis observed.

DISCUSSANT: We are going to present something at the American Thoracic Society, but it is really fairly preliminary. We learned your technique for microdissecting the lung, and exposed animals to carbonyl iron for 1 or 6 hours at 100 mg/m^3, and collected lung tissue samples from the cranial, costolateral, and caudal regions.

Our preliminary findings indicate that there are significantly more carbonyl iron particles deposited in the cranial region compared to the deposition in the caudal region. The costolateral region is sort of intermediate, and it is really hard to differentiate at this point between depositions in the costolateral and the cranial regions. There seem to be differences between the cranial and caudal regions. There are also differences in the macrophage response which relate to the number of particles that are deposited.

DISCUSSANT: I would like to ask a more general question, perhaps for Dr. Ferin, or Dr. Scholander.

I once had a colleague who had learned that the definition of a bronchus, in human terms, is something that has cartilage. You can't call the main bronchi of small animals bronchioles, on the grounds that, except perhaps for the first part, they have no cartilage. The point that I am making is that it is obviously very dangerous to think of the rodent lung as just a very small human lung, because the structure of the airways changes quite remarkably.

Now, the point I really want to make is that during the course of the routine histopathology—except sometimes in mice and less often in rats—you don't see any bronchial mucus glands. There is nothing producing mucus very much beyond the bifurcations here.

And in many animals there are no goblet cells either, so if you are postulating a mucus escalator and all the rest that you were talking about yesterday, from where does the mucus come? The flow by definition must be upward. From where does the mucus come?

The second question is, from where does the mucus come in the model that you have described for us here?

DISCUSSANT: First, it is true that there are no submucosal glands, at least in the rat lung, and that may be true for all rodent lungs. However, there are mucus-producing cells down to the level of some of the larger bronchioles. When you reach the level of the terminal bronchiole, you have the Clara cell, which is the secretory cell, which does produce a surface lining.

Dr. Luchtel has done some extensive studies where he was able to preserve the mucous lining layer through flash-freezing of the lung. Work done at Duke University by Dr. Mercer has also demonstrated that there is a continuous lining layer from the alveolar air spaces, which at that level is a surfactant lining layer extending up to the terminal bronchioles. By the time it reaches the major bronchi of the lobes it is a mucus layer that is up to 1 μm thick. Dr. Luchtel mentioned to me that this is a continuous blanket; it is not disrupted in his observations. So even though there are no submucosal glands, there are cells that populate the airways that will produce the mucus or secretory products that form the surface lining on it.

DISCUSSANT: Well, probably—but certainly if you rely on PAS stains, it is very easy to have a whole series of sections of lung, particularly in hamsters, where you do not see a single globlet cell.

DISCUSSANT: Right. The type of analysis that you need, and that one would like to see done and has been done to a limited extent by Dr. Faulkner, is to characterize the airway cells, the epithelial cells, which populate the airways at different generations. These studies were done at electron microscopic levels of resolution to resolve two types of cells that were present. The PAS stain shows that, as you get further down, most of the cells will be ciliated cells, and you won't have the mucus globlet cells that you see in the trachea.

These inhalation tests have been made with a radioactive substance. I don't know whether it is wrong to assume that, but I believe that it is required to have some kind of a liquid medium. Without the liquid medium you wouldn't be able to transport these particles up.

DISCUSSANT: You indicated that the number of fibers deposited was a function of path length, bifurcation number, and so on. You also gave some characterization of the fiber in that it related the fiber to length. Did you calculate fiber mass?

DISCUSSANT: Yes, we did.

DISCUSSANT: And how did those numbers compare with the deposition characteristics?

DISCUSSANT: This relationship is more fully developed in earlier work that we did in our laboratory (Pinkerton et al., *Lab Invest 55:* 688-695, 1986). It is important to note that fiber mass is determined by the average fiber number, length and diameter. Therefore, these are not independently derived values. Fiber mass demonstrated a high degree of correlation with tissue response, with a correlation coefficient of 0.85 for comparisons of the cranial, costolateral and caudal regions of the rat lung.

DISCUSSANT: Regarding the studies which you did with combined exposure to ozone and asbestos, it was not clear to me whether those animals were returned to an ozone environment after the asbestos exposure.

DISCUSSANT: No. They were maintained in filtered room air. But the exposure to ozone and the exposure to asbestos did not overlap. The animals were exposed to ozone for 6 weeks at EPA, then during the weekend they rested. We then brought them over on Monday and exposed them for 5 hours to asbestos on Tuesday morning. After that, they were maintained in room air.

DISCUSSANT: And when did you observe a threefold greater retention of asbestos fibers in the lungs of the animals?

DISCUSSANT: We looked at the animals immediately after the end of the asbestos exposure to determine the fiber burden and the distribution or deposition pattern for each group of animals, i.e., the air-exposed and the ozone-exposed animals.

There was no difference; there were identical fiber burdens and deposition patterns. We looked at the deposition sites, at first alveolar duct bifurcations, and counted fibers per bifurcation and found no difference at all.

However, after 30 days, we found enhanced retention. When we first did the study, we thought that the enhanced retention in the ozone-exposed animals might have been due to the presence of short fibers, but as we conducted more extensive studies, we found that the size distribution of those fibers that were retained in the lungs after 1 month was the same in the air-exposed and the ozone-exposed groups.

This was interesting, because we originally thought that maybe it was just that the macrophages were not picking up the short fibers and clearing them, but that is not the case.

DISCUSSANT: What did you see light-microscopically after 6 weeks of ozone exposure?

DISCUSSANT: Although I tend to think that I can identify lots of things, I can't tell the difference between an air- and an ozone-exposed animal after 6 weeks of exposure to the ozone.

DISCUSSANT: So the only differences were those in the morphometric measurements? You suggested that there was a modest increase in the relative volume of the alveolar Type I lung cells.

DISCUSSANT: Yes. Those studies were conducted by Dr. Crapo et al., and are part of a study to look at the effects of ozone, using a pattern to mimic the Los Angeles environment. They examined the animals after 1 week, after 3 weeks, and after 3 months of exposure. The slope of the curve that is drawn on that graph is based on multiple time points. The ozone is expressed in parts per million hours of ozone, so it is a cumulative dose, and the results of our study fit on that line. We did not morphometrically measure whether our Type I epithelium had increased by about 20%, but we assumed that it was one of those variables.

DISCUSSANT: In your ozone study did you find similar retention in all areas? Was there the same retention in the cranial region? Did you look at each of the regions in the ozone study?

DISCUSSANT: No. We attempted to do that and found that it was very difficult. We had to take a larger sample size, so what we elected to do was to take a sagittal slice of the lung that was located between the first and the second ventral branch of the left lobe. Then we took the tissue that was peripheral to that. That tissue was located between the cranial and costolateral region.

DR. McCLELLAN: Is that the same region on which Dr. Crapo did his morphometric study, or was it a different region?

DISCUSSANT: If he is following the same procedures as in the past, he takes one slice above the hilus and one slice below the hilus, so he has a combination of the two.

DR. McCLELLAN: I don't recall seeing the data presented. Later, you can comment on your findings and how they fit in with the data that Dr. Ferin presented for Dr. Oberdörster. I think there are some interesting correlations there.

DISCUSSANT: I want to ask you about one of your photomicrographs. You showed a scanning electron micrograph of Mount St. Helens ash deposited in an animal lung. The particles were grouped; they were clumped. Were these particles inside a macrophage?

DISCUSSANT: No, they were impacted on Type I cells.

DISCUSSANT: How do you keep your materials from agglomerating in your aerosol? How do you keep these materials dispersed? It seems to me that what we saw in your SEM was an artifact in your aerosol.

DISCUSSANT: I have not really thought about that. This is the first time that I have ever seen particles in that deposition pattern. I showed you the carbonyl iron. Fiber glass has been widely distributed on the bifurcation; while it is a focal deposition, that is, restricted to the bifurcation, it is nevertheless widely distributed on the bifurcation. I usually do not see clumps.

DISCUSSANT: Is clumping a generic problem? Has anyone else had problems with clumping of particles?

DISCUSSANT: The particles would not have penetrated that far if they were agglomerated in the air because the size of agglomerated particles would have precluded their deposition in the alveolar regions of the lung. Furthermore, particle size analysis, using a cascade impactor, clearly indicated that the Mount St. Helens ash particles were of a respirable size. The agglomerate would have been too big for alveolar deposition.

DISCUSSANT: When I see a very large area like that, and I see 100 particles in one specific area, it seems to me that there is some other force operative besides the normal impaction.

DISCUSSANT: Frankly, the purpose of that micrograph was to demonstrate, basically for myself, that inhaled Mount St. Helens particles deposited on bifurcations. I don't even know what the rest of that particular bifurcation looked like.

DISCUSSANT: What time frame does the micrograph depict?

DISCUSSANT: The time period was immediately after exposure.

DISCUSSANT: How long was the exposure?

DISCUSSANT: A 3-hour exposure, plus maybe 10 to 15 minutes after exposure until the lumps were perfused.

DISCUSSANT: Are you talking about agglomeration or aggregation?

DISCUSSANT: Well, it is my recollection that we had the electron micrograph and we saw a whole pot full of particles in one area.

DISCUSSANT: It was a very high-magnification shot.

DISCUSSANT: Were these lungs fixed through the airways?

DISCUSSANT: No, all of the lungs studied for deposition are fixed through the vasculature.

DISCUSSANT: I don't know what aerosol generation system was used here, but it certainly had a fair amount of electrical charge generated, and therefore probably had a charge neutralizer, did it not?

DISCUSSANT: Well, that particular Mount St. Helens study was done at NIEHS (with a Timbrell generator), but frankly, I have not seen any change in the deposition patterns or the distribution of particles on bifurcations. Using, for example, a K-Tron bin feeder results pretty much in the same distribution.

DISCUSSANT: If, in fact, 100 particles were all agglomerated together, the aerodynamic size would be tremendous. Such a cluster would undoubtedly never make it past the rat's nose. In a 3-hour period an awful lot can happen within the lung in terms of movements of material and so on.

DISCUSSANT: I didn't mention it, because it is very preliminary, but we have now tried to look at the fluid flux of particles in the alveolar regions after a 6-hour exposure versus a 1-hour exposure. As I indicated, after a 1-hour exposure, about 80% of the particles are on the bifurcation or the immediately adjacent alveolar duct. After 6 hours, only about 56% of the particles are there. Many of the particles are on the terminal bronchioles, and they are actually getting swept up. We probably could examine at 15 minutes after exposure; that would probably be better, but I don't think there is much movement of particles within 1 hour. There are no indications.

DISCUSSANT: Are you suggesting that the particles at the interface of the terminal bronchiole level might be interesting because that is an area that is particularly at risk?

DISCUSSANT: Yes. There are no appreciable numbers of recruited macrophages—at least with exposure to carbonyl iron—until 8 to 10 hours after exposure, so even at 6 hours after exposure, we see very few macrophages.

DISCUSSANT: May I display my ignorance? Why a study with Mount St. Helens ash? Is this because it happened to land on your laboratory and you didn't have to pay shipping costs?

DISCUSSANT: Well, it was just a matter of choosing interesting particles.

DISCUSSANT: Of what does Mount St. Helens ash consist?

DISCUSSANT: The crystalline components consisted of plagioclase feldspar and orthopyroxene and feldspar, with smaller amounts of titanomagnetite and hornblende, and 2 or 3% free crystalline silica (quartz, trydimite, or cristobalite).

DISCUSSANT: I think people studied Mount St. Helens volcanic ash because large parts of several Northwestern states were covered with it, and there was a great concern about its respirability and ultimate biological effects.

DISCUSSANT: This material was basically a volcanic glass with crystalline components, including free crystalline silica in the form of quartz, and no one seemed to be terribly concerned about its effects when inhaled.

DISCUSSANT: We did a study on it. Parenthetically, I was scheduled to give a week-long course on inhalation toxicology at Washington State University in Pullman, in the eastern part of the state that year, and it turned out to be about 5 weeks after the volcanic eruption. When the eruption occurred, my mother, who lived in the eastern part of the state, called up to tell us about how dark it got that day because of the ash cloud that had passed over. She then asked whether I was still going to come up in about 5 weeks, and I said, "Well, I assume so."

The next day I got a call from the school and they said they were debating whether to close the school or not. In fact, they finally allowed students the option that if the students felt that they had a medical indication for leaving school—this was just before the final examinations—they could. It was amazing to see how many students felt they had to leave Pullman for medical reasons.

Because I was going to visit there, we were very interested in the volcanic ash, and we did a lot of work in our laboratory. I was able to illustrate every lecture in my inhalation toxicology course with Mount St. Helens ash, whether you wanted to talk about generating aerosols, characterizing areosols, or whatever. But when it came to biological activity, I have to say that the material was way down on the list. In the test tube, in macrophage cytotoxicity studies, you'd have to put in enough to bury them under the stuff to see something. For a while I had five very large trash cans of volcanic ash set aside that my brother collected on a tennis court in Lind, Washington, where it was deposited several inches deep. Much to my dismay, though, I really don't think that it has any further value. I therefore conned somebody else into accepting it as a gift.

DISCUSSANT: Given that it does not appear to activate complement, one might hypothesize, based on the data that we discussed earlier, that it would be cleared more slowly from the lung than innocuous or inactive particles that activate complement. I think your group did some work on that and showed that it was cleared fairly slowly, is that not the case?

DISCUSSANT: I am trying to think, it was several years ago. I will have to look it up.

DISCUSSANT: As to biological effects, we had two exposure concentrations, 1 mg/m^3 and 10 mg/m^3, if I remember correctly. We saw some pretty striking changes at 1 mg/m^3, a lymphoreticular proliferation, which was more than I expected to see. We did not have anything to which to compare it, but I thought there was more of a lymphoreticular proliferation in the subpleural areas and peribronchiolar areas than I anticipated seeing.

DISCUSSANT: Dr. Thomas Martin, here at the medical school in Seattle, did studies with macrophages and the ash, with quartz as a positive control. I do have that paper in my files, and I will be happy to send you a copy.

DISCUSSANT: Going back to your paper, am I recalling that you indicated that you had an inflammatory response in the mice?

DISCUSSANT: Right.

DISCUSSANT: That was greater than that observed in the other three species?

DISCUSSANT: I did not see anything in any of the other species, and that was what was so surprising. We saw an inflammatory response at 24 to 48 hours. Our tissue and lavage samples were collected at various time points, including immediately after exposure, at 6 hours, 24 hours, 48 hours, 8 days, 1 month and sometimes 3 months after exposure. So we generally look at five or six different time points after exposure.

DR. McCLELLAN: And the exposure was at what level again?

DISCUSSANT: 100 mg/m^3.

DR. McCLELLAN: I was struck by that in view of our studies with diesel exhaust as the particulate material. We exposed at 7 mg/m^3, 5 days a week, 7 hours a day. One of the striking things was, as I recall, the lesser inflammatory response of the mouse lungs compared to those of the rat.

DISCUSSANT: Well, when you look at the proteins, cytoplasmic enzymes, and cell counts, there was substantial inflammation in the mice, but it was not greater than in rats. The main difference we saw was following chronic exposure; we did not see in the mice this macrophage aggregation and formation of lesions, focal regions, that we see in rats and other species. The mice had the same amount of material per gram of lung and the material was accumulated in macrophages. The macrophages were fat and full and black, but they were pretty much dispersed. There was less fibrotic response, but there was an inflammatory response in those species, but that in the mouse was not greater than that in the rats.

DISCUSSANT: Frankly, I still almost do not believe the results that I obtained lavaging the mice and seeing such a low percentage of macrophages containing carbonyl iron. I just have no explanation for it. Certainly *in vitro* there is lower phagocytic capacity, but not that much lower. I just have no idea why that is the case. We have repeated this experiment four times.

DISCUSSANT: Which mouse strain did you use?

DISCUSSANT: The first one was CD-1, but I have also looked at the B10.D2/NSNJ, for different reasons, and also included those in there. We found inflammation in the B210NSN, which is the normal mouse, and did not find nearly the number of PMN in the complement-C5-deficient mouse, which suggests to me that complement may have some involvement.

DISCUSSANT: I would like to ask you about the complement activation in the serum in the Mount St. Helens ash study. What kind of aerosol concentration did you use? Did you overdose each of these substances, or how did you do that?

DISCUSSANT: Initially we used several concentrations. We used 5, 10, 15 and 25 mg of particles/ml. What we found was interesting. Zymosan is considered one of the quintessential activators in complement. Normally we get a dose response, but zymosan is so potent that a maximal response was reached at 5% (v/v). What is happening is saturation of the C5 receptors. So for those studies we used 10 mg/ml zymosan, but 25 mg/ml for the other dusts. And for Mount St. Helens ash, our dilutions ranged from 5 to 50 mg/ml.

We tried a greater range of concentrations just to make sure that this was not the reason that it was not activating complement.

DISCUSSANT: This is interesting—that you came to the conclusion to use basically the same concentration, 25 mg, except zymosan and Mount St. Helens ash.

DISCUSSANT: No, we used that for Mount St. Helens ash in these studies, but initially, for pilot studies, we used a greater range to see whether there was a dose that would activate complement.

DISCUSSANT: When you used the wide range, did you get a dose-response type of curve?

DISCUSSANT: At 25 mg/ml we get our maximal dose-response range; that is, if you use 1, 5 and 10% serum, you will get a dose response. With zymosan you have to go to lower concentrations, because you have too much C5A.

DISCUSSANT: So you ended up, with all the others, zymosan and Mount St. Helens, with 25 mg/ml?

DISCUSSANT: Including Mount St. Helens. And Mount St. Helens mimicked the same response as with normal heated serum, because serum spontaneously activates to a lesser degree, just by heating. And just by incubating it as a control with all the other dusts, you actually increased the level of C5A in there.

DISCUSSANT: We recently used a similar dose, and we tested those various particles and came up with various responses. We therefore decided not to go that route, to take 1 and 25 mg, but to compare it to a certain activation of zymosan.

DISCUSSANT: In my experiment, I could not do that. If you use zymosan-activated serum at 10 mg/ml, and 0.5, 1, 5, and 10%, you get, in our system, about 750 cells per migrating high-power field at 1 and 0.5%.

With chrysotile asbestos, which is the next best thing, the most that we ever get, at the high point, is 200 to 300 cells. So we could never equilibrate the other dust particle responses to zymosan. That is why zymosan is always sitting by itself in all of our figures, because it is so much higher than anything else, no matter what concentration of particles in serum it is.

DISCUSSANT: First of all, I believe that the activation has something to do with the surface.

DISCUSSANT: Absolutely.

DISCUSSANT: So the dose does not necessarily correspond to the surface of these various particles that you are using. Therefore, some particles may be much more activating than others if you use dose expressed in milligrams, or mass.

DISCUSSANT: Right.

DISCUSSANT: And if you do not take this into account in your comparisons, then you are really not comparing appropriately.

DISCUSSANT: That is why initially you use three or four different concentrations and hope that one or more of them will fall into the ballpark.

DISCUSSANT: The last question: How high did you go with Mount St. Helens particles?

DISCUSSANT: Well, probably about 40 mg/ml, because, don't forget, you cannot stuff that much material in there; it adsorbs most of the fluid and serum. That certainly is a problem with asbestos. There are so many particles, particularly for silica, at 25 mg/ml, they almost soak up all the serum. Then you really have to spin it down hard just to get half the serum back.

DISCUSSANT: We thought that the enzymes were activating. The one that you are using is not activating. At higher concentrations we obtained a level activational curve. Of course, it was still lower than many of these others.

DISCUSSANT: That is interesting, because my preliminary findings are that titanium dioxide is negative as well.

DISCUSSANT: I find these studies very interesting. I thought one of the objectives of this meeting is the synergism between cigarette-smoking and asbestos fibers. And then during the first day it was mentioned that there is not a good animal model for carcinogenicity. But based on these four species that you have looked at and the types of deposition patterns and the responses you see in macrophages, what would you say is the best species with which to do a carcinogenicity study?

DISCUSSANT: I know they oftentimes use the mouse because of the inflammation problems.

DISCUSSANT: Well, my understanding is that cancer is pretty resistant to this problem. Most of my experiments have focused on fibrogenicity, and I really see carcinogenicity as another ball game.

I would still go with the rat because we are planning on doing *in vitro* human macrophage studies to see whether they respond to the same chemotactic factors. When we described the asbestos work, there was a great similarity between the development of asbestosis in humans and what we found in rats. The lesion in rats was initiated in the same location as in humans, namely in the respiratory bronchiole, the so-called bronchioalveolar junction, the very same region as in the rat, except that humans have three generations of respiratory bronchioles.

One of the advantages of doing acute studies as opposed to chronic studies is that you can monitor early developmental stages of the disease. If you do a chronic study, you take random sections through the lung after a year or two of exposure and find out that the animal has diffuse and progressive pulmonary fibrosis.

However, we believe that asbestosis is initially a focal disease, that it starts at these bronchioalveolar junctions, or alveolar duct bifurcations, and then follows a circumferential pattern. So when you look a year or two later, you just see this diffuse fibrosis. But if you look earlier, you might see these circumferential patterns of fibrosis, which ultimately coalesce as the disease progresses.

In terms of asbestosis, I think that the rat is a good model. In terms of cancer, I just do not know what the advantage of the rat would be over the mouse.

DISCUSSANT: In inhalation studies with cigarette smoke, the problem with all models is that exposures are limited by carbon monoxide concentrations. This makes it impossible to mimic in a laboratory rodent the exposure of a human who smokes, say, 40 cigarettes per 16-hour day.

DISCUSSANT: You are quite correct. You cannot get into the animal model the high doses to which humans expose themselves. With asbestos, we are used to producing tumors in the animals by using 100 times the dose to which humans are exposed. If we only use 10 times that dose we might get a few tumors. I think we would, but we would not have the numbers to produce meaningful statistics. So there is a very big gulf, and I think that this is perhaps one of the most important aspects of the discussion. We do not have a good animal model for cigarette smoke for the reasons you just heard. I would like to ask, are there any possibilities of developing a good animal model for that purpose? If we could talk about that, that would be one of the most important things that would come out of this meeting.

DISCUSSANT: Yes, there is one nice model. You mix cigarette-smoke condensate with beeswax and implant it in the lungs of rats. If you do get the tobacco condensate into the lung, you do get lung tumors, metastasizing epidermoid carcinomas, at relatively low doses: 67 mg condensate produced a tumor incidence of 42%, and 1 mg condensate produced one tumor. I have no idea why we do not get a significant incidence of lung tumors in inhalation studies. It is a big disappointment, but tobacco itself does produce epidermoid carcinomas in the lung, as we have demonstrated in our beeswax implantation study. We are also very successful at producing lung tumors with radon daughters.

DISCUSSANT: One could and should try 16-hours/day, 7-days/week lifespan inhalation exposures. However, normally nobody can or will pay for such a study. With this exposure regimen, you could get quite a dose into the lungs of laboratory rodents. I do not know whether it would be the equivalent of heavy human smoking, but you certainly would deposit significantly more material in the lungs than by exposing just 6 hours a day, 5 days a week.

DISCUSSANT: I think that for such frequent and long exposure, you would have to put the whole animal in the chamber and leave it alone. You probably could do that, but there have always been objections to whole-body exposures because smoke is deposited on the pelt and a lot of material is licked off, and so the dosimetry becomes a bit of a nightmare.

But I daresay you are right, you could construct a system for putting the whole animal in a smoke atmosphere, and this could be done without excessive cost.

DISCUSSANT: You still have to control the carbon monoxide level, keep that down and the cigarette smoke concentration up.

DR. McCLELLAN: Dr. Cross, do you want to comment on radon and cigarette smoke and the extent to which one sees an enhancement of effects of cigarette exposures by radon in the rat?

DISCUSSANT: Actually, I was going to comment under Dr. Oberdörster's paper, concerning this. But I'll pick it up now because there was a flagged item on one of your slides that you showed. It was a question that said radon on smoke particles, question mark. His thesis was that no synergism occurs, and it is only the dose that determines the effects of asbestos and cigarette smoke. Presumably, he assumes that anything that slows clearance increases dose and therefore enhances the risk. Regarding radon and radon daughters, this is not true, because even if you have complete stasis in the lungs, the dose does not increase because of the short half-life. Therefore, Dr. Oberdörster's assumption probably is not applicable to radon and radon daughters.

Cigarette-smoke mixtures with radon daughters present a very complex and confusing situation at the moment. In some earlier studies with smoking dogs, to which Dr. Sterling referred, we alternated cigarette-smoke and radon exposure. In other words, the exposures were given the same day. In the smoking group of dogs we found fewer lung cancers. We looked very carefully afterward as to what the explanation might be. I mean, many years later. We thought that there might be increased numbers of mucus glands, or mucus-producing cells, or increased thickness of the epithelium, but we saw no difference between the two groups, the one exposed to cigarette smoke and the one without smoke exposure. The final conclusion was that it must have been that the group of cigarette-smoking dogs produced more mucus, but we had no specific data related to that.

In follow-up experiments at the COGEMA laboratories in southern France, where rats were exposed to radon first, and then to cigarette smoke, there was a synergistic increase in the number of lung cancers. Now, the synergism observed there did not occur following simultaneous exposure because radon was given first and then cigarette smoke. Thus, the promotional effect of cigarette smoke seems to be evident in some experiments, namely in experiments in which cigarette smoke can promote effects that radiation has initiated.

Now, when that sequence was reversed and cigarette smoke was given first, and then the radon, there was no change compared to effects induced by radon alone. So that again points to a promotional effect of cigarette smoke. At present, we have an initiation/promotion/initiation protocol in our laboratory, where we are trying to determine, hopefully once and for all, what is initiating and what is promoting in these mixtures. We want to test the two-stage model of carcinogenesis with these data. But at the moment we cannot shed any more light on the human smoking question or to what is going on in the animal studies, because we have such a mixture of results. Results appear to depend, to a large extent, I think, on the time sequence of the exposures to radiation and cigarette smoke.

DISCUSSANT: Which agents are being used in your current studies with the two-stage model?

DISCUSSANT: Radon daughters and cigarette smoke.

DISCUSSANT: I would like to comment on the points that have been raised about the inhalation exposures to cigarette smoke. Of course, everyone is quite right. If you go through even crude calculations about the amount of material, particulate material, a moderate to heavy human smoker deposits per gram of lung or per volume of lung over a day's time or a week's time, and compare that with the amounts that were likely to have been deposited in any of the animal studies, you find quite a discrepancy. This is probably one of the few places in the field of toxicology where we underdose the subject.

We are planning a series of studies in which the question of cigarette-smoke interactions with the effects of other materials is a critical part of the program. If one adheres to conventional wisdom, one is puffing cigarettes with a 35-ml puff of 2-second duration once per minute, and you do it in a certain conventional way.

None of those systems, except perhaps with the cigarette in a tracheostomy of a dog, or in a mask, probably comes close to simulating the relationship of the cigarette to the human airway. But in all the other studies, you are no longer dealing with a mass concentration that results in substantial biological effects, which, as we have heard, is probably important. I would certainly agree that this would be important in terms of airway deposition. But now you are dealing with a concentration of particulate material in the air, milligrams per cubic meter, and you are in the realm of the peculiar physicochemical properties of the smoke cloud. Clearly, you changed the chemistry, the temperature, and a lot of other parameters in the smoke.

So, if one is willing to step further out toward less conventional or typical ways of exposing animals to cigarette smoke, yes, you can do whole-body exposures. But if you go through those calculations, it is not unreasonable at all to do whole-body exposures in rodents in very conventional patterns, 6 hours a day, 5 days a week, or 7, something like that.

I think you can strike a balance between mass concentration of cigarette smoke and staying below the toxic levels of CO and nicotine. We have done some preliminary studies and are still in the process of doing that, playing around with these ideas, generating the smoke in different ways, and exposing rodents in different modes.

It has been pointed out by other people that there are ways of characterizing smoke that might be important that we have not used yet. Essentially, we do not really know what is important in that smoke for carcinogenicity although we have some ideas. We do what we can to characterize the material, and we have done some short-term studies to try to characterize the biological response to that material. We found that we can deviate quite a bit from this standardized puffing and exposure profile and not see any significant differences in composition or in biological response in parameters like DNA adducts, lung inflammation, deposition, clearance of other particles, etc.

We are at the point now where we are considering whether or not this unconventional way is the way to go. The sense that I get from the participants here, and certainly my own personal bias, is that it ought to be tried.

DR. McCLELLAN: I was struck by the material presented at the recent Society of Toxicology meeting that came from Battelle-Northwest, and from the R. J. Reynolds laboratory, in terms of cigarette smoke, both conventional cigarettes as well as Reynolds' new "smokeless" cigarettes. I do not recall the dosing regimen there, but certainly those were relatively short-term studies, as I recall, 12 weeks' duration, and they did show substantial lesions in animals exposed to conventional cigarette smoke as compared to the animals exposed to the new smokeless cigarette.

I would be very interested in seeing what the lesions would look like in those animals if those exposures had been continued for 24 to 30 months, similar to what we have recently done in our laboratory and in the other laboratories around the world with these capabilities.

What comes home to me is that cigarette smoke is a relatively low-potency carcinogen, it is just the fact that people take in tremendous quantities of it. In most of our animal systems we have tended to underdose animals and thus, I think, the results are partly related to that.

In those Battelle-Northwest studies with the smokeless cigarettes, what was the smoking regimen, the number of cigarettes, time period per day, and so on?

DR. WEHNER: They were typical subchronic studies, and I would like to point out here that the objective of those studies was limited. They were, of course, not intended to be carcinogenicity studies, but rather a comparison of the relative toxicity of the new "smokeless" cigarette with that of a standard reference cigarette. The dose criterion was total particulate mass (TPM) at concentrations of 0.12, 0.35, and 0.64 mg TPM/L of air. The animals were exposed in modified Battelle-Geneva smoking machines for 1 hour/ day, 5 days/week, for 13 weeks. We conducted two identical studies: first, one with rats and then one with hamsters.

The results in those two species were very similar, with one notable exception: in the rats exposed to the highest concentration (0.64 mg/L) of, as you called it, the smokeless cigarette, the only lesion that we observed was a minimal degree of metaplasia at the base of the larynx. This lesion was not readily apparent, you really had to look hard to find it, and this lesion was not observed in the hamsters.

The rat thus appears to be a more sensitive model in terms of histopathologic changes. Because the histopathologic changes are the most important criteria for this type of test, the rat in this case appears to be preferable to the hamster. The hamster, in turn, appears to be somewhat more sensitive with regard to body-weight changes.

This emphasizes one of the points that I could not make in my verbal presentation due to time limitations, but that I discussed in my paper: when you are looking for an animal model, you have to have clearly in mind the parameters and end points that you want to use and measure as your experimental criteria, and then decide on the most appropriate animal model.

To summarize my answer to your question, we did subchronic studies in both the hamster and in the rat. We observed the lesions that you would commonly expect in cigarette-smoke-exposed animals in the rats and hamsters that were exposed to smoke from a conventional reference cigarette. But with the exception of minimal squamous metaplasia of the larynx in the rat, we did not see any lesions in the animals that were exposed to the new cigarette.

DR. McCLELLAN: I was most interested in the presentation, in the results with the conventional cigarette, because what is of the greatest interest here are the interactions between the materials. That is really the theme of what one is trying to get at. Is there a role for animal studies, or for what I call subanimal models, in trying to help us understand the interactions between exposure to cigarette smoke and other agents.

DISCUSSANT: I do have quite a lot of unpublished experiments in this area, when attempts were made to develop tobacco substitutes. Tobacco in the standard cigarette was used as a positive control.

Different groups of people were using a regimen whereby animals were exposed, I believe for 10 minutes, to smoke, with probably an hour between exposures, once in the morning and again in the afternoon. So the animals were exposed twice for 10 minutes in the morning and twice for 10 minutes in the afternoon, and there were all sorts of presentations as to what the concentrations were. The fact is that there was very little pathology in the lungs of those animals after a reasonable length of time.

Now, other groups were using a different regimen, namely a 30-minute exposure, with 10 minutes in between, and then another 30-minute exposure, a much more intensive exposure. Those animals developed a quite marked and extensive squamous metaplasia throughout the trachea and down into the main bronchi.

So, while exposures were still only for 1 hour a day, some lesions developed which could serve as an end point. I have little doubt that by playing around with this and having enough money to do so, one could get closer to end points associated with the challenge by cigarette smoke in humans. I have no doubt that we would then find out that the rat is the best model, certainly better than the hamster or any other laboratory rodent for this type of lung changes.

DR. WEHNER: I particularly worry about the interruptions of exposure during the week-end, because this provides the opportunity for cell repair. We thus have an entirely different ball game compared to a continuous insult.

DISCUSSANT: Yes, I agree with you. It is always noticeable in these studies that most of the deaths occur on Mondays, after the animals had an exposure-free weekend. When they come back into the chamber on Monday, that's when they die. So it appears that after they had become acclimatized, they rapidly got "unacclimatized" during the weekend. This is the criticism I have for these experiments that have exposures interrupted over the weekend. I think that is far too long a period of exposure-free time, and I think you have wasted your acclimatization efforts that you made before the start of the exposures.

DISCUSSANT: I would like to make a point, just in case there is anyone here who does not know the literature on smoke studies in animals. We are talking here as if long-term smoke inhalation studies producing relevant lesions have not been done, or they have been done and did not pass muster. This is not true.

Dr. Wehner et al. published a very nice paper on a study done at Battelle, Pacific Northwest Laboratories. It is a very nice study—intensive, nose-only exposures, in which smoke-induced lesions were produced (*Toxicol Appl Pharmacol 62:* 1-17, 1981).

And Dr. Kendrick et al. at Oak Ridge published a paper, a number of years ago (*Toxicol Appl Pharmacol 37:* 557-569, 1976). Again, the animals received intensive exposures over their life span, a very nice, competent study. And both of them produced relevant lesions.

What we are talking about is not that there have not been lesions and progressive lesions, but that the end point, in the form of a significantly increased incidence in lung tumors, has not been reached. But there have been some very nice long-term studies done that have produced progressive lesions.

DISCUSSANT: Yes, but the problem with all of these studies is that the focus has been on bronchiolar and alveolar lesions. And there is a dispute as to whether these were really tumors or not. The studies that I referred to earlier were getting end points which are totally different from those. These were getting end points of squamous metaplasia or dysplasia within the trachea, and that is the difference.

DISCUSSANT: The sponsor specified the type of smoking machine to be used in that study. We could not use the machine that we would have preferred to use. It was not fresh cigarette smoke to which the animals were exposed. I consider that a flaw in the experimental approach over which we had no control.

DISCUSSANT: You expressed your concern about week-ends without smoke exposures in animal studies. It is not the number of cigarettes you smoke but the duration. If you have many, many weeks of smoking with 2 days per week off, I doubt that the 2 days off are going to affect matters very much.

DR. WEHNER: But we do not *know* that. And because we do not know for sure, and because human smokers are exposed 7 days a week, we should try to simulate human exposure conditions as closely as possible if we want to investigate their biological effects in an animal model. This postulate appears even more justified in view of the problems we have with the animal models in inducing convincing lesions by cigarette-smoke inhalation. I consider it entirely possible, if not probable, that 2 days of rest after every 5 days of exposure allow for sufficient cellular lesion repair to thwart tumor development, given the fact that we are not dealing with a potent carcinogen. If you want to roll a boulder up a hill but rest and let go of it before you reach the top, it will roll back down, and you will never get it over the crest no matter how long you keep trying.

DISCUSSANT: I have a question on fibers. Have you ever looked in your rats as to whether there are concentrations of asbestos fibers in upper and more proximal airway bifurcations?

DISCUSSANT: I have looked briefly. In one or two generations and the bifurcations below the terminal bronchiole I found enhanced deposition as well. But I would expect that there would be more fiber movement. It is not quite as focal as I see it in the alveolar region, but I certainly did see a number of fibers impacted on bifurcations of small airways.

DISCUSSANT: I would like to correlate your results with a paper that was published by a Japanese scientist, Toshihiko Myojo, in the *Journal of Aerosol Science* (*18*:337-347, 1987). He made a Weibel bifurcation model in an engineering system surrogate to simulate, for instance, Weibel generations three, four, five. He introduced glass fibers into this model and found markedly enhanced deposition occurring right at the carinal ridge. This deposition decreased very sharply immediately downstream, within 2 mm of the carinal ridge. There was a strong peak enhancement in the Weibel generation. With one of my coauthors in the paper presented yesterday, a Hungarian postdoctoral student, I have started developing a model of that. It takes into consideration impaction and sedimentation simultaneously in the equation, and lo and behold, the theory points out that there will be a peak, definitely, at those locations.

DISCUSSANT: We never investigated that high up because that has not been my primary objective. We take some lung tissue and dissect down to the bifurcation, and whatever large airways happen to be there at the time, I will take a casual glance at them, but I really have not carefully looked at them.

I have looked one or two generations proximal to the terminal bronchiole, and I have noticed what appear to be preferential-type depositions. Certainly there are a lot of fibers hanging around, because those are big bifurcations, but I have not really looked proximal to that region.

DISCUSSANT: I wanted to emphasize what has been said about the end point you want. When you look at humans, those with obstructive lung disease have a much higher incidence of lung cancer. But the animals clearly are different. Our model, by rodent standards, does not produce a very high carboxyhemoglobin concentration, but the smoke-exposed animals develop distinct emphysema in 6 months, and that is on 5-days-a-week exposures, with the weekends off. They do not get any identifiable lesion whatsoever in the airways, so you can produce one lesion and completely miss another lesion.

DISCUSSANT: As to Dr. Warheit's paper, volcanic ash perhaps was not as innocuous as it might appear. Dr. Wehner et al. did some inhalation studies on it in rats and observed pulmonary alveolar proteinosis, a disease in which I have been interested for a number of years (*Environ Res 40*:499-517, 1986). So volcanic ash does stimulate something related to the alveolar surface, but apparently it does not stimulate an inflammatory process.

DISCUSSANT: This is only partially correct. In addition to alveolar proteinosis we did, indeed, see an inflammatory response in the form of interstitial and lymphoreticular reactions.

DISCUSSANT: Well, actually what I am talking about is not an inflammatory process. We do not see an increased number of macrophages in the lung; it is simply a redistribution of the population of macrophages from the adjacent areas. That is, the macrophages are sitting in adjacent alveolar spaces or ducts, and they come to those locations. You do not see any influx from the vasculature or the interstitium. And when I said that the Mount St. Helens volcanic ash was not biologically active, actually that is a different issue from toxicity.

I think that it has been demonstrated that with 50 mg/m^3 for a year or two you do get tumors, maybe, but certainly fibrosis. So certainly it is not totally innocuous.

DR. McCLELLAN: Has there been more pulmonary alveolar proteinosis in people in the Northwest since this incident? Is there any information on that? Because you had a very dispersed cloud, for a while, that people must have been breathing. So there was a very fine dust, which could conceivably deposit in the alveoli.

DR. WEHNER: I do not know, but I can speculate. I don't believe that there was an increase in alveolar proteinosis in the population that had been exposed to volcanic ash because people generally were not exposed long enough to sufficiently high concentrations for this to happen. We exposed our animals to very high concentrations for a very long period of time. I personally happen to have been caught in the center of the volcanic ash cloud during the eruption of Mount St. Helens in our cabin in the Cascade Mountains, and common sense told me to stay indoors.

However, the loggers had to go into this area, where for months and actually for years, each time they cut down a tree or drove through this area, there was a tremendous plume of dust. These loggers did not wear any protection, so they were inhaling this resuspended airborne ash at relatively high concentrations for relatively long periods of time. That is why we wanted to investigate in an animal model what might happen under extreme conditions. But I don't think the general population received the type of exposure that would result in proteinosis. We exposed the animals to 5 and 50 mg/m^3—and, as I recall, we didn't see alveolar proteinosis at 5 mg/m^3. We attributed the pulmonary lesions mainly to the free crystalline silica content of the ash, which was about 3 to 4%. Slightly more than half this quantity was quartz, and most of the rest of it was cristobalite.

The best data on human exposure to the volcanic ash and its consequences were summarized by Drs. Buist and Bernstein in the supplement to volume 76 of the *American Journal of Public Health* (March 1986).

DR. McCLELLAN: You talked about the activities of asbestos, and I think you made reference to fiber glass, and everyone asked you what your findings were, how you interpreted them with regard to the potential for fiber glass producing irreversible lesions.

DISCUSSANT: The question initially came up because asbestos activates complement, and carbonyl iron may be even more innocuous than fiber glass. How can I reconcile the fact that they both activate complement, drawing macrophages to the bifurcations? The only answer I could think of, unsupported by data, is that I believe that complement activation and C-5A-generation is a mechanism which essentially brings the macrophages to the particles and perhaps allows them to phagocytize the particles.

After that, I think it is the inherent properties of the fiber or the particle that take precedence in terms of the development of the pathogenesis. That is the only explanation I would have. It is conceivable that particles and fibers that activate complement do not necessarily lead to fibrosis. They may lead simply to clearance. And it is also conceivable that chrysotile and crocidolite may have very different properties once they are phagocytized. There is a whole scenario that has been hypothesized for these possibilities.

DR. McCLELLAN: Let us move on to the Oberdörster and the Mauderly papers dealing with the effect of chronic cigarette smoke on long-term pulmonary clearance.

DISCUSSANT: An interesting problem is presented to us here, which has general implications. Dr. Ferin, Dr. Mauderly, and Dr. Oberdörster all referred to a study by Cohen et al. in *Science* (*204*:514-517, 1979). Now, the Cohen magnetic lung measurement study has been shown to be erroneous. This presents the problem of how to get rid of an invalid study.

The study purports to show that there is a difference in the ratio of dust elimination in the lungs of smokers as compared to those of nonsmokers, with nonsmokers eliminating five times as much dust as do smokers. The question is: Is there a problem with the study and, secondly, has there been a professional evaluation of the conduct of the study, and what was it?

Basically, the magnetometric technique employed by Cohen et al. involves the inhalation of magnetic particles by subjects who are then subjected to strong magnetic fields. The remaining magnetic force (remanence) is then measured to give an index of the amount of magnetic material remaining inside the body. What Cohen et al.

did was to have a number of smoking and nonsmoking subjects inhale large amounts of magnetite and then subject them to strong magnetization.

Cohen et al. overlooked the fact that individuals vary with respect to the viscosity of the content of the lung. Smokers have a lower lung viscosity than nonsmokers. Therefore, the magnetic particles could move around the lungs of smokers and form clusters; this occurred to a lesser degree, or not at all, in nonsmoking subjects.

I reviewed the Cohen et al. study and concluded that the investigators overlooked the fact that, during the magnetization phase of their experiment, iron oxide clusters were preferentially formed in smokers' bronchi because of their high mucus content and consequent low resistance to redistribution of particles. This analysis was reviewed and published (*Appl Phys 52:* 2575-2577, 1981). However, I was not the only one who noticed the error in the Cohen et al. work. A physicist (Reinstein) and an oncologist (Glicksman) did so as well. They then performed an experiment that basically repeated the method of Cohen et al. with various types of viscous materials, using a lung-equivalent physical model. They showed that the lung's viscosity determined the formation of hard-to-eliminate clusters of magnetite under the influence of magnetization.

While there is no simple way to demonstrate the truth of this key assumption *in vivo,* it is possible to show *in vitro* that it must be false and that, in fact, the Cohen et al. experiment itself caused iron oxide dust in smokers' lungs to form hard-to-eliminate clusters.

The Society for Magnetism and Magnetic Materials included a special session on this experiment and its criticism in its meeting in Dallas in 1980. Cohen was invited but refused to come. The reports by myself and by Reinstein and Glicksman were invited by the *Journal of Applied Physics.* The papers were heavily reviewed, also by Cohen, who refused to contribute in the end, and were published.

I might also mention that this type of experiment has been discontinued because it is not in the interest of human subjects to inhale iron dust, even though it is considered an inert material. The point is to include in the record of this symposium the opinion that references to this experiment are subject to question.

DISCUSSANT: There is a lot of discussion and a lot of controversy regarding the Cohen study. I have heard that, and I have looked at the results of the Bohning inhalation study (*Ann Occup Hyg 26:*259-271, 1982), in which radioactively labeled microspheres were used, a totally different technique, in that case. The Bohning study showed results quite similar to those reported by Cohen et al. To the best of my knowledge, the Bohning study seems to be without any major defect.

DISCUSSANT: Well, the question is not whether another study has the same results, the question is whether or not the Cohen study is an acceptable reference.

DISCUSSANT: I think possibly the record of this meeting might show that there are some questions concerning references to Cohen.

DR. WEHNER: The discussions here are being recorded and will be a part of the Proceedings; therefore, your position will be a matter of record.

DISCUSSANT: I think that is quite satisfactory.

DISCUSSANT: Well, again, you can argue with the Cohen study, but I think the chairman is right. There are other studies that support Cohen's results, and you would be much harder pressed to say that it is wrong. We have concluded a study, and there is one done at NIOSH in Morgantown, looking at particle retention in the lungs of cigarette smokers as a function of the number of cigarettes smoked. In both studies there is a clear correlation between particle retention and the amount of smoking, historical amount of smoking.

DISCUSSANT: I did not wish to argue what the data show about dust elimination in smokers' lungs. However, there are a number of studies with contradictory results, and my paper quotes them. In fact, there are a number of studies that summarize the evidence, including one by Dr. Cross, and they agree that the evidence is highly contradictory. I don't think that there is evidence to support the position that dust elimination in smokers is one-fifth that of nonsmokers. I think that is nonsense.

What I want to say is that here is an experiment which makes certain claims that are widely referenced in the literature. However, there were errors made. Thus, we have an erroneous experiment that did not consider all of the variables which it should have, and its results did not seem to follow from the findings, and the findings are contradictory in themselves. One can study the experiment, especially in light of the Reinstein and Glicksman experiment, and quite clearly see that. I really have not met anyone who has read the paper who has not come to the same conclusions.

DISCUSSANT: I would tend to disagree with what has been said. All I can speak to is our approach. Our approach is to go to the literature and find the study of humans that most closely matches the experimental techniques that we apply in rats. Smoking populations are very diverse, they are not homogenous populations at all. So our approach was to look at the study in which the experimental conditions, the hypothesis that was being tested, was most similar, and that is to what I compare the data. Now, I mentioned the Cohen study, and I mentioned this morning that it was controversial. But I thought that people might be curious as to how the rat data matched it, and they seem to match it fairly well.

DISCUSSANT: I think you would match it better if you were to take the Bohning study, rather than the Cohen study, which I understand is not on fiber agglomeration.

DISCUSSANT: The issue is not the 5:1 ratios, the issue is whether or not chronic smoking reduces clearance of particulate material in the lungs. At least that is the issue with which I was dealing.

DR. McCLELLAN: As I understood the Oberdörster paper, it is simply drawing attention to the importance of dose and the extent to which the interactive effects of cigarette smoke and fibers may be associated, not with some special biological phenomenon in terms of interaction, but with an alteration in the dose. It seems to me that this is a very important concept that is put forward. I was struck by the extent to which what I view as very mild lesions in the respiratory tract—in the terms that Dr. Pinkerton referred to them—can have a significant effect on long-term retention of fibers in the respiratory tract of rats. As Dr. Pinkerton noted, he did not see any alterations at the light microscope level, but he did see what I view as a profound effect on long-term clearance of fibers, and that is an important observation and one that does deserve a follow-up. Likewise, I think the Oberdörster paper is an excellent contribution to remind us of one avenue by which interactions can occur.

DISCUSSANT: Maybe the change in macrophage transport processes is actually an indication of pathological changes that follow.

DISCUSSANT: I believe that kinetically they are more sensitive than histology in picking up effects in the lung.

DISCUSSANT: Yes, certainly, if you want to use kinetics as a measure of well-being of that organ's system.

DISCUSSANT: Were all those macrophages observed in the form of small accumulations with brown pigment? And would you care to speculate on the mechanism which impairs clearance? Is it a macrophage function, or is it an airway impairment, or both, or none of the above?

DISCUSSANT: I have no proof of what I am going to say, only bias. First of all, I don't know what the mechanism is; I wish I did. We are doing studies, and we are trying to get at that mechanism and mechanisms of other kinds of clearance impairment. My bias is that it is probably related to the macrophage. If you look at the half-times for clearance via the mucociliary escalator, the reduction in half-time is not so severe that it can account completely for the retention of the material in the lung over a long time. My bias is that it is more of an impact on the ability of that material to move to the elevator, or to whatever pathway it needs, to leave the lungs. My bias is that this occurs largely through phagocytic cells, primarily the macrophages. Because cigarette smoke is known to have effects on macrophage functions *in vitro,* I believe that the effect is largely attributable to the phagocytes, i.e., phagocyte functions. I have no idea how, but that makes sense to me. If the phagocytes were normal, and the mucociliary clearance rates were reduced to a third, the impact on long-term clearance would not be very severe, in my opinon. That does not mean that this ciliary clearance might not be impaired. I think it probably is, we just did not measure it in this study.

DISCUSSANT: Do you have any data on where your radioactive particles end up?

DISCUSSANT: We don't have those data yet from this study. We are still looking at those materials, but we have information from numerous other studies at our laboratory with cerium and similar materials. We know that those particles can move into the interstitium, and we know that even long after exposure you can find some in macrophages on the alveolar lining, and you find some in the interstitium, and you see some moving into the lymph nodes. Those studies did not include smoke-exposed animals. This study here is the first we have done that has, and we are very interested in trying to identify where those particles might be. So I cannot answer that question.

DISCUSSANT: In most studies in which animals are exposed to cigarette smoke you see these collections of gold-brown macrophages near the ends of terminal bronchioles. There are two ways up: either up the mucociliary escalator, or into the lymphatic system. Does anybody know why some go one way, and some the other way, and whether this is a species characteristic or a compound characteristic, or what is going on?

DISCUSSANT: We have two or three people in the laboratory right now who are working on that, using fluorescent beads and several techniques to try to get at the kinetics of particle movement among macrophages. Yes, we know they can go to the cilia, and probably most of them do. A lot of the smoke particles are soluble, and a lot of that material dissolves and leaves, through the blood stream, presumably. We know that particle-laden macrophages and, presumably, smoke-stained macrophages, also move to lymph nodes, which means they get into the lymphatics, and you can see them in the interstitium. The state of the art now is that we know that they go to these places, but nobody knows exactly why or how. Some of the most recent information suggests that indeed there may be a species difference in the predisposition. It appears that the macrophage that ingests a particle in a dog has a greater predisposition to move into the airway wall, or the alveolar wall of the interstitium, than the macrophage in a rat. Rat macrophages appear biased, running toward the cilia. I think that we are going to find that there are species differences in the rate constants for the different pathways. I personally do not believe that there are species differences in the pathways themselves, but probably in the predisposition to take different paths.

DR. McCLELLAN: In the very early stages of those studies we were struck by a marked difference in the accumulation of the material, plutonium, in the tracheobronchial lymph nodes in a dog as compared to a rat. Again, it was not quantitatively different in terms of rates and kinetic models but, qualitatively, the basic biology was similar.

DISCUSSANT: There was a cigarette-smoking study presented here. Did you measure carboxyhemoglobin?

DISCUSSANT: Yes. It was around the 10-to-15% level immediately after smoking seven cigarettes a day, on Friday afternoon, which we presume to be the peak. The clearance half-time is incredibly fast. When you look at it a few minutes or an hour later, it has regressed almost back to baseline. But the peak carboxyhemoglobin level in that study was at around 10 or 12%.

DISCUSSANT: Very shortly I would like to respond to your question about the movement of particles in lymph nodes. From a certain amount of lung burden on, a decrease in the movement of particles in the lymph nodes occurred, very suddenly. In this particular case, in the rat, it was around 800 $\mu g/g$ of lung tissue. We reached that, and suddenly a larger fraction of the total lung burden moved into the lymph nodes than at the previous lower concentration. That was one of the first indications of overload, at least for me. We suggested at that time that it may happen before we become aware of it. If you put too many particles there, those particles—if they are left standing there without being phagocytized by macrophages—have a tendency to be either phagocytized by epithelial cells or move into the interstitial space.

I therefore suggested that the macrophages have too much to do because there are too many particles. Those particles then have a bigger chance when they are free, i.e., not phagocytized, to get into the interstitial space and, subsequently, into the lymphatics. In summary, if you have a large lung burden, those particles will go into the interstitial space without the help of macrophages. I have a histological slide where you see a stream of particles, which have not been phagocytized, in the lymph nodes.

DISCUSSANT: This could account for the longer retention that you observed in your rats. Those smoke-filled macrophages were impaired, and the particles remained at their deposition site longer than they normally would, and eventually they translocated to the interstitium. That would account for a longer half-time in terms of retention.

DISCUSSANT: You focused on the airway clearance variability, which is normal in humans. But you show that there is also increased variability in rats. That is very interesting, because these rats, especially today, are very homogeneous, very similar, very clean, and still you see this individual variation in the lung clearance. Obviously, in human beings this variation has to be larger, much larger.

DISCUSSANT: I agree. I have no explanation for that, but I have a hypothesis: one of the problems I had with this kind of smoking pattern is that puff-by-puff exposure of the rats. Those rats will breathe nicely and regularly until the smoke bolus is introduced. Then, as you watch the breathing patterns, you can see when each puff occurs. Rats would prefer not to smoke, and when they learn that the smoke is only going to be there for 28 seconds, they will hold their breath as much as possible, some rats more than others. So, one hypothesis is that the smoke-dosing might have varied from rat to rat, but I have no measurements of that. This variability in the rat data is very interesting, because you would suppose that you could not get the exposure conditions and the animal characteristics more uniform than you could with laboratory animals, whereas in a human study you have so many variables (different ages, different pack years, some subjects with emphysema, some without), and you expect variation. So it fascinated me that we got variations on the same order of magnitude without those variables, which you could use to suggest that those variables that are so obvious in man may not be so important.

DISCUSSANT: This may have no bearing, but I have read the standard pulmonary pathology texts in which the concept of pleural drift is introduced. According to this concept, particles tend to drift to the pleura. That is where you see asbestos bodies and other changes in asbestos workers. And that is where you get the subpleural fibrosis. Do you see this pleural drift in laboratory animals?

DISCUSSANT: You do to a certain extent, but not as much. Again, we do not know much about that kind of movement of the particles in animals. If you assume that that has to do with mechanical movement, their breathing, we have that in animals and man. And if you assume, as I am inclined to do, that in humans it has a lot to do with lymphatic channels—you also have subpleural lymphatics in animals. But in the rat, which has a very thin pleura, these lymphatic channels are very small compared to man. Now when you expose a rat to small, relatively insoluble particles for a long period of time, you will find these particles all over, but primarily at the terminal bronchiolar alveolar duct junctions and subpleurally. So the answer is, yes, you do see some of that in laboratory animals. I suspect that it may not be as marked as it is in man. That is the extent of my understanding.

DISCUSSANT: Does anybody ever measure lymph flow in animals?

DISCUSSANT: Yes, there are some measurements of lymph flow in animals, but those are largely of the main channels of the large ducts—and that is not going to help us very much. So if we are talking about lymph flow in small rodents, and particularly lymph going toward the periphery, no, there are no measurements to the best of my knowledge.

Edited Transcript of the Discussions of Day 3

Chairman: Dr. A. M. Langer

Papers by the following authors were discussed in this session: Adler, Brody, Kagan, Luchtel, Boatman, Johnson, Coffin (two presentations), Palekar, Langer, and Wasserman.

DR. LANGER: I have been asked to have Dr. Wasserman's paper discussed first, as he has some scheduling problems. Were the cigarettes that you used for the experimental smoke exposures research cigarettes or commercial cigarettes?

DISCUSSANT: The cigarettes were unfiltered, commercially available, 85 mm long, and had 24 mg tar.

DISCUSSANT: In both of your studies, when you talked about pack years of smoking experience, particularly in the asbestos workers (shipyard workers), do you have some information on their current smoking history? For example, 36-pack years: Were they recent, two-pack-a-day smokers, or one-pack-a-day smokers, or what?

DISCUSSANT: They were current smokers. I was not the principal investigator of this study, so I do not remember whether there was a trend in their current smoking habit. They were selected because they were average smokers.

DISCUSSANT: Were they reasonably fit; or retired?

DISCUSSANT: These men were actively working at the time of the evaluation. They were not retired, nor particularly identified as having any lung diseases. They were identified by the Department of Labor as having been exposed to asbestos and that they should be evaluated. So there was no discrimination except by history. Those people who said they never smoked were checked for carboxyhemoglobin values at the time of study. We routinely check carboxyhemoglobin when measuring arterial blood gases. We discovered that, many times, people being evaluated for disability claim that they are not smokers, yet their COHb is elevated to the range of the smoker's.

DISCUSSANT: Did you measure the COHb levels at the beginning and end of each smoking day?

DISCUSSANT: We measured CO at the beginning and end of the exercise test. CO might wash down in concentration as a result of the exercise. The measurements of COHb that I have shown were made at the beginning of the test. The COHb decreased on the smoking day from 6.6 to something like 4.5 at the close of 10 to 15 minutes of exercise.

DISCUSSANT: I think you said that you tried washing out CO with oxygen beforehand. I wonder whether it would have been better to use carbon dioxide, because this might stimulate breathing.

DISCUSSANT: Oxygen competes with CO for the hemogloblin binding site. I do not think that increased ventilation resulting from CO_2 breathing would be more effective than the increased ventilation from exercise in washing out CO from the blood.

DISCUSSANT: Could you tell me the incidence of COPD in asbestos-exposed smokers and nonsmokers? Was there a difference?

DISCUSSANT: We do know that compared to nonsmokers, smokers do have some impairment, even when they are not complaining of dyspnea. The pulmonary-function abnormalities in these smokers were not very great, as shown by the fact that they were not disabled and had active jobs. There were 23 of 73 smokers who had abnormally low FEV values.

DISCUSSANT: How about the nonsmokers?

DISCUSSANT: There were three individuals with reduced FEV_1 values among the nonsmokers.

DISCUSSANT: Your results suggest, then, that asbestos workers who do not smoke do not have COPD?

DISCUSSANT: Yes. It is unlikely. It turned out that two of the three nonsmokers with a reduced FEV_1 had histories of asthma. If you use the forced expiratory volume measurement, 25 to 75%, then none of the nonsmokers were abnormal, but 12 of the smokers were abnormal. We find the FEV_1/VC more sensitive. Three of the 73 nonsmokers had reduced values compared to 23 of the 73 smokers.

DISCUSSANT: Was there any characterization of the exposure to asbestos, either quantitatively or qualitatively?

DISCUSSANT: The best we could do with respect to quantifying asbestos exposure was to determine the number of years of exposure and the intensity of exposure, graded as mild, moderate, or intense. The latter was based on whether or not there was dust visible to the worker. Both nonsmoking and smoking groups had comparable exposure according to this assessment.

DISCUSSANT: Did any of these workers show any radiographic signs of asbestosis?

DISCUSSANTS: Yes. In both groups there were some who had pulmonary fibrosis, as graded by the radiologist according to the ILO classification. There were more who had ILO classification Grades 2 and 3 in the smoking group than in the nonsmoking group, so there was a radiological difference as well as a physiological difference.

DISCUSSANT: You just focused on parenchymal changes?

DISCUSSANT: We focused on parenchymal changes and the radiologist's independent reading on whether the classification was grade 2 or 3. Even when we removed all the subjects with X-ray evidence of pulmonary fibrosis, there was a physiological difference between the smoking and the nonsmoking groups. So, in contrast to the physiological evidence, the X-ray evidence of pulmonary fibrosis was not discriminatory with respect to whether subjects were smokers or nonsmokers.

DISCUSSANT: Were you at all concerned that the shipyard environment may have been too complex a work environment to gauge the two effects individually?

DISCUSSANT: We recognize that this is a limitation. Trying to evaluate people who are exposed to asbestos and also have cigarette-smoke exposure, both of which can be potential contributors to airway obstruction, may not have differentiated between the effects of those two causative agents. But we are often faced with the need to know whether the pulmonary-function impairment is caused by cigarette-smoking or asbestos exposure. That is really why we did this study: we knew that cigarette-smoking can cause airway obstruction; we did not know whether asbestos exposure, by itself, causes physiological changes that reflect airway obstruction.

DISCUSSANT: Yesterday you were describing some of these people as asbestos-exposed and said that they worked in a shipyard setting. But didn't they have occupations other than pipe-laying and insulating?

DISCUSSANT: That was, of course, a different study, conducted here in Seattle.

DISCUSSANT: So these are asbestos workers in shipyards, not just shipyard workers who are exposed to asbestos?

DISCUSSANT: These are shipyard workers exposed to asbestos, but I am sorry, I do not have their specific job descriptions. How actively they are involved with asbestos is indicated by the grading, by the history that I described. In both the smoking and nonsmoking groups there were only three subjects who were graded as having only a slight exposure. The histories were recorded by a trained nurse who has conducted many of these studies. We really depended on the answers given by the individual workers.

DR. LANGER: Let us move to Dr. Adler's paper on his novel culture system.

DISCUSSANT: Have you tested mineral fibers? How did you introduce the mineral fibers into the system? What were your results?

DISCUSSANT: One of the nice things about this system is that you are looking for a response of the epithelial cells to any sort of stimuli. You introduce that particular stimulus, either from above, where you would expect to find mineral fibers, other particulates, and gases that are inhaled; or from below, if you are looking for the effects of the bloodborne substances.

DISCUSSANT: But are you using it with an aerosol? Or how are you exposing the cells?

DISCUSSANT: You can use an aerosol, or just introduce a suspension of particulates.

DISCUSSANT: And then did you put it on top of the cells?

DISCUSSANT: Yes, you put it on top of the cells and see what happens. We have done some studies with asbestos fibers, about a year ago, just to see whether these cells took up asbestos fibers—and they didn't.

DISCUSSANT: How does your culture system compare with fibers in humans regarding the mucus, the viscosity, and other properties of the mucus?

DISCUSSANT: I showed one slide this morning about the biochemical characteristics of the mucus which is produced. It is identical to what is produced by the cells in the culture, as far as we have tested. We are now conducting a study with a group at the University of North Carolina at Chapel Hill concerning the amino acid composition of mucus that is produced by human cells. We are comparing that to the mucus produced by airway explants or mucus in mammals *in vivo,* but we do not yet have the results. As far as the viscous properties and things like that are concerned, it is not an area in which we are interested, and we have not looked at that.

Under the microscope, with proper lighting, these cells look similar to what you see in an explant. In the intact airway you do see cilia beating, and there's no uncoordinated beating. What I meant by coordinated is, you can usually see the change, and you can see waves propagating. You are not looking at individual cilia, but you can certainly follow waves of movement over quite a distance.

DISCUSSANT: I just wonder whether your system would be adaptable for studies of, say, 10 weeks?

DISCUSSANT: I had the growth curves on one of the slides that I did not show this morning. After an exposure of 15 days, the numbers of cells decreased precipitously. So if you are talking about studies of more than 2 to 3 weeks, I would say no.

DISCUSSANT: The University of California, Davis, is using a similar system. In fact, we developed this together; they are using hamster cells. I think they keep the cells going for a longer period of time than I did. But again, I did not really try to keep the cells going for any extended length of time.

DISCUSSANT: Did you try any cells other than trachea cells?

DISCUSSANT: Tracheal and bronchial cells. It is also a very species-specific type of culture system. I used guinea pig cells, and they seemed to work really well. Others use hamster cells, rabbit cells, primate cells, canine cells.

DISCUSSANT: And rat cells.

DISCUSSANT: And rat cells, also, but they do not do nearly as well in this culture system. It is a mystery as to why the guinea pig cells do so well.

DISCUSSANT: It depends on what you are looking for. If you are looking at an end point as to what has happened to the epithelium, and you are interested in looking at the proteinaceous material, I think this is an excellent method. But if you are looking at something like transformation, I don't think it is a good method because, first of all, the cells are from adult samples and, usually, there is a better percentage of transformation with embryonic cells. Also, in embryonic tissue you can get a lot of cells easily, and it is less expensive. So that is another disadvantage of this method over having the embryonic cells. They grow faster, and they have a better proliferation rate. It all depends upon what your end point is, and what you are looking for in the *in vivo* system.

Then again, there are some cell lines which are very useful. In our laboratory we have used V79 hamster lung cells. We have done some cytotoxicity assays, and we have shown a correlation between cytotoxicity and tumorigenesis, so that is a very good assay. The cell line grows very fast, and you can have many passages in your laboratory.

DR. LANGER: Any more points for discussion? If not, let us go on to the presentation of Dr. Brody on the biology and biochemistry of macrophage-derived growth factors.

DISCUSSANT: In the trachea you have a cell turnover value of 1 to 2%. Do you have any idea whether those basal secretory cells are growing—dividing?

DISCUSSANT: In the upper airways the turnover was so low, as you pointed out, that we did not make any attempts to differentiate the various cell types. But that 1 to 2% may have been in basal cells or secretory cells—I can't tell you which.

DISCUSSANT: You indicated that you do your morphometric determinations based on point counting.

DISCUSSANT: Which is nothing more than a statistical grid, a point count based on an interception point of an object.

DISCUSSANT: Rocks have certain structural fabrics. If you do point counts on rocks, occasionally you have to take three sections at right angles—to determine a modal analysis of the mineral content of the rocks. Do you do the same with biological systems where you have structures? Do you take preferred orientations, or do you take several orientations and run them through the point count?

DISCUSSANT: Yes. In other words, you have a block of tissue that you have collected from a specific anatomical region in the lung. In this case, you take the whole left lung of the rat, and you cut a sagittal section, and embed that whole section, about 2 mm thick, in plastic. After it sets, you look at it under transmitted light, and you can see right through it, and you look at the bronchioloalveolar junctions under a dissecting microscope. Then you put that whole section on a warming tray and cut out small blocks of those bronchioloalveolar junction regions. Those blocks are then mounted on the end of a regular plastic block for electron microscopy, and that block then is randomly sectioned. That bifurcation region is randomly oriented; we cannot dictate the angle at which that bifurcation is coming off the end of the bronchiole. Therefore, I am sure that we are getting what could be called random sections; we cannot set it up in any particular direction.

DISCUSSANT: You say it is a relatively homogeneous structure.

DISCUSSANT: Well, no, I am sure it is not.

DISCUSSANT: In reality it is not, but when you cut the sections from blocks that are just randomly oriented, then it is all random.

DISCUSSANT: I would like to interject something. The equations that Weibel uses to establish his volume density and molecular density of the different cell types were based on random orientation.

DISCUSSANT: Yes.

DISCUSSANT: Talking about randomization, you stressed that the changes occurred only at those spots where there are fibers, and the fibers are at the bifurcations. Therefore, you have to be sure that you are really measuring the bifurcation and not something else. How do you determine what is the bifurcation and what is an area beyond a bifurcation?

DISCUSSANT: That is the point that I was making about the fact that you have the whole lung slice. You put that under a dissecting microscope, and you see where the terminal bronchioles enter the alveolar duct—then you cut that out and section it, and take each section and put it under a light microscope and look as you go through that region. You will then come to the bifurcation, as I showed by light microscopy. Now I am going to take the next 20 sections and do the morphometry on that bifurcation.

DISCUSSANT: I wonder whether the plane of the section is really so random. I mean, if you are selecting these alveolar airways—alveolar duct areas—might not there be a preferred orientation just because you tend to recognize those units oriented as you are looking down at them?

DISCUSSANT: Well, it may be, but I don't know how preferential it is. I can tell you, when you look at the light micrographs that come off these sections that go through the bifurcations, you can see the airways coming in at all angles. Sometimes you will hit the bifurcation first and then the airway, and sometimes you hit it where you would like to see it: where you see the entire airway, the whole unit and three or four bifurcations coming off. But that is very unusual. I can also tell you that we cannot dictate which way it is going to go. Therefore, I am not really worried about preferential rather than random orientation.

DISCUSSANT: You showed a picture in which the inhaled fibers were phagocytized by the epithelial cells within a few hours after exposure.

DISCUSSANT: Yes. Actually, it happens during the first hour of exposure. We know that this event occurs very rapidly.

DISCUSSANT: I was very surprised that chrysotile was not phagocytized by the macrophages. Do you think that chrysotile fibers are not incorporated, and that they are just staying there? Or do you think that they can be removed again—cleared?

DISCUSSANT: I believe that they stay there for just a very short time. The evidence that we have is that the transit time is very fast. When you look at the first few hours after exposure, you see most of the asbestos in the epithelium. As you go past 5 to 10 hours after exposure, you see very little asbestos in the epithelium; it is either already in the interstitium, or it has been picked up by macrophages. Occasionally, you will see a macrophage sharing an asbestos fiber with an epithelial cell. That is one way in which those fibers seem to stay around for a long time.

DISCUSSANT: Do you think an asbestos fiber can pass through the epithelium and go into the interstitium?

DISCUSSANT: It happens. You can see that event happening for the next month after exposure. I can show you asbestos in the alveolar epithelium 1 month after exposure. However, I cannot tell you which way the dust is going. That, of course, is one of the real problems, that we do not know whether it is on its way in or out. But certainly during the first few hours, 12 hours after exposure, I would suggest that the dust that we see is going in and heading toward the interstitium. But that seems to be a rapid transit, an active process that we think is actin-mediated. We have shown that there is increased actin associated with the asbestos. Working with Dr. Adler, we took some epithelial cells *in vitro* and put asbestos in them and showed that there is increased active polymerization going on. Apparently there is an active process of transport going on.

DISCUSSANT: The epithelial cells, are they not damaged?

DISCUSSANT: It depends on how you interpret the morphometric data that I showed you. When you look at 48 hours, the data suggest that there are very few alterations in that epithelium. But both the morphometric data and autoradiographic data suggest that something is going on. Now, it depends on how you want to interpret damage. There is no evidence of cell death, but there is very clear evidence of some sort of reparative process going on. The Type-II cells are proliferating; they are in some kind of DNA synthesis. On the other hand, there is a small protein leak. When you lavage the lungs of these animals 48 hours after 1 hour of exposure, there are increased amounts of "protein" in the lavage fluid. We don't know exactly what it is: complement, serum protein, etc. There is more of it in the lungs of animals that have been exposed than in the lungs of nonexposed animals. But when you start looking for cell death, you won't see it. If you look for cell thickening, it is there; autoradiography shows that proliferation is occurring; a protein leak is there; so it depends on how you want to interpret "damage."

DISCUSSANT: This is a more speculative question: Is there cellular damage from cigarette-smoking, for example, if this process would be faster? If the epithelial cells are possibly damaged by cigarette-smoking, how much more is the percent of asbestos damage than the cigarette-smoke damage, that is the question.

DISCUSSANT: I think that, first of all, it is important to separate what goes on in the airways from what goes on in the alveoli. I know that this discussion has taken place before, but the damage to the alveolar epithelium in cigarette smokers, I don't believe, has really been documented. It may not, in fact, really happen. So we have to talk about the airways, and one of the things that we recognized is that there is no uptake of asbestos by the normal airway epithelium. I may have seen it once, but in all the thousands of pictures that I have looked at, I just do not see that happening in normal epithelium. The best data on uptake of particles in damaged epithelium with which I am familar are those of Dr. Brooke Mossman and her group in Vermont. She has taken explants of airway epithelium and then put asbestos fibers on them. And you get this sort of squamous metaplastic type of differentiation, and those cells are very phagocytic for fibers. So I can envision happening what I saw in the diagram in Prof. Pott's presentation. Prof. Pott is suggesting that damaged epithelium may cause fibers to become lodged at the site of damage and that may be an exceptionally good site for particle uptake. But I do not know whether that experiment has actually been done. I think it should be.

DISCUSSANT: I would like to make a generic point, specifically about those papers. First you conduct these very elegant exposures with basically naive animals and look at the pulmonary deposition in the sacrificed animals. Then you extrapolate for the long term. This is really totally unjustified, because by that time you get the disease to the point where the anatomy is different, the elasticity is different, and the air flow is different, so that you might get orders-of-magnitude differences in deposition and clearance, and in a million other things that were observed.

DISCUSSANT: Sure.

DISCUSSANT: I am not saying *you* are doing this, but I think that some people do this. They do a short version of the study on relatively normal tissues, and then extrapolate to the long term, which is, perhaps, totally unjustified.

DISCUSSANT: What you say is correct if you want to know what is going on chronically. But if you want to find out what the initial events are in the mechanisms, you need to start at the beginning or you will never know. You can look at all the diseased animals you want, or at diseased people, and you will never know what is going on.

DISCUSSANT: I know; it was not meant as criticism.

DISCUSSANT: No, I understand; your point is well taken.

DISCUSSANT: But I think there is a danger, which is often forgotten.

DISCUSSANT: I would like to respond in general terms to what you just said. There is a danger, but it depends on the purpose for which you want to use that extrapolation. For example, this question arose because Prof. Pott had advanced his hypothesis that fibers can be trapped in damaged airway epithelium. Now the discussant says, "Oh, because of what I know from past experience, that may be a good possibility." "However," he says, "the experiment was not done, and it should be done." He extrapolated from what is known and said this may be a good idea; it should be proven. I think that in that case, the extrapolation is perfectly legitimate. That is why we are sitting here, and why Dr. Wehner asked us to brainstorm and to advance new ideas. And that is why we do not have our names recorded, so that we can be brave and say some daring things without the risk of being called stupid by posterity.

DISCUSSANT: I agree with you that people want to have practical results for whatever is important from a primary trial, then they make bold extrapolations. That obviously is a dangerous thing to do, I agree with you. However, for the initiation of some kind of ideas or discussions, and particularly ideas for new experiments, it is excellent.

DISCUSSANT: Up to now we only have preliminary results. We instilled in the trachea a small amount of formaldehyde for inducing inflammation of the trachea. After a few days we instilled glass fibers or other mineral fibers. There were six low-dose endotracheal instillations of the fibers. About 4 weeks after the last instillation we killed the animals and collected only the trachea and the main bronchi, without any alveoli. The tissue was ashed, and we counted the fibers. We found a lot of fibers by microscopic examination, but there was no clear difference between the animals which were treated with formaldehyde solution and the other group, which received only fibers. But I think it is clear that over a period of

4 weeks after endotracheal instillation there were fibers in the wall of the trachea. I did not expect this before this experiment, because normally the bronchi should be cleared of the fibers.

DISCUSSANT: Was this observed only in the formaldehyde-treated group?

DISCUSSANT: No, there was about the same amount of fibers in both groups.

DISCUSSANT: Do you think that you would have made the same observation if the animals had been exposed by inhalation?

DISCUSSANT: I don't know.

DISCUSSANT: Dr. Churg and others have shown that you can get small airway disease and even large airway disease when you inject asbestos, and I think that is clear. But I do not know whether any of the inhalation models show airway disease. What I am suggesting is that when you inject the asbestos into the airways, you create the damage, you damage the lining epithelium, and then you get incorporation of fibers into the airway walls.

DISCUSSANT: I believe when you carefully instill a very small amount you do not damage the epithelium.

DISCUSSANT: I don't know exactly; I can only say that 4 weeks after the last instillation, we found a lot of fibers in the trachea and in the bronchi.

DISCUSSANT: I want to make it clear that I think it is a well-taken point that there is one set of experiments that should be done using animals that have certain conditions associated with disease. It would be nice to expose cigarette-smoking animals and animals with pneumonia (as an infection) to particles and see what happens, because that is the real world. On the other side of the coin, if you want to know the initial invasive mechanisms through which a particle causes disease, then you have to start by extrapolating. That is the bind in which we are, and while it might be dangerous, I think that we may have to do that.

DISCUSSANT: At one time, one of the contract research laboratories for which I worked decided that they were going to develop a model for measuring emphysema and that they were going to use the mean linear intercept surface in rats. So they exposed several groups of rats to various agents, some of which, in fact, caused some fibrosis. Now, the question at the end is, how do you harvest the lungs of these animals? What are the rules? Do you ligate the trachea while the lung is still in the chest and measure it, that is, put the whole lung in fixative? Or do you, as was recommended by many people at that time, distend the lung with fixative, using a quick-setting fixative? Well, you are immediately in trouble if you do that, because, for instance, the more diseased the lung, the more difficult it is to distend it with fixative. Consequently, the results of some of these tests were not very much affected by the fibrosis. They were actually the opposite of what you would expect, because it was quite easy to overdistend the normal part of the lung with fixative, but you could not do that to the diseased part. You therefore got precisely the wrong answer to the question posed. Therefore, under certain circumstances, the disease that you are trying to investigate may actually cause you to get exactly the wrong data.

DISCUSSANT: Even when you infuse at a fixed hydrostatic pressure?

DISCUSSANT: Sure.

DISCUSSANT: What he is saying is right. That is why you have to get your morphometric measurements based on some standard linear parameter in the lung, like length of basement membrane, or something like that.

DISCUSSANT: Yes. The trouble is, there are quite a number of papers in the literature which are based on that sort of artefact.

DISCUSSANT: How do you recover the interstitial macrophages and how do you identify them as interstitial macrophages?

DISCUSSANT: The question of interstitial macrophages is a very good one, because there are a lot of people involved in trying to separate that potentially important population of cells. No one believes that they have a pure population of interstitial macrophages, because you can lavage the lungs *ad infinitum* and you will never be able to remove all the alveolar cells. The most effective method seems to be that in which you lavage the lungs first, and then use an enzyme digestion method, chop up the lung, and then use a differential adherence type of selection after you have used a density gradient separation. Now, we skipped the density gradient separation, because with or without that we get this very clear 80% population of very small, highly esterase-positive cells that look, for all the world, like all the other people's cells that they call interstitial macrophages. So that is what we are calling interstitial macrophages; we say they are approximately 80 to 82% pure interstitial macrophages. Now, I cannot prove that, but they are certainly only available after enzymatic digestion; they are highly phagocytic; and they measure about 8 to 10 μm in diameter versus the usual 10 to 20.

DISCUSSANT: Again, hearing Dr. Brody's presentation, I was impressed by the degree of sophistication that we can bring to bear looking at the respiratory tract now, using these contemporary techniques. I am wondering whether, in fact, you have, or you have plans to use, these same techniques looking at respiratory tracts of rodents exposed to cigarette smoke?

DISCUSSANT: No, we do not—that is not one of the things that we have planned. I would dearly love to see that kind of experiment done, because I think it is such a perfectly natural and important thing to do. And I would like very much to know how these deposition patterns and how the development of these lesions occur in the face of a smoke exposure. I think that would be an excellent study, but that is not one of the priorities that we have planned.

DISCUSSANT: Looking at the more recent chapters of your work, again, it continues to focus on the central role of the macrophage in lung diseases. Certainly the macrophage and cigarette smoke would have an important set of interactions.

DISCUSSANT: I agree with that.

DISCUSSANT: I think it is time that we revisit some of the issues of cigarette smoke in the respiratory tract, using these modern techniques that we have at hand now, which were not available in some of the earlier investigations. It seems to me that we are looking at a two-bladed kind of approach. One can take the elegant work that Dr. Brody has conducted on the fiber itself. In addition, you really need the matching counterpart in terms of work with cigarette smoke. And, finally, one needs to bring those two together if we want to understand the nature of the interaction of these materials in influencing the respiratory tract.

DISCUSSANT: It would be fascinating to see whether we could collect the macrophages that are accumulating in the lungs that Dr. Mauderly is showing, and investigate whether they behave like the cells that are exposed to the fibers.

DISCUSSANT: How specific do you think these things at which you are looking are for asbestos?

DISCUSSANT: Well, I showed you that they are not specific for asbestos. Iron, for example, does the same thing as asbestos. And I think cigarette smoke would do just exactly the same thing. The issue is that you can turn on these cells in a variety of different ways. You can activate them just by attaching them to the dish. The data that I showed you on the background production of platelet-derived growth factors (PDGF) were collected after the cells had been sitting on a dish. Now, cells that are suspended, that have never touched plastic, do nothing; they produce no measurable PDGF. So sitting on the dish does a variety of things: it causes the cell to make a whole array of arachidonic acid metabolites, and it causes them to produce PDGF. When you feed them something like iron or asbestos, they take off again. Now, if they have been exposed to cigarette smoke first, that would be another interesting question.

DISCUSSANT: At the beginning of the steps of fibrosis induced by asbestos, should not there not be some specificity for asbestos?

DISCUSSANT: Well, the other point I made was that when you look at the *in vitro* exposure to the two kinds of particles versus the *in vivo* exposure, you get the same levels. But then, when you look at the macrophages collected from animals at varying times after inhalation exposure—and I did not show you the data because they were too good to believe; I am going to have to do a couple of more tests before I believe it—the level of PDGF produced by the asbestos-exposed animals remained elevated for a week. The PDGF from the iron-exposed animals came down by 48 hours and stayed down for the rest of the week. Now, what I am suggesting is that you can get an initial nonspecific response, but what the nature of the dust is, and how it is handled in the lung, and how well it is cleared, and how long it stays around may be the key factors. Our future studies are designed to do the right *in situ* hybridization and immunocytochemistry to find out where the substance is being produced, and which cells are making it, and how long it stays around.

DISCUSSANT: Could that not also be explained on the basis of dose-response between the iron particles and the asbestos on those areas affected?

DISCUSSANT: Well, dose-response is a very important issue that has been hard to resolve. We know that doses of both iron and asbestos are sufficient to attract similar numbers of macrophages to the bifurcations; those are the basic exposures that we use. The dose is measured by a biological response. Now, if we were to conduct appropriate dose-response studies in terms of the numbers of fibers or spheres inhaled, that would be a very good experiment; but we have not done that.

DISCUSSANT: So for now, there is really nothing in these data suggesting that the macrophage response is specific for asbestos in particular?

DISCUSSANT: I would say it is not. I would say that the nature of the fibrotic response is more relevant to where the production of the growth factors is, and how much of it gets there.

DISCUSSANT: The isolation of the macrophages by enzymatic digestion, one would think, might have some adverse effect of the enzymes on the macrophages . Was the amount of growth factor produced by the alveolar macrophages the same as that produced by the interstitial macrophages?

DISCUSSANT: Absolutely. We have a manuscript in press comparing the interstitial-macrophage-conditioned medium to the alveolar-macrophage-conditioned medium, on a per DNA basis: they are the same. Apparently, the enzymatic treatment lets them sit in a culture for 24 hours to sort of catch up. Maybe, if we studied the cells right away after they come out of the animal, they might be different, but we let them "equilibrate."

DISCUSSANT: Don't you think that you lose a lot of cells during those 24 hours?

DISCUSSANT: No, very few. They seem to be hardy. In fact, they seem to be hardier than the alveolar cells and are less likely to lyse over time.

DISCUSSANT: Now, there is a question of dose. I believe, of course, that the dose is very important. However, it is getting even more complicated as we look into that in more detail: how to express the dose? Even the dose for an individual cell can be expressed in various ways. We are used to expressing the dose in micrograms per whatever; that may be good for a solute, but not necessarily for particles. For example, as we mentioned in connection with the overloading of animals, there is now a tendency to express the particles in volume because one very light, big particle can fill up the macrophage completely.

DISCUSSANT: We conducted a study where we asked whether or not C5-deficient animals would be any different than C5-normal animals. They were not. Now, our original hypothesis was that they would be different, but I don't want to get into that because that is another story.

DISCUSSANT: You did do a complement study?

DISCUSSANT: Yes, we did do a complement study. The data from that study for the asbestos-exposed animals were the same as those from any other study we have done, and the same as those from the unexposed controls. But that is at 48 hours after exposure. By 1 month after exposure, C5-deficient animals (which have depressed macrophage responses) also exhibit less interstitial disease.

DISCUSSANT: I have thought about microcalcifications, and I wanted Dr. Davis to comment on that. How frequently do you see microcalcifications?

DISCUSSANT: They are in $33 \pm 5\%$ of the bifurcations, as determined by morphometry.

DR. LANGER: The next paper is "The Effects of Amphibole and Serpentine Asbestos Inhalation on the Distribution and Functional State of Alveolar Macrophage Subpopulations," by Dr. Kagan et al.

DISCUSSANT: We had been working with fractions, with density fractions in populations. Some of our earlier studies had shown that when we looked at alveolar macrophages in unfractionated populations, this was purely the expression of IA antigens. We were not looking during exposures, but we exposed animals for a month, then we looked at the expression of IA, at 3 months and 6 months after the cessation of exposure in one group of animals. And in the other group of animals, I think it was about 15 to 18 months after exposure. Those times were selected because we were doing some other studies, we finished that study and had some animals left and said, "Hey, let's look at some other things." And, in fact, we found expression of IA in two different strains of rats. There was an enhanced expression; enhanced in the sense that there were greater numbers of IA-positive cells in the crocidolite-exposed animals as long as 15 to 18 months after exposure, but this was not seen in the chrysotile-exposed animals. In the 3- to 6-month group, the percentage in chrysotile-exposed animals was higher than in sham-exposed but not nearly as high as in crocidolite-exposed animals. This is consistent with what we are saying: Those results may be due to differences either in clearance or differential solubility, or the lack thereof, between amphibole and serpentine asbestos.

DISCUSSANT: We are talking about a hypothesis which concerns the role of the macrophage and, perhaps, interactions. I have a fairly clear idea of the sequence of events which you see during the course of a long-term study. You see the accumulation of these small, particle-laden macrophages very early in the disease, occurring in the region of the terminal bronchioles, and subsequently you see other lesions developing at that site. But just concentrating on the macrophages, in the very early stages, they don't stay. Later on they pick up ions. And then you start to see a mixture of healthy, pigment-laden macrophages, and dying macrophages which swell to considerable size. As they swell, they are less and less alive, and eventually they die. If you have a fairly good understanding of the sequence in time, over many months, of what happens to these smoke-particle-laden macrophages, you don't have to have any comparable experience with asbestos. But if we are thinking of interactions, I would like to know, does the same sort of thing happen, is it the same sort of sequence? Somebody said that the half-life of the macrophage is perhaps as long as 80 days. Now is that true only for "unburdened" macrophages, or is it also true for macrophages containing dusts and other materials? Is an interaction between materials possibly killing the macrophages? Or is tobacco smoke, for some reason, killing macrophages and creating problems for this reason? What information, what data base, do we have about this?

DISCUSSANT: Well, I can answer part of your question. In earlier studies that Dr. Brody and I did together, we looked at the distribution patterns of crocidolite and chrysotile asbestos in the rat lung. The animals were exposed for 1 month, and then we monitored them for up to 16 months, generally by performing lavage and necropsies, and looked at the distribution of the particles. The lesion that Dr. Brody observed within 24 to 48 hours is seen as long as 15 months or more after the cessation of exposure. The alveolar duct bifurcations are thickened; there are macrophages around. In another study that we did, just looking at the lavage cells of such exposed animals as long as 18 months after exposures, 60% of crocidolite-exposed animals still had crocidolite in their lungs. But we never saw chrysotile, and this we ascertained by transmission electron microscopy. And what does that tell us about the half-life of the macrophage? I cannot tell you, but it certainly would suggest that, obviously, there is recycling. We therefore are dealing with the effects of not just inhalation exposure but with what is deposited and "in residence" in the lungs and what is being recycled. This process continues all the time. I contend that one can certainly extrapolate that to the human exposure situation, because when I was in South Africa at one institute, I saw the lungs of about 600 asbestos workers during a 5-year period. It was fascinating to see the lungs of a mine worker, the lower lobes, with classical asbestosis that the village policeman could diagnose. Now these are people who had their exposure in the past and they had long since been removed from exposure. In the nonfibrotic areas you see a distinct desquamated interstitial pneumonitis, just a pouring-out of an exudative reaction of alveolar macrophages full of fibers that you could see with a light microscope (it was done with light microscopy) and asbestos bodies galore. So, obviously, this process must be continually recycling, and I guess that this would probably create the basis for perpetuation of the lesion. Whatever growth factor you want to talk about, be it PDGF or IA-1 or TNF or whatever, I guess if those fibers are not being removed, the stage is set for perpetual release. Of course, you could say to me, well, if you did not see any chrysotile fibers, what is going on there? I cannot answer that. In the South African context, virtually all the people had mixed occupational exposures, and usually it was chrysotile and/or crocidolite exposure. So I do not know, but the mechanisms seem to be somewhat the same. I can also tell you that we had looked at the release of chemoattractants, not complement-derived, from macrophages. Alveolar macrophages were releasing chemoattractants for other alveolar macrophages, following crocidolite or chrysotile exposure. And once again, we plotted this with time. There was always greater release of chemoattractants, based on the SDS profile. They had molecular weights different from those reported by Dr. Brody. I don't think they were complement-derived. Nevertheless, results from both chrysotile and crocidolite looked almost identical compared with the controls, and yet, where is the chrysotile? There was no chrysotile in the macrophages, and yet the factors are being released. There is obviously a lot more to it than the presence of fibers within cells.

DISCUSSANT: Dr. Pinkerton's studies with chrysotile in rats show a good interstitial population of macrophages with chrysotile fibers.

DISCUSSANT: In our study, we found chrysotile in the interstitium, but a lot of crocidolite was located within the alveolar macrophages. It really is strange that the alveolar macrophages in the chrysotile-exposed animals are producing chemoattractants, and yet there is no evidence of the fibers.

DISCUSSANT: We actually found some of these foamy macrophages that you are describing, in fact, with crocidolite.

DISCUSSANT: Right. The interesting thing is, as Harrington showed years ago *in vitro,* that chrysotile was more cytotoxic to macrophages than crocidolite. Yet when you look at the viability of cells obtained by lavage in those two different chrysotiles, they are probably about 95% viable, just the same as you see with the sham-exposed controls. Now that does not exclude the possibility that a lot of the cells have been lysed and that we have preselected obviously viable cells.

DISCUSSANT: Not only that, but a viable cell does not mean that the macrophage can perform all the functions that it should perform. The scenario that you described with cigarette smoke, and the point that Dr. McClellan was making earlier, suggest that the experiment needs to be done, because these macrophages are coming up there as a result of cigarette smoke. Then you have to ask the question, to what has the animal been exposed? Because now the macrophages are responding in a very different way. Instead of sitting around normally as they would in the alveolar space or on the alveolar duct surface, now they are primed, and they are going through a variety of changes that you have described. And then, what happens if they get into asbestos? To find the answer to this question would be a great experiment. Actually, it has been done, but the questions have not been asked of those cells.

DISCUSSANT: I do feel a bit of concern when we use the term cytotoxic for a macrophage that becomes foamy after, perhaps, several months. That development seems to be totally different from the cytotoxicity that one sees in that short a time. These foamy macrophages seem to have a cell body which is 50 times bigger than normal; they are quite enormous, they are a physical lesion, as distinct from a physiological state.

DISCUSSANT: There is a possibility of reducing foamy macrophages by the use of certain drugs. I did that, and in these macrophages the clearance of titanium dioxide was completely, absolutely stopped. Those macrophages could not take part in clearance. When you discontinue the drug shortly after inhalation of TiO, particle clearance increases again because the clearance is only temporarily blocked by the drug. And I am not sure whether new macrophages are performing the clearance or whether the old macrophages are recovering. After a certain time period, clearance is almost the same in those two groups, but at the beginning, during the first 2 or 3 weeks, clearance was absolutely stopped. Thus, even foamy macrophages might clear up, but our findings indicate that those macrophages are not functioning, at least not for clearance.

DISCUSSANT: I just want to point out that Dr. Kagan's point about chemotactic factors in these macrophages is a very interesting one. It turns out that the growth factors, particularly platelet-derived growth factor and transforming growth factors beta, are very potent chemotactic factors for the macrophages.

DR. LANGER: The two papers by Dr. Luchtel and Dr. Boatman are now open for discussion.

DISCUSSANT: You showed some data that fascinated me. That bar graph showed the percentage of macrophages with one or more particles and the percentage of macrophages with more than five phagocytized particles. You had quite a number of macrophages with more than five aluminum oxide particles. With quartz, however, you had an increase in macrophages with particles, but few of them had phagocytized more than one quartz particle. That is how I understood your data. That may mean that one particle (i.e., quartz) is toxic to a macrophage, which therefore can no longer phagocytize, whereas with aluminum oxide the macrophage is free to phagocytize as many particles as it likes. That is an attractive idea, but this was 1 month after exposure. I would be interested in your conjecture about the general validity of that idea: how the fact that we were looking at a "snapshot" 1 month after exposure might impact on whether that idea is or is not true.

DISCUSSANT: I would agree that the quartz particle is more toxic and that the macrophage would not tend to phagocytize a lot of them. Or, if it did, it would die, and you would have to start all over with another macrophage and go from there. I don't really have any further conjecture about that.

DISCUSSANT: That is a hypothesis that could be generated from the data: macrophages can "eat" only one or two quartz particles, and then that's it. But they can "eat" many more of less noxious particles. Probably nobody would argue much with that. Yet the data at which we were looking came from 1 month after exposure. So maybe we were not looking so much at differences in phagocytosis but at differences in survival. I just wonder, do you make anything of that?

DISCUSSANT: Well, I sort of put it together with the data from the fiber-epoxy composite exposures, which were more similar to those for quartz uptake than to those for aluminum oxide uptake. In general, few of the macrophages from the rats exposed to the fiber-epoxy composites had multiple particles in them. Usually there was just one particle per macrophage. This indicated to me that these composite particles were toxic because the macrophages were responding more like those in the quartz exposure than those in the aluminum oxide exposure.

DISCUSSANT: Could the availability of particles have been a factor? I mean, we are talking as if there is an infinite number of particles available for them to work on. What I was trying to put into context is, how can we interpret that?

DISCUSSANT: If animals were exposed to respirable fractions of these various dusts—they were all on the order of, or close to, a median diameter of 1 μm—I would assume that roughly equal numbers of particles are deposited in the lung in each case.

DISCUSSANT: But that was a month ago.

DISCUSSANT: Yes.

DISCUSSANT: Last week I was told by a trustworthy fellow that the life span of a macrophage is about 30 days.

DISCUSSANT: I was going to suggest that the answer to the problem might well be turnover. If you start off with one particle that makes the macrophage sick so that it does not take up any more particles, then you choke the macrophage and it releases the first particle. The macrophage then picks up another particle and goes through this cycle one more time, a second time, a third time, etc.; something like that.

DISCUSSANT: I think one of the most important things that we have to do in phagocytosis studies is to keep the ratio the same from one study to the other and one particle to the other. Otherwise, if you upset that ratio, if the ratios are not the same, you should not expect to get the same results and a good comparison between the two.

DISCUSSANT: The ratio of what?

DISCUSSANT: The ratio of the number of particles you want to be phagocytized to the number of macrophages present.

DISCUSSANT: I am wondering whether you can tell us more about the epoxy material? We had a discussion at the coffee break regarding the epoxy. Of what did this material consist?

DISCUSSANT: I do not have any more information on the composition of these materials than what I presented in the table. The exact composition is proprietary information. The only information that we could get about their organic compounds was for those that volatilized from the material and collected under isothermal conditions. We did not do anything specific to identify the fiber types, except to look at them under the light microscope. There was an opaque type of fiber which seemed to be the carbon fiber or graphite fiber, and then there were these clear fibers, which we assumed to be fiber glass. There was also a very small proportion of very thin fibers. In general, both the fiber glass and the carbon fibers were fairly thick, on the order of 7 to 10 μm in diameter, but we also saw these very thin ones. We do not know the specific identity of those very thin fibers. We did not characterize them, other than just looking at them under the light microscope.

DISCUSSANT: What is the abrasive used on those cutting devices? Diamond dust?

DISCUSSANT: I guess it depends on exactly what kind of operation it is. I am not sure that you need to have an abrasive for all of those operations, like a particular cutting or sawing operation. I was not present when they did the machine operations on them. We had an industrial hygienist who collected them, and I do not know what kinds of abrasive may have been used.

DISCUSSANT: Did you show some data for the compounds? Did you burn these materials, or some of these materials?

DISCUSSANT: I really do not know that much about it. That work was done by Dr. David Kalman, an analytical chemist in our laboratory. It is a method of heating the material, eluting the organics, and then identifying them.

DISCUSSANT: There are data coming out of Canada on these plastic-type materials, according to which cyanide gas is formed at combustion. Did you find anything like that?

DISCUSSANT: No.

DISCUSSANT: Did you look for low-molecular-weight products?

DISCUSSANT: No, not to my knowledge.

DISCUSSANT: There are several things that are important in these kinds of situations, depending on what you are cutting, or grinding, or routing, and how you are doing it. You may perform these procedures dry, or you may do them wet. In addition, the geometry of the cutting tool markedly affects particle size. It also depends on what you are doing and how you are doing it, because the surface oftentimes is resin-rich. Therefore, one has to be very careful in identifying what the off-gassing in a particular situation would be.

DISCUSSANT: That is why I am asking whether it is a fair comparison. What happens if you have a table listing components of these things, and your rug catches fire, or something like this? Nowadays, a lot of these exotic plastics are being used in just about everything.

DISCUSSANT: In some ways, the findings were very similar to what I have seen in a variety of reinforced plastic applications. The refined fiber was interesting because some of the agents to keep the resin from separating can be an asbestos material. While you cannot find it when you sample the air, the question stuck in my mind, was there nevertheless some of this material present? Was there enough of it that, when you administer it intratracheally, you would see interstitial fibrosis?

DISCUSSANT: This is one of the problems of substituting for asbestos. The substitute materials are very good at forming what we call a "green mold," when you are first trying to get the materials to stick together to create some type of composite material. With the "good" material, everything sticks to it, and you are not able to work with it.

DISCUSSANT: Well, ordinarily you do not do that with fiberglass-reinforced plastic, but you can use an asbestos as a fixotropic agent. The other question I had was with regard to a silica filler. In some plastics, it is not uncommon to have a precrystalline silica filler. That could raise a question, because you can get enough of this material airborne when you work with a filled plastic. We have to watch that, from the standpoint of just plain, old-fashioned silicosis.

DISCUSSANT: How stable are these epoxy fillers? Do they break down or just stay there?

DISCUSSANT: Apparently, they are stable, because we readily see these particulates after a month in the lungs. I want to clarify one point that you made. Isothermal desorption is done at 250°C. There is not any kind of ignition process there; it is just heating and then measuring the gases as they come off.

DISCUSSANT: Why was there such a big weight difference between the animals that you treated with the aluminum oxide and the animals treated with the composite materials?

DISCUSSANT: I don't know; that was very surprising to us. We did not expect any weight difference.

DISCUSSANT: I was wondering whether it may have something to do with the nutrition, or maybe with the animals being used. What was the weight at the beginning of the exposures?

DISCUSSANT: They were all approximately 200 g to start with.

DISCUSSANT: And they did not gain weight?

DISCUSSANT: No, they did not gain weight as well as the controls. Both the saline control and the aluminum oxide control were approximately 400 g; they roughly doubled in weight during the experiment. By comparison, the groups exposed to the composite materials or to quartz had mean body weights between 300 and 350 g.

DISCUSSANT: There is a tremendous weight difference.

DISCUSSANT: A relatively nonspecific stress on a continuing basis has this effect. In virtually all the long-term tobacco-smoking experiments, the smoke-exposed animals gained much less weight than the controls. It is a relatively common nonspecific response to certain types of stress. In inhalation studies, for example, the animals are put in a chamber for 6 hours, and they do not get any food while they are in there. When you compare the results, you will see differences in weight between untreated controls, sham-exposed controls, and the exposed animals. If the material has a smell or taste that is unpleasant to the animals, you have another confounding variable. There are many alternative explanations for these weight differences, but they are very consistent across each of the groups. I would guess that it is a general artefact in the system, which is somehow giving rise to something which the animals perceive as stress. I would not have thought it was a specific response.

DISCUSSANT: Did you measure the feed consumption during this study?

DISCUSSANT: No. We started with all the animals at the same weight, and we observed that the composite groups did not gain weight at the same rate as the controls.

DISCUSSANT: What about quartz?

DISCUSSANT: The quartz-exposed and the composite-exposed groups were similar in their lack of weight gain compared to the saline and aluminum oxide control groups.

DR. LANGER: Now we will proceed to Dr. Johnson's paper.

DISCUSSANT: You mentioned that you looked at the erionite samples. You recovered the erionite from the lungs and then did an elemental analysis. Did you also look at their particle size to see whether they were bigger?

DISCUSSANT: Not yet, no.

DISCUSSANT: Because erionite is very fragile, I would suspect that the fibers may be split in the lungs. The average diameter of the erionite fibers in the lungs may then be smaller than the diameter of the airborne fibers before inhalation and deposition in the lungs.

DISCUSSANT: That is possible. We are progressing with the findings.

DISCUSSANT: We notice that very strikingly with the fibers of actinolite. Actually, what you are effectively getting through this process is a larger dose in the lungs.

DISCUSSANT: I have a question about the diagnostic criteria for mesothelioma. You showed some very impressive lesions, but you also showed some very unimpressive lesions. And I wondered what are your in-house rules, your rules for saying something is a mesothelioma and something is not? You showed in one of your early slides a trivial lesion under the pleura, such as I see many times in untreated control animals as they get older. This is a rather crucial point, because for many types of neoplasm there is a hyperplastic precursor, and pathologists have argued for years where the borderline is between hyperplasia and tumor. One of those lesions that you showed I thought was a mesothelioma, but about the other two, I wondered, on the basis of that evidence. With reference to that point, in experiments that we did with mice—with amosite, particularly—we got mesotheliomas. Most of those mesotheliomas were really only mesothelial tissue that was papilliferous, metastasizing all over the place. There were some of the fibrous kind, but the ones that you illustrated, what were they?

DISCUSSANT: I demonstrated two epitheliomas, and one sarcomatous tumor.

DISCUSSANT: What you described as an epithelial variety certainly did not look like it to me. I am not a rat mesotheliologist, but, certainly from the standpoint of human pathology, that lesion looked like a typical spindle-cell type. It looked not at all like the lesion that Dr. Palekar showed with her cell lines. Again, comparing the lesions with those induced in humans, I also thought that what you showed as a very focal nodular lesion looked to me, in many respects, analogous to a localized fibrosarcomatous lesion that you see in humans, especially because it was on the visceral pleura. You also showed a lot of fibroblasts in some of the earlier lesions. I wondered whether this was not just the next, excessive stage of whatever factors were involved in fibroblast proliferation, using a localized neoplastic lesion.

DISCUSSANT: I accept that. But I did show epithelial lesions, using electron microscopy.

DISCUSSANT: I was going to say roughly the same thing. I think from the slides shown, it is very difficult, if that was the only evidence, to say positively that these are mesotheliomas as distinct from vigorous pleural reaction. But, of course, your follow-up, part of the same study, was 100%. So I have no difficulty in accepting these, for that reason alone, as mesotheliomas. In terms of these tumors, one had grade 2, and I think that is evidence in that one case, and the other tumor had multiple focal tumors. The epithelial ones tend to be very discrete and well-delineated, whereas the primary sarcomatous ones tend to be slightly more diffuse focally over more than one area.

DISCUSSANT: What percent of the total tumors in your study were epithelial or sarcomatous, or both?

DISCUSSANT: In the one I presented here, or in the one that Dr. Wagner and I did previously?

DISCUSSANT: Both.

DISCUSSANT: Erionite-induced tumors generally tend to be more sarcomatous. The chrysotile-induced tumors that we have seen before tend to be slightly more epithelial.

DISCUSSANT: The cells that killed the rat were very similar to those focal proliferations. When we saw hyperplasia, certainly in the area of that one, it was superimposed on a fibrous sort of plaque. It was one or two cellular layers deep, and the cells were very loosely organized—basal cell tumors. It was very cellular and very well organized.

DISCUSSANT: Where we saw hyperplasia, it was diffuse, one or two cell layers deep but not very well organized. The tumors were very distinct and distinctly similar.

DISCUSSANT: Why did the animals die? From the severity of the lesion?

DISCUSSANT: They were sick and could not breathe; therefore we killed them for humanitarian reasons and necropsied them.

DISCUSSANT: So they did not have asbestosis or mesothelioma? Was fibrosis part of the picture that killed them?

DISCUSSANT: No. The fibrosis—

DISCUSSANT: Part of the reason you killed them was because they were sick, or was it purely related to the tumor?

DISCUSSANT: I think the fibrosis was between a score of 3 and 4 in severity. In the rats examined by Dr. Johnson, the fibrosis score was also between 3 and 4, on average. The erionite-exposed rats had a very similar score to those exposed to crocidolite. I do not believe that fibrosis was the major complication. The tumors were so extensive in the pleural cavity that at least one lesion had broken through to the peritoneal cavity. These were large, spreading tumors, and most of our rats looked very ill.

DISCUSSANT: Because of the importance attached to the finding of mesothelioma in humans, this is determined by litigation here in the United States. There must be half a dozen stains used to distinguish mesothelioma from other tumor types.

DISCUSSANT: Is this type of staining ever done on a routine basis in animals? You have mucin stains, hyaluronic acid stains, keratin stains, and all those other stains. What is the routine staining procedure in animals to distinguish these tumors from other tumors?

DISCUSSANT: There are stains with hyaluronic acid which are used by Dr. Wagner quite frequently. For these rats that Dr. Wagner used, it was mainly H&E. That was his usual way of diagnosing them, and he used conventional criteria of pattern recognition.

DISCUSSANT: You have got to check all the tumors by serial dissection, or how do you know what percent of them are mesotheliomas? Sometimes 30% of them, and perhaps half of the carcinomas, are invading the pleural cavity. If you do proper histology you see that they are metastasized lesions within the lung tissue.

DISCUSSANT: Do you have the same confusion with adenocarcinoma as with mesothelioma?

DISCUSSANT: I don't think it is a confusion, because the pattern of adenocarcinomas in rats is very characteristic.

DISCUSSANT: Could we ask Dr. Coffin to comment on his diagnostic criteria because he is producing mesotheliomas?

DISCUSSANT: I am not a pathologist who looks at the slides, but I have often listened to the discussions of these specialists, and I think sometimes there is some confusion about the diagnosis. Therefore my question is, when you show your slides to some other pathologists, are you sure that no one would find carcinomas?

DISCUSSANT: In the older experiments, the slides had been shown to about five different authorities. Dr. Wagner was thrilled by these carcinomas, and there was very little evidence of malignant change in the nonepithelial cells.

DISCUSSANT: Bronchiolar—

DISCUSSANT: —bronchioloalveolar hyperplasia—and then the tumor formation. I do not know whether the animals tend to die very early, before the possibility of developing carcinoma. On the other hand, these tumors were primarily on the pleura, and they did not migrate into the lung tissue. There was no evidence in any of these tumors of extension into the lung tissue.

DISCUSSANT: Obviously, a lot of these tumors originate on visceral pleura—

DISCUSSANT: Not in my animals, but I do not remember that. I think there were some in the original experiment. I would have to go back and look, but as you say, they were predominantly visceral.

DISCUSSANT: You mentioned the number of particles and fibers and certain dimensions. These dimensions have basically been established by intraperitoneal inoculation. Very few tumors have ever been induced by inhalation. Do you believe now, from the process that you have done, that possibly those are not the right dimensions for optimal mesothelioma induction by inhalation?

DISCUSSANT: No, I am still a strong believer in Stanton's dimensions. I think his test picks up those fiber dimensions. It does not pick up other parameters, like surface properties. I think it is a good test for fiber-size-related lesions, which are usually mesotheliomas. However, it does not tell you anything about surface chemistry.

DISCUSSANT: With regard to Dr. Stanton's work, we have to remember with what he was working when he developed his classic theory. The other day, we talked about the so-called Stanton fiber and the fact that the material on which Stanton developed his thesis had a rather wide variety of fibers, both in length and diameter. It was a statistical rendering that identified the most probable fiber size to cause mesothelioma. In a number of discussions with Dr. Stanton, he often said, "I can't really tell; it is around 1 μm or less in diameter and about 60 μm long." It seems to be based on the experiments that they were conducting. Now that does not necessarily come through in the paper that he wrote. I want to pitch this out for information, having known the fellow who supplied it.

DISCUSSANT: Well, we want to know the material that produces 100% mesothelioma by inhalation, and there is nothing that would have made us guess when we looked at erionite. Nobody looked at erionite and said, this a hot new fiber. We are using new fibers in society; we are constantly introducing new materials, and I don't know whether we are going to be interested in what kind of surprises the new materials will present. People who are going to change to new materials do not know whether these new materials may be worse than the ones that they are replacing.

DISCUSSANT: The data that were presented at the Montreal meeting showed that erionite and crocidolite were just about indistinguishable by size distribution, but the number of tumors induced by inhalation were very different.

DISCUSSANT: That does not mean to say that size is not important.

DISCUSSANT: There were two erionites, I know, in use: a commercial one that was made from the same chemistry—and one from New Zealand, which was of similar composition.

DISCUSSANT: The really important experiment now is to determine whether it is the short or the long erionite fibers which cause 100% tumors. You have got to determine the correct dimensions.

DISCUSSANT: Well, I think that whatever that is may have something to do with the induction of fibrosis, and I half-suspect that they are linked in some way.

DISCUSSANT: Just a few remarks about the pathology of mesothelioma. We intended to present a pathology paper in this session, but Dr. Sagartz did not have enough time to prepare it, so we withdrew it. That paper would have described our intratracheal studies; the mesotheliomas are induced by the intratracheal injection. We have not counted them, we are doing it blindly at this point. Our criterion for a mesothelioma, especially the fibrous ones, is whether or not it invades other tissues and spreads. Because we let our animals die spontaneously or kill them in the moribund stage, we do not find too many small tumors, except in those animals that died of pneumothorax. There we do find small tumors. We find that the erionite tumors differ from the asbestos tumors in that they seem to arrive *de novo* from the pleura. We see some that are kind of pleural in their origin, and we see some that are pedunculated and which appear to be derived from the submesothelial tissues. They are surrounded by a columnar epithelium which is more or less contiguous with the mesothelium, and they frequently have acini in the center, and connective tissue. Further tumor development now can go either way: (a) the connective tissue can take over and the tumors develop, go into a mesenchymal type and spread, and they can invade the lung—not truly the lung tissue, but the septa; or (b) they can develop into epithelial tumors and you have a tubulopapillary tumor. Now, this is one type of tumor we see. In addition, we see another type which is papilla-like in the beginning, all the way down, a great, high papillary tumor, spreading. Then again, we see a third type which we call a highly vacuolated mesothelioma. It looks rather innocuous when you look at it, but it is very malignant, it spreads fast, and it can be either mesenchymal or tubulopapillary.

I believe that the one that Dr. Johnson showed was a small, submesenchymal fibrosis. I do not believe he intended to imply that this was a genuine mesothelioma. You probably had tumors elsewhere in that particular case, but I think you are going to be a little hard-pressed to call that a mesothelioma just on its own. In that case, I don't think we have too many problems with lesions induced by erionite. The problems comes with chrysotile, where you have so much granuloma, and to distinguish the granuloma from a mesenchymal tumor, this is my problem.

DISCUSSANT: We do not get any granulomas, because we do not inject intrapleurally.

DISCUSSANT: These are by inhalation, so—

DISCUSSANT: Yes. Well, we don't see them with erionite, either.

DISCUSSANT: Does anybody know something about the durability and the capability of the splitting of erionite in the body?

DISCUSSANT: I do not think it happens.

DISCUSSANT: Why do you think it does not happen?

DISCUSSANT: I think that the erionite fiber that you see is an ultimate fiber. I don't think that it breaks down like chrysotile, which is composed of fibrils. Chrysotile does not break down further than to the stage of fibrils.

DISCUSSANT: What about the dissolution?

DISCUSSANT: That is a different story. When you look at zeolite particles recovered from tissues, it is almost impossible to obtain a selected area diffraction on these materials because they are being damaged. They explode, and the structure disintegrates.

DISCUSSANT: When we look at the crocidolite and chrysotile in lungs in our pathology slides, we have no problem seeing the fibers, but we can hardly see erionite fibers.

DISCUSSANT: We see them, but they are small.

DISCUSSANT: Very small.

DISCUSSANT: How are you looking at this, by SEM?

DISCUSSANT: No. By light microscopy.

DISCUSSANT: That is very, very difficult. One of the questions that I had to ask you is whether some of these erionite particles were not contaminated with mordenite, because some of those very large fibers look more like mordenite than erionite.

DISCUSSANT: We did not see any large fibers with erionite.

DISCUSSANT: Well, in one of your studies, there was a very thin erionite fiber and a very large one. We did not observe any very wide or very long erionite fibers. When you inject the material into the pleural cavity, you see a lot of big crocidolite, but it is only a very small percentage of the total, so they stand out.

DISCUSSANT: We saw some coarse fibers like that in our sample, but the analysis identified it as erionite.

DISCUSSANT: Did you do any lung-burden studies?

DISCUSSANT: We are in the process of doing one. Preliminary results suggest the burden to be about half a million fibers per gram of dry tissue.

DISCUSSANT: Why did you use intrapleural injection, in view of the fact that intraperitoneal injection is a much more sensitive test?

DISCUSSANT: Well, first of all, I think that Dr. Wagner was using intrapleural injection in his erionite study, and we had to ask ourselves whether or not we wanted to duplicate his work, because we are using the same material. We also find that the intrapleural space is a lot simpler to deal with than the peritoneal space, because there are fewer complications there, and we don't have all these walls and intestines to contend with. The intrapleural space is a pretty clean system, that is why we used it. We did not know whether some increase in sensitivity in the intraperitoneal test system would give us that much of an advantage over the intrapleural test if we assume that it is 10% or 20% more sensitive.

DISCUSSANT: Oh no, I think the difference is much larger.

DISCUSSANT: You also injected smaller amounts of about 0.5 mg, but you show that there are only results for 16 mg, if I understood you correctly?

DISCUSSANT: No, we had dose responses from 0.5 up to 32 mg; we had effects at the lower dose ranges. I do not disagree with you; both you and Dr. Davis obtained very good results with the intraperitoneal test. But we have been using the intrapleural test, which has also been used by many other investigators. We started with it, and I guess maybe we are stuck with it. We can reproduce the differences with it, and we get dose responses. And certainly with the erionite, our problem is not to get increased sensitivity but less sensitivity. We got down to the 0.5-mg level, and we got practically 100% tumors. We had a flat response with that, so we would probably have to go on down several orders of magnitude below that to get the proper dose responses. I agree with you that the intraperitoneal injection is more sensitive, I guess because you have a greater amount of epithelial tissue to deal with. But we are of the opinion that we do not need the increased sensitivity in our situation.

DISCUSSANT: Do you believe that you get more false positives because the peritoneal test is more sensitive?

DISCUSSANT: No.

DISCUSSANT: What is the advantage of using one over the other?

DISCUSSANT: I think that we have two points of consideration. One is that the pleural cavity is the site in which we are interested. On the other hand, intraperitoneal injections pose no problem at all, the test is more sensitive, and you can spot the tumor earlier than in the pleural cavity. The point is that either one is a pretty artificial technique. Once you have accepted that, I don't think it matters which one you use.

DISCUSSANT: I am not sure I am getting past the first question. My first argument for the interperitoneal application—about 20 years ago—was that it is possible to inject a higher dose. When you inject 10 mg or more intrapleurally, I think you will have some lumps, and you cannot expect an exact dose-response relationship. We have injected a lot of dusts in higher quantities, 100 mg perhaps, which showed no positive effects after the injection. This model is so sensitive that a substance which has no positive effect after intraperitoneal injection of a high dose probably poses no risk, and therefore does not need to be regulated. I think that this is an important argument for this practice. The model is sensitive, and up to now we have no arguments regarding false-negative results.

DISCUSSANT: It is not so much the false-negative results, it is the false-positive results that may be troublesome. It is so sensitive that it reflects any biological activity.

DISCUSSANT: Please tell me an example of a wrong positive result.

DISCUSSANT: I think we have the wrong model for investigating the biological effects of glass fibers. It is not possible to administer a dose of glass fibers which is high enough to induce tumors. In the experiments which were done, the number of man-made mineral fibers was much lower in comparison with the number of crocidolite fibers to which the animals were exposed. The tumor rate in the lungs of rats after exposure to crocidolite was very low, less than 10%. Consequently, when you have a fiber which has only a fraction of the carcinogenic potency of crocidolite you cannot expect positive results. I therefore think it is a wrong model, because we all know that crocidolite is a very strong carcinogen in man. But after exposure of rats to a very high dose of crocidolite, only a very low tumor rate was observed.

DISCUSSANT: I don't know to which type of tumors you are referring. I would like to interject here that we exposed hamsters chronically by inhalation to 23 mg/m^3 chrysotile asbestos, and we saw a substantial number of tumors which, however, were not malignant; they were benign lung adenomas. Nevertheless, we did manage to produce a significant amount of tumors, some of them malignant, by inhalation.

DISCUSSANT: Dr. Coffin, it is the crocidolite that causes the problem. There are five studies with crocidolite which did not show a significant tumor rate, and this is the difficulty.

DISCUSSANT: I think here, in general, is one of the bad points about the UICC samples. The amphibole produced samples with fibers that were too short; we have the evidence. We have administered UICC preparations of amosite by inhalation and observed tumors only very, very rarely. Doing the same experiment with a much longer fiber preparation, we get 25% tumors. I don't think it is the crocidolite that has proved unsuccessful in experimental animals, I think it is that one sample. I would love to use a raw crocidolite sample in an experiment with animals, using generation techniques that would really result in long fibers. It has not been done.

DISCUSSANT: No. We had another experiment with longer fibers that was carried out by Dr. Muhle, and there was also a very low effect. I think there is a large difference between rats and man. The fibers do not persist long enough in rats, and therefore we underestimate the carcinogenic potency of fibers based on results from inhalation experiments in rats. By injection we can administer a high amount in 1 minute at the starting point of the experiment, and we see the tumors after 2 or 2½ years. When we expose the animals to the dust by inhalation, it takes at least half a year until the essential amount of dust has accumulated in the lungs to produce a tumor. We don't have this time in the animal toxicity experiments.

DISCUSSANT: You have already given me a partial explanation, but I am having a lot of trouble tracking the conversation here. It seemed that most of it was addressing a test system for determining tumorigenicity of materials, independent of the route of delivery of the material. I come from a perspective where, ultimately, risk modeling is most important. It seems to me that the inhalation route is the most important way. And then, it could be that the rat is not the right model, because you can't keep the material in the lung long enough. The problem is extrapolating from that situation to man.

DISCUSSANT: I think that fibers are not "normal" carcinogens, and this is the difference. I think we cannot extrapolate conclusions which we draw from experiments with, for example, diesel exhaust, to the fiber problem. Because with fibers we have additional factors which are very important, namely the persistence of the fibers in the lungs and their variation in size. The biological effects of some agents happen in seconds, but in fibers they need many years.

DISCUSSANT: My position in this is that I accept that there is a place for the intraperitoneal or intrapleural injection tests, but when it comes to trying to relate this to human risk, I think you cannot possibly use it or rely on it. For one thing, it is clearly a relatively unquantified test for the various reasons that Dr. Pott has outlined. And you cannot use an unquantified test in predicting carcinogenic risk.

It is a general principle of toxicology that you do have to try to use a realistic route of administration. There may be exceptions to this, but they have got to be spelled out before you depart from that principle. So as a preliminary screening test, yes, by all means use intraperitoneal and intrapleural tests, but in the end, you have got to do an inhalation study. And if there is a discrepancy between your intrapleural and interperitoneal results and your inhalation results, surely you have to spend some time asking why.

But I would have thought there was perfectly adequate information in the literature that you can produce tumors with crocidolite. I just don't think that it is justifiable to use crocidolite as a reason to use an intrapleural or intraperitoneal test. One should not think, or even contemplate, judging human risk on the basis of an unrealistic administration. That is my position.

DISCUSSANT: My experiment was with crocidolite, and I think the one who chose it was Dr. Wagner in 1974. But in the study with erionite, which he published in '82 or in '83, he also used crocidolite. And he did not, or could not, show tumors at the same concentration as before. In other words, he could not reproduce the results of his own study. This is the only one I know in which this happened. I think that we are taking the attitude that the results were not conclusive. I think that the animals were of the same age as the erionite-exposed animals.

DISCUSSANT: Perhaps that is the explanation.

DISCUSSANT: Crocidolite takes longer to induce tumors.

DISCUSSANT: I am not sure, but I think there was an age comparison, and the erionite animals died early, so you would not expect any lung carcinomas.

DISCUSSANT: Did Dr. Wagner kill the crocidolite animals at the same time?

DISCUSSANT: I don't know, but I believe they were of similar age; I think he killed the control rats at 18 months.

DISCUSSANT: I have a question for Dr. Roe. Do you accept that a fiber is the carcinogenic agent? If not, what additional data do you want to convince you that a fiber which is long enough and thin enough, and which is durable—that such a fiber is carcinogenic?

DISCUSSANT: I accept that some fibers have been shown to cause cancer, and therefore it is justifiable to regard them as carcinogenic. However, simply to conclude that an agent is a carcinogen is not necessarily very helpful.

Let me explain what I mean. I have produced malignant cancers by feeding lactose to rats. It is therefore just as correct to conclude that lactose is a carcinogen as it is to conclude that asbestos is a carcinogen. However, merely to find a way of demonstrating that something is carcinogenic, irrespective of how unrealistic the situation may be, does not make much sense to me. In my lactose experiments, the rats were fed 20% lactose over a long period, which is unrealistic. That is why I maintain that just to say something is, qualitatively, carcinogenic is a reasonably useless piece of information. Cancer has been produced simply by injecting distilled water subcutaneously into rats, and also by injecting aqueous glucose if the osmotic pressure is not close to physiological. There is no great merit in such studies. If you put fibers directly into the peritoneal cavity or pleural space, and get tumors, you have achieved carcinogenesis. But you have not shown that under realistic conditions of exposure, e.g., by inhalation, there is any carcinogenic risk. On the other hand, it is not without interest that some materials introduced directly into, say, the pleural space induce tumors and others do not. An insight into why some substances do and some do not might be useful in understanding the mechanism. One of the points I wish to emphasize is that the mere production of a tumor by putting something in an animal by an unrealistic route is of very dubious relevance to testing for a carcinogenic hazard.

DISCUSSANT: If you have a fiber which is only about 10% as carcinogenic as crocidolite when injected intrapleurally, you cannot reasonably expect a positive effect in an inhalation experiment. The question is, do you think that the risk which is presented by this fiber to man is an acceptable risk?

DISCUSSANT: I think you have to do the right experiment, with a realistic route of exposure and a realistic exposure dose to find out. One can produce a high incidence of tumors with 20% lactose, but I am still drinking milk, which has a much lower concentration of lactose.

DISCUSSANT: It is a very difficult problem. But largely I would side with Dr. Roe that, in the real world, you have got to make a judgment about whether a material that you have identified as a potential hazard to animals has an effect on human beings. Extrapolating to man from tumor experiments in animals is risky in any case, even if you get tumors by administering the materials by a realistic route. If you cannot do that, then I think you are on very shaky ground indeed. It is especially difficult to interpret weak or borderline results. But it should be possible to detect significiant carcinogenic potential under realistic conditions of exposure if enough trouble is taken to perfect the methodology of both exposure and evaluation.

DISCUSSANT: You will probably have to use more animals and higher doses.

DISCUSSANT: One of the things that I think might be helpful is to define the question that you are trying to answer. One question is: Is the material, and we have been talking about fiber glass, is it under any circumstance a carcinogen? That is one question. Another question is: Is it a carcinogen under circumstances in which it is likely to be used or misused?

In my view, it is essential to relate one's findings to lung loading. One of the problems that always comes up is to be able to generate an aerosol in the laboratory that is respirable by the rodent on a consistent basis over a long enough period of time. Can one get enough test material into the lower respiratory tract and keep it there long enough to produce tumors? A French investigator, whose name escapes me, achieved a lung loading with glass fibers of something like 6 x 10^6 fibers per gram of dry lung weight. The study in lung loading conducted at Los Alamos was, I believe, around 2 x 10^6 mg/g of dry lung weight. This would suggest that these investigators were able to deposit a large number of fibers in the animals' lungs—many, many more than one would see in humans from a workplace environment, where we are quibbling over whether we are seeing fibers in the second, third or first decimal place.

DISCUSSANT: Which work environment is that? Manufacturing environment?

DISCUSSANT: I am talking about both the manufacturing environment and the user environment.

DISCUSSANT: Just one more point, and that concerns the Ames test. This is a fairly crude exercise in the sense that they have tested compounds in various animal systems over reasonable lengths of time. Where there is a tumor yield, they have not been particular about the route of administration that was used, as far as I can remember. For any one substance, there might be a variation in dose by one or, possibly, two orders of magnitude, for which you get a 50% tumor yield. This goes across species, across laboratories, and across all sorts of substances. So I think that one has to understand that one's animal model, even if it is a realistic model, has maybe a tenfold variation in sensitivity and rarely more than that. But when you are looking at laboratory evidence, where you have got a factor of 10^6, then you really are wasting your time to do any more toxicology on those animals. I think if you have done a study with an unrealistic route of administration, then you surely have an obligation to go back and look at it by a realistic route of administration. If you really have done this, and you have gone way beyond a 100-fold difference in model sensitivity, and you are still getting absolutely nothing, you can probably rely on your earlier results as being misleading. That is a sort of general principle. Certainly if you have got a thousandfold, ten-thousandfold, a hundred-thousandfold difference in exposure concentrations, then you would certainly be wasting your time to carry out further tests.

DISCUSSANT: I was just wondering about the general validity of the intraperitoneal and the intrapleural injections. It is pretty well established that they are sensitive tests, but what about their specificity? How specific is it in showing a noncarcinogenic fiber to be noncarcinogenic? In other words, do you ever get a negative result with the intrapleural or intraperitoneal injections?

DISCUSSANT: Well, only with a few very big fibers, only with a few fiber samples with dimensions that are really enormous. I don't know of any what I would call "normal" fibers as being negative in those tests.

DISCUSSANT: You were just talking about false positives. I know one false-positive case, and that is the ability to induce mesothelioma in laboratory animals with anthophyllite, which does not cause any human mesotheliomas. I think that would be a false positive, because among the Finnish anthophyllite workers there is not a single case of mesothelioma. But anthophyllite can and does produce mesotheliomas in laboratory animals following exposure by the intraperitoneal, intrapleural, or intratracheal routes.

DISCUSSANT: From where did you get the attapulgite sample? Was that provided by one of the mining companies?

DISCUSSANT: Yes. From the Angle Bar.

DISCUSSANT: Did they prepare this material for you?

DISCUSSANT: Yes, they did.

DISCUSSANT: Was it heated?

DISCUSSANT: I don't know how they prepared it.

DISCUSSANT: Did you ask them?

DISCUSSANT: I don't think that they picked out all the long fibers, if that is what you mean.

DISCUSSANT: No, we are not saying that. Did they anneal it? Did they heat it?

DISCUSSANT: Well, maybe they did; I don't know.

DR. LANGER: Let us proceed now to Dr. Palekar's paper.

DISCUSSANT: You have looked at one type of cell, the V79. Would you not want to look at the chromosome aberrations in other types of cells before being able to conclude whether you are getting a true carcinogenic effect?

DISCUSSANT: We are also looking at mesothelial cells from Fischer-344 rats. We did not present the data here because the experiments are incomplete. We have two cell lines; one we bought commercially, and the other one we established in our own laboratory. We are looking at two end points, cytotoxicity and chromosomal changes. We have observed chromosmal aberrations and changes in chromosome numbers in the cells exposed to mineral fibers.

DISCUSSANT: What about the test cells which are commonly used, such as human lymphocytes, and Chinese hamster ovary cells?

DISCUSSANT: In our laboratory we have examined various other cell types such as sheep erythrocytes, rabbit alveolar macrophages, and Chinese hamster ovary cells, in addition to the V79 cell line. We tried to correlate hemolysis or cytotoxicity with tumorigenesis of mineral fibers. Our data indicate that in the V79 cytotoxicity assay there was a correlation between tumorigenesis and cytotoxicity. We did not observe this with other cell lines.

DISCUSSANT: What is the origin of V79 cells?

DISCUSSANT: The line is derived from the Chinese hamster lung.

DISCUSSANT: They are not tumor cells, though?

DISCUSSANT: No. They are not tumor cells.

DISCUSSANT: Are you troubled by the observation that there is no correlation between the erionite, chrysotile, crocidolite, and the cytogenetic changes that you see in the cells?

DISCUSSANT: Well, I was at first. One of the aspects at which we have been looking in our laboratory, because we have a contract with EPA, is developing some short-term, predictive bioassays. We are constantly looking for correlations. We have a very good animal model in our laboratory. Our *in vivo* studies showed that erionite was much more tumorigenic than chrysotile and crocidolite. So when we looked at cytotoxicity studies and also at cytogenetic studies, we were disturbed that we did not observe similar correlations in them.

We realized that these correlations were made per mass dose. Because a fiber is an etiological factor, or at least a very important factor in cellular—or biological—interaction, we decided to look at the *number* of fibers per sample and to correlate our results not just per mass dose, but also per dose in number of fibers. Our correlation then turned out to be very good with cytogenetic studies and also with cytotoxicity studies. There are fewer erionite fibers than crocidolite fibers per equivalent mass dose. The chrysotile and crocidolite samples were UICC samples, and the number of fibers we reported correlate very well with those reported by Timbrell a long time ago for the UICC samples. We therefore have a good reason to believe that the number of fibers we reported in the erionite sample is accurate.

DISCUSSANT: Based on those observations, do you believe that the Stanton hypothesis is oversimplified, based on dimensions or surface properties?

DISCUSSANT: There are many factors here that we have to consider. It is not that simple. Stanton took one type of fiber glass and looked at the various size distributions. In his experiment, the variability was minimal, whereas we are looking at chrysotile, crocidolite, and erionite, three different types of fibers. We cannot simplify and just say that it is only the size that is responsible for biological effects. There are other factors that have to be considered, such as number of fibers, surface characteristics, surface area, etc.

Erionite appears to be much more reactive, showing higher tumorigenesis, cytotoxicity or cytogenetic changes, than those observed with asbestos, when the mass dose is converted to the dose in number of fibers.

DISCUSSANT: What is the mechanism by which the presence of a fiber might damage chromosomes?

DISCUSSANT: Dr. Kagan asked me a similar question earlier. His question was whether I can identify a mineral fiber as an initiator or as a promoter. It is not as easy as in skin carcinogenesis, where there is experimental evidence showing that you need an initiator and a promoter. Here we find a different ball game.

The mechanism of mineral fiber tumorigenesis is poorly understood. Some people believe that the asbestos fibers followed by abnormal growth may be the cause. Others believe that asbestos is a promoter. There is no evidence suggesting that asbestos is mutagenic. However it does induce chromosomal aberrations and aneuploidy. Thus it has also been speculated that asbestos interacts with microtubules or other cytoskeletal proteins active during division. We have found numerous chromosomal changes in the cells exposed *in vitro* to mineral fibers and also in the cell lines derived from tumors induced with mineral fibers. Out of 13 cell lines examined, 10 had chromosome #1 abnormality. The significance of this cannot be judged at this time; however, I would like to mention that the *Ha-ras* oncogene is known to be located on rat chromosome #1.

DISCUSSANT: If it is the mechanical interaction of the cell with the fiber, then, if I understand correctly, that means that the aneuploid cell was in contact with the fiber at the time of division? Is a physical contact between that cell and any fiber necessary at that time?

DISCUSSANT: The observations made with electron microscopy and scanning electron microscopy have shown that the fibers penetrating the cell sometimes can be in contact with the nucleus. At this time we do not know whether this contact is necessary. It is not yet known how many cells are needed to induce a tumor; maybe it is just one cell. There is contact, but we do not yet know whether that is necessary.

DISCUSSANT: I was just wondering whether there is any way that you could extrapolate, from the numbers of cells that you have in culture and the numbers and dimensions of fibers, whether or not there could have been a contact.

DISCUSSANT: Well, it would be difficult, but as I showed earlier, erionite was least reactive, and chrysotile was the most reactive per mass dose. When we examined anaphases, we observed that there was missegregation at all dose levels of chrysotile, whereas the percent of missegregations was minimal for erionite and crocidolite. Just looking at these data, it appears that, yes, probably because chrysotile has many more fibers per mass dose, we saw these changes.

DISCUSSANT: Have you tried any experiments in which you used condensate products on asbestos?

DISCUSSANT: No, I have not.

DISCUSSANT: Now we have the last paper, by myself and Dr. Nolan, Inorganic Particles in Cigarettes and Cigarette Smoke. Any questions?

DISCUSSANT: You talked about the composition of ash, but unless I missed it, you did not talk about the materials coming through the cigarette that might be inhaled.

DISCUSSANT: That part of it was not presented. We had a smoking machine and collected condensate on filters, and we had to ash the filters and redisperse the materials. We do see some of the salts, we do see an occasional clay—silica particles, very small quantities, in the submicrogram range—that is just what comes through in an unfiltered cigarette; not very much.

DISCUSSANT: Is that where the kaolinite comes from?

DISCUSSANT: I do not know how in the world they saw so much kaolinite. I just do not understand that experiment. It is reported in the literature; it is obviously an observation, but I do not understand it. I cannot explain it on the basis of my own work.

DISCUSSANT: Kaolinite is an aluminum silicate; it is a very common clay mineral in the southern part of the U.S.

DISCUSSANT: Tobacco stalks are very sticky. If you harvest the crop on a very dry day and you have a lot of dust, you can incorporate a lot of soil particles. In fact, some farmers like that, because they get paid by the weight of the tobacco, so they wait for a very dry day to harvest tobacco because they make more money. It is a very difficult material to get off.

DISCUSSANT: The reason for my asking is that we have looked at particles that we get from research cigarettes, which are the only type with which we work, and we see a very small number of supermicron particles that range anywhere from 1 up to maybe 20 μm in size, without any particular size distribution.

DISCUSSANT: They are probably a part of the crystallization process.

DISCUSSANT: If you smoke a 2R1 cigarette using the standard puff, you get 10 to 12 puffs. You will see this large-particle phenomenon mostly in the first puff, and subsequently it will decrease. We have never seen these large particles after the fourth puff, and if you puff the cigarettes without burning them, you get the same results. So obviously, this material is entrained, and it is in the cigarettes' debris, but we have not characterized it as to what it might be. I am just curious to know what some of that debris might be.

DISCUSSANT: I don't know.

DISCUSSANT: With which cigarette did you work?

DISCUSSANT: The one I am talking about is the 2R1.

DISCUSSANT: Is that filtered or nonfiltered?

DISCUSSANT: It is nonfiltered; it is a blend of flue-cured, burley, and oriental tobaccos, and it is high tar and high nicotine. It was developed about 10 years ago—or longer than that. The most modern of the Kentucky reference cigarettes, 1R4F, which is a filtered, low-tar, and low-nicotine product, matches today's average cigarette pretty closely. You raised a question this morning about the cigarette that Dr. Wasserman had used in his study. It was a commercial cigarette; he did not remember the brand. He used, I believe, an 85-mm cigarette with 1.4 mg nicotine, and 24 mg tar.

DISCUSSANT: Have you ever seen asbestos in any tobacco smoke, or have you ever looked?

DISCUSSANT: We do not know. We have done only a very small amount of work looking at these particles by EM, and we find some particles that look fibrous. In other words, they are long and thin. We have not characterized them at all, but they are not droplets. These large-debris particles are very heterogeneous. Some are chunks, and some are fibers because of their aspect ratios.

DISCUSSANT: How do you collect these particles?

DISCUSSANT: We blow clean air through the cigarette and collect the material on filters immediately after we have lighted the cigarette. You must ash the filter, and you have got to dissolve the organic material.

DISCUSSANT: I thought that you puff the cigarette but don't light it, is that right?

DISCUSSANT: We have collected these particles from both lit and unlit cigarettes.

DISCUSSANT: We dry-puff the cigarette to see whether we get the same results as from a lit cigarette, and we find that we do get the same results. The amount of this material that we are observing is very small, but we know the material is there. We have not been particularly concerned about it.

DISCUSSANT: I was wondering—just to throw out an idea here—about the potential for interaction with zeolite and tobacco smoke. I think it could be either positive or negative. There are probably more negative than positive aspects. But in the gas state, for instance, the CO_2 and the NO would be removed. There may be some tiny organic molecules in tobacco smoke that I don't know about that could also be removed. And then there is a potential for interaction with a carcinogen like asbestos, which I think should be considered.

DISCUSSANT: Sure.

DISCUSSANT: Not that it is perhaps a practical matter, because there are not very many people exposed to erionite or the other zeolites, I guess, but I think it is something to consider, especially from the protection angle, e.g., for use in filters.

DISCUSSANT: Well, not to worry lots of people, but zeolites are used extensively in detergents as a water softener.

DISCUSSANT: They also put zeolite in animal feeds, and in soil additives, and many other things. It is also used as an anticaking agent and for cleaning up hazardous waste.

DR. LANGER: Any other reassuring statements?

In that case, I want to thank you very much, and we will see you tomorrow.

Edited Transcript of the Discussions of Day 4

Moderator: Dr. A. P. Wehner

DR. WEHNER: Good morning, Ladies and Gentlemen. We would like to take this time now for the chairmen to give some reflections and comments. Would the chairman of the first day, Dr. Roe, please start.

DR. ROE: Thank you, Mr. Chairman.

The facts that seem to be firmly established are: (1) that the combined effects of human exposure to asbestos and cigarette smoke on lung-cancer risk are more than additive; (2) that there are, theoretically, numerous mechanisms which might be implicated in this apparent interaction; and (3) that there are serious obstacles to investigating the possible mechanisms of interaction. In particular, there is no reliable and easy-to-use laboratory model for producing lung cancers of the types seen in humans by exposing animals to tobacco smoke by inhalation. Despite all the research that has been undertaken, there is a need for further investigation of particle deposition, clearance, and the involvement of macrophages. This is particularly true in the case of chronic exposure to noxious agents after disease processes have already begun.

In the case of asbestos, the relationships between pulmonary fiber load, fibrosis, and cancer risk remain obscure and are subjects for further investigation and debate. Still to be explained is the fact that many more fibers are deposited and remain in nonciliated parts of the lung than in ciliated areas, yet cancers seem to arise much more often in the parts of the respiratory tree that are normally ciliated.

Physicochemical data suggest that airway epithelium is normally well protected from lipid-soluble carcinogens, such as polycyclic aromatic hydrocarbons (PAH), by a three-layered barrier of surfactant on top of gel and sol phases of aqueous mucus. But questions remain: Do particles break down natural defenses by piercing these barriers, thereby allowing PAH, or other carcinogens, to reach epithelial cells? How important is penetration by fibers into the epithelial lining of the respiratory tract? If this is important, why should penetration by a few fibers in a large airway be so much more dangerous, in terms of cancer risk, than massive fiber penetration in the lung parenchyma?

There are many different types of cells lining airways and alveoli as well as a wide variety of supportive mesodermal cells. Fibrosis in the lung parenchyma, irrespective of whether it is the result of asbestosis or some other disease process, seems to be positively associated with increased lung-cancer risk. But questions remain: How and why, in the case of asbestos, does fibrosis in the lung parenchyma predispose to cancers arising in the main airways?

At one time it was widely held that a majority of lung cancers in persons with asbestosis arise peripherally in the lower lobes and are adenocarcinomatous in type. Has the picture changed in some way as a consequence of the fact that reduced exposure has led to asbestosis occurring—and killing—subjects at an older age? Nowadays, the picture appears to be that one cannot distinguish between the spectrum of lung cancers seen in persons exposed only to asbestos and that seen in persons exposed only to cigarette smoke. Although we have a lot of information about precancerous changes in the bronchial epithelium of smokers and of asbestos workers who are smokers, this information seems to be wholly lacking for nonsmoking asbestos workers. One of the most important and unnecessary gaps in the presently available data base is a survey of the airway epithelia of nonsmoking asbestos workers to see whether the metaplastic and dysplastic changes observed in heavy smokers and thought to be precancerous in nature also occur in response to asbestos. If such changes do not occur in response to asbestos exposure in nonsmokers, then there must be real doubt as to whether tobacco smoke and asbestos act at the same target sites and on the same cells. If their targets are different, then some of the postulated theories for interaction must be unlikely.

The basis is questionable for the view that the activities of tobacco smoke and mineral dusts, including asbestos, are strictly multiplicative in relation to lung-cancer risk. A survey of the published evidence suggests that the relationship may be somewhat less than multiplicative. The uncertainty arises because the epidemiological basis for such calculations is heavily dependent on a very limited data base in the case of lung cancer in nonsmokers, whether or not they are exposed to asbestos.

Understandably, the greatest attention has been paid to interactions which lead to cancer as the final end point. However, this is clearly an unjustifiably limited approach. In animal experiments, exposure to dusts and/or cigarette smoke has been associated with prolonged survival as compared with unexposed controls. This prolongation of survival is usually due to the delayed onset of diseases caused by overnutrition (e.g., amyloid disease in hamsters; nephropathy, and mammary, pituitary, and other endocrine tumors in rats). Body weight gain provides an index of overnutrition in relation to this picture in rodents. The longer-surviving dust- and/or smoke-exposed animals usually gain less weight than the nonexposed controls. There is no clear evidence that these apparently beneficial effects of exposure in rodents are mirrored in humans. Nevertheless, there is clearly a need to pay more attention than hitherto to end points other than neoplasia.

Diagnostic criteria for lung neoplasia and mesothelioma vary between laboratory animals and humans and among different pathologists. It is therefore somewhat hazardous to rely on data reported by different investigators in different laboratories in relation to small differences in the apparent neoplastic potency of different test materials. In particular, in the case of mesothelioma, there seems to be a need to discuss the distinction between hyperplastic, precancerous, benign, and malignant neoplastic lesions.

It is easy to see that animal tests involving the intrapleural and intraperitoneal routes have some role to play in screening dusts for carcinogenic potential. However, positive results should not be used to predict risk to humans. Their main value is to indicate a need for further, more realistic, testing. *(Editor's note: Some participants disagreed with the position reflected in the last two sentences.)*

I would therefore summarize the present situation and the current state of our knowledge as follows: for two exposure agents to act synergistically they have to act on the same target. All in all, it seems unlikely that asbestos and cigarette smoke share the identical group of targets in the lung. Asbestos seems to have more targets in the lung parenchyma, with fibrosis as a precancerous state, while cigarette smoke has more targets in the bronchial epithelium. Insofar as the effects of exposure to asbestos and cigarette smoke in relation to lung-cancer risk are clearly more than additive, though probably not really multiplicative, it is reasonable to assume that there is some overlap in targets.

I came to the symposium vaguely hoping that it might be possible to identify a single target for both agents and to speculate with regard to the basis of synergism for that target. I will leave with a fairly clear idea that both agents have multiple targets, that some of these targets are shared, and that there is almost certainly not just one mechanism, but a wide variety of different mechanisms by which interaction occurs.

DR. WEHNER: Thank you, Dr. Roe, for your cogent and concise summary.

I would now like to give the floor to Dr. McClellan.

DR. McCLELLAN: Cigarette smoke and asbestos are two of the best-characterized risk factors that adversely affect human health. It might be tempting to suggest that our current level of knowledge on this subject is such that no further research is required on either of these materials. In support of this view, for example, the risks of cigarette-smoking are reasonably well understood, and it is a personal choice whether to smoke and incur the associated risk. In the case of asbestos, our level of understanding is sufficient for establishing controls to limit human exposures.

My alternative view is that we need to improve our knowledge of the mechanisms by which cigarette-smoking and asbestos exposure cause diseases of the respiratory tract. This improved knowledge may then lead to a better understanding of the mechanisms by which other potentially toxic airborne materials act. This might include materials to which human exposures are limited, or even new materials to which people have not yet been exposed. For either of these situations, we must obtain data from animal experiments, because it is not possible to obtain human data directly as a basis for making decisions about appropriate exposure limits. To be specific, the study of mechanisms of disease induction by cigarette smoke may give insight on the extent to which exposure to other combustion products may produce disease. In a similar vein, understanding the mechanisms by which asbestos produces disease may elucidate the potential of other fibers to cause disease.

I have already stated that we know a great deal about cigarette-smoking and asbestos exposure as risk factors. Most of the information on cigarette-smoking has been derived from epidemiological studies or direct chemical observations on people. The contributions from studies conducted with laboratory animals have been much more limited. The situation with regard to the relative contributions from studies of people versus laboratory animals is only marginally different for asbestos.

Studies in which laboratory animals were exposed to cigarette smoke failed to yield a remarkable increase in respiratory tract cancers, in contrast to the high incidence observed in people who smoke. We must therefore ask: Is this related to the experimental approaches used, the low carcinogenic potency of cigarette smoke (smokers inhale and deposit kilograms of cigarette tar over many years, yet only about 1 in 10 develops lung cancer), or to some other factor? Recently, Mauderly et al. (*Fundam Appl Toxicol 9:* 208-221, 1987) observed that exposure of F344 rats to high levels of diesel exhaust soot for up to 2½ years caused an excess incidence of lung cancer, most of which occurred after 2 years of exposure. The exposure and observation period was longer than that in most cancer bioassay studies, which may have been an important factor in identifying diesel exhaust as a low-potency carcinogen in the rat.

Cuddihy et al. (*Environ Sci Technol 18:* 14A-21A, 1984) noted that short-term assays suggested that cigarette smoke and diesel soot have similar carcinogenic potency. Based on this information, it seems appropriate to evaluate the feasibility of conducting a 2½-year cigarette-smoke cancer bioassay using current inhalation exposure methodology. In addition, modern molecular and cellular biology techniques could be used to explore the pathogenesis of respiratory tract injury and, possibly, lung-cancer induction. If successful, these methods would provide a more rapid, less costly tool for studying the combined effects of cigarette smoke and exposure to other agents, such as fibers. Certainly, our human experience with the combined effects of smoking and asbestos emphasizes the need for combined exposure studies in the laboratory with many materials. The major obstacle to such studies today is the lack of a suitable experimental model.

The approach I have advocated involves a blending of epidemiology, whole-animal experimentation, and studies using molecular and cellular systems. It is critical that we integrate the complementary information that can be acquired within each of these specialized areas. This meeting, which has brought together scientists from each of these areas, is a positive step toward achieving such integration.

One approach that can be especially useful toward that end is to orient risk assessment toward linking exposure → dose → response. Within this risk-oriented framework, it is especially important to investigate the effect of dose at the level of cells and, indeed, molecules. Examples of this type of thinking were evident in this symposium. Dr. Oberdörster, for example, called attention to the possibility that synergistic effects may be mimicked by an alteration in dose by concurrent exposure to multiple agents.

Data obtained using sophisticated new *in vitro* techniques can be used in combination with information obtained in the whole animal. This is important because cancer development in the individual is a very complex process, going well beyond the molecular and cellular level and involving other elements of the body.

Without question, mechanistic toxicology has much to contribute in the coming years. We need to direct our efforts toward elucidating the mechanisms of action of toxic materials. In that regard, I am reminded of the story of the inebriated man who lost his car keys. Let us call him George. When his friend Sam left the tavern, he observed George on his hands and knees under a lamppost. Sam inquired what George was doing. He replied that he was looking for his car keys, whereupon Sam agreed to help him find the keys. After about 15 minutes of searching in vain, Sam said, "Tell me again, where did you lose the keys?" George responded, "Oh, down the street a way." Sam was aghast. "Then why in hell are we looking here?" George responded, "Because the light is better here."

My concern is that we may be spending a lot of time in toxicology looking for mechanisms of action where the light is so good—at high exposure levels in whole-animal studies, and even higher concentrations in *in vitro* systems. The mechanisms of action at these high levels, regardless of how elegantly they are studied, are not necessarily relevant to the exposure levels typically encountered by people. I am confident that a risk-assessment orientation can direct our mechanistic toxicology away from the bright light that surrounds past investigations and into the areas where the light may be dimmer but the payoffs high in terms of relevant information. This will require that scientists build on past results but also be willing to take chances by using new techniques and approaches to tackle old problems, such as understanding the effects of smoking and exposure to fibers.

DR. WEHNER: Thank you, Dr. McClellan, for your eloquent summary. May I now ask Dr. Langer to present his summary and comments.

DR. LANGER: Drs. McClellan and Roe have done an admirable job summarizing the presentations in their sections and adding their own perspectives. The interaction of particles and cigarette smoke will occupy us for some time to come.

As a mineralogist, or physical scientist, I have my own perception of the field. I am particularly wary of the pitfalls associated with material characterization and the interpretation of data pertaining to recognizing the hazards of inorganic dusts. Frankly, the concept that a single mineral or inorganic dust is invariant is incorrect.

In our own laboratory, we have observed that the lack of correlation which plagues many of the "simple" *in vitro* test systems is the direct result of variations in the important physicochemical properties, including surface chemistry, of the test dusts. A range in critical properties dictates a similar range in biological potential. Dr. Nolan's paper on the surface properties of the titania polymorphs and their membranolytic behavior supports this argument. We believe that these principles apply to all varieties of inorganic dusts and all biological systems.

Allow me to approach the papers presented in my session as a physical scientist rather than as a biologist. I accept full responsibility for any misinterpretation of the biological data. What does the physical scientist perceive as important?

- The successful development of an *in vitro* test system which more closely mimics the structure and function of the human airways appears to be a major contribution to the field. Dr. Adler and his colleagues are exploring the area of liquid (biological medium)/gas interface. After all, human epithelium is in contact with gases in the lung. Wouldn't this be a more appropriate way to explore the interaction of inhaled dusts and cigarette smoke than in an immersed cell-culture system? The shortcomings associated with this technique were discussed in some detail. The issue is that development of the assay may overcome many of the artifacts of the more "normal" cell culture, where target cells are entirely submerged in a biological "soup." Even if all the data which may be obtained from an intact animal cannot be retrieved with this model, this assay may emerge as a critical screening technique, or even as a specific target system for the study of inflammation or acute insult to the small airways. The preliminary results, which focused on the survival of intact segments of animal bronchioles, appear promising.

- The research community continues to explore the development of meaningful, reliable *in vitro* test systems for screening compounds. How can we predict the toxicity and/or carcinogenicity of compounds to which humans are exposed, using models a bit more sophisticated and complex than an Ames test? Dr. Palekar and her colleagues are having success with the V79 Chinese hamster lung cell, which appears to yield results compatible with those obtained in more complex systems. Listening to her presentation, I wondered whether the elusive "tier test system" could be developed so that results obtained in *in vitro* systems could be used to predict biological outcome in intact animals. The interest in these models is pragmatic: Can the Environmental Protection Agency ban asbestos and asbestos-containing products in the United States on the basis of the supposition that asbestos substitutes are "safe?" By no means have all of the asbestos substitutes been tested in animals by inhalation, and many of the *in vitro* tests have limited value when extrapolated to humans. Of course, the bottom line is that animal studies consume a considerable number of resources, because they require a long time to complete. Obviously, biologically meaningful *in vitro* test systems are urgently needed to screen hundreds of new inorganic materials which appear in the workplace almost daily. If a tier testing program could be developed, then the limited inhalation toxicology resources of the United States could be used on a targeted group of compounds. Dr. Palekar's work is very important; it serves the dual role of being a practical instrument of assay and, at the same time, elucidates mechanisms of damage to cells by noxious agents.

- Dr. Brody presented some facinating data, obtained in his laboratory, concerning mechanisms of cell-cell communication.

It has long been suspected that there is some "factor" which permits the alveolar macrophage to communicate with the fibroblast after the macrophage has been damaged by some inhalant. This stimulation appears to be the key to fibrogenesis. Dr. Brody and his colleagues are exploring the role of specific (platelet-derived) growth factors in this process. Questions have been raised concerning the specificity of these chemical messages: Are the communication paths and end points generic, or are they specific for mineral dusts? How does one explain the range in anatomical sites for fibrotic lesions that develop after asbestos exposure, compared to, for example, quartz dust exposure? Is the model developed for asbestos fibers universally applicable to all mineral dusts? How would this model respond to complex mixtures of dust? Regardless of the questions raised, the model is elegant and should be pursued with the resources it deserves.

- Dr. Kagan's presentation covered the pulmonary macrophage population. Its range and variety of surface markers, and its evolution with time after dust challenge underscore the complexity of this cell line. As the presentation was made, I could not help but think that most (if not all) *in vitro* systems which make use of these cells produce results which represent an averaging of data. Individual subpopulations of macrophages may respond to mineral dusts differently; they may have different functions, and different degrees of importance for the biological host. I can easily understand that a range of results is obtained on a number of animal species regarding the systemic effects of mineral dusts. Dust/macrophage derangement/immune response may vary according to the nature of the macrophage population. Obviously, we have to learn more about this critical cell line.

In conclusion, there are two crucial issues on which I would like to comment:

First, materials used in test systems *of any kind* must be properly and thoroughly characterized, including expressed surface area, particle number per mass of dust, size distribution (for fibers, length, diameter, aspect ratios), surface chemistry (expressed chemical functionalities, bonding character, crystallinity, state of hydration, surface charge), and bulk properties. Perhaps surface defects and fractal number may be important. After an investigator thoroughly understands the material he wishes to use experimentally, he may have to re-characterize the substance if it requires *manipulation* for use. This may be critical if the compound is ground, crushed, heated, or reacted with another material. Do dust generators used in inhalation studies produce alterations in the physicochemical properties of the test dust? And, lastly, after exposed animals, cells, etc., die, would it not be informative to re-analyze recovered dusts to see what was retained, in which form, in the biological system, especially in animal lungs? Are there some minerals or compounds, or some subpopulations of the specimen, which are preferentially retained? I am thinking specifically of the problem of mixed asbestos fiber exposure and the preferential retention of amphiboles in human lungs. The implications of such observations are many; the conclusions one may draw will have profound societal effects.

Second, speaking as a mineralogist, with no biological axe to grind, it is of great importance to also perform animal testing by a route of exposure other than inhalation. I submit to you that results from such tests are biologically meaningful even though dose-response data and extrapolation to human risk are very limited. Animal experimentation, by any route of administration, has limitations, but we do not have the resources to test by inhalation the vast numbers of new compounds which continue to enter our environment.

Medical specialists and epidemiologists involved in the study of human populations are hard-put to discriminate between effects produced by agents in the workplace and those produced by cigarette smoke. I believe it is important for all of us to contribute to the understanding of the interaction of complex mixtures. We must resolve whether "work kills smokers or smoking kills workers." This will involve the efforts of the many disciplines represented at this workshop.

And with that, Mr. Chairman, I will stop.

DR. WEHNER: Thank you, Dr. Langer, for your illuminating comments as a physical scientist—albeit one with considerable biological knowledge and experience—which add a fresh perspective to the problems at hand.

I will take this opportunity to volunteer a couple of comments of my own.

I fully agree with Dr. Roe and Dr. Langer that we should not fall into the trap of looking for the *one* mode of action or the one method that should solve our problems. Most biological problems are too complex to lend themselves to simple solutions. Multifactorial problems demand that we take into consideration all of the various interacting factors.

Most of us have been aware of this complexity for quite some time. The problem is, how do we reduce that very complex situation to some practical experiment in the laboratory in terms of logistics and, last but not least, in terms of funding? These are problems with which we will have to continue to wrestle.

Regarding Dr. McClellan's comment, I agree with him, too. One important direction is to look at the effect of low-level dose exposures. But here again, I am reminded not of a drunkard searching for his car key, but of a mother with six young children who, worn to a frazzle, runs to her doctor in desperation: "Doctor, I am close to a nervous breakdown, please help me, I don't know what to do any more." And the doctor looks at her thoughtfully, examines her carefully, and then nods and says sagely: "Yes, you should take it easy."

(General laughter)

The problem is, again, how do we reduce the investigation of chronic low-dose exposures of humans to multiple agents to practical laboratory reality?

We know that we cannot conduct so-called megamouse experiments. Therefore it has been accepted by a wide majority of toxicologists to compensate for this inability by increasing the dose for a smaller number of animals. For one reason or another, this "compensatory" increase in dose almost always seems to be interpreted as the maximally tolerated dose, which, of course, results in an overloading of the animals.

What can we do to investigate the effects, for example, of indoor air pollution, where we are dealing with very low concentrations of multiple toxic agents over a life span, other than perhaps using state-of-the-art equipment in *in vitro* studies to obtain some basic data? But in the generally accepted and normally conducted inhalation studies, as you do them in your laboratory, as we do them in our laboratory, how does one go about simulating chronic human exposures to low doses of multiple toxic agents without compensating by higher aerosol concentrations for the relatively low number of animals?

And finally, of course, there is the problem with which all of us have to wrestle, the shortcomings of almost any model. The only answer I have, and this is not much of a consolation, is that it is better to have a model that is as good as we can reasonably make it, than to have no model at all. With that, I yield.

DISCUSSANT: Let me expand a little bit on it. I think the direction in which we have been moving, very appropriately, with the whole-animal studies, is that of trying to better understand what the dose is. We heard this from Dr. Langer when, referring to fiber-exposed animals, he postulated not only characterization of the mass, but also the physicochemical characteristics of the particles that are retained in the lungs of the animals.

During the last 5 years, we have seen a very few studies, some in our laboratory, some in Dr. Muhle's laboratory, where the lung burden for particulate material was characterized. So we now start to get an understanding of that relationship between exposure and dose and we can understand whether the kinetics are behaving in a "linear" or "nonlinear" way.

That is the kind of information about which we are talking. Using that as a jumping-off point, the message is that, whenever possible, we need to use multiple exposure levels and multiple dose levels. I think that, for example, the usefulness of some of the techniques that Drs. Brody, Warheit, Pinkerton, and others have been employing has now been demonstrated. Many of those studies were conducted at single exposure levels. Now let's start to look at lower concentrations to find out whether these have the same interrelationships occurring in terms of the mechanisms in these very complex processes that involve interactions between various cell types and a whole host of mediator compounds.

I think it is that kind of insight that needs to be linked to the whole-animal system. I don't think that there is much hope in terms of what we can do regarding the difficulty and possibility of studying the effects of low-level exposure in even hundreds of animals when we want to make extrapolations to hundreds of thousands of people.

DISCUSSANT: Let me make just one comment. I think there is a theoretical danger here, and it probably doesn't apply so much to mineral fibers, but it is possible that none of the causative agents is still present in the tissue from where cancers arise. A good example of this would be the mineral hydrocarbon carcinogenesis in the kidney of the mouse. The agents which cause the cancer produce cell necrosis and the target cells largely disappear, and a series of changes occurs. And then very late in the game, real cancers appear. But there is no way in which, halfway through that process, you could look for the retained dose of anything in the kidney; it is not there.

Now, in the case of the lung, when you expose animals to mineral fibers, you assume that you get some sort of end point later, and you further assume that what is there and the nature of what is there is directly related to the end point. Well, it depends upon whether anything has happened in the meantime. There may have been agents which have passed through, such as substances on the fibers, which have been leached out and metabolized. They have done their DNA damage and are gone, and you cannot find them. So there is theoretically a danger here that prior conditions cannot necessarily be characterized by what you find at the time of the end point. You are probably on much safer ground with fiber carcinogenesis than with anything else in this area. But, in general, we are dealing with lots of different materials, and it may not always be possible to determine prior events by analyses at the time of the end point.

DISCUSSANT: I know that we should probably discuss today those bigger issues of where we go from here, but I really cannot leave before I get this off my chest. And that is, regarding the risk factors and the relative risk which we have discussed, especially during the first day. The risk factors for modern cigarette smoke and for various other exposures, like asbestos and other materials, arsenic, and so on, show that, in some instances, the relative risk factor is lower in cigarette smokers than in nonsmokers. But by the same token, we find that there is the same situation with arsenic or asbestos. In some instances, the relative risk factor is lower for those who are exposed to arsenic or asbestos. This would suggest that, as cigarette smoke can be protective, asbestos exposure can also be protective.

It is only a game that we play with these numbers. Therefore I was asking myself, where is the mistake made in this line of thinking, because obviously we reject the notion that asbestos exposure or arsenic exposure is protective. Because I am not the statistician who prepared and presented these papers, I could not really point my finger to where the mistake was made, why the relative risk usage led to obviously erroneous results.

I think the problem is that the dose is not considered in these simple calculations. Probably this relative risk assessment can be used in instances where risk factors are compared with the dose. But in this situation, I believe it cannot be used because we can come to the conclusion that asbestos or arsenic is protective.

DR. WEHNER: Let me comment on that, please. I don't think anybody here would claim a beneficial effect for a toxic agent in general. I addressed this point in my full paper, but I could not do it in the limited time available for the verbal presentations. I presume that people who speak along a similar vein mean to make some of the points that I want to make, and that is, very simply, that we have to be careful with the interpretation of results.

It is, for example, well known that several agents that are recognized as toxic in higher concentrations have a reverse effect at very low doses. Now, whatever kind of adjectives one wants to attribute to this phenomenon is up to individual people. I prefer not to attribute any adjectives to it but merely to draw attention to the phenomenon as such, which is known as hormesis. Hormetic effects have been observed with selenium, with active immunization, and even with radiation. Last year the prestigious Health Physics Society devoted an entire meeting to radiation hormesis. There is ample evidence that very low doses of radiation have effects opposite to those that are generally recognized at high doses. This is contrary to what we would expect, but as scientists we should not disregard it just because it does not fit our concepts. I believe that Dr. Sterling wanted to make a similar point a couple of days ago. We certainly do not want to say that cigarette smoke is protective or asbestos inhalation is protective. Nevertheless, there are phenomena, such as increased mucus production following tobacco-smoke inhalation, that may locally offer what could be called a certain "protective" effect. These phenomena deserve attention, if for no other reason than that the mode of action, if we can decipher it, may help us to better understand biological mechanisms—protective or harmful, whatever the case may be—of other agents.

DISCUSSANT: I don't have any problem with what you said. I was not referring to that. I was referring to where you calculated relative risk using ratios from the risk factors. If one determines that a low dose of radiation has a protective effect, that is one thing. I agree that this could be so. I personally once published that SO_2 at a low concentration stimulated clearance. I know that it is possible, that a low concentration has a stimulating effect at the beginning but goes on to have a depressing effect if the concentration is increased or exposure is prolonged. That is known to be so in many cases, including, for example, in radiation. So I am not having any problem with that. I am having a problem drawing a conclusion based on some observational data which are incorrect, and they are probably incorrect because not all relevant factors have been taken into account. The point is this—the relative risk from smoking may be different in the asbestos worker than in the nonasbestos worker. Similarly, the relative risk from abestos may be different in smokers and nonsmokers. One cannot simply take data from one situation and apply them to the calculation of relative risk in another situation.

DISCUSSANT: Let me make another point to make my position completely clear. My point is academic. I can perfectly well accept that if somebody says, "I don't want to hear the word 'protective,' " that's fine. I don't need to use that word. We all know that the data for lung cancer incidence in nonsmoking asbestos workers are based on very few cases. And we all know that lung cancer is not only relatively rare in nonsmokers but that the spectrum of types of the disease differs between smokers and nonsmokers. This surely means that we should be very cautious about accepting the all too simple concept that asbestos increases lung-cancer risk by a factor of 5, smoking increases it by a factor of 10, and, therefore, it is reasonable to expect exposure to both agents to increase risk by a factor of 50.

DISCUSSANT: I would agree that models such as some of those described in the literature are presently helping us to understand the mechanisms behind disease that may be induced by gases and/or by particles. I also agree with Dr. McClellan that it is important for us now to test our theories in experimental animals and that in such experiments we should use concentrations that are more relevant to human environmental exposures.

We now have methods by which we can look at specific sites and specific cells in the lung. It is important to realize that the lung is not a homogeneous organ, that there are many different types of cells that make up the lung, and that the lung is designed in such a way that there are going to be specific sites where these particles and gases are going to be deposited, as has been shown by many of the presentations at this meeting. We now have methods to look at and treat the lung, not as a homogeneous organ but in terms of specific sites where deposition may occur. We can focus our attentions on those areas. It is important to recognize the types of cells that are present in those areas where deposition takes place, and to realize that these cells may have different types of metabolism, they may produce different types of secretion. All these points are very important, and this consideration gives credence to some of the models, the theoretical models, that were presented here, showing how substances may translocate from the mucus blanket to underlying epithelial and interstitial compartments. Many of those models make sense, because biologically we know that those substances are present in the area concerned. We should be just as concerned with characterizing the sites of deposition accurately as with the nature of the aerosols to which humans and experimental animals are exposed.

DISCUSSANT: Absolutely.

DISCUSSANT: Many speakers have sought to relate biological effects to the mass of deposited particulate matter (e.g., expressed as mg/m^3 or $\mu g/L$). However, it appears that, in the case of fibers, the active agent is the fiber and not the weight of the sample. I don't understand why no studies are done which relate number of fibers, rather than mass, to the biological activities.

I also think that the various types of mineral fibers are different from one another. They don't differ just in the size of the fiber, but their surface characteristics are different. There are very few studies which relate surface quality to biological activity. Papers were presented yesterday about erionite, chrysotile, and crocidolite. However, these fibers are altogether different in their mineral properties. We don't see much in the literature that relates a fiber's surface area, surface charge, or surface structure (e.g., the presence of surface pores, as in the case of erionite) to its biological activity. I suggest that far more attention should be paid to this.

DISCUSSANT: I agree with you. As to your first point, I think it is just so much simpler to define the concentration by milligrams per cubic meter than it is to count fibers. Nevertheless, I agree it should and must be done. As to your second point, I think it is absolutely necessary that anybody who works with fibers nowadays—as compared to 20 years ago, when we had not refined our concepts and perceptions of biological experiments with fibers—defines the surface area and other characteristics of the fiber.

DISCUSSANT: It is essential to have fiber counts established by random spot sampling distribution. But from a practical point of view, for inhalation studies, one needs to control dust particle concentration every day. To do it by mass is no trouble at all. To do it by light microscopy is a bit more trouble. To do it by electron microscopy, and to do that every day, is a lot of trouble. Therefore, the approach that we have adopted is to decide on a mass that equilibrates to the fiber number we want, and to verify the fiber number estimates once a week, or once a fortnight, perhaps, while determining the daily aerosol concentrations by mass. That is purely a practical reason for that approach.

DISCUSSANT: There is another point. It is very important to determine what happens to these mineral fibers in the lung, not only the retention and location, but whether they split or are dissolved. There are very few studies on that.

DISCUSSANT: I agree with you that for routine measurements one should take the mass measurement, but I believe that Dr. Palekar would say that the relationship has to be established. Now, even if the number of fibers relating to the mass varies from day to day by plus or minus 20 or 40%, that isn't so bad, that is a relatively small variation under the given circumstances. What we want to know is, is it 10,000 fibers, 50,000 fibers or 200,000 fibers. I think we basically agree on that point.

DISCUSSANT: I was wondering about Dr. Roe's statement that the multiplicative effect indicates that two agents are affecting the same target. As an example, with cigarette-smoking and asbestos, I could think of a scenario in which the agents affect two different targets but nevertheless have a multiplicative effect. This is getting back to this point that was made the first day, that although asbestos seems to deposit in the lower parts of the lung, most lung cancers arise in larger airways near the hilum. One could speculate that although asbestos deposits in the lower part of the lungs, cigarette-smoking affects clearance mechanisms in the larger airways and thereby sensitizes bronchial epithelium, so that asbestos fibers, instead of being cleared, stay around and cause more damage than in nonsmokers.

DISCUSSANT: Let me make myself clear. When I used the word "target," perhaps it was misleading. I did not necessarily mean a structural target. What I meant was that the mechanisms by which the two agents act have to meet at some point. They have to affect the same anatomical target. In this sense, what you say might be right.

The problem, as I see it, is that, on the one hand, Dr. Churg has published a paper saying that the spectrum of lung cancers is similar in smokers and asbestos workers. On the other hand, it is clear to me that this has not always been so. Historically, the cancers associated with asbestosis were mainly in the lower lobes, and they were mainly adenocarcinomas; whereas those in smokers are mainly squamous and mainly in the main airways. Also, many people here have said that fibrosis is important in relation to asbestos cancer. By contrast, there is no clear evidence that fibrosis is important in relation to lung cancer in cigarette-smokers. This suggests to me that quite different mechanisms are involved.

One other point: Chrysotile fibers split longitudinally after lodging in the lungs. This changes the mass-fiber count ratio and makes comparisons with exposure to crocidolite fibers, which do not split, difficult.

There is just one more thing I wanted to say: if you investigate a fiber, let's take, for example, a mineral fiber which has a carcinogenic potency of about only 10% of crocidolite, it would be very difficult to demonstrate this in an inhalation experiment. Yesterday I heard the statement that intraperitoneal injection could yield a false-positive result. I think part of that problem is that nobody knows whether it is a false positive or not, because it is unknown whether it is a carcinogen for humans.

One problem is that the length of crocidolite fibers in the UICC standard material is less than that to which asbestos workers have been exposed. This may have reduced the apparent carcinogenic potency of inhaled crocidolite in the rats. Irrespective of the results of studies in rats, there is no evidence that exposure to glass fibers enhances lung-cancer risk in man. We cannot even be sure whether exposure increases the risk of noncancerous lung disease.

DISCUSSANT: Are you talking about extruded glass or rock wool? If you are talking about extruded glasses, I would agree with you. If you are talking about mineral rock wool, I would disagree.

DISCUSSANT: The data that we presented yesterday show the correlations between the human cancers, including the incidence of mesothelioma and human exposure, and the type of fibers used, which were chrysotile, crocidolite, and erionite. This was, of course, an intrapleural study, and the results were based on the number of fibers introduced, not on fiber mass.

Based on fiber mass, we found that crocidolite was inferior to chrysotile in tumor induction. But based on the number of fibers, we found that, yes, the number of tumors was greater for crocidolite than for chrysotile, which is what we see in humans following natural exposure.

So I don't think that we had an inferior system for testing the crocidolite, and I do believe that there is considerable merit to these exposures in the biocavities. We cannot just dismiss this test system lightly with the argument that it is an artificial system. The ability to produce tumors in the pleural cavity or in the peritoneal cavity probably does not depend so much on the relationship of the passage of the fiber through the lung as had been claimed with chrysotile, but on the intrinsic ability of those fibers to produce tumors when they get there, regardless of how you put them in.

DISCUSSANT: I was calculating the relative densities for chrysotile and crocidolite, and you would have a 60% difference in fiber numbers, just based on the difference in the relative densities of those fibers. You therefore have to normalize on the basis of the number of fibers.

DR. WEHNER: We better push the agenda ahead and raise the question, where do we go from here?

DISCUSSANT: I am sorry that Dr. Cross is not here, because I wanted to comment on his statement. It is important, not only for fiber glass, but for any other material that is characterized or studied, to characterize its physicochemical properties under varying circumstances.

When people compare asbestos to glass fibers, they oftentimes compare them on a fiber-per-fiber basis. I don't think that this is always applicable. I will use fiber glass as an example. In the large majority of glass fibers, and in mineral-wool-sized fibers, the fiber, as it is taken into the body, won't fracture into further, smaller filaments, whereas the crocidolite will. Therefore, the effective dose may be different than the airborne concentration as sampled by industrial sampling methods.

Further, many of the industrial sampling methods in use have been developed for asbestos, and they work well for asbestos, because the concentrations are often higher. As one of my hygienists characterized it one time, "Our present methods of sampling glass fibers in the air are just slightly better than a wet finger in the wind."

I think this is probably true, because, for a given sample, if you count it in the morning, you can get one figure, and if you count it in the afternoon, you can be off by 20%. Now, when you are dealing with the very low concentrations that we see in most man-made mineral fibers, including fiber glass, a numerical difference of one fiber can change an estimate of airborne fiber concentration by an order of magnitude, e.g., from the second to the third decimal place, and we may be "measuring" further with a pencil than we can as far as true sensitivity goes.

I think these factors are extremely important to keep in mind when you take into consideration what I will call the practical risk of the materials. Again, I reiterate what I said yesterday, and that is, let us be sure of the question that we want answered: Does the material have any carcinogenic potential under any circumstances? That is one question.

The second question, which I think is very important to keep in mind even for basic scientists, is: Does the material under practical use have any projected misuse conditions which demonstrate a hazard from either cancer or noncancer, and if so, what is the rough indicator as to how serious that hazard is?

DR. WEHNER: Okay. Where do we go from here?

DISCUSSANT: I would just like to remind people that at one time experimentalists used to put this sort of material subcutaneously into rats and got a whole lot of data, to which nobody now, at least hardly anybody, would give any credence at all. You can very easily get sarcomas with a wide variety of substances, including glucose, and nobody believes that this is real.

So this is a route of administration which is more artificial than intraperitoneal, less artificial than intratracheal injection, but still, it is the same phenomenon. This is really the background of my concern, that you should not use results of this type of study for quantitative risk assessment. You should only use this type of study as some sort of a screening test, which can tell you whether you should do a more meaningful study. I just wanted to point this out.

DISCUSSANT: Stating what to me is obvious, we do not have a good inhalation model for cigarette-smoke carcinogenesis. This fact has been discussed at considerable length and there have been certain suggestions. One is to use whole-body exposure tolerated at maximal concentrations.

This is obviously a route to go. I think we would agree that perhaps it could be done. The point is this: To validate such models would take 3 to 4½ years. I would therefore like to pose the question, should we go, stepwise, into such an experiment before we think of combined exposures to asbestos and cigarette smoke? Or are we so sure that we might get interesting results with combined exposures that it would be worthwhile to start combining immediately in an attempt to produce this model of mixing cigarette smoke with fibers? Rats exposed to tobacco smoke, rats exposed to asbestos, rats exposed to both of them. That would be something we would like to do if we could trust the cigarette-smoke model. Is it worth gambling at this stage or, say, in 3 or 4 years?

DISCUSSANT: I think you could waste a huge amount of money if you went straight into a long-term study of this kind. But there are quite a lot of data that I know of that show bronchial epithelial changes in 7 or 8 weeks from really heavy exposure to smoke. Therefore I would have thought that it would be justifiable to do relatively short-term studies, using the very much better methods that are now available—certainly in relation to fiber deposition or fiber penetration and macrophage clearance. I think it would be worth doing that with much heavier cigarette-smoke exposures and slightly unrealistic methods. But it would be really risky to do a long-term study initially.

DISCUSSANT: This is going back to the first day. I think Dr. Martonen's paper on the deposition characteristics of cigarette smoke under conditions that pertain to human smoking is very interesting. It does suggest that we may have been underestimating the dose to the bronchial tree in the human, which is extremely difficult to attain from the conditions of smoking experiments that are carried out in animals. I am looking forward to reading his theoretical assessment when the paper is published.

I think it is very important to administer as many dosages as it takes for animals to experience the same order of magnitude of exposure as humans.

The radon experience in animals tends to reinforce this point. In the case of radon, we have very good experience at Battelle, and in France: If you irradiate the animal at about the same level as you do in the human case you get very much the same response to the radiation. This applies also to longer-lived particulates of plutonium. And again, in this case, we have Dr. McClellan's point that we can use the animal experiments to extrapolate to the human on the basis of a common and rational scale, namely, extrapolation of absorbed dose from one radionuclide to another. We have the human experience of cancer from radium; from this we can infer the risk of exposures to actinides.

DISCUSSANT: The test system of tumorigenesis and a realistic model for extrapolating risks to man have been discussed, but the concentration at which a fiber is deemed to be safe by artificial injection into these systems may not, in fact, be safe by the inhalation route. So it is necessary to use inhalation exposures as a fall-back, final procedure to give the new materials a clean bill of health.

The fact that tumors are produced in man, but not so easily by inhalation experiments in the rat with cigarette smoke, does not disqualify the rat lung *per se*. There are obviously other factors that have not been accounted for adequately. Man is also exposed to other carcinogens and promoters to which rats in the laboratory are not exposed. Humans, therefore, have a complex exposure regimen.

This, in part, may be the reason why cigarette smoke, when administered by the inhalation route, has not been tumorigenic in rats. It also points to the relatively weak carcinogenicity of cigarette smoke in comparison with radiation exposure.

Lifetime exposure of rats to indoor radon concentrations is sufficient to produce tumors, but practical cigarette-smoking regimens are not. I repeat that, perhaps, by comparison, fibers are also weak carcinogens by the inhalation route. The point that Dr. Muhle has made is that you need a relatively strong carcinogen to detect the effect with a reasonable number of rats in an experiment. In contrast to the laboratory rat, man is exposed, in addition, to other carcinogens and promoters, particularly radon and cigarette smoke, which are common elements in the induction of cancer in the population where we do see lung cancers.

DISCUSSANT: I have a basic question how to design further experiments. How, on a scientific basis, should we approach a situation when somebody goes to court claiming compensation for exposure to harmful agents. In cigarette-smoke-related litigation, it is difficult to prove harmful health effects in a specific human individual by reference to animal experiments. Someone may say that results in animals are just a correlation, not proof. I don't know how they will be used in court. Can they prove anything?

DR. WEHNER: May I volunteer an answer, and I invite others to do likewise. Let me preface this by saying that we here in the United States are a more litigious society than you in Germany. Therefore we have perhaps a bit more experience in dealing with court situations. My personal opinion is that, in court, we should leave the extrapolation of our results in animal studies to humans and the legal arguments to others. We should concentrate on designing the best possible experiments, conduct them with state-of-the-art equipment and interpret the results conservatively. If we are invited as court experts, my advice is to say, okay, this is what we did, this is how we did it, and those are the results in such-and-such an animal model, period.

DR. McCLELLAN: I agree. In terms of the design of experiments we can relate that to an earlier comment made by Dr. Davis, suggesting that perhaps the time has now come to launch a long-term study in which one is looking at the effects of cigarette smoke, asbestos, and the combined agents.

Then Dr. Roe indicated that he would be somewhat cautious launching such a combined exposure study right away. But I think there is an intermediate point. We now have seen a whole host of assays or approaches available to us to assess injury and repair in the intact animal. Much of this has come from our *in vitro* studies, but we can now proceed to take a look at damage to the DNA and at the role of oncogenes, which we have not really discussed at all here, as to how that fits into this picture.

There are things that could be done on a shorter-term basis. Although they fall short of the absolute parameter assessments that we would like to see in lung cancer, I think in most scientific circles they would certainly be considered as important aspects of the process of carcinogenesis.

We ought to be focusing on better understanding of those short-term results, with the anticipation that, at some point in time, we will be able to establish the linkage to the end point of absolute concern, and that is lung-cancer induction. I think we have to get smarter in designing those studies and doing the sorts of things that you are talking about, Dr. Wehner, but then thinking very critically about what kinds of measurements we are going to make on these tissues and materials from those intact animals.

DR. WEHNER: Certainly, that was included in my definition of good experiments: state-of-the-art procedures and equipment and conducting all the ancillary tests that make for a complete investigation of a given problem, not just shoving animals in a chamber and then killing them after 24 months.

DR. McCLELLAN: I think another important point comes from the experience in our laboratory, Dr. Muhle's laboratory in Hannover, the Battelle laboratory, and the Japanese. All four groups were working with diesel exhaust. In those studies we identified chronic exposure to high concentrations of diesel exhaust as producing a low-potency carcinogenic response. But it was only when those studies were continued beyond the 24 months used in the typical bioassay that the results were really most clearly evident.

In the study for which Dr. Mauderly was responsible in our laboratory, approximately 80% of the lung tumors were observed after 24 months. The question is open as to whether the 20% tumor incidence that was observed at 24 months and earlier would have been sufficient to indicate a clearly positive result.

We can't exclude the possibility that, if we sacrificed at 24 months and 1 day, all of those other tumors might well have been evident in those animals, but it is probably unlikely. That emphasizes, again, the need to look at true lifespan observations in these studies of low-potency carcinogens.

DR. WEHNER: Of course, in trying to do what needs to be done I find a continual occupational hazard in our field, namely the lack of funds and, sometimes, bureaucrats who try to tell us how to do our work.

DR. McCLELLAN: Well, I think that is a very real difficulty, particularly in this area, because I think that the prevailing view is that, well, we really know almost all there is to know about cigarette-smoking and asbestos exposure, so why spend any more money? I think the key there is to try to educate our fellow scientists and others to understand that the real payoff in these areas does not relate just to understanding these two agents, but to develop a level of understanding that can be applied to other materials.

But, you see, that is an educational process that we all need to undertake with all scientists that sit on peer groups that are going to judge allocations of funds.

DISCUSSANT: Yes, but we should not underestimate the seriousness of not having a good animal model for tobacco smoke. There really is no limit to the number of percentages that you can measure in the short term, and we have seen some fine papers here on measuring various parameters, and good observational papers. But we are really a long way from knowing what even the anatomical targets are in both asbestos and tobacco-smoke carcinogenesis. We have ideas but, as I have said earlier, there are things you can do in the short term. The hazard of this is that what you are measuring may, in fact, have little relationship to the end point. You really need to have a system where you can produce something which is a surrogate or a meaningful form of lung cancer, and then you can work backwards.

When you have that information, you can work back to the short term and then probably develop some meaningful short-term bioassays. But if you try to play around with the short-term bioassays first, you really don't know whether they are relevant. They might be relevant to some other lung disease, or they might be irrelevant, but you don't really know unless you can get the end point that you want.

DISCUSSANT: Well, you put us in a "Catch-22 situation." Earlier, you argued that we were not ready to launch into the life-span study of these agents, and now you come back and argue that we should be very cautious doing the short-term studies.

DISCUSSANT: I was answering two different questions. One is, would it be right to try to get the money to do a long-term experiment, on the basis of present knowledge. My instinct tells me that you would be wise to do a several-week study first and get some data, and then embark on the long-term experiment, rather than go straight into it.

DISCUSSANT: Well, I think we are actually getting around to the same path. I agree with you that to incorporate into shorter-term studies some of our contemporary measurements of genetic injury, of cell injury, and so on will provide a stronger argument.

DR. WEHNER: The standard solution in a situation like that would be to form a committee.

(General laughter)

More seriously, an international committee, with the best minds pooling their input, could probably come up with some useful recommendations and guidelines.

DISCUSSANT: The road we need now is to develop long-term animal lung carcinogenesis by cigarette smoke. There is no way of doing that except going into the full life-span study.

What I was really saying was, while you are doing that, are you going to risk adding exposure to asbestos and everything else to the cigarette-smoke exposures at the same time? Let's forget that issue for the moment. Is there a way out? You highlighted the fact that it is very serious that we do not get a lot of tumors from inhaled cigarette smoke in animals. I can see no way out of that problem.

DR. WEHNER: But there are a lot of things that you can do along the way. You can start your full life-span study and periodically kill some animals and subject them to appropriate tests and examinations to monitor onset and development of treatment-induced changes.

DISCUSSANT: The truth of the matter is that it would not add very much if you tried a new approach to administering a high dosage of tobacco smoke. We have the technology of exposing animals to dust, and it would not actually add a great deal. We know a lot about how to generate the dust, we know how much to expose, it's just adding a few groups. So, my answer to you is, if you have reached the point at which you feel confident enough to embark on a new cigarette-smoke study with higher dosage, then by all means, add some groups with asbestos, because it is not going to add much in terms of efforts. That is not the weakness. The weakness is the tobacco-smoke side.

DR. WEHNER: Because many of you have to leave in 5 minutes to catch the bus to the airport, I would like to conclude the discussions with a few comments and reflections.

A good number of the presentations during the last 3½ days did, indeed, offer new ideas on the interaction of inhaled mineral fibers and cigarette smoke. Others, as expected, dealt with more peripheral but nevertheless interesting and pertinent topics in either of the two fields.

You may recall that I said in my opening statement that we might not be able to resolve ever a single one of the issues that are challenging us, but that we surely would debate them. And I think we did this rather successfully.

We had a good mix of participants from various disciplines, representing academia, government agencies, industry, and research institutes, and we had good discussions. So I believe that, basically, we achieved our goal and perhaps even went somewhat further than we could have hoped for when we started.

It could, perhaps, be said that we did not focus enough on interaction. I don't think that there was a lack of focus. I believe that this impression—if it existed at all—was merely due to the fact that not enough information on the interaction processes exists. This lack of information and the intention of getting talks on this subject started was what gave birth to the idea of having this conference in the first place.

I would like to express my hope that the Proceedings of this symposium/workshop, which will include the edited anonymous discussions, will become a useful source of information and a stimulus for further investigations, not only for the participants of this meeting, but also for all of our colleagues who are interested in the biological interaction of inhaled mineral fibers and cigarette smoke.

Finally, I would like to thank all of you: the participants, for having come and for having contributed to the discussions; the speakers, for having taken the time to prepare presentations; and the chairmen, seasoned veterans of many international meetings, for guiding our symposium.

Many of you have graciously volunteered rather flattering comments on various aspects of this meeting. For this I am truly grateful. But let me assure you, it was your presence and your participation that made this meeting what it turned out to be, and I think we can call it a solid success. Personally, I received much more from you than I was able to give to this meeting.

With this rather unscientific concluding note, I declare this symposium closed, and I wish you a safe and pleasant trip home.

Postsymposium Comments

Editors note: Those participants who, upon further reflection, wished to submit further comments on topics discussed during the symposium, were encouraged to do so with the understanding that these comments would be published under their names in a Postsymposium Comments Section of the Proceedings.

Comments from Dr. Martonen and his coauthor, Dr. Hofmann:

We believe that an issue to be addressed in future research is the integral effect of naturally occurring radionuclides in cigarette smoke. Because they are inherent in the smoke, their presence and biological effects cannot be ignored. However, in most research endeavors, including most of those presented at this symposium, the known effects of radioactive materials, e.g., ^{210}Pb (Martell, *Proc Natl Acad Sci USA 80:* 1285-1289, 1983; Cross, *Health Phys 46:* 205-208, 1984; Martonen and Hofmann, *Radiat Protect Dosim 15:* 225-232, 1986), are not considered. This unavoidable, confounding influence of inherent potentially toxic substances may, we suggest, be a considerable factor in the carcinogenicity of cigarette smoke. Since the radioactive components of smoke are intrinsic, their carcinogenic effects—if not recognized—may mask interpretation of laboratory results attempting to identify mechanisms of cancer evolution. The role of radioactive materials must be accepted, and concomitant complicating factors must be addressed in future scientific investigations.

Cigarette-smokers are continuously exposed to ambient radon progeny in residences and in the workplace . It has recently been estimated that 8 to 25% of all current lung cancer deaths in the U.S. population are attributable to past radon progeny exposure (Puskin and Yang, *Health Phys 54:* 635-643, 1988). Therefore, the cumulative effect of inhalation exposure to radon progeny and chemical or radioactive carcinogenic components of smoke is an issue to be investigated. The synergistic influences of radionuclides that are not present in smoke *per se,* but to which smokers are routinely exposed, must be included in research efforts related to the initiation and promotion of cancer (Stranden, *Phys Med Biol 24:* 921-930, 1979; James et al., *Proceedings 5th Congress IRPA, vol. 2,* pp. 1045-1048, Pergamon Press, Oxford, 1981; Martonen et al., *Health Phys 52:* 213-217, 1987). It is conceiveable that, at low doses, the exposure of epithelial cells to radon progeny may be the controlling factor in tumor induction. Whereas in scientific research on radionuclide topics these synergistic effects are routinely considered, these complicating effects seem to be ignored in experiments specific to cigarette smoke. We suggest that such synergistic influences be incorporated in future research vectors.

Comments from Prof. Pott:

When, and within which limitations, is it permissible to extrapolate from results obtained in unrealistic animal models (e.g., intraperitoneal or intrapleural injections) to humans exposed to a given agent(s) by inhalation? This question gave rise to lively discussions during the symposium and prompted me to submit the following postsymposium comments which summarize my viewpoint.

The problem, defined by the foregoing question, pertains especially to man-made mineral fibers and cigarette smoke. Inhalation experiments with either agent are not producing significant numbers of lung tumors even though there is good epidemiological evidence for a significant lung tumor incidence following exposure to high concentrations of certain thin natural mineral fibers (that remain and do not dissolve in the lungs) or cigarette smoke.

There are explanations why inhalation experiments with cigarette smoke or crocidolite in the rat are so ineffectual. This ineffectual model forces us, in my opinion, to rely on routes of administration other than inhalation to obtain results on which qualitative—and, under certain circumstances, even a "semiquantitative"—risk assessment can be based. I believe that the formalistic insistence on results from inhalation experiments, especially with mineral fibers, cannot be sufficiently justified either scientifically or from the viewpoint of preventive medicine.

Summarizing comments from Dr. Wehner:

Having "relived" the symposium and discussions by editing the Proceedings, I am perhaps in a better position than most participants to evaluate in retrospect the results of this endeavor with regard to its stated objectives.

In several ways the organizational and technical approach to the symposium was unconventional: A limited number of selected scientists, from a variety of disciplines and backgrounds, convened by invitation in a think-tank-like atmosphere to tackle vexing technical and scientific problems. Emphasis was on informality and on the development of knowledge in lively discussions during the workshop sessions, for which more time had been scheduled than for formal presentations. No pertinent subject was taboo. Rational speculation was encouraged. The names of the discussants were deleted in the Proceedings to stimulate the expression of new ideas without the potential for later embarrassment.

Problems whose complexity has defied solution and puzzled some of the brightest scientific minds for a couple of decades cannot, of course, be solved in a single meeting. However, participants presented new techniques and results and advanced fresh hypotheses on mechanisms of the biological interaction of inhaled mineral fibers and cigarette smoke. This will stimulate new thinking and research to contribute to the resolution of the problems challenging us.

The vigorous discussions raised interesting questions and provided a treasure trove of responses and comments. The information developed in these discussions should be of considerable interest to all individuals and institutions involved in investigating the biological interaction of inhaled mineral fibers and cigarette smoke. The discussions also focussed on the gaps in our knowledge in this field, thereby pointing the way to future research objectives.

Against this background and based on the feedback from many participants, the symposium/workshop was an unqualified success. Attention has been focussed on important biomedical issues that affect millions of people. I do hope that support will continue for further scientific research in this field.

List of Participants

Kenneth B. Adler, Ph.D.
Department of Anatomy,
Physiological Sciences,
and Radiology, 204400
School of Veterinary Medicine
North Carolina State University
4700 Hillsborough Street
Raleigh, NC 27606

Piergiuseppe Agostoni, M.D.
Instituto di Cardiologia
Universita di Milano
Milano
ITALY

Dr. Scott Appleton
Senior Toxicologist
R. J. Reynolds Tobacco Company
Winston-Salem, NC 27102

Arnold R. Brody, Ph. D.
Group Leader,
Pulmonary Pathology
Laboratory of Pulmonary
Pathobiology
National Institutes of
Environmental Health Sciences
P. O. Box 12233
Research Triangle Park, NC 27709

Prof. John Butler, M.D.
Division of Pulmonary and Critical
Care Medicine
University of Washington School of
Medicine
Mail Stop RM 12
Seattle, WA 98195

Ching-Hong Chen, Ph.D.
Northwest Lipid Research Clinic
Department of Medicine
Harborview Medical Center
326 Ninth Avene
Seattle, WA 98104

Prof. Andrew Churg, M.D.
Department of Pathology
University of British Columbia
Health Sciences Centre
2211 Wesbrook Mall
Vancouver, BC V6T 1 W5
CANADA

David L. Coffin, V.M.D.
U. S. Environmental Protection
Agency
Health Effects Research Laboratory
Mail Stop 50
Research Triangle Park, NC 27711

Fred T. Cross, Ph.D.
Biology and Chemistry Department
Battelle, Pacific Northwest
Laboratories
P. O. Box 999
Richland, WA 99352

Gerald E. Dagle, D.V.M., Ph.D.
Biology and Chemistry Department
Battelle, Pacific Northwest
Laboratories
P. O. Box 999
Richland, WA 99352

J. M. G. Davis, M.A., Sc. D
Head, Pathology Branch
Institute of Occupational Medicine
Roxburgh Place
Edinburgh EH8 95U
GREAT BRITAIN

Prof. Juraj Ferin, M.D., Ph.D.
Department of Biophysics
School of Medicine and Dentistry
University of Rochester
Rochester, NY 14642

Donald E. Gardner, Ph.D., D.A.T.S.
Northrop Services, Inc.
P. O. Box 12313
Research Triangle Park, NC 27709

Per Gerde, Ph.D.
Department of Chemical Engineering
Royal Institute of Technology
S 100 44 Stockholm
SWEDEN

Neil F. Johnson, Ph.D.
Lovelace Inhalation Toxicology Research Institute
P. O. Box 5890
Albuquerque, NM 87185

Prof. Elliott Kagan, M.D., M.R.C. Path.
Department of Pathology
Georgetown University School of Medicine
3900 Reservoir Road N.W.
Washington, DC 20007

Jon L. Konzen, M.D.
Vice President, Medical Affairs
Owens Corning Fiberglas
Fiberglas Tower
Toledo, OH 43659

Arthur Langer, Ph.D.
Environmental Sciences Laboratory
Applied Sciences Institute of the City
University of New York at Brooklyn College
Flatbush Avenue
Brooklyn, NY 11210

Daniel Luchtel, Ph.D.
Department of Environmental Health
School of Public Health
University of Washington
Seattle, WA 98195

Ted Martonen, Ph.D.
Inhalation Toxicology Division
Health Effects Research Laboratory
Mail Drop 82
U.S. Environmental Protection Agency
Research Triangle Park, NC 27711

Joe L. Mauderly, D.V.M.
Lovelace Inhalation Toxicology Research Institute
P. O. Box 5890
Albuquerque, NM 87185

Roger O. McClellan, D.V.M.*
President/Director
Lovelace Inhalation Toxicology Research Institute
P. O. Box 5890
Albuquerque, NM 87185

Owen R. Moss, Ph.D.
Manager, Inhalation Technology and Toxicology Section
Battelle, Pacific Northwest Laboratories
P. O. Box 999
Richland, WA 99352

Dr. Hartwig Muhle
Head, Inhalation Research Department
Fraunhofer Institut f. Toxikologie und Aerosolforschung
Nikolai-Fuchs-Str. 1
D 3000 Hannover 61
FEDERAL REPUBLIC OF GERMANY

---

*Present address: Chemical Industry Institute of Toxicology, P. O. Box 12137, 6 Davis Drive, Research Triangle Park, NC 27709

Robert P. Nolan, Ph.D.
Environmental Sciences Laboratory
Applied Sciences Institute of the City University of New York at Brooklyn College
Flatbush Avenue
Brooklyn, NY 11210

Prof. Gilbert Omenn, M.D., Ph.D.
Dean, School of Public Health and Community Medicine
University of Washington
Seattle, WA 98195

Lalita D. Palekar, Ph.D.
Northrop Services, Inc.
P. O. Box 12313
Research Triangle Park, NC 27709

Kent E. Pinkerton, Ph.D.
Department of Anatomy
School of Veterinary Medicine
University of California
Davis, CA 95616

Prof. Dr. med. Friedrich Pott
Medizinisches Institut für Umwelthygiene
Universität Düsseldorf
Auf'm Hennekamp 50
D 4000 Düsseldorf 1
FEDERAL REPUBLIC OF GERMANY

Francis J. C. Roe, D.M., D. Sc., F.R.C. Path.
19 Marryat Road
Wimbledon Common
London, SW19 5BB
GREAT BRITAIN

Peter Scholander, Ph.D., M.D.
Department of Chemical Engineering
Royal Institute of Technology
S 10044 Stockholm
SWEDEN

William S. Simmons, Ph.D.
Director, Smoking & Health
R. J. Reynolds Tobacco Company
Winston-Salem, NC 27102

Dorsett D. Smith, M.D.
4310 Colby Avenue
Everett, WA 98203

Prof. Dr. Theodor D. Sterling
School of Computing Science
Faculty of Applied Sciences
Simon Fraser University
Burnaby, BC V5A 1S6
CANADA

David B. Warheit, Ph.D.
Haskell Laboratory for Toxicology and Industrial Medicine
E. I. duPont de Nemours & Co.
P. O. Box 50
Elkton Road
Newark, DE 19714

Prof. Karlman Wasserman, M.D., Ph.D.
Chief, Division of Respiratory Physiology and Medicine
Harbor-UCLA Medical Center
1000 West Carson Street
Torrance, CA 90509

Alfred P. Wehner, D.M.D., Sc. D., Cand. Med., D.A.T.S.
Biology and Chemistry Department, MS K4-16
Battelle, Pacific Northwest Laboratories
P. O. Box 999
Richland, WA 99352

Author Index